The Cerebral Cortex of the Rat

The Cerebral Cortex of the Rat

edited by
Bryan Kolb and Richard C. Tees

A Bradford Book
The MIT Press
Cambridge, Massachusetts
London, England

This book was typeset in Palatino by DEKR Corporation and printed and bound in the United States of America.

Library of Congress Cataloging-in-Publication Data

The Cerebral cortex of the rat / edited by Bryan Kolb and Richard C. Tees.

   p.   cm.
   "A Bradford book."
   ISBN 0-262-11150-0. — ISBN 0-262-61064-7 (pbk.)
   1. Cerebral cortex—Physiology. 2. Rats—Physiology. I. Kolb,
Bryan, 1947–   . II. Tees, Richard C.
QP383.C46   1990   89-48302
599.32'33—dc20   CIP

Contents

Contributors

Vlastimil Bracha
Institute of Physiology
Czechoslovak Academy of
Sciences
Prague, Czechoslovakia

J. Jay Braun
Department of Psychology
Arizona State University
Tempe, Arizona

Jan Bures
Institute of Physiology
Czechoslovak Academy of
Sciences
Prague, Czechoslovakia

David P. Carey
Department of Psychology
University of Western Ontario
London, Ontario, Canada

Anthony J. Castro
Department of Anatomy
Stritch School of Medicine
Loyola University of Chicago
Maywood, Illinois

John K. Chapin
Department of Physiology and
Biophysics
Hahnemann University
Philadelphia, Pennsylvania

Nadja-Dorothee Dausch
Anatomical Institute
University of Cologne
Cologne, Federal Republic of
Germany

Paul Dean
Department of Psychology
University of Sheffield
Sheffield, England

Stephen B. Dunnett
Department of Experimental
Psychology
University of Cambridge
Cambridge, England

Melvyn A. Goodale
Department of Psychology
University of Western Ontario
London, Ontario, Canada

Janice M. Juraska
Department of Psychology
University of Illinois
Champaign, Illinois

Andries Kalsbeek
Netherlands Institute for Brain
Research
Amsterdam, The Netherlands

Jack B. Kelly
Laboratory of Sensory
Neuroscience
Department of Psychology
Carleton University
Ottawa, Ontario, Canada

Bryan Kolb
Department of Psychology
University of Lethbridge
Lethbridge, Alberta, Canada

Chia-Sheng Lin
Department of Physiology and
Biophysics
Hahnemann University
Philadelphia, Pennsylvania

Edward J. Neafsey
Department of Anatomy
Stritch School of Medicine
Loyola University of Chicago
Maywood, Illinois

John G. Parnavelas
Department of Anatomy and
Developmental Biology
University College London
London, England

Richard C. Tees
Department of Psychology
University of British Columbia
Vancouver, British Columbia,
Canada

Harry B. M. Uylings
Netherlands Institute for Brain
Research
Amsterdam, The Netherlands

Cornelius H. Vanderwolf
Department of Psychology
University of Western Ontario
London, Ontario, Canada

Corbert G. Van Eden
Netherlands Institute for Brain
Research
Amsterdam, The Netherlands

Ian Q. Whishaw
Department of Psychology
University of Lethbridge
Lethbridge, Alberta, Canada

Andreas Wree
Anatomical Institute
University of Cologne
Cologne, Federal Republic of
Germany

Karl Zilles
Anatomical Institute
University of Cologne
Cologne, Federal Republic of
Germany

Preface

The idea of putting together a volume on the neocortex of the rat arose from (1) our belief that a book on the state of knowledge of the structure and function of the neocortex of the rat would be useful to neuroscientists, and especially behavioral neuroscientists; and, (2) our frustration in trying to locate information about the rat's neocortex, especially information from fields that we were not actively studying ourselves. Although we felt that such a volume could be an important contribution, we approached the project with some concern because we were uncertain as to how the idea of a volume on the *rat's* neocortex would be received. There is probably more known about the structure and function of the brain of the laboratory rat than any other species, yet there has been a peculiar reluctance by neuroscientists in general, and those working on primates and carnivores in particular, to consider the neocortex of the rat as being worthy of study. As we approached potential contributors, we were pleasantly surprised, however, as we found great enthusiasm for the idea. Indeed it soon became clear that we would have difficulty in including detailed discussions on every relevant topic, or in including chapters on other forms of cortex, including especially the limbic cortex and hippocampus. As a result, although our coverage of the rat cortex is extensive, it is not complete, and we recognize this. We were guided by comments of reviewers of the proposed volume who felt that discussion of these structures, especially the hippocampus, would best be left to more specific volumes and by our bias toward including information that is directly relevant to behavioral studies.

The following twenty-five chapters are organized into six parts: (I) introduction to the rat as an appropriate species, (II) organization of the rat cortex, (III) motor functions of the neocortex, (IV) sensory cortex, (V) association cortex, and (VI) plasticity of the neocortex. The first five parts emphasize structural, physiological, and behavioral organization of different cortical areas, whereas the last part focuses on variables that influence the basic structural and physiological properties of the cortex.

The authors were asked to write broadly about their topics and to provide an overview of information about each topic. They were discouraged from presenting details of individual experiments, but were encouraged to be integrative and to speculate. It is our hope that by doing so the chapters will allow readers to get a general picture of the structure and function of the rat's neocortex and to appreciate the larger questions that the authors believe are the important ones.

We would like to thank the authors for their efforts and for agreeing to the sometimes extensive revisions that were recommended by our reviewers, who usually were other contributors. We would especially like to thank Ian Whishaw, who eagerly read about half of the chapters and was supportive throughout the project. We also would like to thank our secretaries, Adria Allan and Mirana Yu, for their efforts. Finally, we would like to thank Fiona Stevens at The MIT Press for her patience and enthusiastic support of this book.

Bryan Kolb and Richard Tees
Lethbridge, Alberta, and Vancouver, British Columbia

I   Introduction

1 The Rat as a Model of Cortical Function

Bryan Kolb and Richard C. Tees

The use of nonhuman species as models of cerebral functioning in humans dates back at least to Flourens (1823), who is usually credited as being the father of experimental brain research. Flourens was particularly interested in the claims of Gall and Spurtzheim that psychological processes were localized in the cortex. He found that ablation of various parts of the brain of chickens, pigeons, dogs, and other animals led to a general loss in behaviors such as feeding, walking, and wing flapping. Furthermore Flourens noted that if the damage was not too severe, the behavioral loss seemed to show almost complete recovery. He concluded that the observed restitution of function was due to the activity of the remaining brain and surmised that any surviving remnant of cortex could fulfill all cortical functions.

It is generally recognized that Flourens's experiments undermined the basis of phrenology for they clearly did not support the idea of localized functions. Although Flourens's studies are largely of historical interest today, the methodological problem of how to generalize about human brain function from the study of nonhuman animals remains. Flourens generalized from wing flapping in pigeons to psychological processes in humans, a conclusion requiring a leap of faith that few people would be willing to make today.

The publication of *Descent of Man* by Darwin in 1871 can probably be taken as the beginning of the widespread interest in nonhuman subjects as a way to study psychological processes in humans. In his book Darwin argued that human and animal minds were similar and that differences were quantitative, not qualitative. Thus for Darwin there was a continuum of mental complexity; humans differed in degree but not in kind from other animals.

Darwin's novel hypothesis led to the development of comparative psychology, in which learning as well as behavior in general was investigated. Demonstration of unexpected mental capacities in nonhuman subjects clearly influenced neurology, and in 1915 Luciani included a description of the behavior of various brain-damaged laboratory animals in his text, *Human Physiology*.

Today it is generally assumed that most mental processes in humans rely heavily on the dominant characteristic of the mammalian brain, namely, the neocortex. Because it is reasonable to assume that the evolution of neural structure is closely tied to behavior, the apparent correlation between the extent of cortical development and the superior cognitive capacity of primates, especially in *Homo sapiens*, has led to the belief that cognitive complexity is closely linked to cortical complexity. Presumably, if we are to understand the nature of human perception, cognition, or consciousness, the answers will be found in the investigation of structure and function of the human neocortex. Unfortunately, direct study of cortical morphology and function in humans is currently impractical for ethical reasons. Moreover, even if we could study it directly, the human cortex may be too complex a structure to understand without knowledge established as a result of prior work on simpler cortical systems. The ideal animals are usually seen to be lower primates, such as rhesus macaques, and in fact the anatomy, physiology, chemistry, and behavior of macaques has been studied extensively. Once again, however, we must recognize practical problems. Aside from the ethical issue of using members of an advanced species that are frequently trapped in the wild, there are further questions related to cost effectiveness, our ability to effectively analyze the behavior of animals that are difficult to handle, and the difficulty in studying complex cortical systems without prior experiences garnered from studying simpler cortical circuitry.

It is the thesis of this book that the laboratory rat provides a useful alternative to the primate and can serve as an important model of mammalian cortical function. Its study is not only economical but its cortical structure appears to be simpler than that of primates, and it is certainly possible to do a more thorough behavioral analysis for the rat than for most other laboratory mammals. The rat is not appropriate for all questions about cortical functioning in humans, however, so some of the issues surrounding cross-species generalizations are considered briefly.

1.1   Model Systems in Behavioral Neuroscience

Evolutionary theory is central to comparative neuroscience, and its fundamental tenets are certainly consistent with the proposition that information learned from the study of nonhuman species may be used to understand human brain-behavior relations. It must not be assumed, however, that research on any species will be equally useful in answering all questions. The choice of species obviously depends on the nature of the problem under study. There are three principal lines of comparative research in behavioral neuroscience, and for each of them a species can be chosen for different reasons. These include: (1) studies designed to describe the phylogenetic development of the brain, (2) studies directed toward understanding the basic mechanisms of brain function, and (3) studies designed to produce models of human neurological disorders.

Studies of Phylogenetic Development

Here particular species are chosen because of their phylogenetic relationships. It is assumed that understanding the phylogenetic development of the brain is important if we are to make meaningful inferences about brain function in humans. Experiments with rats, cats, and monkeys do not permit many inferences regarding evolutionary development of the human brain because these species do not form an evolutionary sequence; rats were never ancestral to cats, nor cats to monkeys. All these species evolved independently from a common ancestor, and many aspects of cortical organization are likely to be examples of parallel evolution. To draw inferences regarding the evolutionary development of the brain, it is necessary to choose closely related species that constitute what Hodos and Campbell (1969) have termed a quasi-evolutionary sequence. For example, in the study of the phylogenetic development of auditory processing, Ravizza and Belmore (1978) used opposums, hedgehogs, tree shrews, bushbabies, macaques, chimpanzees, and humans. Each succeeding species is believed to have evolved from a species something like the one listed before it. In this sense rat-cat-monkey comparisons are meaningless (see Hodos and Campbell 1969), and rats would be an inappropriate choice in these circumstances.

On the other hand rats may be a valid choice for different types of phylogenetic studies. There are about 3000 species of rodents worldwide, living in habitats ranging from the tropics to near the poles. These species occupy a considerable range of ecological niches including arboreal, aquatic, and burrowing environments. Further there is quite a range in the social structure, diet, maternal investment, and so on in different species. Indeed interspecies variation is sufficient that taxonomists have identified three suborders of rodents, roughly corresponding to squirrellike rodents and beavers, mouselike rodents (gerbils, mice, voles, rats), and other rodents (porcupines, agoutis, guinea pigs). In view of this variation it is reasonable to predict that careful comparison of animals (including rats) from the rodent order might well give clues to questions about phylogenetic development of brain and behavior in mammals generally. Additionally, correlations between differences in cortical organization and behavioral adaptations to particular niches can reasonably provide a way of testing hypotheses regarding cortical function and organization. For example, if the prefrontal cortex is hypothesized to play a major role in the control of social behavior, then it is reasonable to ask whether highly social rodents might have a prefrontal structure different from that of more solitary animals. Because so much is known about the brain and behavior of rats relative to other rodents, it makes sense to use rats as a basis for comparative studies of rodent brain and behavior relations.

Studies of Basic Mechanisms

Species can also be chosen in studies of basic mechanisms because they provide an advantage in studying a particular problem. Perhaps the classic example is Harvey's study of the circulatory system of the fish. By using the fish as a model, Harvey was able to demonstrate that the blood is transferred by the heart from veins to arteries. The advantage of the fish was that it lacks the secondary circulation of the blood to the lungs, which obscured the realization that the function of the heart is the same in all vertebrates (Diamond and Chow 1962).

In neuroscience the goal of this type of work is to determine how behavioral or neural mechanisms work in relatively simple cases. Thus neurophysiologists may choose to study the neural activity of giant nerve fibers because the nerve is so large and accessible. Similarly investigators may wish to investigate synaptic plasticity in the abdominal ganglia in *Aplysia*. There is a limit of simplicity of the nervous system beyond which certain problems are not usefully studied, however. Thus, although *Aplysia* may provide an interesting model for certain questions about simple associative learning, it is unlikely to represent a sensible model of human memory. It can be argued that this is best studied in an animal with a cortical mantle because there is little doubt that both neo- and paleocortical structures play a central role in human memory (e.g., Kolb and Whishaw 1985a) and because the complexity of cortical circuitry is qualitatively different from that of *Aplysia*. To take an extreme analogy, it seems unlikely that understanding the role of calcium flux in synaptic change will lead directly to our understanding of the brain-behavior relations in language. There are, then, levels of simplicity of the nervous system that define the suitability of a species. Studies of the basic processes of neocortical functioning (and by implication cognitive processes requiring neocortex) will require that animals be chosen that have a neocortex. In this sense the rat may be an acceptable model for analyzing neocortical organization at the anatomical, chemical, physiological, and behavioral levels. It is certainly simpler in organization than the rhesus monkey, and it may be possible to establish basic principles of cortical organization that normally are obscured by the volume of neocortex and the complex cortical interconnections that characterize the neocortex in the primate. Indeed there appear to be basic cortical zones common to all mammals (see section 1.4), and it is reasonable to suppose that much can be learned about the basic organization of the mammalian cortex by studying the relationships between these areas in the absence of new, and probably species-specific, cortical regions.

One difficulty with choosing any mammal to use as a model of cortical function is that each species has a unique behavioral repertoire that permits the animal to survive in its particular environmental niche. There is therefore the danger that neocortical organization is uniquely patterned in different species in a way that reflects the unique behavioral adaptations of different species. Warren and Kolb (1978) considered this problem, but noted that although the details of behavior may differ somewhat, mammals share many similar behavioral traits and capacities. For example, all mammals must detect and interpret sensory stimuli, relate this information to past experience, and act appropriately. Similarly all mammals appear to be capable of learning complex tasks under various schedules of reinforcement (Warren 1977), and all mammals are mobile and have developed mechanisms for navigating in space. The details and complexity of these behaviors clearly vary, but the general capacities are common to all mammals. Warren and Kolb (1978) proposed that behaviors and behavioral capacities demonstrable in all mammals could be designated as *class-common* behaviors. In contrast, behaviors that are unique to a species and that have presumably been selected to promote survival in a particular niche are designated as *species-typical* behaviors. The distinction between these two types of behavior can be illustrated by the manner in which different mammals use their forelimbs to manipulate food objects. Monkeys will grasp objects with a single forepaw and often sit upright, holding the food item in one paw, to consume the food. Rats too will grasp objects with one forepaw and then typically transfer the food to mouth, assume a sitting posture, transfer the food back to both forepaws, and then eat. In contrast, cats or dogs tend to use the forepaw to hold the food item on the surface. All mammals use the forepaws to manipulate food (or other items), and this is a class-common behavior. The details vary from species to species, however, and these are species-typical behaviors. (The similarity in the reaching responses of different mammals, especially rats and monkeys, is discussed in more detail by Bures and Bracha in chapter 9.)

Kolb and Whishaw (1983) pursued the concept of class-common versus species-typical behaviors and further considered the question of whether class-common behaviors have class-common neural substrates. They noted that there is no guarantee that just because mammals have class-common behaviors, they have not independently evolved solutions to the class-common problems. There is little evidence in support of this notion, however. Neurophysiological stimulation, evoked potentials, and lesion studies reveal a similar topography in the motor, somatosensory, visual, and auditory cortices of the mammals—a topography that provides the basis for the class-common neural organization of fundamental capacities of mammals, or at least of placental mammals. Similarly we shall see throughout this book that there are remarkable parallels between the basic neurochemical and neuroanatomical structure of the rodent and primitive cortex, which again suggests a basic class-common neural circuitry.

Models of Neurological Disorders

In this type of comparative work, the aim is to produce a particular disorder, or a condition that simulates it, and then to manipulate different variables to try to understand the nature of the disorder and to test potential treatments. This can provide a focus for basic research on a more general issue as well as on a particular problem. A contemporary example can be seen in the research on disorders of memory. By damaging the hippocampal system in a variety of ways, many investigators have been able to show a severe amnesia and have used this amnesic syndrome as a model of human amnesia (e.g., Sutherland, Whishaw, and Kolb 1983, Sutherland and Arnold 1987, Whishaw 1987). For example, in the course of his studies Sutherland has shown that there are interesting parallels between this syndrome and the medial temporal lobe syndrome as seen in patient H. M. Thus it appears that there is a finite period of retrograde amnesia and a severe anterograde amnesia (e.g., Sutherland and Arnold 1987). It is now possible to use the model to evaluate the efficacy of drug treatments that are hoped to be useful in human memory loss such as dementia resulting from Alzheimer's disease as well as to evaluate theoretical models of mnestic systems in the human brain (Mishkin and Appenzeller 1987). A significant advantage of the rat in such studies is that it is possible to evaluate the large number of animals that are needed for neurochemical, histological, and physiological experiments as well as to evaluate both memory and other abilities in a large number of behavioral situations. Such studies would be impractical in cats or monkeys.

1.2   The Rat as a Laboratory Species: Defensible Choice or Bad Habit?

The laboratory rat obviously plays a prominent role in neuroscience research and is probably the most widely used subject in neuroscience research. The choice of the rat for scientific research has been the subject of some controversy, especially in behavioral work, however, because its origin as a laboratory subject has led some investigators to suggest that it is an indefensible choice as a representative mammal (e.g., Lockhard 1968). It is therefore worthwhile to consider the history of the rat in laboratory research.

The laboratory rat is a domesticated version of *Rattus norvegicus*. According to Lockhard (1968), albino forms of wild *R. norvegicus* were noted in England in 1822 and presumably occurred elsewhere. During the 1800s a popular sport in England and France was rat baiting, in which rats were trapped and placed in large numbers (e.g., 200) in a pit with a terrier. Spectators bet on the time taken by the terrier to kill the last rat. According to Richter (1954), albino rats were kept by animal fanciers and kept for breeding purposes, and the first laboratory use of albino rats, which were tamer than pigmented wild rats, was by Philipeaux in 1856. Crampe began breeding experiments with albino rats around 1880, and Donaldson established a colony at the University of Chicago in 1893 from a group of Crampe's rats. This colony later formed the basis of the stock at the Wistar Institute and formed the stock used in the behavioral experiments at Watson and Carr.

According to Munn (1950), Stewart first used the wild gray rat at Clark University in 1894 to study the effect of alcohol, diet, and barometric changes on animal behavior. Because the gray rat proved difficult to handle, Stewart switched to the white rat in 1895, and the first psychological studies of these animals began at Clark soon after when Small and Kline began the first maze studies in about 1898. Watson began his studies at Chicago in about 1901, and when Carr joined Watson in learning studies in 1908, the white rat had become established as a subject for psychological investigation (Munn 1950). In 1915 Donaldson published *The Rat*, which had as a major theme the physiological similarities between rats and humans. By the 1920s the rat had become a favorite species for the study of learning by psychologists. In fact Lashley's (1929) extensive examination of the effects of cortical lesions as well as anatomical structure in rats and monkeys led to the use of rats as the major laboratory species in physiological psychology, a tradition that continues today.

It seems a fair guess that the animals originally chosen for the Chicago colony were a biased sample of *R. norvegicus*: they were albino, they were from Crampe's selected colony, and they derived from stock that had been trapped. Boice (1966) has noted that rat trapping is not a random process because hungry, timid, small, and low-social-status *R. norvegicus* are the most likely to enter traps. According to Lockhard (1968), Crampe's breeding experiments showed that an albino female mated with a wild male transmitted three mutant genes: *c* (albino), *a* (nonagouti), and *h* (hooded). Donaldson's rats proved homozygous for these same genes. Thus the nonagouti (black) and hooded (black or brown and white) rats are derived from albino rats, differing from the albino only in that they have pigment.

The criticism of the rat as a defensible choice for laboratory study has come largely from investigators who have suggested that the process of domestication of the laboratory rat has led to the use of an "unnatural" or "degenerate" animal (e.g., Boice 1971, Lockhard 1968). Furthermore it has been suggested that the process of domestication has significantly changed the physiology of the laboratory rat (e.g., reduced brain size, reduced adrenal size) and that because the laboratory rat continues to be domesticated, it is not stable as a physiological subject. That is, a sample of laboratory rats taken in the 1930s would differ significantly from those of today, making it difficult to reach conclusions that can be generalized to rats, let alone other species. Although a legitimate concern a decade of research by Boice (e.g., 1981a,b) suggests that the apprehension was unfounded. Laboratory rats appear to show the potential for all behaviors characteristic of the wild type, and domesticated rats are capable of assuming a feral existence without difficulty, much like domestic cats. Furthermore, although it does appear that domestic rats have smaller brains than their feral cousins, this is true of virtually every domesticated animal. In any event we know that raising laboratory rats in complex environments increases brain size (see chapter 21 by Juraska). The one clear difference between wild and domesticated rats is the superior performance of the latter in laboratory paradigms, which is likely due to their reduced emotionality produced in response to the artificial test apparatus used in such studies. In sum there seems to be little reason to assume that the basic behavioral or cerebral organization of the domestic rat has been changed in any fundamental way by domestication.

1.3   Analysis of Behavior of the Laboratory Rat

A detailed description of the behavior of the rat is beyond the scope of this book, but it is fundamental to studies of the cortical organization of the rat. Clearly the cortex evolved to produce new behaviors, and it is only in the context of behavior that the organization of the cortex will eventually make sense. The most extensive contemporary reviews of the behavior of the laboratory rat are by Barnett (1963) and by Whishaw, Kolb, and Sutherland (1983). Whishaw and colleagues described a neuropsychological assessment battery for the rat that provides an example of a new technology that is developing for the study of behavior in the rat (table 1.1). Adoption of this technology is not yet widespread, and acceptance faces several obstacles.

First, there is the notion, which dates back to the 1920s, that rats should be tested in a single task and then killed, while additional rats are tested in other tasks. Thus, as Lashley and others began to do lesion studies using the rat, they were influenced by the view of behaviorism that the behavior of animals was uniquely influenced by experiences and that intersubject variation was due largely to differences in environmental experiences (e.g., Lashley 1929). In this context it was reasonable to suppose that studies of decorticated rats would best be done on subjects with no previous experiences in psychological studies. Behavioral study of naive adult rats usually involved a single test of learning, and then the animal was killed. Although classic behaviorism no longer plays a role in neuroscience, the idea that animals should be studied on a single task remains. Furthermore behavioral and anatomical studies are frequently performed on different animals, rather than making more direct correlations between brain and behavioral measures.

Second, the naive belief that a single behavioral test would provide an adequate measure of potentially complex brain-behavior relations has also contributed to a "one-behavioral-test" assessment literature.

Table 1.1 Behavioral Assessment of the Rat: A Partial Summary of Features of
Behavior for Examination

Measure	Specific Feature
Appearance	Body weight, core temperature, eyes, feces, fur, genitals, muscle tone, pupils, responsiveness, saliva, teeth, toenails, vocalizations.
Sensory and sensorimotor behavior	Response to stimuli of each sensory modality presented both in home cage and in novel place such as open field
Posture and immobility	Behavior when spontaneously immobile, immobile without posture or tone; tonic immobility or animal hypnosis; environmental influences on immobility
Movement	General activity, movement initiation, turning, climbing, walking, swimming, righting responses, limb movements in different activities such as reaching or bar pressing, oral movements such as in licking or chewing, environmental influences on movement
Species-typical behaviors	All species-typical behaviors such as grooming, food hoarding, foraging, sleep, maternal or sexual behavior, play, and burying.
Learning	Operant and respondent conditioning and learning sets, especially including measures of spatial learning, avoidance learning, and memory

For details, see Whishaw et al. 1983.

There is little doubt, however, that single behavioral measures provide
very biased estimates of behavior. For example, Kolb and Whishaw
(1981) found that animals with damage to the prefrontal cortex at 7 days
of age showed sparing of learned behaviors relative to animals operated
on as adults, but the same animals were grossly impaired at various
tests of species-typical behaviors. Furthermore additional studies
showed that even the sparing on learned behaviors was task dependent
(e.g., Kolb and Whishaw 1985b). Thus, if we are to develop an understanding of brain-behavior relationships for the cortex, it will be necessary to do extensive behavioral analyses in the same animals. The rat
is a particularly good animal for this purpose for it is possible to perform
tests of both species-typical and learned behavior in the laboratory.

Third, there is a strong bias in favor of limiting behavioral analysis
to easily quantified measures involving learning and memory. Unfortunately such assessments ignore most of the behaviors that the cortex

evolved to support (Warren 1972) and that are presumably class common.

Fourth, studies of animal behavior have suffered from the presumption of many investigators that the behavior of any species is easy to assess, especially in comparison with assessing the physiological, chemical, or anatomical characteristics of the animals' central nervous system. In fact behavior is more difficult to study. Such an assessment is possible, however, and an advantage of the rat is that because it is so well suited to laboratory study, it is possible to establish a standard behavioral taxonomy and take appropriate and representative measures.

One of the unfortunate effects that inadequate behavioral assessment has had on the field of neuroscience is that many neuroscientists appear to be distrustful of behavioral observations, and they have developed the erroneous belief that behavioral work is not really relevant or necessary for an understanding of the operation of the nervous system. This is an odd proposition in view of the fact that the brain's function is to produce behavior. In addition, there is an idea held by many neuroscientists that behavior cannot be useful in understanding brain function because the brain is so redundant that the behavioral consequences of brain alterations are often trivial, if there are any at all. This idea too is simply wrong. If the behavioral observations fail to find a change after some neural manipulation, it is almost certain that the behavior measured was inappropriate. There can be little doubt that different behavioral patterns are supported by different neural systems, and a detection of a behavioral change requires that the appropriate behaviors be monitored. A major advantage of the rat is that with it one can, in principle, do a thorough behavioral analysis. Such studies are impractical in larger animals such as cats and monkeys. Furthermore a major advantage of the rat is that more is already known about its behavior than about the behavior of any other laboratory species, and as the behavioral technology develops, it ought to be possible to reach conclusions regarding brain-behavior relations that will not be possible in the near future by using animals such as rhesus monkeys.

1.4 General Principles of Cortical Organization

Before beginning a detailed examination of the characteristics of the rat cortex, it is worthwhile to consider it in the general context of the cortex of other mammalian species. Such a comparison allows a better picture of the relative complexity of the rat cortex and highlights the similarities and differences between the rat and other species, especially those with more neocortex. Our review is brief, and the reader is directed to discussions by Kaas (1987a,b) for more extensive reviews of cortical evolution and organization in mammals.

Subdivisions of the Cortex

One of the principal characterisics of the neocortex is that it can be subdivided on a variety of cytoarchitectonic, neurochemical, electrophysiological, and other criteria into discrete cortical regions. It is usually assumed that these regions have a unique set of functions, even if they are not yet known. Although early anatomists appeared to believe that there would be clear homologies in these regions in different species, there is little agreement on this, in large part because of the variability across mammals. Thus there is great variation in gross features such as size, shape, and the relative volume of tissue devoted to particular functions (e.g., vision) in different species, in addition to variation in histological structure in regions that would appear to have similar functions. Nonetheless there are several principles of cortical organization that appear to be class common, at least with respect to the placental mammals, which includes all mammalian species except marsupials and monotremes. (In the following discussion we use mammal to mean placental mammal.)

1. Mammals have some cortical fields in common. Kaas (1987a) suggests that all mammals have primary and secondary visual fields (V-I and V-II), primary and secondary somatosensory fields (S-I and S-II), at least a primary auditory cortex (A-I), a region of posterior temporal cortex with input from V-I that is probably visual in function, taste cortex, prefrontal cortex (PFC) related to the dorsal medial nucleus of the thalamus, several subregions of limbic cortex related to the anterior and lateral dorsal thalamic nuclei, and a strip of "transitional" cortex that probably relates neocortical fields with the amygdala and hippocampus (see figure 1.1). The major differences across species include not only the number of other cortical fields, which are largely associated with visual, auditory and somatosensory sublields, but also the size of the class-common subfields. Indeed Kaas concludes that the "evolutionary advance in cortical organization is marked by increases in the numbers of unimodal sensory fields, not by increases in multimodal association cortex, as is traditionally thought."

2. The boundaries between areas are sharply defined. There remains considerable disagreement over the number of distinct areas in any given species, but Kaas (1987a) concludes that the cortical boundaries in all mammals are so sharp that one field changes to the next in about 100 μm. Interestingly there is a historical view that there are sharp borders between fields in the cortex of "advanced" species, such as monkeys, but the borders are indistinct in more primitive species, such as rats. There is not compelling evidence to support this distinction, as the various studies of Zilles (chapter 4) have clearly shown. Furthermore tangential sections of the somatosensory cortex of the rat are now often used as an example of the clarity and distinctness of cytoarchitectonic boundaries.

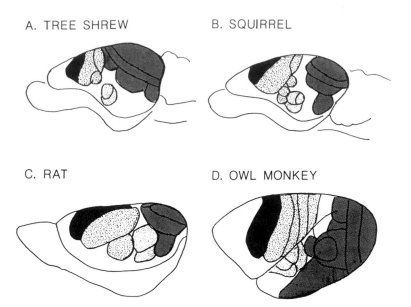

A. TREE SHREW   B. SQUIRREL

C. RAT   D. OWL MONKEY

Figure 1.1 Schematic drawings of four different mammalian brains. The figure illustrates the similarity in general organization across different mammals, but also shows that the number and location of subfields in different sensory modalities is species specific. The lightest stippling shows the auditory areas, the heavier stippling shows the somatosensory areas, the gray shows the visual areas, and the black shows the motor areas. The white regions include various other cortical regions. The drawings of the tree shrew, squirrel, and owl monkey are adapted from Kaas 1987b.

3. The cortex is composed of distinct columns that are relatively constant in width (Bugbee and Goldman-Rakic 1983) and, with the exception of binocular visual cortex, in cell number (Roekel et al. 1980). The major differences between species is in the number of columns in given regions, the number of connections between and within columns, and the thickness of the cortex. In general the greater the number of columns and intrinsic connections, the thicker the cortex.

4. Cortical areas are extensively interconnected. Analyses of species as diverse as rats and monkeys have shown that cortical fields are extensively interconnected, especially within modalities. There may be consistent general patterns of connections across species, such as a prefrontal-parietal connection, but this has not been demonstrated. Furthermore careful study of the connections of the sensory regions of even relatively closely related species, such as rhesus monkeys and owl monkeys, suggests that there is considerable variability in the details of these connections. In addition there is substantial variability in the details of thalamocortical (e.g., Diamond 1982) and other cortico-cortical connections. We cannot exclude the possibility that there is some general rule for these latter connections, however. For example, there are always corticohippocampal, corticoamygdalo, and corticostriatal con-

nections, although again there are significant interspecies differences (e.g., Amaral 1987).

In sum there are four class-common features of the mammalian cortex—multiple areas, sharp boundaries, columnar organization, and multiple interconnections—both with other cortical areas and the hippocampus, striatum, and amygdala. There are significant species differences as well, however, including the number and size of cortical areas, the extent of intracolumnar connections, and the details of cortico-cortical and cortico-subcortical connections. It is tempting to speculate that the neural basis of class-common behaviors will be found associated with the class-common similarities of the cortex, whereas the basis for differences in species-typical behavioral patterns will be found in the significant differences in cortical organization; but this must remain a working hypothesis.

References

Amaral, D. (1987). Anatomy of memory. In *Handbook of Sensory Physiology: Central Nervous System*. Vol. II. Washington, D.C.: American Physiological Society.

Barnett, S. A. (1963). *The Rat: A Study in Behavior*. London: Methuen.

Boice, R. (1971). On the fall of comparative psychology. *American Psychologist* 26:858–859.

Boice, R. (1981a). Captivity and feralization. *Psychological Bulletin* 89:407–421.

Boice, R. (1981b). Behavioral comparability of wild and domestic rats. *Behavior Genetics* 11:545–553.

Bugbee, N. M., and Goldman-Rakic, P. S. (1983). Columnar organization of corticocortical projections in squirrel and rhesus monkeys: Similarity of column width in species differing in cortical volume. *Journal of Comparative Neurology* 220:355–364.

Diamond, I. T. (1982). The functional significance of architectonic subdivisions of the cortex: Lashley's criticism of the traditional view. In J. Orback (ed.), *Neuropsychology after Lashley*. Hillsdale, N.J.: Erlbaum Associates, pp. 101–136.

Diamond, I. T., and Chow, K. L. (1962). Biological psychology. In S. Koch (ed.) *Psychology: A Study of a Science*. Vol. 4. New York: McGraw-Hill, pp. 158–241.

Flourens, P. (1823). Recherches physiques sur les proprietes et fonctions du system nerveux dans les animaux vertebres. *Archives Generales de Medecine* 2:231–274.

Hodos, W., and Campbell, C. B. G. (1969). Scalae naturae: Why there is no theory in comparative psychology. *Psychological Review* 76:337–350.

Kaas, J. H. (1987a). The organization of neocortex in mammals: Implications for theories of brain function. *Annual Review of Psychology* 38:129–151.

Kaas, J. H. (1987b). The organization and evolution of neocortex. In S. P. Wise (ed.), *Higher Brain Functions*. New York: John Wiley & Sons, pp. 347–378.

Kolb, B. and Whishaw, I. Q. (1981). Neonatal frontal lesions in the rat: Sparing of learned but not species-typical behavior in the presence of reduced brain weight and cortical thickness. *Journal of Comparative and Physiological Psychology* 95:863–879.

Kolb, B., and Whishaw, I. Q. (1983). Problems and principles underlying interspecies comparisons. In T. E. Robinson (ed.), *Behavioral Approaches to Brain Research*. New York: Oxford University Press, pp. 237–263.

Kolb, B., and Whishaw, I. Q. (1985a). *Fundamentals of Human Neuropsychology*. 2nd ed. New York: W. H. Freeman and Co.

Kolb, B., and Whishaw, I. Q. (1985b). Earlier is not always better: Behavioral dysfunction and abnormal cerebral morphogenesis following neonatal cortical lesions in the rat. *Behavioural Brain Research* 17:25–43.

Lashley, K. S. (1929). *Brain Mechanisms and Intelligence*. Chicago: University of Chicago Press.

Lockard, R. B. (1968). The albino rat: A defensible choice or a bad habit? *American Psychologist* 23:734–742.

Luciani, L. (1915). *Human Physiology*. London: Macmillan.

Mishkin, M., and Appenzeller, T. (1987). The anatomy of memory. *Scientific American* 256 (6):80–87.

Munn, N. L. (1950). *Handbook of Psychological Research on the Rat*. Cambridge, MA: Riverside Press.

Ravizza, R. J., and Belmore, S. (1978). Auditory forebrain: Evidence from anatomical and behavioral experiments involving human and animal subjects. In R. B. Masterton (ed.), *Handbook of Behavioral Neurobiology*. New York: Plenum Press.

Richter, C. P. (1954). The effects of domestication and selection on the behavior of the Norway rat. *Journal of the National Cancer Institute* 15:727–738.

Roekel, A. J., Hiorns, R. W., and Powell, T. P. S. (1980). The basic uniformity in structure of the neocortex. *Brain* 103:221–224.

Sutherland, R. J., and Arnold, K. (1987). Anterograde and retrograde effects on place memory after limbic or diencenphalic damage. *Society for Neuroscience Abstracts* 13:1066.

Sutherland, R. J., Whishaw, I. Q., and Kolb, B. (1983). A behavioral analysis of spatial localization following electrolytic, kainate- or colchicine-induced damage to the hippocampal formation in the rat. *Behavioral Brain Research* 7:133–153.

Warren, J. M. (1972). Evolution, behavior, and the prefrontal cortex. *Acta Neurobiologiae Expermentalis* 32:581–594.

Warren, J. M. (1977). A phylogenetic approach to learning and intelligence. In A. Oliverio (ed.), *Genetics, Environment and Intelligence*. Amsterdam, Elsevier, pp. 37–56.

Warren, J. M., and Kolb, B. (1978). Generalization in neuropsychology. In S. Finger (ed.), *Recovery from Brain Damage*. New York: Plenum Press, pp. 36–48.

Whishaw, I. Q. (1987). Hippocampal, granule cell and CA3-4 lesions impair formation of a place learning set in the rat and induce reflex epilepsy. *Behavioural Brain Research* 24:59–72.

Whishaw, I. Q., Kolb, B., and Sutherland, R. J. (1983). The analysis of behavior in the laboratory rat. In T. E. Robinson (ed.), *Behavioral Approaches to Brain Research*. New York: Oxford University Press, pp. 141–211.

II Organization of the Neocortex

2 Organization of the Neocortex of the Rat

Bryan Kolb

The organization of neural structures can be inferred from several types of analyses, including (1) embryology, (2) architecture, (3) biochemistry, (4) connectivity, (5) physiological properties, and (6) behavioral correlates. Each provides information that is used throughout this volume, but to provide a general overview, we have included five chapters in part II that focus on the general organization of the rat cortex, with emphasis on anatomical organization. These chapters include a discussion of cortical development, architectonic divisions of the cortex, and electrophysiological activity of the cortex. In this chapter I provide background to these chapters and add information that would otherwise not be covered, especially including a discussion of the connections of the rat's neocortex.

2.1 Developmental Studies

At first look the mammalian neocortex appears almost hopelessly complex with its wide range of cell types, the complexity of its connections, the intricacy of its laminar organization, and its biochemical organization. One way to approach such a complex system is to take advantage of many new techniques in developmental neurobiology (cf. Rakic and Goldman-Rakic 1982). Moreover it is possible to "simplify" the organization of the cortex by analyzing systematically how this system is constructed in different stages embryologically, including cell birth, cell migration and differentiation, dendritic growth, axonal growth, synapse formation, and the subsequent pruning of cell numbers and connections by a "selective" process of cell death. Of course if the functional organization of the cortex is to be understood, it will be necessary to determine how distinct cytoarchitectonic regions are put together and how they come to influence the organization of other areas. For example, we will need to know how areas that have a representation of the external world, such as in primary sensory cortices, come to have this representation and how other structures, such as the prefrontal cortex, come to access this information to construct cognitive representations of space.

Work on the development of the rat cortex really began in the late 1950s as Hicks and D'Amato took advantage of radiation as a lesion tool and tritiated thymidine as a label to map the positions of migrating neural cells in rats (e.g., Hicks and D'Amato 1961, 1968, Hicks, D'Amato, and Lowe 1959). In their extensive studies they showed that although cortical cell division was largely complete at birth in rats, migration continued well into the first postnatal week. At about the same time research with other species, notably the mouse, began to report similar findings (e.g., Angevine and Sidman 1961), and it became clear that, contrary to conventional wisdom, the cortex followed an inside-out developmental sequence such that layer VI forms first, followed by the more superficial layers. Subsequent work by several groups (e.g., Berry 1974, Jones 1981, Bayer and Altman 1987, Rakic 1984) has led to further advances in our understanding the process of cortical development. Chapter 3 by Uylings, Van Eden, Parnavelas, and Kalsbeek summarizes the older work and adds significant new information to the story. Although there have been thorough studies of the connections of restricted regions, especially the somatosensory cortex (e.g., Ivy and Killackey 1982), what remains to be described for the rat is the development of cortico-cortical connections.

2.2 Architectural Studies

Although the rat was used extensively in brain-behavior studies by Lashley (1929) and his contemporaries beginning in the 1920s, the first systematic description of the cortical areas of the rat was not published until Krieg's descriptions in the late 1940s. Krieg felt that the "close study of a simple cortex would be fundamental to an understanding of the human cortex" (Krieg 1946b, p. 268), and he first attempted to identify cortical regions in the rat and then to determine their correspondence to those in primates. In fact in his reports Krieg borrowed the nomenclature of Brodmann and labeled cortical areas in the rat on the basis of presumed homologies to primates. This may have been a sensible way to start, but it was based largely on physical location (e.g., prefrontal as most anterior, visual as most posterior), which has proved unreliable. For example, Krieg assumed that the prefrontal equivalent in rodents would be at the frontal pole. On the basis of thalamocortical and cortico-cortical connections, we now know this to be in error; the prefrontal cortex lies in two areas—one medial and one ventrolateral (see chapter 18 by Kolb).

Recently Zilles and his coworkers (e.g., chapter 4 and Zilles 1985) have provided a more objective quantification of cortical structure by using a computer-controlled image analyzer to identify areal and laminar differences in measures such as cell packing density and myelin density. Such a procedure has allowed a more objective parceling of the rat cortex, which is significantly different from Krieg's in certain respects (see table 2.1 for nomenclature). Chapter 4 provides a further refinement of Zilles's (1985) and Zilles and Wree's (1985) descriptions, providing further information on cortical areal and laminar organization, as well as on the laminar differences of different regions. In addition Zilles, Wree, and Dausch extend the observations in chapter 5 as they describe areal and laminar distribution of various putative neurotransmitters as well as the results of systematic work using a sulphide silver method of Timm, which shows clear areal distinctions in the cortex.

A major advantage of Zilles's studies is that they provide a nomenclature that is independent of previous nomenclature in other species. Thus Zilles's terminology is alphanumeric to denote gross regions (Fr = frontal, Par = parietal, Oc = occipital, Cg = cingulate, Te = temporal, etc.) or to denote traditionally used terms (e.g., AI = agranular insular, RSA = retrosplenial agranular). Numbers are used to supplement the alphabetic characters and denote apparent functional subregions. For example, Oc1 and Oc2 refer to primary and secondary visual areas, respectively. In view of the advantages of Zilles's nomenclature, it has been used as much as possible throughout the book. We have taken the liberty of grouping the cortical regions into the following putative functional groupings, both for purposes of considering the connections and for discussions in other chapters.

1. *Prefrontal cortex*   This includes all the tissue that receives projections from the dorsal medial thalamic nucleus (MD). It is separated into several subregions on the basis of its architectonics and connections: (a) an anterior cingulate area (including Cg1, Cg2, Cg3), (b) the "shoulder region" (Fr2), which has been a proposed homolog of the arcuate cortex (Brodmann's area 8) of the monkey, (c) an orbital prefrontal area (LO, VLO, MO), and (d) an anterior perirhinal region of agranular insular cortex (AI). Infralimbic cortex (IL) is included as prefrontal cortex because Divac and associates (1978) found it to receive MD afferents.

2. *Motor cortex*   This refers principally to the primary motor cortex, which is Zilles's Fr1 and Fr3, as well as the forelimb and hindlimb representations, FL and HL, respectively.

3. *Somatosensory cortex*   The somatosensory regions Par1 and Par2 represent the primary and secondary somatosensory "ratunculi" described by Woolsey (1958). The visceral cortex (Vi) is identified separately. Little is known of its connections, but it can be presumed to be similar to Par1 and Par2.

4. *Visual cortex*   Traditionally the visual cortex of the rat is considered to include Krieg's areas 17, 18, and 18a, which Zilles has subdivided into several regions (see Zilles's figure 4.3). The homologies between areas 18 and 18a in the rat and peristriate areas in the monkey remain uncertain (see chapter 12 by Dean), but it seems likely that these regions have visual functions, as does Zilles's area Te2 (see chapter 19), so they are grouped as "visual cortex."

5. *Auditory cortex*   The auditory cortex includes at least area Te1 and

Table 2.1 Comparison of Krieg's Cytoarchitectonic Regions with those of
Zilles

Zilles's area	Krieg's area
Fr1	4, 10
Fr2	8
Fr3	4, 10
FL	3, 4
HL	3
AID	11
AIV	11
AIP	13
PRh	35
Vi	10
Par1	3
Par2	2
VLO	51
LO	51
IL	25
Cg1	24
Cg2	23
Cg3	32, 24
RSG	29a, b, c
RSA	29d
Oc2M	18a
Oc1	17
Oc2L	18
Te1	39, 40, 41
Te2	20, 36
Te3	14

probably Te3, both of which are associated with the medial geniculate nucleus. It is possible that area Te2 also has some auditory function as it may receive projections from the medial geniculate nucleus in addition to the lateral posterior nucleus of the thalamus.

6. *Posterior association cortex*   On the basis of both anatomical and behavioral evidence, it appears possible to identify a posterior parietal regional that corresponds roughly to Krieg's area 7 (e.g., Kolb and Walkey 1987). Zilles includes this area in visual regions Oc2L and Oc2M, but concedes that there may be grounds for considering it as functionally separable. We consider it as a separate area for the purpose of discussion, but it should remain a working hypothesis (see chapter 19).

7. *Associative insular cortex*   Guldin and Markowitsch (1983) argued that the cortex in the rhinal fissure, which Zilles calls perirhinal cortex, and the cortex just above it, which Zilles calls Te3, Te2, should be considered associative (insular) cortex. They suggest that part or all of this cortex should be considered analogous to the insular cortex of the primate. The connections of the perirhinal cortex itself have been studies by Deacon and Associates (1983), who suggested that this region is analogous to von Bonin and Bailey's TF, TG, and TH of perirhinal cortex in the monkey.

2.3   Cortical Connectivity

The cortex is characterized both by intrinsic connections, which cross laminae in all areas, as well as by its connections to (1) other cortical areas, (2) other forebrain areas, including especially the striatum, amygdala, and hippocampus, (3) diencephalic areas, especially the thalamus, and (4) various midbrain, cerebellar, pons, and spinal regions. The thalamic projections are perhaps the most systematically studied and are reviewed in detail in a major book on the thalamus (Jones 1985). Many of the brainstem projections are considered in detail in the sensory and motor chapters of parts III and IV. There is reason to suspect that the forebrain connections of the cortex may provide important clues to the functional dissociation of different cortical areas and to the functions of cortical areas, so we provide an overview of these data.

Cortico-Cortical Connections

The details of cortico-cortical connectivity have led to important insights into the functional organization of the cortex of the monkey (e.g., Goldman-Rakic 1988, Pandya and Yeterian 1985). Although there have been many studies of specific pathways in rats, we are unaware of any previous attempt to summarize the cortico-cortical connections in the rat. Using a fiber degeneration method, Krieg (1947, p. 282) was unable to demonstrate many cortico-cortical connections and concluded that "there is little evidence of inter- or intraareal association fibers" in the rat. Subsequent degeneration studies (e.g., Leonard 1969) also failed to find corticocortical connections in the rat, but more recently transport techniques (including fluorescent dyes, tritiated amino acids, and horseradish peroxidase) have shown extensive connections in the rat. Figure 2.1 summarizes much of the published information on the cortico-cortical connections of the rat (for more details, see Wise and Donoghue 1986, Miller and Vogt 1984, Vogt and Miller 1983, Beckstead 1979, Guldin and Markowitsch 1983, Kolb and Walkey 1987, Reep et al. 1984, Kolb, Gibb, and van der Kooy 1989).

Several general principles can be identified in the data in figure 2.1. First, it is evident that, in contrast to the conclusions of previous degeneration studies, there are extensive cortico-cortical connections in the rat. Second, several prefrontal regions have extensive connections with the secondary visual areas. Only the Fr2 area has auditory and somatosensory inputs as well, much as in the arcuate cortex of the monkey (Reep et al. 1984). Third, the motor and somatosensory regions are interconnected, and the motor cortex is connected with the orbital prefrontal region and the supplementary region Fr2 (Krieg's area 8, AGm of Donoghue and Wise 1982). There is, however, no direct input from the medial prefrontal zone (Cg1, Cg2, Cg3). Fourth, both the somatosensory (Par1) and the secondary auditory area (Te3) connect with secondary visual area (Oc2L), which may imply a multimodal function of this tissue. Further the Par1 connection to visual areas is selective because the "eye area" projects to Oc2M and Oc2L regions. Fifth, although it is not shown in figure 2.2, at least part of nearly every neocortical area has reciprocal connections with the perirhinal cortex (see table 2.2). The connection is especially heavy from prefrontal regions and represents a major route to the hippocampal and amygdaloid

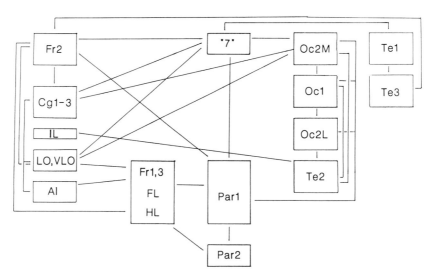

Figure 2.1 A summary of the cortico-cortical connections in the rat (abbreviations as in Zilles's figure 4.3.

Table 2.2 Summary of Perirhinal Afferents and their Principal Thalamic Associates in Rat and Monkey

Rat		Monkey	
Cortical Source	Thalamic Associate	Cortical Source	Thalamic Associate
Cg3, AI, VLO	MDm	Orbital	MDm
Fr2, Fr1, Fr3, FL	M1, VL	Periarcuate	MD1
Cg1, Cg3	MD1, AM	Anterior cingulate	MDm, AM
RSA, RSG	AM, AV, LD	Posterior cingulate	AM, AV, LD
7, Par1	LP, L, MGBc, PoM	Inferior parietal	PuM, LP, P
Te1, Te3	MGBm, MGBc	Temporal, insular	MGBd, VPi, PuM
Te2	LP	Inferotemporal	PuI

Adapted from Deacon et al. 1983.

formations (Deacon et al. 1983). Deacon and colleagues (1983) have suggested that this cortex is analogous to the monkey's perirhinal cortex and the cortex in the posterior parahippocampal gyrus immediately caudal to the termination of the rhinal sulcus (von Bonin and Bailey's areas TH and TF). Table 2.2 shows the striking parallel between the perirhinal afferents and their thalamic associates in the two species. In both species the projections have a clear topographic organization and are likely to have a significant role in associating neocortical and allo-cortical areas. There is virtually nothing known of the function of this tissue, although the projections to the hippocampal formation suggest some role in memory or spatial functions.

In summary recent findings have made it clear that the rat cortex has extensive cortico-cortical connections, especially with the prefrontal cortex. It seems likely, however, that the initial difficulty in demonstrating these connections with degeneration techniques reflects the fact that the connections are less extensive than those of primates and carnivores; many of those cortico-cortical connections can be seen using degeneration techniques.

There is another type of cortico-cortical connection that has not been extensively studied—the callosal connection. In contrast to the ipsilateral cortico-cortical connections, callosal connections can be seen easily with traditional degeneration studies, as summarized in figure 2.2. As in cats and monkeys these connections are extensive, but do not include connections of primary visual cortex or certain regions of the motor and somatosensory cortex.

Medial Temporal Connections
On the basis of conventional use with the primate brain, the medial temporal region can be considered to consist of the amygdaloid complex, including the amygdaloid nuclei and periamygdaloid cortex, and the hippocampal formation, including the subiculum, entorhinal cortex,

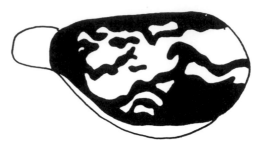

Figure 2.2 Organization of the callosal connections in the rat. The dark areas indicate areas of callosal projection (adapted from Akers and Killackey 1978).

dentate gyrus, and Ammon's horn. The presumed role of these structures in various cognitive and emotional processes makes their connections with distinct neocortical regions of particular importance. Although most cortical areas have access to the amygdala and associated structures via the perirhinal cortex, the amygdaloid complex has reciprocal projections with much of the prefrontal regions (Cg2, Cg3, IL, AID, AIV, LO, and VLO). There are further connections through the MD of the thalamus, with which both systems are connected (Krettek and Price 1977).

The hippocampal formation has extensive neocortical connections via the perirhinal region as well as via the posterior cingulate cortex, as well as direct prefrontal connections arising from Cg3 and IL regions (cf. Amaral 1988, Ferino, Thierry, and Glowinski 1987, Swanson 1981). Again this implies a closer functional relation between hippocampal and prefrontal regions than with other neocortical areas.

Corticostriatal Connections

The neocortex constitutes a major source of afferents to the caudate-putamen (striatum), but, in contrast to most other cortical connections, these are not reciprocal. The corticostriatal connections have three important characteristics. First, they are topographic in the sense that different cortical sensory regions project to different striatal regions (Faull, Nauta, and Domesick 1986, Veening, Cornelissen, and Lieven 1980). For example, the visual projections are largely to the ipsilateral dorsomedial striatum. In contrast auditory projections are primarily to the caudal striatum (figure 2.3). Second, the cortical projections overlap with projections from their own major thalamic nuclei. For instance, the medial geniculate and auditory cortex project to the same region of the striatum. Third, the prefrontal cortex (Cg1–Cg3, MO, LO) has extensive bilateral projections to the striatum that overlap with the sensory (Ferino et al. 1987) and motor projections. These projections are not as heavy to the dorsolateral region of the striatum, and they extend ventrally into the white area in figure 2.3. Fourth, corticostriatal connections

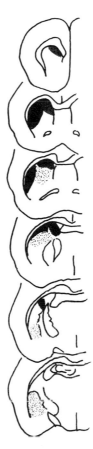

Figure 2.3 Summary of corticostriatal connections of the motor (black), visual (gray), somatosensory (dark stippling), and auditory (light stippling) cortex in the rat. Borders of different projections are approximate. Prefrontal connections are not shown because they overlap with the sensory and motor projections. Perirhinal projections are largely in the white region.

from individual cortical fields "respect" histochemically distinct regions. Thus it has been shown histochemically that the striatum is composed of patches that are acetylcholinesterase-poor and dopamine- and opiate-rich, surrounded by a matrix that is acetylcholinesterase-rich and dopamine- and opiate-poor (Gerfen 1984, 1985). Recently Donoghue and Herkenham (1986) showed that Cg3 projects bilaterally to striatal patches, whereas Cg1/3, and Fr1/3 regions project bilaterally to the matrix (figure 2.4). Furthermore parietal and visual regions (Par1, Oc1) project ipsilaterally to the matrix. The unique pattern of certain prefrontal projections implies that this region has a unique contribution to striatal activity. Furthermore the relation between prefrontal (patch) and sensory (matrix) inputs may allow for "interactions" between sensory and prefrontal regions. This "associative" arrangement complements the direct sensory inputs into the prefrontal cortex and the sensory and

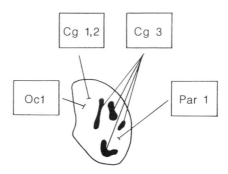

Figure 2.4 Schematic drawing contrasting the corticostriatal projections from the prefrontal regions Cg3 and Cg1,2, as well as the sensory projections. The Cg3 projections are bilateral to the patches; the Cg1,2 projections are bilateral to the matrix; the other projections are largely unilateral.

prefrontal interactions in the perirhinal cortex. Perhaps each of these associative areas plays a unique role in sensorimotor processing, possibly forming the basis of distinct memory systems.

2.4 Electrophysiological Activity

The neocortex of the rat has not been a favorite of electrophysiologists, in part because of its small size relative to the recording apparatus and in part because of the tendency to use animals with more elaborated sensory systems (especially visual) for electrophysiological studies. There is a significant literature on slow wave recording in the rat neocortex, however, which has proved particularly valuable in understanding the role of nonspecific ascending systems in the neocortex. Vanderwolf summarizes in chapter 6 the results of such studies and provides an important comparison with the hippocampus, which has been studied much more extensively in the rat.

References

Ackers, R. M., and Killackey, H. P. (1978). Organization of corticocortical connections in the parietal cortex of the rat. *Journal of Comparative Neurology* 181:513–538.

Amaral, D. (1988). Memory: Anatomical organization of candidate brain regions. In *Handbook of Physiology V*. Washington: American Physiological Association, 211–294.

Angevine, J. B., and Sidman, R. L. (1961). Autoradiographic study of cell migration during histogenesis of cerebral cortex in the mouse. *Nature* 192:766–768.

Bayer, S. A., and Altman, J. (1987). Directions in neurogenetic gradients and patterns of anatomical connections in the telencephalon. *Progress in Neurobiology* 29:57–106.

Beckstead, R. M. (1979). An autoradiographic examination of corticocortical and subcortical projections of the mediodorsal-projections (prefrontal) cortex in the rat. *Journal of Comparative Neurology* 184:43–62.

Berry, M. J. (1974). Development of the cerebral neocortex of rat. In G. Gottlieb (ed.), *Aspects of Neurogenesis*. New York: Academic Press, 7–67.

Deacon, T. W., Eichenbaum, H., Rosenberg, P., and Eckmann, K. W. (1983). Afferent connections of the perirhinal cortex in the rat. *Journal of Comparative Neurology* 220:168–190.

Divac, I., Kosmal, A., Bjorklund, A., and Lindvall, O. (1978). Subcortical projections to the prefrontal cortex in the rat as revealed by horseradish perioxidase technique. *Neuroscience* 3:785–796.

Donoghue, J. P., and Herkenham, M. (1986). Neostriatal projections from individual cortical fields conform to histochemically distinct striatal compartments in the rat. *Brain Research* 365:397–403.

Donoghue, J. P., and Wise, S. P. (1982). The motor cortex of the rat: Cytoarchitecture and microstimulation mapping. *Journal of Comparative Neurology* 212:76–88.

Faull, R. L. M., Nauta, W. J. H., and Domesick, V. B. (1986). The visual cortico-striato-nigral pathway in the rat. *Neuroscience* 19:1119–1132.

Ferino, G., Thierry, A. M., and Glowinski, J. (1987). Anatomical and electrophysiological evidence for a direct projection from Ammon's horn to the medial prefrontal cortex in the rat. *Experimental Brain Research* 65:421–426.

Ferino, F., Thierry, A. M., Saffroy, M., and Glowinski, J. (1987). Interhemispheric and subcortical collaterals of medial prefrontal cortical neurons in the rat. *Brain Research* 417:257–266.

Gerfen, C. R. (1984). The neostriatal mosaic: Compartmentalization of corticostriatal input and striatonigral output systems. *Nature* 311:461–464.

Gerfen, C. R. (1985). The neostriatal mosaic. I. Compartmental organization of projections from the striatum to the substantia nigra in the rat. *Journal of Comparative Neurology* 171:369–386.

Guldin, W. O., and Markowitsch, H. J. (1983). Cortical and thalamic afferent connections of the insular and adjacent cortex of the rat. *Journal of Comparative Neurology* 215:135–153.

Hicks, S., and D'Amato, C. J. (1961). How to design and build abnormal brains using radiation during development. In W. S. Fields and M. M. Desmond (eds.), *Disorders of the Developing Nervous System*. Springfield, Il.: Thomas, 60–97.

Hicks, S., and D'Amato, C. (1968). Cell migrations to the isocortex of the rat. *Anatomical Record* 160:619–633.

Hicks, S., D'Amato, C., and Lowe, M. J. (1959). The development of the mammalian nervous system. I. Malformation of the brain, especially the cerebral cortex, induced in rats by radiation. II. Some mechanisms of the malformations of the cortex. *Journal of Comparative Neurology* 113:435–469.

Ivy, G. O., and Killackey, H. P. (1982). Ontogenetic changes in the projections of neo-cortical neurons. *Journal of Neuroscience* 2:735–743.

Jones, E. G. (1981). Development of connectivity in the cerebral cortex. In F. O. Schmitt, F. G. Worden, G. Adelman, and S. G. Dennis (eds.), *The Organization of the Cerebral Cortex.* Cambridge, MA: MIT Press, 199–236.

Jones, E. G. (1985). *The Thalamus.* New York: Plenum Press.

Krettek, J. E., and Price, J. L. (1977). Projections from the amygdaloid complex to the cerebral cortex and thalamus in the rat and cat. *Journal of Comparative Neurology* 172:687–722.

Kolb, B., Gibb, R., and van der Kooy, D. (1989). Development of the neocortex in the hemidecorticate rat. (Manuscript in preparation.)

Kolb, B., and Walkey, J. (1987). Behavioural and anatomical studies of the posterior parietal cortex in the rat. *Behavioural Brain Research* 23:127–145.

Krieg, W. J. S. (1946a). Connections of the cerebral cortex. I. The albino rat. A. Topography of cortical areas. *Journal of Comparative Neurology* 84:221–275.

Krieg, W. J. S. (1946b). Connections of the cerebral cortex. I. The albino rat. B. Structure of the cortical areas. *Journal of Comparative Neurology* 84:277–321.

Krieg, W. J. S. (1947). Connections of the cerebral cortex. I. The albino rat. C. Extrinsic connections. *Journal of Comparative Neurology* 86:267–393.

Lashley, K. S., (1929). *Brain Mechanisms and Intelligence.* Chicago: University of Chicago Press.

Leonard, C. M. (1969). The prefrontal cortex of the rat. I. Cortical projection of the mediodorsal nucleus. II. Efferent connections. *Brain Research* 12:321–343.

Miller, M. W., and Vogt, B. A. (1984). Direct connections of rat visual cortex with sensory, motor, and association cortices. *Journal of Comparative Neurology* 226:184–202.

Pandya, D. N., and Yeterian, E. H. (1985). Architecture and connections of cortical association areas. In A. Peters and E. G. Jones (eds.), *Cerebral Cortex.* Vol. 4. New York: Plenum Press, 3–62.

Rakic, P. (1984). Defective cell-to-cell interactions as causes of brain malformations. In E. S. Gollin (ed.), *Malformations of Development: Biological and Psychological Sources and Consequences.* New York: Academic Press, 239–285.

Rakic, P., and Goldman-Rakic, P. S. (1982). Development and modifiability of the cerebral cortex. *Neurosciences Research Program Bulletin* 20:430–612.

Reep, R. L., Corwin, J. V., Hashimotok, A., and Watson, R. T. (1984). Afferent connections of medial precentral cortex in the rat. *Neuroscience Letters* 44:247–252.

Swanson, L. W. (1981). A direct projection from Ammon's horn to prefrontal cortex in the rat. *Brain Research* 217:150–154.

Veening, J. G., Cornelissen, F. M., and Lieven, P. A. J. M. (1980). The topical organization of the afferents to the caudatoputamen of the rat. A horseradish peroxidase study. *Neuroscience* 5:1253–1268.

Vogt, B. A., and Miller, M. W. (1983). Cortical connections between rat cingulate cortex and visual, motor, and postsubicular cortices. *Journal of Comparative Neurology* 216:192–210.

Wise, S. P., and Donoghue, J. P. (1986). Motor cortex of rodents. In E. G. Jones and A. Peters (ed.), *Cerebral Cortex*. Vol. 5. New York: Plenum Press, 243–290.

Woolsey, C. N. (1958). Organization of somatic sensory and motor areas of the cerebral cortex. In H. F. Harlow and C. N. Woolsey (eds.), *Biological and Biochemical Bases of Behavior*. Madison: University of Wisconsin Press.

Zilles, K. (1985). *The Cortex of the Rat. A Stereotaxic Atlas*. Berlin: Springer-Verlag.

Zilles, K., and Wree, A. (1985). Cortex: Areal and laminar structure. In G. Paxinos (ed.), *The Rat Nervous System*. Vol. 1. New York: Academic Press, 375–415.

3 The Prenatal and Postnatal Development of Rat Cerebral Cortex

Harry B. M. Uylings, Corbert G. Van Eden, John G. Parnavelas, and Andries Kalsbeek

The development of the cerebral cortex consists of a series of intriguing processes that lead to the structure that is vital for integrating sensory inputs and for cognitive and behavioral functions (see other chapters of this book). Although the cerebral cortex can be divided, on the basis of structural and functional features, into different cortical areas, its general uniformity and cellular composition across regions and species is conspicuous (e.g., Rockel, Hiorns, and Powell 1980). The differences between cortical areas appear to be based mainly on variations in connectivity patterns, which induce the differences in functions. In the early seventies it was thought that nearly all was known on the morphological formation of the cortical layers (Boulder Committee 1970). Over the last two decades, however, research has led to changes in many concepts of development applying morphological and molecular biological techniques to the study of the ontogenetic development. In this chapter we focus on the present knowledge concerning the formation of the cerebral cortex: the generation and migration of neurons, ingrowth of fibers and the specification of the different cortical areas, the occurrence of transient structures during corticogenesis, the differentiation of dendrites, and the postnatal increase in size of the cerebral cortex. We also briefly discuss factors that interfere with cortical development.

3.1 Formation of the Cerebral Cortex

Fetal Lamination and Cell Generation

Different definitions are used in the literature to indicate the timing of the prenatal development of the rat. Most studies concerned with prenatal development of nervous system define the night of mating as E0 and the following day, i.e., the day on which sperm is first noticed in vaginal smears, as E1 (e.g., Hicks and D'Amato 1968, König, Roch, and Marty 1975, Rickmann, Chronwall, and Wolff 1977, Raedler and Raedler 1978, Van Eden 1986, Miller 1987, Cavanagh and Parnavelas 1988a, Kalsbeek et al. 1988). Another system of description, used less frequently in the neuroembryology of the rat, is that proposed by Witschi

(1962). This system, in which the age is expressed in days after fertilization, has been used by a number of authors, e.g., Derer (1979); Beaudoin (1980); Gardette, Courtois, and Bisconte (1982); and Floeter and Jones (1985). In this system counting starts eight hours after copulation, and consequently the day of first presence of sperm in vaginal smear is called E0. To avoid confusion, we use here the former, which is the most frequently applied system.

The adult rat neocortex contains about 34 million neurons,[1] which are generated mostly during the last ten days of gestation (e.g., Rickmann, Chronwall, and Wolff 1977, Raedler, Raedler, and Feldhaus 1980, Miller 1988). Thus it is estimated that on average about 2400 cortical neurons are formed per minute in the second half of the prenatal period, although the mitotic activity in the telencephalon during this period is not constant (Raedler et al. 1980). In fact the actual number might be higher because cell death also occurs in the cerebral cortex during normal development (e.g., Finlay and Slattery 1983, Luskin and Shatz 1985).

The specialized ectodermal structure from which the central nervous system originates is the neural plate. At E10 to E11 the neural plate in the rat starts to fuse to form the neural tube, which closes at E12 (Witschi 1962; see also figures 3.1 and 3.2). At this time three brain vesicles are discernible, viz., prosencephalon, mesencephalon, and rhombencephalon (figure 3.3), which at E12 to E13 transform into five brain subdivisions, viz., the two telencephalic vesicles, diencephalon (interbrain),

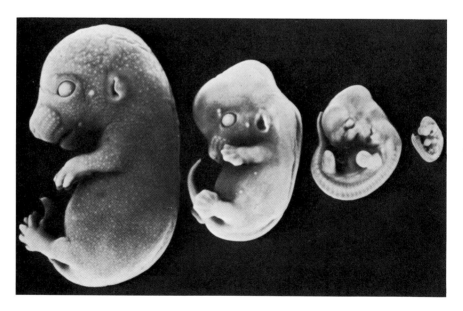

Figure 3.1 Rat fetuses at different prenatal stages. From right to left: E12, E14, E16, and E18. At E16 the whiskerfield pattern around the nose is already visible. (From Beaudoin 1980. Used with permission from Academic Press, Inc.)

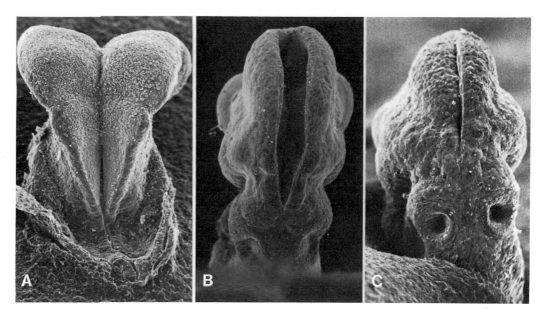

Figure 3.2 Three successive stages of neural tube closure in mouse embryo. The last tube openings are at the cranial, anterior, and posterior neuropores. The cavities in C are ear placodes, i.e., primordium of the inner ear. (The SEM photographs of in vitro embryos are reproduced with the permission of Dr. R. E. Poelman, Laboratory of Anatomy, University of Leyden.)

mesencephalon (midbrain), metencephalon (pons, cerebellum), and myelencephalon (brainstem).

The cerebral cortex originates from the wall of the neural tube as an extension of the two telencephalic vesicles. During the earliest stages of development of the telencephalon, the wall of the neural tube shows a homogeneous structure. Mitotic spindles of dividing germinal cells are only visible close to the ventricle or inner membrane (e.g., Sauer 1935). After mitosis synthesis of DNA occurs in the nuclei of the germinal cells as they move away from the ventricle within the cytoplasmic processes, which are connected with both the inner and the outer membrane of the neural tube. After DNA synthesis the nucleus returns to the ventricle to start the configuration of mitotic spindles. This nuclear movement is called *interkinetic nuclear migration* and has been confirmed with different techniques (see, e.g., chapter 2 in Jacobson 1978). The cell cycle time (i.e., the time of cycle of DNA synthesis and mitosis) of rat cerebral cortical germinal cells is 11 hours at E12 and gradually increases to about 19 hours at E18 and afterward (Waechter and Jaensch 1972; see table 2.1 in Jacobson 1978). On the basis of these data, we roughly estimate that in the rat the number of germinal cells needed for the generation of about 2400 cortical neurons per minute must be about 1.5 million to 2.8 million. If glial cells arise from different stem cells, a much higher number of germinal cells will be present. Since the

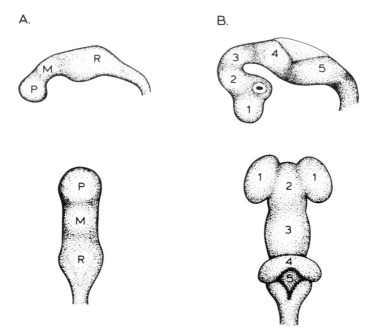

Figure 3.3 (A) The "three brain vesicle" stage of development. P = prosencephalon (forebrain); M = mesencephalon (midbrain); R = rhombencephalon (hindbrain). (B) The "five brain vesicle" stage of development. 1 = telencephalon (endbrain); 2 = diencephalon (interbrain); 3 = mesencephalon (midbrain); 4 = metencephalon (afterbrain: pons and cerebellum); 5 = myelencephalon (brainstem). The ring structure in 2 is the optic cup. The upper figures of A and B are lateral views; the lower figures are dorsal views.

publication by Waechter and Jaensch (1972) and especially Levitt, Cooper, and Rakic (1981, 1983), it has generally been thought that glial cells and neurons arise from different stem cells. This is still a matter of discussion even with the new techniques in which retroviruses are used to determine cell lineage (for review of this debate, which has a long history, see Rickmann and Wolff 1985). Using these techniques, Walsh and Cepko (1988) have suggested that cerebral glial cells and neurons share a common progenitor, whereas Sanes (1989) supports the notion of different progenitor cells for E13.

From E13 the neural wall of the telencephalon loses its homogeneous structure, and fetal lamination evolves. At E13 the plexiform primordium (PP) begins to form in the most lateral part of the neural wall of the telencephalon (figure 3.4), which borders the developing striatum and paleocortex. In this outer zone of the cerebral wall, tangential fibers enter shortly before the arrival of the first cortical neurons (e.g., Marin-Padilla 1971, Raedler and Raedler 1978). The cells in the PP are different in shape from those in the ventricular zone. Among the PP cells are the prospective Cajal-Retzius cells (Figure 3.5) and polymorphous cells.

The Cajal-Retzius neurons are generated in the ventricular zone between E11 and E15, with a peak at E13 (König et al. 1977, Raedler and

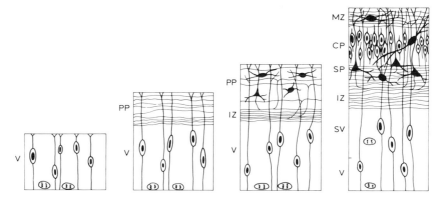

Figure 3.4 A scheme of four different stages in fetal lamination of the cerebral wall. V = ventricular zone; PP = plexiform primordium (preplate); IZ = intermediate zone; MZ = marginal zone; CP = cortical plate; SP = subplate; SV = subventricular zone. The horizontal Cajal-Retzius cells in the MZ and the subplate neurons in SP are cogenerated. The few neurons that are more differentiated, which obliquely traverse the CP, probably belong to the same population.

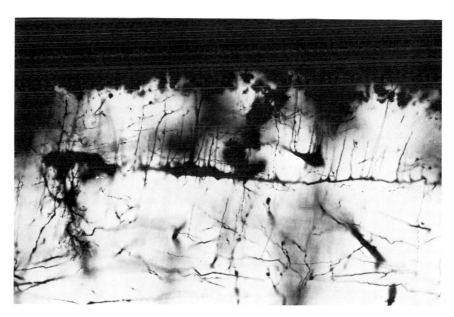

Figure 3.5 A horizontal Cajal-Retzius cell from newborn human cerebral cortex in a Golgi-rapid-stained section. (Reproduced with permission of Dr. L. Mrzljak, Section of Neuroanatomy, University of Zagreb.)

Uylings et al.: Prenatal and Postnatal Development

Raedler 1978). The PP is visible with a two-day lateromedial growth gradient; i.e., two days later, at E15, the PP is also present in the medial wall of the telencephalon. The different growth gradients for the mouse brain are indicated in figure 3.6 (Smart 1984), and these are more or less comparable with those in the rat brain. Note that the lateromedial growth gradient (i.e., maturation of the lateral part of the cerebral wall is more advanced than the more medial part) is much greater (a two-day difference) than the anterior and posterior growth gradient. The growth of the cerebral wall itself starts from the ventricular zone (VZ) in a more or less radial fashion (see below).

The interkinetic nuclear migration is not a persisting phenomenon because at E15 mitotic spindles appear just below the PP in the dorsal part of the cerebral wall (figure 3.7). In the PP polymorphous cells are found below the Cajal-Retzius cells. The oldest cells are thought to be more superficially located than the cells that are generated later in the VZ (Raedler and Raedler 1978). This still has to be established, however, in view of the overlap of the generation periods of Cajal-Retzius cells and polymorphous cells. The PP, sometimes called *preplate* (Rickmann and Wolff 1981, Smart 1983, Stewart and Pearlman 1987), is separated in two zones, viz., the marginal zone (MZ) and the subplate (SP) (Kostovic and Molliver 1974), by the formation of the cortical plate (CP) at E15 to E17. At E15 the very first cells of the cortical plate are visible in the most lateral part of the cortex at the border with the developing striatum and paleocortex and, two days later, at E17 in the medial wall of the telencephalon. Consequently the growth gradients of the CP are similar to those of the PP. Later at E21 the difference in maturation

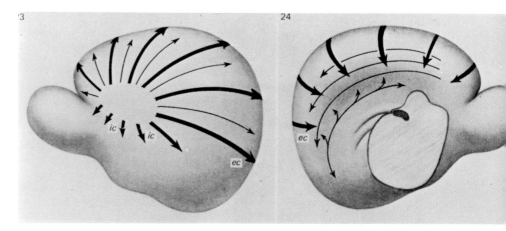

Figure 3.6 Growth gradients of the plexiform primordium (PP) layer are indicated by thin arrows; those of the cortical plate layer are indicated by thick arrows. The left figure depicts the lateral view, the right one the medial view of an E16 mouse brain. ic = insular cortex; ec = entorhinal cortex. (Reproduced with permission from Smart (1984). Histogenesis of the mesocortical area of the mouse telencephalon. *J. Anat.* 138:537–552. Cambridge University Press.)

Organization of the Neocortex

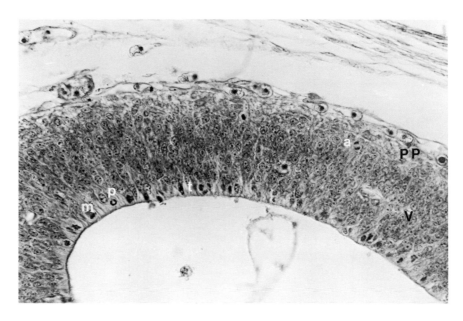

Figure 3.7 The dorsal part of the cerebral wall of an E15 rat fetus. In this part of the fetal laminae visible are the plexiform primordium (PP) and the ventricular zone (V). Note that at this stage the mitotic spindle figures are also found in the upper part of V and not only around the ventricle. The different mitotic phases visible are prophase (p), metaphase (m), anaphase (a), and early telophase (t). Nissl stain.

between the lateral and medial part of the cerebral wall is less clear. The CP is characterized by its densely packed, vertically arranged cells (figure 3.8). From the CP the cortical layers VIa to II are later formed (see below).

Before the CP becomes visible, the subventricular zone (SV) is discernible above the VZ, approximately at E15 (e.g., Raedler et al 1980, Rakic 1982, and figure 3.4). The SV is a cell-dense zone in which mitotic spindles are present. In the SV the somata are mainly vertical, but the radial rows of somata visible in the VZ are lost. The border of the SV and the intermediate zone (IZ) contains tangential cells, which are clearly visible in sections stained with an antibody against γ-aminobutyric acid (GABA). At E15, however, this GABAergic cell group is located in what is considered the lower part of the IZ (Van Eden et al. 1989). Above the SV and below the PP, and later the SP, the IZ is discernible. This is especially clear in GABA-stained sections (Van Eden et al. 1989), in conformity with the scheme of Rakic (1982), but earlier than reported by Raedler and coworkers (1980). The IZ later becomes the subcortical white matter, also called the fetal white matter, although the myelination does not start until several days after birth. Originally the IZ contains a somewhat lower cell density than do the SV and VZ. In addition to radially migrating neurons, it contains tangentially oriented somata, which are somewhat smaller than those in the SV and

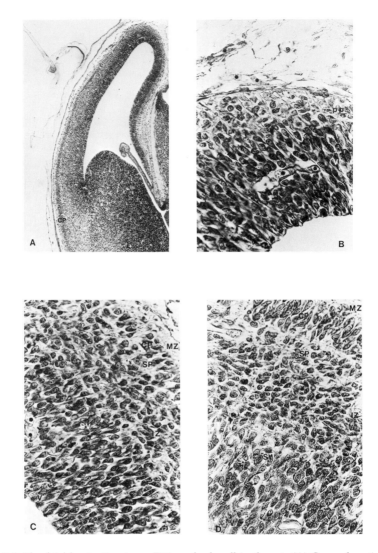

Figure 3.8 The fetal lamination in an E16 cerebral wall in the rat. (A) Coronal section of one hemisphere, which shows the lateral extension of the cortical plate (CP). (B) Dorsal part of the cerebral wall: two laminae are visible, viz., PP and V. At this stage blood cells still contain a nucleus. (C) Dorsolateral part of the cerebral wall; contains a marginal zone (MZ), a two-cell-layer-thick cortical plate (CP), subplate (SP), intermediate zone (IZ), and the subventricular (SV) and ventricular (V) zones. (D) The lateral part contains the same fetal laminae as in (C). Here the CP is about four cell layers thick; the border between SP and IZ is clearer. Nissl stain.

the SP (see figure 3.8) and tangentially running fibers. After a few days the IZ is relatively poor in cells and contains tangentially oriented glial processes (Gadisseux and Evrard 1985), an increasing number of tangential axonal fiber bundles, and radially migrating neurons. The IZ is not a homogeneous fetal zone (note the different sublaminae in figure 3.9). In the literature the borders between VZ and SV and between SV and IZ are defined differently (cf. Raedler et al. 1980, Marin-Padilla 1971, Gadisseux and Evrard 1985, Reynolds and Møllgård 1985, Luskin and Shatz 1985). For example, if the distinction between SV and IZ is defined by stating that mitotic spindles do not occur in the IZ, the border between SV and IZ will be located higher in the neural wall than if the distinction is defined by stating that bundles of tangential fibers occur only in the IZ (see figures 3.9 and 3.10A).

The CP cells start to be generated at E13, with a peak in the genesis at E16 to E17 (in Wistar and Long-Evans rats; see Berry and Rogers 1965, Raedler et al. 1980, Miller 1988). The generated CP cells migrate from the (sub)ventricular zone into the CP at an estimated rate of 15

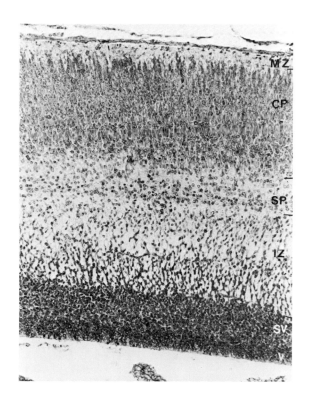

Figure 3.9 The fetal lamination of the cerebral wall in an E18 rate. For abbreviations, see figure 3.4. Note that the IZ is not a homogeneous layer at this stage. Nissl stain. (Photo taken from a preparation lent by Dr. P. Voorn, Free University, Amsterdam.)

Uylings et al.: Prenatal and Postnatal Development

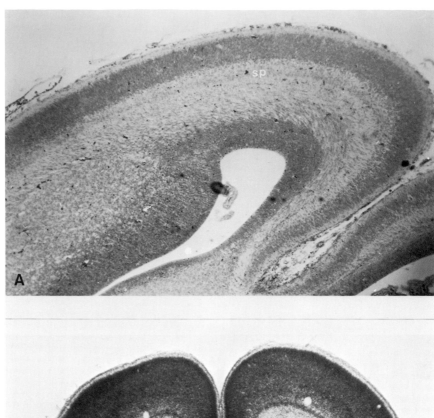

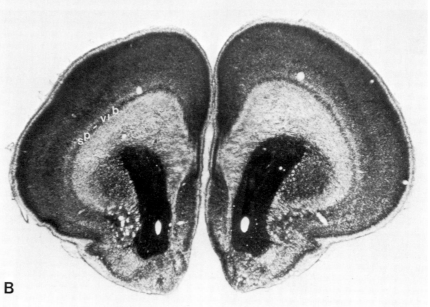

Figure 3.10 The cerebral wall in an E19 (A) and a newborn, P0, rat (B). The subplate becomes discernible as layer VIb. The upper part of layer VIb is poor in cell somata in the dorsal and dorsolateral part of the wall, but not in the medial and lateral cortex.

Organization of the Neocortex

μm to 30 μm per hour (Hicks and D'Amato 1968). Many detailed studies of neurogenesis in the rat cerebral cortex (e.g., Berry and Rogers 1965, Hicks and D'Amato 1968, Brückner, Mares, and Biesold 1978, Raedler et al. 1980, Miller 1985) have reported that neurons that are generated earlier are deposited in the lower CP layers, whereas those generated later are deposited in the more superficial layers (with the exception of layer I), i.e., inside-out development (figure 3.11). There has been some disagreement nonetheless with regard to the pattern of genesis of cortical nonpyramidal neurons. Some authors (Chronwall and Wolff 1981, Wolff, Chronwall and Rickmann 1983) have reported that the position of nonpyramidal neurons is not related to their date of generation; they are diffusely distributed throughout all cortical layers. Others (Miller 1985, 1986a, Fairen, Cobas, and Fonseca 1986, Cavanagh and Parnavelas 1988a,b), however, have confirmed the inside-out pattern of genesis of the nonpyramidal neurons. Nearly all rat cortical neurons are generated before birth, with the exception of only a few layer IV neurons (Kaplan 1981). In primates all neocortical neurons are generated long before birth (Rakic 1988). A number of glial cells, too, are generated before birth in the rat cerebral cortex. In early prenatal development radial glial cells and, somewhat later, nonradial astrocytes are generated at the same time as are cortical neurons (e.g., Rickmann and Wolff 1985, Gadisseux and Evrard 1985). The number of astrocytes increases until the second or third week after birth in the cortical gray matter (Ling and Leblond 1973, Parnavelas et al. 1983), whereas it increases contin-

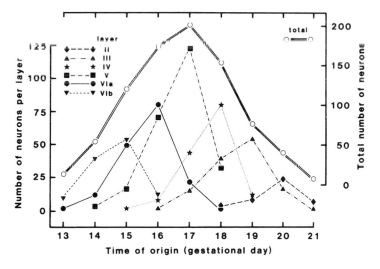

Figure 3.11 Time of origin of cortico-cortical projection neurons in rat visual cortex, determined by means of a double-labeling technique. The neurons were counted in four 375-μm-wide vertical strips of cortex. The dates of birth of local circuit neurons in a particular layer are similar to those of the cortico-cortical projection neurons (Miller 1985). (Reproduced with permission from Miller (1988), in A. Peters and E. G. Jones (eds.): *Cerebral Cortex*. Vol. 7, pp. 133–175. New York: Plenum Press.)

uously in the white matter (Sturrock 1986). Oligodendrocytes are the last type of glial cells to appear. They grow in significant numbers in the corpus callosum immediately before the onset of myelination at postnatal day 12 (Valentino and Jones 1982, Sturrock 1976).

Migration of Neurons

Neurons migrate from the VZ toward their destinations in the cerebral cortex, passing through the different fetal zones. These cells are thought to move along radial glia fibers (Rakic 1972, 1988) more or less radially (see figures 3.4 and 3.12). Cortical neurons produced by a small number of progenitor cells migrate along the same radial glial fibers toward a similar part of the neocortex. The radially directed migration of cortical neurons has recently been discussed by Sanes (1989) on the basis of recent studies that used the technique of retrovirus-mediated gene transfer to examine cell lineage. Afferent fibers from a number of subcortical sites and from other cortical areas temporarily stay in the SP

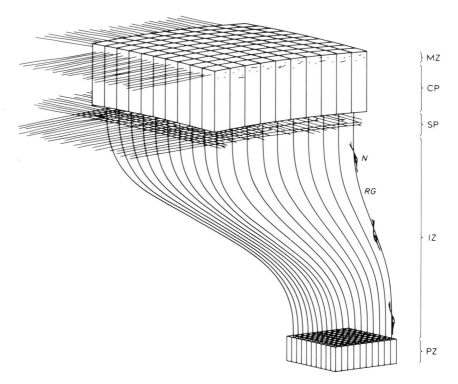

Figure 3.12 This scheme illustrates the radial unit hypothesis (Rakic 1988, Smart and McSherry 1982). Neurons (N) generated by a proliferative unit of the proliferation zone (PZ), i.e., the ventricular and subventricular zones, migrate along the same radial glia (RG) toward a particular cortical columnar zone. Each neuron migrating toward the cortical plate (CP) passes the subplate zone (SP). The SP contains thalamic and other subcortical and cortico-cortical fibers that have transient synaptic contacts with subplate neurons. The cortical zones with the earliest synaptogenesis are SP and MZ. In the marginal zone (MZ) fibers of many subcortical transmitter systems traverse and have synaptic contacts. (Modified from Rakic 1988.)

Organization of the Neocortex

and the MZ before entering the CP (Molliver, Kostovic, and Van der Loos 1973, Kristt and Molliver 1976, König and Marty, 1981, Lund and Mustari 1977, Wise and Jones 1978, Schlumpf, Shoemaker and Bloom 1980, Crandall and Caviness 1984, Van Eden 1986). This period is commonly called the waiting period in the literature, which gives an erroneous impression of passivity during the active processes such as synaptogenesis with SP and MZ neurons. In this period neurons that migrate toward the upper parts of the CP pass these afferent fiber systems. It may be that cortical afferents at this stage of development modulate the neurons in SP and thereby other developmental events (see also Shatz, Chun and Luskin 1988). The radial-unit hypothesis (Smart and McSherry 1982, Rakic 1988) postulates that proliferative units (i.e., a small number of stem cells) produce cohorts of neurons, which migrate columnlike along radial glia. These proliferative units thus specify the destination of cell cohorts in the cortex, which leads to the cortical parcellation. The parcellation of the cortex into cytoarchitectonically different areas is most probably also regulated by the differences in the afferent, e.g., thalamic, input. In this respect it is of interest that glial fibers demarcate the cortical vibrissal barrelfield before the earliest detectable changes in neuronal density (Cooper and Steindler 1986) and that removal of the thalamocortical afferents just after birth, before they reach their definitive distribution, prevents the formation of the cortical barrelfield (Wise and Jones 1978). In Rakic's radial-unit hypothesis the lateral expansion of the cerebral cortex relative to the VZ is accounted for by scaffolding of the radial glial fibers. In contrast, however, the observations of Gadisseux and Evrard (1985) point to another possibility to account for the cortical lateral expansion. They have observed that during the early stages of development in the mouse cerebral wall, the radial glial fibers remain grouped in fascicles of 4 to 8 fibers through all fetal laminae, including CP, but at E17 these fibers appear isolated. That is, they become completely defasciculated in the CP. This defasciculation can lead to 4 to 8 times more routes for migrating neurons.

Early in development, migration has also been observed without the contact guidance by radial glial fibers (e.g., Shoukimas and Hinds 1978, Zagon, McLaughlin, and Rogers 1985). Recent studies also point to extracellular matrix molecules, such as the adhesive glycoprotein fibronectin, as forming the migratory pathway of cellular processes (Stewart and Pearlman 1987, Chun and Shatz 1988). Plasma proteins are also thought to be involved in migration and differentiation of neurons (e.g., Reynolds and Møllgård 1985, Cavanagh and Møllgård 1985). Thus for migration of neurons both "contact" guidance and "biochemical" matching appear to be important.

Growth of Fiber Systems into Cerebral Wall
In a recent review Hankin and Silver (1986) have suggested that the modern theories of axonal guidance can be regarded as a synthesis of

the well-known contact guidance theory of Weiss (1968) and the chemoaffinity hypothesis of Sperry (1963). According to the former, growing fiber tips (i.e., growth cones) are guided in their course by their contacts with surrounding structures. The chemoaffinity hypothesis proposed that growing axons are guided by a chemical matching system between specific axons and chemical cues along the pathways of outgrowth and target-derived cues. Interesting in this respect is the formation of the corpus callosum, which has been studied both in the mouse by Silver and colleagues (Hankin and Silver 1986) and in the rat by Jones and colleagues (Valentino and Jones 1982, Floeter and Jones 1985). In the mouse a glial system, called the glial sling, guides the first callosal fibers from one hemisphere to the other at their initial fusion point (above the caudal septal region), whereas another glial system, the corticoseptal barricade, appears to form a barrier to the growing callosal fibers in each hemisphere at the growing edges of the corpus callosum. Both glial systems consist of primitive astrocytes and GFAP-positive radial glial cells (Hankin and Silver 1986, Poston et al. 1988). In the rat the glial sling is not present as a clear structure, or at least Valentino and Jones (1982) did not report its presence. In the rat we observed that the meninges of the two telencephalic walls fuse at E16 and E19 and the GABA-immunoreactive fibers then cross the midline of the corpus callosum to the contralateral hemisphere (Van Eden and Uylings, unpublished data, 1988), as was previously indicated to occur with some cortical axons (Valentino and Jones 1982, Floeter and Jones 1985). Around birth the advancing front of the callosal fibers is at the midlateral level of the contralateral hemisphere, and at postnatal day 4 or 5 they start to invade the cortical layers (Floeter and Jones 1985). The callosal fibers are formed first by neurons in layers V and VI, and after birth a second stratum of callosal fibers is formed superficially to the already existing stratum by neurons in layer III (Floeter and Jones 1985). As callosal axons grow into the contralateral hemisphere, corticofugal axons project to a number of subcortical structures. These fiber systems are probably not guided by the same growth cues because the different fiber systems intersect.

Well before the formation of callosal connections, monoaminergic and thalamocortical fibers reach the cortical anlage, although these fiber systems follow different growth patterns. It is likely that the thalamocortical and other subcortical fibers modulate the size and growth of different cortical fields during critical or sensitive periods (e.g., Wise and Jones 1978, Rakic 1988, Kalsbeek 1989). The dopamine-containing fibers are found to reach the anlage of the lateral neocortex at E15 (Kalsbeek et al. 1988), and like thalamocortical axons they initially run in the SP until birth, arriving at this position at E16 (figure 3.13). On the other hand both the noradrenergic and the serotonergic fibers (figure 3.13) arrive at E17 and run in both the SP and the MZ until birth (for references, see Parnavelas et al. 1988). The noradrenergic and ser-

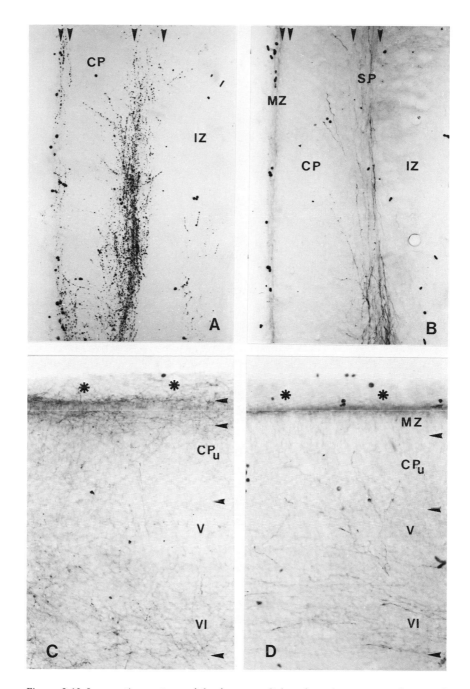

Figure 3.13 Innervation pattern of the future medial prefrontal cortex at embryonic day 20 (A,B) and postnatal day 1 (C,D). Dopaminergic fibers (B,D) are prenatally restricted to the subplate and enter the lower cortical layers, i.e., layers VI and V, around birth. Serotonergic fibers (A,C), however, are found in both the marginal zone and the subplate before birth and invade the cortical plate from both sides. CPu = (upper) cortical plate; IZ = intermediate zone; MZ = marginal zone; SP = subplate; V and VI = developing cortical layers V and VI; ** = the side of the vibratome section, not an extra cortical layer.

otonergic fibers penetrate all cortical areas at birth and reach an "adult" density and fiber pattern at approximately one month and three weeks of postnatal life, respectively (Levitt and Moore 1979, Lidov and Molliver 1982). The cortical dopaminergic fibers become restricted mainly to the prefrontal and entorhinal cortex when they invade the CP of these cortical areas at birth. They reveal an adult density and pattern of innervation by postnatal day 60 (Kalsbeek et al. 1988). The thalamocortical fibers begin to enter the cortex at birth and the few days thereafter (Van Eden 1986, Lund and Mustari 1977, Wise and Jones 1978). At birth the thalamocortical fibers from the different thalamic nuclei have an organization in the SP that is topologically equivalent to the adult organization (Crandall and Caviness 1984, Herkenham 1980). Thus, in contrast with the noradrenergic and serotonergic fibers, the thalamocortical and dopaminergic fibers have a regional specification. It is still unknown what chemo-contact-guiding factors determine the migration of fibers of specific cell groups to different cortical regions over such a long distance, although positional and chemical cues are likely (e.g., Hankin and Lund 1987, Udin and Fawcett 1988).

In contrast to the monoaminergic systems, the cholinergic system appears to develop largely postnatally in the cerebral cortex (Dinopoulos et al. 1989) and attains the adult state by the end of the second postnatal week. In the rat cerebral cortex ChAT-positive neurons and ChAT-positive axons are found from approximately postnatal day 11 (Parnavelas et al. 1988) and arise in the basal forebrain, especially the nucleus basalis and parts of the diagonal band nuclei. One exception is that *transient* ChAT-positive fibers in the rat cortex are visible later and reach mature density considerably later than the acetylcholinesterase (AChE)-positive fibers (e.g., Clinton and Ebner 1988), perhaps because the AChE staining is not a specific marker for cholinergic fibers.

Very early in development GABAergic neurons can be observed in the PP (Van Eden et al. 1989) and, from E16 GABAergic neurons and fibers, are present in all fetal laminae (i.e., VZ to MZ). The majority of these neurons and fibers are transiently found in the MZ as well as in the SP and IZ (figure 3.14) (Wolff et al. 1984, Van Eden et al. 1989, Lauder et al. 1987), and a number of SP neurons, which at E17 are mainly GABAergic, have "callosal" axons (see above; Van Eden et al. 1989, Shatz, Chun and Luskin 1988). From the septal region, GABAergic fibers enter the medial rat cortex at E17 (Van Eden et al. 1989). The maturation of the GABAergic immunoreactivity in the cerebral cortex is nearly accomplished by the end of the fourth week (Wolff et al. 1984, Binneveld, Uylings, and Kalsbeek; unpublished report, 1988).

Data on the development of neuropeptidergic fiber systems in the cerebral cortex are scanty. The majority of the papers deal with the development of peptidergic neurons rather than peptidergic fibers (e.g., Parnavelas et al. 1988).

Finally, a number of neurotransmitter systems are thought to influ-

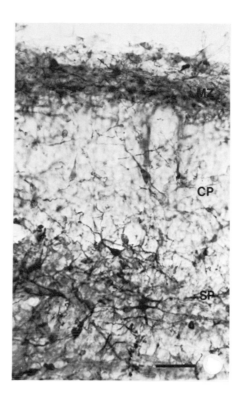

Figure 3.14 GABAergic neurons and fibers in cerebral cortex of an E18 rat. The majority of these neurons and fibers are found in the MZ and SP. The length of the bar is 50μm.

ence the plasticity of the cerebral cortex during development (e.g., Mattson 1988). For example, the monoamines that develop before the onset of neurotransmission have been implicated in the control of neural tube closure and myoblast differentiation (e.g., Lauder and Krebs 1986). Noradrenaline has been implicated in the maintenance of neuronal plasticity (Kasamatsu 1983), although recently this view has been challenged by the observations that acetylcholine is also a crucial factor involved in the ocular dominance plasticity (Bear and Singer 1986, Bear, Cooper and Ebner 1987, Gu and Singer 1988; see also Brenner and Mirmiran 1988). Dopamine (e.g., Kalsbeek 1989) and GABA (e.g., Spoerri 1987, Mattson 1988, Van Eden et al. 1989) are also thought to have a neurotrophic function in neuronal development.

Transient Structures during Development
The presence of transient structure appears to be a characterisic feature of normal development. The fetal lamination changes completely during development, so that after birth the various zones that are present during early development either acquire different characteristics or have disappeared. The transient features of the SP and MZs have recently been studied in considerable detail. For example, a study of the developing cat visual cortex by Luskin and Shatz (1985) showed that the

Uylings et al.: Prenatal and Postnatal Development

majority of the SP neurons die after birth, although this is still an open question for the rat cerebral cortex. Thus Nissl preparations show a gradual transition of the SP into layer VIb in the rat (see figures 3.9 and 3.10). Furthermore Reep and Goodwin (1988) recently have observed a survival of a large number of SP neurons at 3 weeks of postnatal age, although Al-Ghoul and Miller (1989) used tritiated thymidine labeling and the transient presence of Alz-50 immunoreactivity to show that the large majority of SP neurons die between postnatal day 5 and day 30. The beginning of this period coincides with the start of the invasion of the CP by subcortical and callosal axons, which leave the SP at this stage. Lushkin and Shatz (1985) also claim that the majority of the MZ neurons die during development in the cat, but this too is controversial. The fate of the Cajal-Retzius cells in this zone has been the subject of debate for nearly a century, and in the rat Parnavelas and Edmunds (1983) have shown that at least some of these neurons transform to nonpyramidal neurons rather than degenerate.

Cell death is a prominent factor within restricted periods during normal development in many brain regions (e.g., Cowan et al. 1984, Breedlove 1984, Fawcett 1988). The occurrence of neuronal death in cerebral cortex, however, has been the subject of debate. Neuronal death has been reported as part of the normal development of cortical layers in the hamster (Finlay and Slattery 1983), mouse (Heumann and Leuba 1983), and cat (Price and Blakemore 1985). Finlay and Slattery (1983) reported that neuronal death is more pronounced in medial than in lateral cerebral cortex, and Windrem and colleagues (1988) have hypothesized that thalamic afferents control the cortical cell number (see also Wise and Jones 1978). However, in recent experiments involving neonatal damage to the thalamocortical afferents to the medial prefrontal cortex, no indications were found for a massive cell death (Van Eden, Kalsbeek, and Uylings 1987). A confirmation of neuronal death in the developing cerebral cortex by unbiased stereological techniques that do not imply assumptions on cell shape and size (e.g., Braendgaard and Gundersen 1986) will be important. Combined immunocytochemical-autoradiographic studies have shown a transient expression of neurotransmitters in the developing cortex (e.g., Parnavelas and Cavanagh 1988, Wahle and Meyer 1987). In one such study on the development of somatostatin (SRIF)-containing neurons (Cavanagh and Parnavelas 1988), it has been suggested that the diminishing SRIF expression in the rat visual cortex may be due to cell death rather than cessation of SRIF production (Parnavelas and Cavanagh 1988). Finally, cell death of glial cells is reported to occur in the corpus callosum in neonatal mice (Hankin and Silver 1986), and macrophages are found in the developing rat corpus callosum (Floeter and Jones 1985).

In many systems axonal collaterals are eliminated during normal development, generally after the phase of cell death (e.g., Innocenti 1988, Ivy and Killackey 1981, Van Eden, Kros, and Uylings 1990). Transient structures in normal postnatal development are also indicated by excess growth of the volume of cortical regions such as the prefrontal cortex (Van Eden and Uylings 1985; see figure 3.15), of size of dendrites, and of number of synapses (Huttenlocher et al. 1982, Parnavelas et al. 1978, Blue and Parnavelas 1983a,b). This is discussed in the next section.

3.2 Postnatal Development

Postnatal Growth of Cerebral Cortex[2]
The postnatal growth of rat cerebral cortex, excluding the hippocampus, is shown in figure 3.16. These data on fresh weights are based on two litters per age group, each age group consisting of eight male and eight female Wistar rats. On day 30 a clear difference in weights of cerebral cortices of male and female rats can be seen, and there is little change after day 60, when adult values are reached. The volumetric growth pattern of cortical regions frequently shows a relatively short period in which there is an excess of particular cortical areas, which is often different for different cortical regions (see figure 3.15 and Van Eden and Uylings 1985, Zilles 1978). Therefore, in growth graphs of the entire cerebral cortex, such an excess growth is not apparent (see figure 3.16; see also Wingert 1969 for data on mice). When the cerebral cortex data

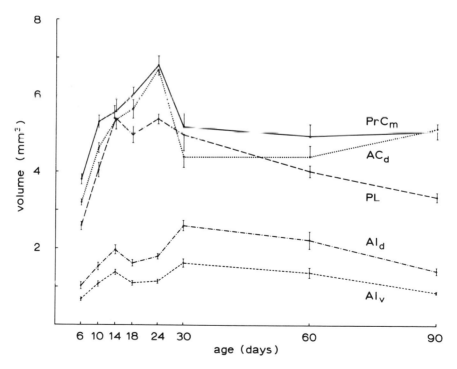

Figure 3.15 Volumetric development of five prefrontal cortical areas in the rat, corrected for shrinkage. (Adapted from Van Eden and Uylings (1985), *J. Comp. Neurol.* 241:268–274.)

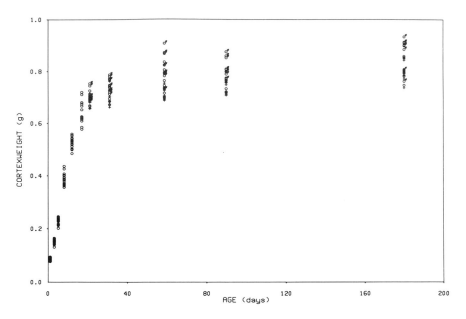

Figure 3.16 The development of rat cerebral cortex weight versus postnatal age.

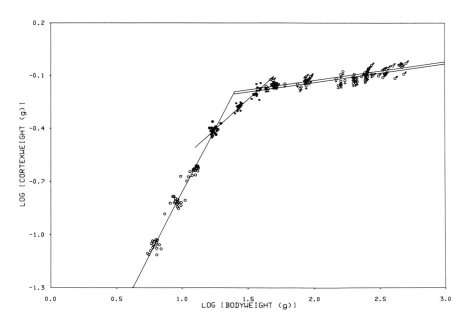

Figure 3.17 The development of rat cerebral cortex versus body weight. Open circles indicate individual rats of day 1, day 3, and day 5 groups. Closed circles indicate individual rats of day 8, day 12, and day 17 groups. The male and female symbols indicate individual male and female rats of day 21, day 30, day 60, day 90, and day 180 groups.

are compared with the body weight data (see figure 3.17), three different phases are noted. (Similar phases have been described in the relations between the entire brain and body weights of Wistar rats (Uylings, Hofman, and Matthijssen 1987).) The first phase of rapid growth is from birth until day 8. It can be described by

$$\log CW = \log 0.006 + 1.43 \log P \quad (r = 0.99),$$

in which CW is the fresh weight in grams of the cerebral cortex, and P is the body weight in grams. The transitional phase, from day 8 until day 17, is described by

$$\log CW = \log 0.056 + 0.67 \log P \quad (r = 0.97),$$

and the mature phase, from day 17 until day 180, is described by

$$\log CW = \log 0.45 + 0.11 \log P \quad (r = 0.8).$$

In the last phase the two regression lines for the male and female rats (figure 3.17) do not differ significantly (for the statistical methods, see Uylings, Van Eden, and Hofman 1986b, Uylings et al. 1987).

The data on cerebral cortex weight versus brain weight from day 1 to day 180 do not reveal a linear relation, although they are highly correlated ($r = 0.98$). The data of the day 60, day 90 and day 180 groups deviate. Furthermore the regression line for the days 3 through 8 groups, with the equation

$$CW = -0.07 + 0.56E \quad (r = 0.99),$$

deviates significantly from the one for the days 8 through 30 groups, which has the equation

$$CW = 0.01 + 0.46E \quad (r = 0.99),$$

(E is fresh brain weight.) Figure 3.18 indicates that after day 30 the relative proportions of brain regions still change considerably in the day 60, day 90, and day 180 groups. Our rat data are fairly comparable with what has been reported for the mouse (Wingert 1969).

Finally, these data on cerebral cortex weights indicate that, when comparing experimental and control groups, body weight has to be taken into account and that the use of sample ratios can be misleading (Uylings et al. 1986b). For a practical example, see Uylings et al. 1987.

Cerebral Asymmetry during Postnatal Development
The rat cerebral cortex appears to be asymmetric (e.g., Diamond 1987, Kolb et al. 1982, Van Eden, Uylings, and Van Pelt 1984) both during development and in adulthood. For example, Diamond (1987) found that male Long-Evans rats show a significantly greater cortical thickness in the right hemisphere as compared with the left one and that this difference is visible from day 6. This result was consistent because the thickness of Krieg's area 2 (Par1) was the sole exception among the seven cortical regions measured and because there was a significant

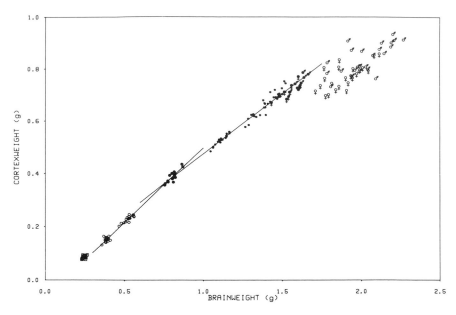

Figure 3.18 The development of rat cerebral cortex versus brain weight. For symbols, see caption to figure 3.17.

right-over-left difference in area 2 at two ages, viz., on days 185 and 400. In female Long-Evans rats, however, no significant differences in thickness were found between the right and left hemispheres in nine cortical regions measured during development and adulthood (Diamond 1987). The occurrence of this sexual dimorphism in cortical thickness has been confirmed by Stewart and Kolb (1988) for the adult Sprague-Dawley rat. Furthermore the studies by Stewart and Kolb (1988) and Fleming and colleagues (1986) indicate that, in the perinatal period, the testicular hormones especially suppress the enlargement of the left cerebral cortex, which causes the right-over-left difference in cortical thickness in male rats. Both prenatal stress (Fleming et al. 1986) and perinatal gonadectomy (Stewart and Kolb 1988) lead to the disappearance of asymmetrical cortical thickness in male rats, without affecting the cortical thickness of female rats. This is in agreement with part of Geschwind and Behan's hypothesis (1982) that states that testosterone in the human fetus results in a reduction in the growth rate of the left hemisphere. Sex differences and the influence of sex steroid hormones may be different for different brain regions. For example, the presence of testosterone prevents cell death in the spinal motor nucleus (e.g., Breedlove 1984), and there is a difference in sexual dimorphism with regard to dendritic response to environmental conditions between the visual cortex and the hippocampus (Juraska 1984). Diamond (1987) has reported that neonatal ovariectomy leads to a greater cortical thickness, to the extent that a right-over-left asymmetry in cortical thickness arises, whereas neonatal gonadectomy does not alter the cortical asymmetry in male Long-Evans rats (Diamond 1987). This influence of sex hormones has not been confirmed for the Sprague-Dawley rat by Stewart and Kolb (1988). More detailed studies on this subject are necessary for more definitive conclusions. The cortical thickness can be indicative for cortical size changes, but measurements have to be performed according to a set of rules for comparing homologous regions (Uylings, Van Eden, and Verwer 1984).

Particularly in developmental studies, volume of cortical regions is preferred to cortical thickness as a measure, because the relative size and position of different brain regions change during development. In a volumetric study of the development of the rat prefrontal cortex, corrected for shrinkage, Van Eden and coworkers (1984) observed that in Wistar rats cortical asymmetry changes during development (figure 3.19), indicating a differential growth of the right and left prefrontal cortex in rats at certain times (for this developmental phenomenon in the human cerebral cortex, see also Thatcher, Walker, and Giudice 1987). We have also observed a significant right-over-left asymmetry in male but not female orbital prefrontal cortex at day 90 (figure 3.20), but a left-over-right asymmetry in the medial prefrontal cortex (see figure 3.19). In the medial prefrontal cortex of Wistar rats, a left-over-right asymmetry in dopamine content also has been found by De Bruin and colleagues (in preparation) (see also Slopsema, Van der Gugten, and De Bruin 1982). In the human left- or right-handedness is correlated with some, but not all asymmetrical brain/cerebral functions (e.g., Kimura and Harshman 1984, Butler 1984). In the rat neonatal tail posture may be analogous to human left- or right-handedness. Neonatal tail

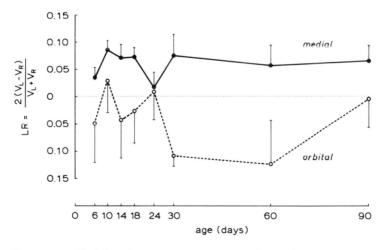

Figure 3.19 The left-right asymmetry in volume of medial and orbital prefrontal cortex in rat changes during development. This is indicated by the lateralization ratio (LR). The volume of left (V_L) and right (V_R) hemisphere is corrected for differential shrinkage with age. The bars indicate the SEM values. (Adapted from Van Eden, Uylings, and Van Pelt (1984), *Dev. Brain Res.* 12:146–153.)

Uylings et al.: Prenatal and Postnatal Development

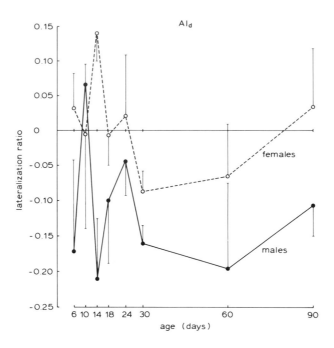

Figure 3.20 Relative lateralization (RL) of the dorsal agranular insular area (AI_d) of the rat dorsal prefrontal cortex during development. The bars indicate the SEM values. (Reproduced from Van Eden, Uylings, and Van Pelt (1984), *Dev. Brain Res.* 12:146–153.)

posture appears to be different for different rat strains and to be affected by prenatal testosterone treatment (e.g., Ross, Glick, and Meibach 1981, Rosen et al. 1983). These data suggest the possibility of differences in brain asymmetry for different rat strains.

Postnatal Development of Cortical Dendrites
Much of the volume of the cerebral cortex is taken up by dendrites. At birth both cortical pyramidal and nonpyramidal cells have very small dendritic trees. Consequently the maturation of dendrites of neurons in the cortical layers II through VI is mainly a postnatal phenomenon. On the other hand the cortical pyramidal projection neurons have long axonal processes descending from many cortical areas, e.g., visual cortex (Stanfield and O'Leary 1985) and prefrontal cortex (Van Eden et al. 1990, Joosten and Van Eden 1989) to, among other regions, spinal cord and brainstem. Different hypotheses on dendritic development have been proposed: (1) neurons located in ontogenetically older layers mature earlier, (2) projection (pyramidal) neurons mature earlier than local-circuit (nonpyramidal) neurons, and (3) larger cells differentiate before smaller cells (e.g., Jacobson 1978, Lund 1978). Qualitative studies (Parnavelas et al. 1978, Hedlich and Winkelmann 1982) and quantitative studies (e.g., Wise, Fleshman, and Jones 1979, Parnavelas and Uylings 1980, Jursaka 1982, Miller 1988, Petit et al. 1988) on cortical dendritic development have modified these hypotheses. The cortical region in

which the dendritic development has been studied most extensively is the rat visual cortex (Parnavelas et al. 1978, Parnavelas and Uylings 1980, Juraska 1982, Hedlich and Winkelmann 1982, Miller 1988). In an extensive time series, Miller (1988) examined only the soma size and the number of dendrites, whereas Juraska (1982) and we examined dendritic variables such as total dendritic length, radial distance of terminal tips, number of dendritic segments. In addition we distinguished small and large layer V pyramidal cells. From these studies we may conclude that initially (at birth) the state of maturation differs between neurons in ontogenetically different layers. The layer V pyramidal neurons are more advanced than the layer III pyramidal neurons (Wise et al. 1979, Miller 1988). The phase of rapid dendritic growth is after the ingrowth of subcortical and callosal fibers, i.e., between day 6 and days 16 to 18 for layer IV and III/II neurons, and especially between days 10 and 18 (figures 3.21 and 3.22). The maximum values are attained at day 18, irrespective of layer, type and size of the neuron. In the rapid

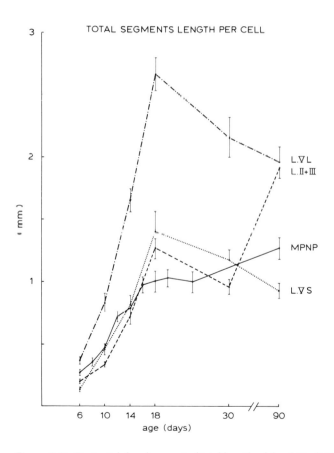

Figure 3.21 Postnatal development of total length of dendritic field of a neuron, measured in Golgi-Cox–stained sections. L.V₁ = large layer V basal dendrites; L II+III = layers II/III basal dendrites; LVs = small layer V basal dendrites of pyramidal neurons; MPNP = dendrites of layer IV, multipolar nonpyramidal neurons. Bars indicate SEM values.

Uylings et al.: Prenatal and Postnatal Development

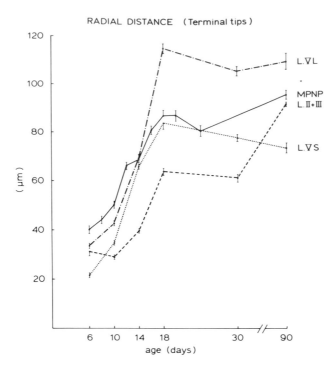

RADIAL DISTANCE (Terminal tips)

Figure 3.22 Postnatal development of the average radial distance of uncut terminal dendritic tips. For abbreviations, see figure 3.21. Bars indicate SEM values.

growth phase, the length of the dendrites of the large layer V pyramidal neurons grows three times faster than that of the multipolar nonpyramidal cells. In this period the average length of the basal dendritic field of the large layer V pyramidal cells and of a single basal dendrite increases by about 190 μm and 35 μm per day, respectively, whereas the average length of the multipolar nonpyramidal dendritic field and of a single dendrite increases by about 65 μm and 11 μm per day, respectively (figures 3.21, 3.22). In view of the limitations due to shrinkage and cutting, these data can only indicate the magnitude of growth (Uylings, Ruiz-Marcos, and Van Pelt 1986a). This dendritic growth seems slower than the axonal growth rate of 490 μm to 590 μm per day of frog and chick neurons (Katz, George, and Gilbert 1984). Because the developmental figures for the radial distance and total length of all dendrites per cell are similar to those of uncut individual terminal segments, we may be confident about the detected period of rapid growth (Parnavelas and Uylings 1980, Uylings et al. 1986a). The initial dendritic increase is accounted for mainly by the increase in branching and length of terminal segments. From day 10 onward the increase in dendritic size of large layer V pyramidal cells is caused mainly by increase in length of individual terminal segments. The same applies to other cortical neurons from day 14 onward.

The early outgrowth of dendrites during the first postnatal week occurs before the ingrowth of afferent fibers and can be genetically determined or induced by the outgrowth of its axon (Mrzljak et al. 1988). SP and MZ neurons may also influence this process. Afferent fibers influence the rapid growth phase of dendrites and synapses. For example, Kalsbeek, Matthijssen, and Uylings (1989) have shown that neonatal depletion of the afferent dopaminergic fibers to the medial prefrontal cortex induces reduced branching of the basal dendrites of layer V pyramidal neurons, which results in a 30 percent reduction in the total length of the basal dendritic field. Efferent cortical fibers also modulate the growth of neurons, as indicated by Ramirez and Kalil (1985). In their study on sensorimotor cortex neurons in the hamster, they have found that before the age of 11 days layer V pyramidal neurons grow independent of axotomy of the pyramidal tract. After this time neuronal growth is arrested by axotomy, whereas adult axotomy results in a large reduction of pyramidal cell size. Throughout life the pattern of cortical dendrites may be influenced by, among other things, environmental factors (see chapter 21 by Juraska and, e.g., Uylings et al. 1978).

Analysis of various developmental stages (Uylings et al. 1983) has shown that the dendritic structures of layer II/III pyramidal neurons and layer IV multipolar nonpyramidal neurons are compatible with topological tree predictions based on random bifurcation along the terminal segments only. On the other hand basal dendrites of pyramidal neurons and dendrites of nonpyramidal neurons have different topological tree structures (e.g., Van Pelt, Verwer, and Uylings 1986).

To date no study has reported a difference in dendritic size between the left and right homologous cortical brain regions (Bruch et al. 1988), although on the basis of the size differences between the left and right cortex (see above), this might be expected. The difference in size between left and right cortex might also be induced by a different number of neurons.

The outgrowth of dendrites and of axons is guided by the activities of their growth cones during pre- and postnatal development. Growth cones are dilations of terminal tips or of segments from which small filopodia and lamellipodia protrude and retract (e.g., Letourneau 1986). Growth cones are dynamic structures responsible for (directing) the elongation of neuronal fibers, for navigation through the nervous system to the target area, and for branching and recognition of the target tissue (for recent reviews on this topic, see Letourneau 1986, Lockerbie 1987, Raper et al. 1988, Stirling and Summerbell 1988).

Postnatal Development of Synapses
Although there are synaptic specializations between neurons in the rat cerebral cortex before birth (e.g., König and Marty 1981, Wolff 1978), synapse formation and maturation is mainly a postnatal event. At birth both asymmetrical (type I) and symmetrical (type II) synapses are pres-

ent (Kristt and Molliver 1976, Wolff 1978, Blue and Parnavelas 1983a,b), but type I synapses form the overwhelming majority throughout postnatal life. A very large increase of synapses in the rat cerebral cortex occurs during the second and third postnatal weeks (Blue and Parnavelas 1983a,b, Miller and Peters 1981). This increase coincides with the steep increase in spine formation on the dendrites of pyramidal and nonpyramidal neurons (Parnavelas et al. 1978, Wise et al. 1979, Miller 1988). In all developing and adult rats, the cortical axospinous synapses are predominantly type I (Blue and Parnavelas 1983a). The development curves for type I and type II synapses differ considerably, and both curves appear to be different from that of dendritic development (e.g., Blue and Parnavelas 1983b). Type II synapses appear to grow considerably in number after the first postnatal week and decrease in density after day 20, suggesting elimination of type II synapses (Blue and Parnavelas 1983b). In the small group of axosomatic synapses, type II synapses form the majority after the first postnatal week (Blue and Parnavelas 1983a, Bähr and Wolff 1985). Expressing the data in total number of synapses per human occipital cortex, Huttenlocher and colleagues (1982) found a significant reduction in number of synapses between eight months and eleven years of age. At the age of eight months, they have estimated a total number of about 3500 billion synapses in the human visual cortex, which decreased to 2100 billion synapses at the age of eleven years. On day 28 the synapses in rat visual cortex appear qualitatively indistinguishable from synapses identified in adult cerebral cortex (Blue and Parnavelas 1983a,b).

The study of Müller and coworkers (1984) in the rabbit visual cortex indicates that the receptive surface of day 20 pyramidal neurons is not smaller than that of adult pyramidal neurons, whereas the nonpyramidal receptive surface still increases after day 20. This study suggests that, in contrast to dendritic development, the development of the receptive surface of nonpyramidal neurons attains its adult level later than that of the receptive surface of pyramidal neurons.

Blue and Parnavelas (1983a) emphasized in their report that particularly during the first eight days of life postsynaptic specializations are seen without any specialized appositions. These observations suggest that postsynaptic sites in the cerebral cortex develop before presynaptic specializations and that they may induce the synapse formation.

For quantification of synapses it is relevant that new techniques have been developed that are, among other things, independent of synaptic shape and orientation (e.g., Braendgaard and Gundersen 1986).

3.3 Interference of Cortical Development

In previous sections we have described when during normal development excess numbers of neurons, neuronal fibers, and/or synapses occur in different periods and when they are reduced later in development. This temporary excess growth may provide the nervous system with additional flexibility. This flexibility would require less genetic information concerning the billions of nerve connections to be formed and would create a nervous system that is capable of being less vulnerable to deleterious influences. Especially in early development the cerebral cortex is sensitive to deleterious influences, such as ionizing radiation (Hicks and D'Amato 1978), alcohol exposure (Miller 1986b, Cadete-Leite et al. 1988), hypoxia, opioid exposure (e.g., Zagon and MacLaughlin 1986), and cortical lesion (e.g., Kolb and Tomie 1988). The review by Hicks and D'Amato (1978) on the effects of ionizing radiation clearly shows a differential sensitivity related with the stage of development. Irradiation with 1.5 Gray (Gy; 1 Gy = 100 rad) on the twelfth day of gestation produces a devastating damage to the cerebral hemisphere, i.e., massive cell death and malformation. In the late fetal period an irradiation with as little as 0.3 Gy was sufficient for inducing ectopic location of neurons and to alter individual differentiation of cortical neurons. After birth the sensitivity of the cerebral cortex to irradiation changes rapidly. Irradiation with 4 Gy induces no acute cell death or detectable alteration of the differentiation of cortical neurons in 7-day-old-rats. In 2-month-old-rats no acute effects of 10 Gy were observed; one year later, however, some proliferation of perivascular connective tissue cells were found in the cortex (Hicks and D'Amato 1978). The effect of ionizing radiation depends on dose and age but also on brain region (e.g., Hicks and D'Amato 1978, Schmidt and Lent 1987) and the sensitive periods are different for cerebral cortex and cerebellum. The phase of cell proliferation appeared to be particularly sensitive, which is also the case when the organism is exposed to alcohol (e.g., Miller 1986b, 1987, Tavares, Paula-Barbosa, and Cadete-Leite 1987, Cadete-Leite et al. 1988). Prenatal exposure to ethanol affects the proliferation and migration of cortical neurons. Thus it reduces the number of neurons generated, delays the generation period, and leads to a distortion of the "normal" final position of cortical neurons as it is described in the inside-to-outside patterns previously mentioned (Miller 1986b). In prenatal exposure to alcohol the corticospinal neurons that are generated later show permanent differences in their corticospinal connections. The normal process of reduction of exuberant corticospinal projections was affected in the ethanol-exposed rats (Miller 1987).

Chronic postnatal alcohol consumption also leads to cell death, especially in those brain regions in which postnatal neuronal proliferation occurs, viz., cerebellum, hippocampus, and olfactory bulb (e.g., Tavares et al. 1987, Cadete-Leite et al. 1988). In the medial prefrontal cortex no cell reduction was established after 6 to 18 months of postnatal chronic alcohol consumption (Tavares and Cadete-Leite, in preparation). Exposure to alcohol also affects the neuronal differentiation (e.g., Cadete-Leite et al. 1988). The size of the effect is not the same for each cortical area. In the rat, for example, there is a difference between the fascia dentata and the medial prefrontal cortex (Cadete-Leite et al. 1990). Cell proliferation and maturation is also affected by opioids. Curiously endogenous opioids appear to be natural trophic factors in brain development, but brain development is retarded by exposure to exogenous opioids (e.g., Zagon, McLaughlin, and Zagon 1984, Zagon and McLaughlin 1986, 1987, Hauser, McLaughlin, and Zagon 1987).

Until recently a prevailing idea concerning the plasticity of the nervous system, that of the cerebral cortex in particular, was that the earlier the lesion was inflicted on the cortex, the better the recovery. In view of the data now available, this hypothesis appears to be too simplistic (e.g., Schneider 1981, Kolb 1987, Kolb and Tomie 1988). For example, neonatal bilateral removal of rat frontal or parietal cortex affects cortical thickness and behavior more severely than do the lesions executed on postnatal day 10, which in their turn were also less disruptive than similar lesions in adulthood (e.g., Kolb 1987). On the other hand rats with complete neonatal removal of the neocortex of one hemisphere have a thicker cortex, and performed better behaviorally than rats with similar lesions executed on postnatal days 5 or 10 or in adulthood (Kolb and Tomie 1988).

The development of the cerebral cortex can be enhanced by environmental enrichment (Uylings et al. 1978, Renner and Rosenzweig 1987, chapter 21 by Juraska). The period of "flexible response" to environmental enrichment appears to be a lifespan long, although the cortical alterations seem to be smaller at a later age. In conclusion, it is difficult to formulate general rules on the flexibility or sensitivity of the rat cerebral cortex. This flexibility or plasticity will differ for different deleterious and advantageous influences and for the different phases of development during which they occur (see chapter 21 by Juraska and chapter 23 by Kolb).

3.4 Summary

This chapter reviews the pre- and postnatal development of the rat cerebral cortex. It deals with the formation of the (fetal) cortical lamination, neuronal generation, and migration to the cortex. Emphasis is given to specifying the timing of the different prenatal processes. The growth of subcortical and callosal fiber systems in the cerebral cortex is described, as well as hypotheses on neuronal outgrowth and target finding, and the role of transmitter systems in cortical development.

Different aspects of postnatal maturation of the rat cerebral cortex are considered, such as the volumetric growth, asymmetry of the cerebral cortex, the dendritic growth, and synaptogenesis. The last section of this chapter deals with factors like ionizing radiation, alcohol consumption, and lesions that interfere with the development of the cerebral cortex.

Notes

We thank Dr. Marion E. Cavanagh (University College, London, UK) for her comments on this paper, Ms. M. A. H. Matthijssen for her technical assistance, Mr. A. Janssen for typing and correcting the manuscript, Mr. H. Stoffels for his graphic work, and Mr. G. Van der Meulen for his photographic assistance.

1. This estimate was made during the 3rd International Practical Course on Morphometry and Stereology in Neurosciences, Aarhus (Denmark), August 22–26, 1988.

2. In staging the postnatal development, the day of birth is generally called day 0. This definition is used throughout this chapter.

References

Al-Ghoul, W. M., and Miller, M. W. (1989). Transient expression of Alz-50 immunoreactivity in developing rat neocortex: a marked for naturally occurring neuronal death? *Brain Res.* 481:361–367.

Bähr, S., and Wolff, J. R. (1985). Postnatal development of axosomatic synapses in the rat visual cortex: morphogenesis and quantitative evaluation. *J. Comp. Neurol.* 233:405–420.

Beaudoin, A. R. (1980). Embryology and teratology. In H. J. Baker, J. R. Lindsey, and S. H. Weisbroth (eds.), *The Laboratory Rat. Vol. II. Research Applications.* New York. Academic Press, pp. 75–101.

Bear, M. R., Cooper, L. N., and Ebner, F. F. (1987). A physiological basis for a theory of synapse modification. *Science* 237:42–48.

Bear, M. F., and Singer, W. (1986). Modulation of visual cortical plasticity by acetylcholine and noradrenaline. *Nature* 320:172–176.

Berry, M., and Rogers, A. W. (1965). The migration of neuroblasts in the developing cerebral cortex. *J. Anat.* 99:691–709.

Blue, M. E., and Parnavelas, J. G. (1983a). The formation and maturation of synapses in the visual cortex of the rat. I. Qualitative analysis. *J. Neurocytol.* 12:599–616.

Blue, M. E., and Parnavelas, J. G. (1983b). The formation and maturation of synapses in the visual cortex of the rat. II. Quantitative analysis. *J. Neurocytol.* 12:697–712.

Boulder Committee (1970). Embryonic vertebrate central nervous system: revised terminology. *Anat. Rec.* 166:257–262.

Braendgaard, H., and Gundersen, H. J. G. (1986). The impact of recent stereological advances on quantitative studies of the nervous system. *J. Neurosci. Meth.* 18:39–78.

Breedlove, S. M. (1984). Steroid influences on the development and function of a neuromuscular system. In G. J. De Vries, J. P. C. De Bruin, H. B. M. Uylings, and M. A. Corner (eds.), *Sex Differences in the Brain. Prog. Brain Res.* 61:147–170. Amsterdam: Elsevier.

Brenner, E., and Mirmiran, M. (1988). Function of noradrenergic innervation of the rat brain: coping with the unexpected. *Brain Dysfunction* 1:57–70.

Bruch, L., Ebert, A., Schulz, E., and Wenzel, J. (1988). Quantitativ-neurohistologische Untersuchungen an Lamina V- und Lamina III-Pyramiden-neuronen der Regio praecentralis agranularis der Ratte. Zu Fragen der Lateralisation. *J. Hirnforsch* 29:461–472.

Brücker, G., Mareš, V., and Biesold, D. (1978). Programmed cell formation in the rat's developing visual cortex. Autoradiographic studies. In G. Dörner and M. Kawakami (eds.), *Hormones and Brain Development*. Amsterdam: North Holland-Elsevier, pp. 285–292.

Butler, S. (1984). Sex differences in human cerebral function. In G. J. De Vries, J. P. C. De Bruin, H. B. M. Uylings, and M. A. Corner (eds.), *Sex Differences in the Brain. Prog. Brain Res.* 61:443–455. Amsterdam: Elsevier.

Cadete-Leite, A., Alves, M. C., Paula-Barbosa, M. M., et al. (1990). Quantitative analysis of basal dendrites of prefrontal pyramidal cells after chronic alcohol consumption and withdrawal in the adult rats. (Submitted).

Cadete-Leite, A., Tavares, M. A., Uyling, H. B. M., and Paula-Barbosa, M. (1988). Granule cell loss and dendritic regrowth in the hippocampal dentate gyrus of the rat after chronic alcohol consumption. *Brain Res.* 473:1–14.

Cavanagh, M. E., and Møllgård, K. (1985). An immunocytochemical study of the distribution of some plasma proteins within the developing forebrain of the pig with special reference to the neocortex. *Dev. Brain Res.* 17:183–194.

Cavanagh, M. E., and Parnavelas, J. G. (1988a). Development of somatostatin immunoreactive neurons in the rat occipital cortex: a combined immunocytochemical-autoradiographic study. *J. Comp. Neurol.* 268:1–12.

Cavanagh, M. E., and Parnavelas, J. G. (1988b). Neurotransmitter differentiation in cortical neurons. In J. G. Parnavelas, C. D. Stern, and R. V. Stirling (eds.), *The Making of the Nervous System*. Oxford: Oxford University Press, pp. 434–453.

Chronwall, B. M., and Wolff, J. R. (1981). Nonpyramidal neurons in early developmental stages of the rat neocortex. *Biblthca Anat.* 19:147–151.

Chun, J. J. M., and Shatz, C. J. (1988). A fibronectin-like molecule is present in the developing cat cerebral cortex and is correlated with subplate neurons. *J. Cell Biol.* 106:857–872.

Clinton, R. J., Jr., and Ebner, F. F. (1988). Time course of neocortical graft innervation by AChE-positive fibers. *J. Comp. Neurol.* 277:557–577.

Cooper, N. G. F., and Steindler, D. A. (1986). Lectins demarcate the barrel subfield in the somatosensory cortex of the early postnatal mouse. *J. Comp. Neurol.* 249:157–169.

Cowan, W. M., Fawcett, J. W., O'Leary, D. D. M., and Stanfield, B. B. (1984). Regressive events in neurogenesis. *Science* 225:1258–1265.

Crandall, J. E., and Caviness, V. S. (1984). Thalamocortical connections in newborn mice. *J. Comp. Neurol.* 228:542–556.

Derer, P. (1979). Evidence for the occurrence of early modifications in the 'glia limitans' layer of the neocortex of the reeler mutant mouse. *Neurosci. Lett.* 13:195–202.

Diamond, M. C. (1987). Sex differences in the rat forebrain. *Brain Res. Rev.* 12:235–240.

Dinopoulos, A., Eadie, L. A., Dori, I., and Parnavelas, J. G. (1989). The development of basal forebrain projections to rat visual cortex. *Exp. Brain Res.* (in press).

Fairén, A., Cobas, A., and Fonseca, M. (1986). Times of generation of glutamic acid decarboxylase immunoreactive neurons in mouse somatosensory cortex. *J. Comp. Neurol.* 251:67–83.

Fawcett, J. W. (1988). Retinotopic maps, cell death, and electrical activity in the retinotectal and retinocollicular projections. In H. G. Parnavelas, C. D. Stern, and R. V. Stirling (eds.), *The Making of the Nervous System*. Oxford: Oxford University Press, pp. 395–416.

Finlay, B. L., and Slattery, M. (1983). Local differences in the amount of early cell death in neocortex predict adult local specialization. *Science* 219:1349–1351.

Fleming, D. E., Anderson, R. H., Rhees, R. W., Kinghorn, E., and Bakaitis, J. (1986). Effects of prenatal stress on sexually dimorphic asymmetries in the cerebral cortex of the male rat. *Brain Res. Bull.* 16:395–398.

Floeter, M. K., and Jones, E. G. (1985). The morphology and phased outgrowth of callosal axons in the fetal rat. *Dev. Brain Res.* 22:7–18.

Gadisseux, J. F., and Evrard, P. (1985). Glial-neuronal relationship in the developing central nervous system. *Dev. Neurosci.* 7:12–32.

Gardette, R., Courtois, M., and Bisconte, J.-C. (1982). Prenatal development of mouse central nervous structures: time of neuron origin and gradients of neuronal production. A radioautographic study. *J. Hirnforsch.* 23:415–431.

Geschwind, N., and Behan, P. (1982). Left handedness, association with immune disease, migraine, and developmental learning disorder. *Proc. Nat. Acad. Sci. USA* 79:5097–5100.

Gu, Q., and Singer, W. (1988). Blockade of muscarinic receptors prevents ocular dominance plasticity of kitten striate cortex. *Eur. J. Neurosci.* (suppl.) 1:S271.

Hankin, M. H., and Lund, R. D. (1987). Role of the target in directing the outgrowth of retinal axons: transplants reveal surface-related and surface-independent cues. *J. Comp. Neurol.* 263:455–466.

Hankin, M. H., and Silver, J. (1986). Mechanisms of axonal guidance. The problem of intersecting fiber systems. In L. W. Browder (ed.), *Developmental Biology*. Vol. 2. New York: Plenum Press, pp. 565–604.

Hauser, K. F., McLaughlin, P. J., and Zagon, I. W. (1987). Endogenous opioids regulate dendritic growth and spine formation in developing rat brain. *Brain Res.* 416:157–161.

Hedlich, A., and Winkelmann, E. (1982). Neuronentypen des visuellen Cortex der adulten und juvenilen Ratte. *J. Hirnforsch* 23:353–373.

Herkenham, M. (1980). Laminar organization of thalamic projections to the rat neocortex. *Science* 207:532–535.

Heumann, D., and Leuba, G. (1983). Neuronal death in the development and aging of the cerebral cortex of the mouse. *Neuropathol. Appl. Neurobiol* 9:297–311.

Hicks, S. P., and D'Amato, C. J. (1968). Cell migrations to the isocortex in the rat. *Anat. Rec.* 160:619–634.

Hicks, S. P., and D'Amato, C. J. (1978). Effects of ionizing radiation on developing brain and behavior. In G. Gottlieb (eds.), *Studies on the Development of Behavior and the Nervous System*. New York: Academic Press, pp. 36–72.

Huttenlocher, P. R., De Courten, C., Garey, L. J., and Van der Loos, H. (1982). Synaptogenesis in human visual cortex—evidence for synapse elimination during normal development. *Neurosci. Lett.* 33:247–252.

Innocenti, G. M. (1988). Loss of axonal projections in the development of the mammalian brain. In J. G. Parnavelas, C. D. Stern, and R. V. Stirling (eds.), *The Making of the Nervous System*. Oxford: Oxford University Press, pp. 319–339.

Ivy, G. O., and Killackey, H. P. (1981). The ontogeny of the distribution of callosal projections in the rat parietal cortex. *J. Comp. Neurol.* 195:367–389.

Jacobson, M. (1978). *Developmental Neurobiology*. 2nd ed. New York: Plenum Press, 562 pp.

Joosten, E. A. J., and Van Eden, C. G. (1989). An anterograde tracer study on the development of corticospinal projections from the medial prefrontal cortex in the rat. *Dev. Brain Res.* 45:313–319.

Juraska, J. M. (1982). The development of pyramidal neurons after eye opening in the visual cortex of hooded rats: a quantitative study. *J. Comp. Neurol.* 212:208–213.

Juraska, J. M. (1984). Sex differences in developmental plasticity in the visual cortex and hippocampal dentate gyrus. In G. J. De Vries, J. P. C. De Bruin, H. B. M. Uylings, and M. A. Corner (eds.), *Sex Differences in the Brain. Prog. Brain Res.* 61:205–214. Amsterdam: Elsevier.

Kalsbeek, A. (1989). *The Role of Dopamine in the Development of the Rat Prefrontal Cortex*. Ph.D. thesis, University of Amsterdam. Meppel: Krips Repro, 218 pp.

Kalsbeek, A., Matthijssen, M. A. H., and Uyling, H. B. M. (1989). Morphometric analysis of prefrontal cortical development following neonatal lesioning of the dopaminergic mesocortical projection. *Exp. Brain Res.* (in press).

Kalsbeek, A., Voorn, P., Buijs, R. M., Pool, C. W., and Uylings, H. B. M. (1988). Development of the dopaminergic innervation in the prefrontal cortex of the rat. *J. Comp. Neurol.* 269:58–72.

Kaplan, M. S. (1981). Neurogenesis in the 3-month-old rat visual cortex. *J. Comp. Neurol.* 195:323–338.

Kasamatsu, T. (1983). Neuronal plasticity maintained by the central norepinephrine system in the cat visual cortex. In J. M. Sprague and A. N. Epstein (eds.), *Progr. Psychobiol. and Physiol. Psychology*. Vol. 10. New York Academic Press, pp. 1–112.

Katz, M. J., George, E. B., and Gilbert, L. J. (1984). Axonal elongation as a stochastic walk. *Cell Motility* 4:351–370.

Kimura, D., and Harshman, R. A. (1984). Sex differences in brain organization for verbal and non-verbal function. In G. J. De Vries, J. P. C. De Bruin, H. B. M. Uylings, and M. A. Corner (eds.), *Sex Differences in the Brain. Prog. Brain Res.* 61:423–441. Amsterdam: Elsevier.

Kolb, B. (1987). Recovery from early cortical damage in rats. I. Differential behavioral and anatomical effects of frontal lesions at different ages of neural maturation. *Behav. Brain Res.* 25:205–220.

Kolb, B., and Tomie, J.-A. (1988). Recovery from early cortical damage in rats. IV. Effects of hemidecortication at 1, 5 or 10 days of age on cerebral anatomy and behavior. *Behav. Brain Res.* 28:259–274.

Kolb, B., Sutherland, R. J., Nonneman, A. J., and Whishaw, I. Q. (1982). Asymmetry in the cerebral hemispheres of the rat, mouse, rabbit and cat: the right hemisphere is larger. *Exp. Neurol.* 78:348–359.

König, N., and Marty, R. (1981). Early neurogenesis and synaptogenesis in cerebral cortex. *Biblthca Anat.* 19:152–160.

König, N., Roch, G., and Marty, R. (1975). The onset of synaptogenesis in rat temporal cortex. *Anat. Embryol.* 148:73–87.

König, N., Valat, J., Fulcrand, J., and Marty, R. (1977). The time of origin of Cajal-Retzius cells in the rat temporal cortex. An autoradiographic study. *Neurosci. Lett.* 4:21–26.

Kostovic, I., and Molliver, M. E. (1974). A new interpretation of the laminar development of cerebral cortex: synaptogenesis in different layers of the neopallium in the human fetus. *Anat. Rec.* 178:395.

Kristt, D. A., and Molliver, M. E. (1976). Synapses in newborn rat cerebral cortex: a quantitative ultrastructural study. *Brain Res.* 108:180–186.

Lauder, J. M., and Krebs, H. (1986). Do neurotransmitters, neurohumors, and hormones specify critical periods? In W. T. Greenough and J. M. Juraska (eds.), *Developmental Neuropsychobiology*. New York: Academic Press, pp. 119–174.

Lauder, J. M., Han, V. K. M., Henderson, P., Verdoorn, T., and Towle, A. C. (1987). Prenatal ontogeny of the GABAergic system in the rat brain: an immunocytochemical study. *Neuroscience* 19:465–493.

Letourneau, P. C. (1986). Regulation of nerve fiber elongation during embryogenesis. In W. T. Greenough and J. M. Juraska (eds.), *Developmental Neuropsychology*. New York: Academic Press, pp. 33–71.

Levitt, P., Cooper, M. L., and Rakic, P. (1981). Coexistence of neuronal and glial precursor cells in the cerebral ventricular zone of the fetal monkey: an ultrastructural, immunoperoxidase analysis. *J. Neurosci.* 1:27–39.

Levitt, P., Cooper, M. L., and Rakic, P. (1983). Early divergence and changing proportions of neuronal and glial precursor cells in the primate cerebral ventricular zone. *Dev. Biol.* 96:472–484.

Levitt, P., and Moore, R. Y. (1979). Development of the noradrenergic innervation of neocortex. *Brain Res.* 162:243–259.

Lidov, H. G. W., and Molliver, M. E. (1982). An immunohistochemical study of serotonin neuron development in the rat: ascending pathways and terminal fields. *Brain Res. Bull.* 8:389–430.

Ling, E. A., and Leblond, C. P. (1973). Investigation of glial cells in semithin sections. II. Variation with age in the numbers of the various glial cell types in rat cortex and corpus callosum. *J. Comp. Neurol.* 149:73–82.

Lockerbie, R. O. (1987). The neuronal growth cone: a review of its locomotory, navigational and target recognition capabilities. *Neuroscience* 20:719–729.

Lund, R. D. (1978). *Development and Plasticity of the Brain*. New York: Oxford Press, 370 pp.

Lund, R. D., and Mustari, M. J. (1977). Development of the geniculocortical pathways in rats. *J. Comp. Neurol.* 173:289–306.

Luskin, M. B., and Shatz, C. J. (1985). Studies of the earliest generated cells of the cat's visual cortex: cogeneration of subplate and marginal zones. *J. Neurosci.* 5:1062–1075.

Marin-Padilla, M. (1971). Early prenatal ontogenesis of the cerebral cortex (neocortex) of the cat (*Felis domestica*): a Golgi study. I. The primordial neocortical organization. *Z. Anat. Entwickl.-Gesch.* 134:117–145.

Mattson, M. P. (1988). Neurotransmitters in the regulation of neuronal cytoarchitecture. *Brain Res. Rev.* 13:179–212.

Miller, M. W. (1985). Cogeneration of retrogradely labelled cortico-cortical projection and GABA-immunoreactive local circuit neurons in cerebral cortex. *Dev. Brain Res.* 23:187–192.

Miller, M. W. (1986a). The migration and neurochemical differentiation of γ-aminobutyric acid (GABA)-immunoreactive neurons in rat visual cortex as demonstrated by a combined immunocytochemical-autoradiographic technique. *Dev. Brain Res.* 28:41–46.

Miller, M. W. (1986b). Effects of alcohol on the generation and migration of cerebral cortical neurons. *Science* 233:1308–1311.

Miller, M. W. (1987). Effect of prenatal exposure to alcohol on the distribution and time of origin of corticospinal neurons in the rat. *J. Comp. Neurol.* 257:372–382.

Miller, M. W. (1988). Development of projection and local circuit neurons in neocortex. In A. Peters and E. G. Jones (eds.), *Development and Maturation of Cerebral Cortex*. Vol. 7, Cerebral Cortex. New York: Plenum Press, pp. 133–175.

Miller, M. W., and Peters, A. (1981). Maturation of rat visual cortex. II. A combined Golgi-electron microscope study of pyramidal neurons. *J. Comp. Neurol.* 203:555–573.

Molliver, M. E., Kostović, I., and Van der Loos, H. (1973). The development of synapses in the human fetus. *Brain Res.* 50:403–407.

Mrzljak, L., Uylings, H. B. M., Kostović, I., and Van Eden, C. G. (1988). Prenatal development of neurons in the human prefrontal cortex: I. A qualitative Golgi study. *J. Comp. Neurol.* 271:355–386.

Muller, L. J., Verwer, R. W. H., Nunes Cardozo, B., and Vrensen, G. (1984). Synaptic characteristics of identified pyramidal and multipolar nonpyramidal neurons in the visual cortex of young and adult rabbits. A quantitative Golgi-electron microscope study. *Neuroscience* 12:1071–1087.

Parnavelas, J. G., and Cavanagh, M. G. (1988). Transient expression of neurotransmitters in the developing neocortex. *Trends Neurosci.* 11:92–93.

Parnavelas, J. G., and Edmunds, S. M. (1983). Further evidence that Retzius-Cajal cells transform to non-pyramidal neurons in the developing rat visual cortex. *J. Neurocytol.* 12:863–871.

Parnavelas, J. G. Bradford, R., Mounty, E. J., and Lieberman, A. R. (1978). The development of non-pyramidal neurons in the visual cortex of the rat *Anat Embryol.* 155:1 14.

Parnavelas, J. G., Luder, R., Pollard, S. G., Sullivan, K., and Lieberman, A. R. (1983). A qualitative and quantitative ultrastructural study glial cells in the developing visual cortex of the rat. *Phil. Trans. R. Soc. Lond.* B301:55–84.

Parnavelas, J. G., Papadopoulos, G. C., and Cavanagh, M. E. (1988). Changes in neurotransmitters during development. In A. Peters and E. G. Jones (eds.), *Development and Maturation of Cerebral Cortex*. Vol. 7, Cerebral Cortex. New York: Plenum Press, pp. 177–209.

Parnavelas, J. G., and Uylings, H. B. M. (1980). The growth of non-pyramidal neurons in the visual cortex of the rat: a morphometric study. *Brain Res.* 193:373–382.

Petit, T. L., LeBoutillier, J. C., Gregario, A., and Libstug, H. (1988). The pattern of dendritic development in the cerebral cortex of the rat. *Dev. Brain Res.* 41:209–219.

Poston, M. R., Fredieu, J., Carney, P. R., and Silver, J. (1988). Roles of glia and neural crest cells in creating axon pathways and boundaries in the vertebrate central and peripheral nervous systems. In J. G. Parnavelas, C. D. Stern, and R. V. Stirling (eds.), *The Making of the Nervous System*. Oxford: Oxford University Press, pp. 282–313.

Price, D. J., and Blakemore, C. (1985). Regressive events in the postnatal development of association in the visual cortex. *Nature* 316:721–724.

Raedler, E., and Raedler, A. (1978). Autoradiographic study of early neurogenesis in rat neocortex. *Anat. Embryol.* 154:267–284.

Raedler, E., Raedler, A., and Feldhaus, S. (1980). Dynamical aspects of neocortical histogenesis in the rat. *Anat. Embryol.* 158:253–269.

Rakic, P. (1972). Mode of cell migration to the superficial layers of fetal monkey neocortex. *J. Comp. Neurol.* 145:61–84.

Rakic, P. (1982). Early developmental events: cell lineages, acquisition of neuronal positions, and areal and laminar development. In P. Rakic and P. S. Goldman-Rakic (eds.), *Development and Modifiability of the Cerebral Cortex, Neurosci. Res. Prog. Bull.* 20:439–451.

Rakic, P. (1988). Specification of cerebral cortical areas. *Science* 241:170–176.

Ramirez, L. F., and Kalil, K. (1985). Critical stages for growth in the development of cortical neurons. *J. Comp. Neurol.* 237:506–518.

Raper, J. A., Chang, S., Kapfhammer, J. P., and Rathjen, F. G. (1988). Growth cone guidance and labelled axons. In J. G. Parnavelas, C. D. Stern, and R. V. Stirling (eds.), *The Making of the Nervous System.* Oxford: Oxford University Press, pp. 188–203.

Reep, R. L., and Goodwin, G. W. (1988). Layer VII of rodent cerebral cortex. *Neurosci. Lett.* 90:15–20.

Renner, M. J., and Rosenzweig, M. R. (1987). *Enriched and Impoverished Environments. Effects on Brain and Behavior. Recent Research in Psychology.* New York: Springer Verlag, 134 pp.

Reynolds, M. L., and Møllgård, K. (1985). The distribution of plasma proteins in the neocortex and early allocortex of the developing sheep brain. *Anat. Embryol.* 171:41–60.

Rickmann, M., Chronwall, B. M., and Wolff, J. R. (1977). On the development of nonpyramidal neurons and axons outside the cortical plate: the early marginal zone as a pallial anlage. *Anat. Embryol.* 151:285–307.

Rickmann, M., and Wolff, J. R. (1981). Differentiation of 'preplate' neurons in the pallium of the rat. *Biblthca Anat.* 19:142–146.

Rickmann, M., and Wolff, J. R. (1985). Prenatal gliogenesis in the neopallium of the rat. *Adv. Anat. Embryol. Cell Biol.* 93:1–104.

Rockel, A. J., Hiorns, R. W., and Powell, T. P. S. (1980). Basic uniformity in the structure of the cerebral cortex. *Brain* 103:221–243.

Rosen, G. D., Berrebi, A. S., Yutzey, D. A., and Denenberg, V. H. (1983). Prenatal testosterone causes shift of asymmetry in neonatal tail posture of the rat. *Dev. Brain Res.* 9:99–101.

Ross, D. A., Glick, S. C., and Meibach, R. C. (1981). Sexually dimorphic brain and behavioral asymmetries in the neonatal rat. *Proc. Natl. Acad. Sci. USA* 78:1958–1961.

Sane, J. R. (1989). Analysing cell lineage with a recombinant retrovirus. *Trends Neurosci.* 12:21–28.

Sauer, F. C. (1935). Mitosis in the neural tube. *J. Comp. Neurol.* 62:377–405.

Schlumpf, M., Shoemaker, W. J., and Bloom, F. E. (1980). Innervation of embryonic rat cerebral cortex by catecholamine-containing fibers. *J. Comp. Neurol.* 192:361–376.

Schmidt, S. L., and Lent, R. (1987). Effects of prenatal irradiation on the development of cerebral cortex and corpus callosum of the mouse. *J. Comp. Neurol.* 264:193–204.

Schneider, G. E. (1981). Early lesions and abnormal neuronal connections. *Trends Neurosci.* 4:187–192.

Shatz, C. J., Chun, J. J. M., and Luskin, M. B. (1988). The role of the subplate in the development of mammalian telencephalon. In A. Peters and E. G. Jones (eds.), *Development and Maturation of Cerebral Cortex*. Vol. 7, Cerebral Cortex. New York: Plenum Press, pp. 35–58.

Shoukimas, G. M., and Hinds, J. W. (1978). The development of the cerebral cortex in the embryonic mouse: an electron microscopic serial section analysis. *J. Comp. Neurol.* 179:795–830.

Slopsema, J. S., Van der Gugten, J., and De Bruin, J. P. C. (1982). Regional concentrations of noradrenaline and dopamine in the frontal cortex of the rat: dopaminergic innervation of the prefrontal subareas and lateralization of prefrontal dopamine. *Brain Res.* 250:197–200.

Smart, I. H. M. (1983). Three dimensional growth of the mouse isocortex. *J. Anat.* 137:683–694.

Smart, I. H. M. (1984). Histogenesis of the mesocortical area of the mouse telencephalon. *J. Anat.* 138:537–552.

Smart, I. H. M., and McSherry, G. M. (1982). Growth patterns in the lateral wall of the mouse telecephalon. II. Histological changes during and subsequent to the period of isocortical neuron production. *J. Anat.* 134:415–442.

Sperry, R. W. (1963). Chemoaffinity in the orderly growth of nerve fiber patterns and connections. *Proc. Nat. Acad. Sci. USA* 50:703–710.

Spoerri, P. E. (1987). GABA mediated development alterations in a neuronal cell line and in cultures of cortical and retinal neurons. In D. A. Redburn and A. Schousboe (eds.), *Neurotrophic Activity of GABA during Development*. New York: Alan R. Liss, pp. 189–220.

Stanfield, B. B., and O'Leary, D. D. M. (1985). The transient corticospinal projections from the occipital cortex during the postnatal development of the rat. *J. Comp. Neurol.* 238:236–248.

Stewart, G. R., and Pearlman, A. L. (1987). Fibronectin-like immunoreactivity in the developing cerebral cortex. *J. Neurosci.* 7:3325–3333.

Stewart, J., and Kolb, B. (1988). The effects of neonatal gonadectomy and prenatal stress on cortical thickness and asymmetry in rats. *Behav. Neural Biol.* 49:344–360.

Stirling, R. V., and Summerbell, D. (1988). Motor axon guidance in the developing chick limb. In J. G. Parnavelas, C. D. Stern, and R. V. Stirling (eds.), *The Making of the Nervous System*. Oxford: Oxford University Press, pp. 228–247.

Sturrock, R. R. (1976). Light microscopic identification of immature glial cells in semithin sections of the developing mouse corpus callosum. *J. Anat.* 122:521–537.

Sturrock, R. R. (1986). Postnatal ontogenesis of astrocytes. In S. Fedoroff and A. Vernadakis (eds.), *Development, Morphology and Regional Specialization of Astrocytes*. Vol. 1, Astrocytes. New York: Academic Press, pp. 75–103.

Tavares, M. A., Paula-Barbosa, M. M., and Cadete-Leite, A. (1987). Chronic alcohol consumption reduces the cortical layer volumes and the number of neurons in the rat cerebellar cortex. *Alcoholism: Clin. Exp. Res.* 11:315–319.

Thatcher, R. W., Walker, R. A., and Giudice, S. (1987). Human cerebral hemispheres develop at different rates and ages. *Science* 236:1110–1113.

Udin, S. B., and Fawcett, J. W. (1988). Formation of topographic maps. *Ann. Rev. Neurosci.* 11:289–327.

Uylings, H. B. M., Hofman, M. A., and Matthijssen, M. A. H. (1987). Comparison of bivariate linear relations in biological allometry research. *Acta Stereol.* 6/III:467–472.

Uylings, H. B. M., Kuypers, K., Diamond, M. C., and Veltman, W. A. M. (1978). Effects of differential environments of plasticity of dendrites of cortical pyramidal neurons in adult rats. *Exp. Neurol.* 62:658–677.

Uylings, H. B. M., Ruiz-Marcos, A., and Van Pelt, J. (1986a). The metric analysis of three-dimensional dendritic tree patterns: a methodological review. *J. Neurosci. Meth.* 18:127–151.

Uylings, H. B. M., Van Eden, C. G., and Hofman, M. A. (1986b). Morphometry of size-volume variables and comparison of their bivariate relations in the nervous system under different conditions. *J. Neurosci. Meth.* 18:19–37.

Uylings, H. B. M., Van Eden, C. G., and Verwer, R. W. H. (1984). Morphometric methods in sexual dimorphism research on the central nervous system. In G. J. De Vries, J. P. C. De Bruin, H. B. M. Uylings, and M. A. Corner (eds.), *Sex Differences in the Brain. Prog. Brain Res.* 61:215–222. Amsterdam: Elsevier.

Uylings, H. B. M., Verwer, R. W. H., Van Pelt, J., and Parnavelas, J. G. (1983). Topological analysis of dendritic growth at various stages of cerebral development. *Acta Stereol.* 2:55–62.

Valentino, K. L., and Jones, E. G. (1982). The early formation of the corpus callosum: a light and electron microscopic study in fetal and neonatal rats. *J. Neurocytol.* 11:583–609.

Van Eden, C. G. (1986). Development of connections between the mediodorsal nucleus of the thalamus and the prefrontal cortex in the rat. *J. Comp. Neurol.* 244:349–359.

Van Eden, C. G., Kros, J. M., and Uylings, H. B. M. (1989). Development of the rat prefrontal cortex its size, connections with thalamus, spinal cord and other cortical areas. *Prog. Brain Res.*, (in press).

Van Eden, C. G., and Uylings, H. B. M. (1985). Postnatal volumetric development of the prefrontal cortex in the rat. *J. Comp. Neurol.* 241:268–274.

Van Eden, C. G., Kalsbeek, A., and Uylings, H. B. M. (1987). Effects of thalamic lesions on the development of the prefrontal cortex in the rat. Proc. Satellite Symposium 2nd IBRO world congress "Cellular Thalamic Mechanisms," Verona, Italy.

Van Eden, C. G., Mrzljak, L., Voorn, P., and Uylings, H. B. M. (1989). Prenatal development of GABAergic neurons in the neocortex of the rat. *J. Comp. Neurol.* 288 (in press).

Van Eden, C. G., Uylings, H. B. M., and Van Pelt, J. (1984). Sex-difference and left-right asymmetries in the prefrontal cortex during postnatal development in the rat. *Dev. Brain Res.* 12:146–153.

Van Pelt, J., Verwer, R. W. H., and Uylings, H. B. M. (1986). Application of growth models to the topology of neuronal branching patterns. *J. Neurosci. Meth.* 18:153–165.

Waechter, R. V., and Jaensch, B. (1972). Generation times of the matrix cells during embryonic brain development: an autoradiographic study in rats. *Brain Res.* 46:235–250.

Wahle, P., and Meyer, G. (1987). Morphology and quantitative changes of transient NPY-ir neuronal populations during early postnatal development of the cat visual cortex. *J. Comp. Neuro.* 261:165–192.

Walsh, C., and Cepko, C. L. (1988). Clonally related cortical cells show several migration patterns. *Science* 241:1342–1345.

Weiss, P. A. (1968). *Dynamics of Development: Experiments and Inferences*. New York: Academic Press, 624 pp.

Windrem, M. S., Jan de Beur S., and Finlay, B. L. (1988). Control of cell number in the developing neocortex. II. Effects of corpus callosum section. *Dev. Brain Res.* 43:13–22.

Wingert, F. (1969). Biometrische Analyse der Wachtumsfunktionen von Hirnteilen and Korpergewicht der Albinomaus. *J. Hinforsch.* 11:133–197.

Wise, S. P., Fleshman, J. W., and Jones, E. G. (1979). Maturation of pyramidal cell form in relation to developing afferent and efferent connections of rat somatic sensory cortex. *Neuroscience* 4:1257–1297.

Wise, S. P., and Jones, E. G. (1978). Developmental studies of thalamocortical and commissural connections in the rat somatic sensory cortex. *J. Comp. Neurol.* 178:187–208.

Witschi, E. (1962). Development: rat. In P. L. Altman and D. S. Dittmer (eds.), *Growth Including Reproduction and Morphological Development*. Washington: Fed. Am. Soc. Exp. Biol., pp. 304–314.

Wolff, J. R., (1978). Ontogenetic aspects of cortical architecture: lamination. In M. A. B. Brazier and H. Petsche (eds.), *Architectonics of the Cerebral Cortex*. New York: Raven Press, pp. 159–173.

Wolff, J. R., Böttcher, H., Zetzsche, T., Oertel, W. H., and Chronwall, B. M. (1984). Development of GABAergic neurons in the rat visual cortex as identified by glutamate decarboxylase-like immunoreactivity. *Neurosci. Lett.* 47:207–212.

Wolff, J. R., Chronwall, B. M., and Rickmann, M. (1983). "Diffuse deposition mode" provides rat visual cortex with nonpyramidal and GABA-ergic neurons. *4th Intern. Congr. Intern. Soc. for Developm. Neurosci., Abstr.*, p. 54.

Zagon, I. S., and McLaughlin, P. J. (1986). Opioid antagonist-induced modulation of cerebral and hippocampal development: histological and morphometric studies. *Dev. Brain Res.* 28:233–246.

Zagon, I. S., and McLaughlin, P. J. (1987). Endogenous opioid systems regulate cell proliferation in the developing rat brain. *Brain Res.* 412:68–72.

Zagon, I. S., McLaughlin, P. J., and Rogers, W. E. (1985). Neuronal migration independent of glial guidance: light and electron microscopic studies in the cerebellar cortex of neonatal rat. *Acta Anat.* 122:77–86.

Zagon, I. S., McLaughlin, P. J., and Zagon, E. (1984). Opiates, endorphins, and the developing organism: a comprehensive bibliography, 1982–1983. *Neurosci. Biobehav. Rev.* 8:387–403.

Zilles, K. J. (1978). Ontogenesis of the visual system. *Adv. Anat. Embryol., Cell Biol.* 54:1–138.

4 Anatomy of the Neocortex: Cytoarchitecture and Myeloarchitecture

Karl Zilles

The neocortex of the rat shows a considerable degree of differentiation into functionally and anatomically specialized subunits. These cortical areas are characterized by their predominant function as either motor, sensory, or associative regions. This subdivision is accompanied by anatomically demonstrable differences in the laminar and cellular composition. Motor and associative areas are characterized by a small or absent internal granular layer, which has been designated as layer IV (Brodmann 1909). Sensory areas have a more obvious layer IV, which is the major target of the ascending thalamocortical fibers from specific relay nuclei of the thalamus. These differences in laminar structure, visible in Nissl-stained sections, were the main criterion for the earliest attempts at neocortical mapping (Droogleever Fortuyn 1914, Krieg 1946, Svetukhina 1962). Considerable discrepancies between the different maps can be found. Additional methods were accordingly introduced to establish a broader and more reliable basis for mapping the areal structure of the neocortex. Degeneration (e.g., Krieg 1947), tracing (e.g., Krettek and Price 1977) and electrophysiological (e.g., Welker 1971) studies as well as histological and histochemical methods have enlarged the basis for neocortical subdivisions. Architectonical studies can be further improved by quantitative observations with morphometric techniques, including image analysis (Zilles et al. 1980, Schleicher et al. 1986). All methods together permit an integrative approach for the study of neocortical architecture. This chapter discusses the areal and laminar structure of the neocortex, mainly on the basis of histological and tracing techniques. Chapter 5 summarizes histochemical, immunohistochemical, and neurotransmitter receptor studies relevant for the neocortical architecture in the rat.

4.1 Definition of the Neocortex

The mammalian neocortex is conventionally defined as the phylogenetically youngest part of the brain with a more or less uniform, six-layered structure. Compared with the highly variable laminar structure of the phylogenetically older paleo- and archicortex, the neocortex appears to be more homogenous. Thus the term *allocortex* was coined to designate paleo- plus archicortex, and the term *isocortex* was coined as a synonym for neocortex (Vogt and Vogt 1919). Brodmann (1909) used the terms *homogenetic* and *heterogenetic* cortices for iso- and allocortex. These two largest parts of the cortex are separated by transitional cortical areas with more isocortical-proisocortex (Stephan 1963)—or more allocortical-periallocortex subdivided into periarchi- and peripaleocortex (for review, see Stephan 1975)—structures. Figure 4.1 shows the distribution of iso-, periallo- and allocortical areas in the rat forebrain. The isocortex covers most of the dorsal, a major part of the lateral, and minor parts of the medial and basal aspects of the rat brain. The allocortex and the respective transitional areas completely surround the isocortex. The delineation of proisocortical from isocortical areas is very difficult in the rat. Therefore both subdivisions are summarized as iso- or neocortex in this chapter. The nomenclature of the cortical areas is based on previous publications on the rat cortex (Zilles 1985; Zilles and Wree 1985), with some minor modifications. Periallocortical areas are included only in the present discussion because the functional or morphological context requires their description.

4.2 Cellular Composition

The primary visual cortex (Oc1) of the rat is the most extensively investigated neocortical area regarding cell types and their laminar distribution. It can be regarded with minor modifications as a model for the whole neocortex. Hedlich and Werner (1988), Hedlich and Winkelmann (1982), Peters and Kara (1985a,b, 1987), Peters and colleagues (1985,

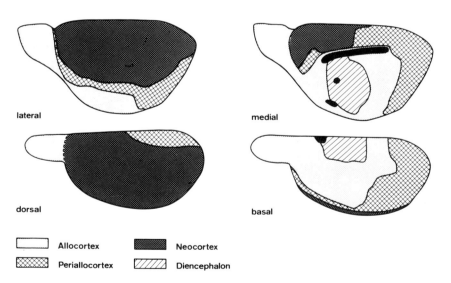

Figure 4.1 Left hemisphere of a rat brain with the position and extent of the neocortical, allocortical, and periallocortical parts in lateral, medial, dorsal, and basal views.

1987), Werner (1981), and Werner and colleagues (1979, 1982, 1985) have published a series of observations based on Golgi, Golgi-EM, Nissl-stain, and morphometrical analyses that gives a rather complete picture of the cellular basis of neocortical cytoarchitecture. The cortical neurons can be subdivided into projection and local circuit nerve cells (interneurons) regarding their axonal extent. Large cells with a high proportion of cytoplasm compared with the nucleus are found in both groups. A further criterion, which can be related to the projectional/interneuronal classification, is the density of dendritic spines. Only the projection neurons have a great amount of spines (except the enigmatic multiangular cells in layer 1), whereas the interneurons possess a low spine density or no spines at all. Table 4.1 gives a survey of the neuronal cell types.

The vast majority of neurons in the rat's visual cortex is represented by pyramidal cells (71 percent, Werner et al. 1985; 85 percent to 97 percent, Peters and Kara 1985a, 1987, Peters et al. 1985). The difference between the two groups of investigators can be explained by a differing definition of the spiny stellate cells (Lund 1984). Peters and Kara (1985a) apparently include these cells as star pyramids in their pyramidal cell class, whereas Werner and coworkers (1985) list these cells as a separate class, but closely related with the classical pyramids. This difference in classification is important in layer IV, because here Werner and coworkers (1985) enumerate 7 percent pyramids and 87 percent spiny stellates. Peters and Kara (1985a) counted 90 percent pyramids in this layer. If the data of Werner and coworkers (1985) are recalculated according to Peters and Kara's (1985a) classification, 92 percent of the cells in layers II through VI are pyramidal cells. Pyramidal cells can be identified by their round to oval or triangular cell body (major axis 10 μm to 19 μm, minor axis 8 μm to 14 μm; Werner et al. 1979), a high cytoplasmic/nuclear ratio, a round nucleus, a strong apical dendrite and several basal dendrites with numerous spines, a long axon, and only symmetrical synapses on their cell bodies. The spiny stellate cells differ

Table 4.1 Neuronal Cell Types in the Neocortex of the Rat

Spine-rich Neurons	Spine-poor or Spine-free Neurons
Pyramidal cells	Cells with a high cytoplasmic nuclear ratio
Spiny stellate cells	Basket cells
Multiangular cells of layer 1	Neuroglioform cells
	Cells with a low cytoplasmic nuclear ratio
	Bipolar cells
	Double bouquet cells
	Chandelier cells
	Martinotti cells

from pyramids in having a low cytoplasmic/nuclear ratio, no clearly identifiable apical dendrite and a lower degree of dendritic polarization. Spine-rich multiangular cells, which have a high cytoplasmic/nuclear ratio, have been described in layer I. These cells need to be further characterized in the rat. The bipolar cells (Hajós et al. 1988a,b, Peters 1984b) have a very small cytoplasmic rim surrounding a vertically folded nucleus and two vertically oriented dendritic shafts. The cell body is spindle-shaped ("fusiform cells") with a major axis of 15 μm to 25 μm and a minor axis of 9 μm to 12 μm (Peters and Kara 1985b, Werner et al. 1979). The axon originates frequently from one of the dendrites. Symmetrical and asymmetrical synapses are found on the soma. The dendrites are free of spines, but dendritic varicosities can be seen on the terminal branches in layers I and II (Hajós et al. 1988a,b). The most typical features of the fusiform bipolar cells is the strictly vertical arrangements of dendrites and axons within a small cylindrical space (Morrison et al. 1984). These neurons are the most numerous nonpyramidal cells (4 percent of all cortical neuronal profiles).

All other nonpyramidal neurons together account for 6 percent (Peters and Kara 1985b). The double bouquet cells (Hedlich and Winkelmann 1982, Somogyi and Cowey 1984) also have a low cytoplasmic/nuclear ratio and sparsely spinous to spine-free dendrites. Like the bipolar fusiform cells the dendrites originate from the upper and lower poles of the cell bodies and are vertically arranged. The dendrites branch into tufts, which are also vertically arranged. The axon has several main vertical collaterals and arborizations in layers II through V with axonal varicosities. The cell bodies are mostly found in layers II and III. The axonal features separate these cells from the chandelier cells (see below).

The chandelier cells (Hedlich and Winkelmann 1982, Peters 1984a, Peters et al. 1982, Somogyi 1977, Szentágothai 1975, Werner et al. 1985) have a low cytoplasmic/nuclear ratio. Two or more dendrites originate from the upper and lower poles of the soma, producing tufts of ascending and descending, sparsely spinous dendrites. Peters and Kara (1985b) consider these cells as bitufted or multipolar cells, with the latter having spherical or elongated dendritic trees. The axons of the chandelier cells form a laterally spread plexus and bear the boutons on the terminals in vertical strings. This arrangement gave the name *chandelier*. These boutons form symmetric synapses. The cell body of the chandelier cell is observed as having symmetric and asymmetric snapses (Peters et al. 1982). Most of these cells are located in layers II and III.

The Martinotti cells (Fairén et al. 1984, Feldman and Peters 1978, Hedlich and Winkelmann 1982, Marin-Padilla 1984, Werner 1981, Werner et al. 1979) of the rat are most frequently found in layers III and IV, but also in more superficial and deeper layers. The soma is elongated with a low cytoplasmic/nuclear ratio. The sparsely spinous dendrites originate at the poles of the cell body. The axon leaves at the upper pole or from an ascending dendrite and takes an ascending course ending with numerous terminal fanlike branches in layer I. Axonal collaterals ascend and descend and have numerous varicosities. According to Szentágothai (1978), the Martinotti cells may contribute asymmetrical synapses in layer I on dendritic spines of pyramidal cells. On the other hand Marin-Padilla and Marin-Padilla (1982) have suggested an inhibitory action on the dendritic bouquets of the pyramidal neurons. About 0.7 percent of all cortical neurons in the rat are Martinotti cells (Werner et al. 1982).

About 3.4 percent of the nonpyramidal neurons have a high cytoplasmic/nuclear ratio and comprise the basket cells and neuroglioform cells (Werner et al. 1982, 1985). The basket cells have a round to oval cell body that can be found throughout layers II through VI (Hedlich and Winkelmann 1982, Jones and Hendry 1984). These neurons are multipolar and have smooth dendrites. The short axon bears numerous boutons and has horizontally or obliquely oriented branches (Werner et al. 1985) that end in pericellular nests of terminal branches ("baskets") around the cell bodies of pyramidal cells. The axons of such smooth or sparsely spined cells have been found with and without a myelin sheath in the rat (Peters and Proskauer 1980). The neuroglioform cell (Jones 1984) was demonstrated in the rat cortex by Hedlich and Werner (1988) and Somogyi and associates (1984). These cells have a small, irregularly shaped cell body with dense dendritic and axonal plexus in the immediate neighborhood of the perikaryon. The sparsely spinous dendrite forms a radial dendritic field. The varicose axons branch mostly within the dendritic domain. Neuroglioform cells are found in layers I through VI of the rat cortex.

Figure 4.2 gives a survey of the neuronal types in the rat visual cortex demonstrated with a Golgi impregnation method. An excellent review of the different cell types of the rat visual cortex in electron microscopy has been published by Peters (1985).

4.3 Principles of Cortical Connectivity

The principle connections of a neocortical area are described here because they are of major importance for the understanding of the laminar structure. Each neocortical sensory area receives afferent fibers from specific thalamic nuclei (e.g., Oc1 receives input from the dorsal nucleus of the lateral geniculate body). They terminate in layer IV and the lower layer III (Herkenham 1980, Ribak and Peters 1975). In addition to this main target for thalamocortical input, additional endings, with a much lower density, are found in layers I and VI (from ventromedial and intralaminar thalamic nuclei). This pattern was demonstrated in neocortical areas that have an inner granular layer (sensory areas). In areas without or with a poorly developed layer IV, the main target of thalamocortical input are layers I and III. Most of these specific afferents in layers III and IV are found to establish asymmetric synapses on dendritic

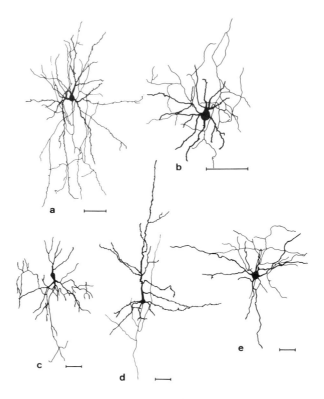

Figure 4.2 Neuronal cell types in the neocortex of the rat. (a) Spiny stellate cell in layer IV. (b) Neuroglioform cell in layer IV. (c) Chandelier cell in layer II. (d) Pyramidal cell in layer IV. (e) Basket cell in layer IV. (f) Spiny multiangular cell in layer I. (g) Martinotti cell in layer III. (h) Double-bouquet cell in layer II. (i) Fusiform bipolar cell in layer III. These cells have been redrawn from different sources and slightly modified to emphasize the characteristics of the different cell types (a from Werner et al. 1979, b from Hedlich and Werner 1988, c through from Hedlich and Winkelmann 1982, and i from Hajos et al. 1988).

spines (83 percent to 88 percent) and dendritic shafts (12 percent to 15 percent) (Peters and Feldman 1976, Schober and Winkelmann 1977) of pyramidal and nonpyramidal neurons (Peters et al. 1979, Peters and Kimerer 1981). The terminals in layers I and VI synapse primarily with dendritic spines (Peters and Saldanha 1976). The cortex is reciprocally connected with the thalamus. The origin of these corticothalamic fibers are the pyramidal cells of layer VI. Nonreciprocal connections to thalamic nuclei (e.g., ventral nucleus of the lateral geniculate body) originate from layer V pyramidal cells. The callosal connections (Cipolloni and Peters 1979, Cusick and Lund 1981, Isseroff et al. 1984, Ivy et al. 1984, Olavarria and van Sluyters 1983, 1985, Olavarria et al. 1984, Rieck and Carey 1984, Sarter and Markowitsch 1985, Wree et al. 1985, 1986, Záborsky and Wolff 1982) of the rat cortex are homotopic (between symmetrical loci in both hemispheres) or heterotopic (between asymmetrical loci in both hemispheres). Within Par1 interdigitating, complex

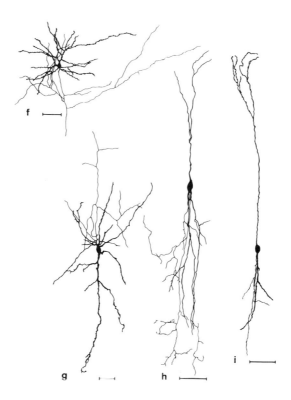

patterns of callosal and specific thalamocortical terminals were demonstrated. The perikarya that give rise to callosal fibers and the terminals of these fibers are described in coronal sections as columns or strips and in tangential sections as patches of variable shape. Areas free of callosal connections are found as granular regions between the dysgranular callosal fields of Par1. The perikarya projecting to the other hemisphere are mostly pyramidal cell bodies concentrated in layers II to III and V to VI. Layer IV contains no or only a few callosal neurons. This corroborates the complementarity of the thalamocortical and callosal systems on the laminar level. The terminals of axons coming through the corpus callosum are found in all layers, but they are most densely packed in layers I to III and V to VI in many cortical areas.

The shape of such terminal fields appears in frontal sections as an hourglass with a maximal width of 250 μm to 750 μm. The location of perikarya in layers II and III and of terminal fields tend to coincide in cases of homotopic projections, but the callosal cell bodies in layer V often form continuous bands and are, therefore, also found outside terminal fields of callosal afferent fibers.

The cell bodies and terminal fields of cortico-cortical association projections between areas of the same hemisphere or through the heterotopic callosal system show a laminar pattern very similar to that found in the homotopic callosal system (Donoghue and Parham 1983, Isseroff et al. 1984, Miller and Vogt 1984).

The long descending fiber systems to the spinal cord, cranial nerve nuclei, and pons originate from large pyramidal cells in the lower layer V (Bates and Killackey 1984, Leichnetz et al. 1987, Leong 1983, Leong et al. 1984, Miller 1987). Another long cortical efferent pathway terminates in the tectum of rats. The cell bodies of these corticotectal axons belong also to the large pyramids of layer V, which are distinguished by apical dendrites extending into layer I (Schofield et al. 1987).

Efferent cells projecting to the claustrum are found in layer VI. The claustrocortical afferent fibers also terminate in this layer (Carey and Neal 1985).

A major connectivity exists between the cortex and the caudate-putamen complex. The cell bodies of the efferent corticostriate axons are localized predominantly in the upper layer V. A few cells are found in the lower layer V, and occasionally there are also some cells in layers III and VI. These cells were identified as pyramidal cells projecting to the ipsilateral caudate-putamen, but 6 percent to 14 percent of these cells in the frontoparietal cortex terminate additionally with axon collaterals in the contralateral striatum (McGeorge and Faull 1987).

All these findings show that the agranular and subgranular layers (I through IV) of the rat neocortex are mainly concerned with input, whereas the infragranular layers (V through VI) are predominantly engaged with cortical output.

4.4 Cingulate Cortex

The cingulate cortex of the rat comprises the areas Cg1, Cg2, Cg3, and IL (figures 4.3 and 4.4). The whole region represents a transitional field varying from more isocortical to more allocortical features. Cg1 through Cg3 can be identified as medial prefrontal cortex (Beckstead 1976, 1979, Divac et al. 1978a,b, Domesick 1969, 1972, Kretteck and Price 1977, Leonard 1969, 1972, Markowitsch and Guldin 1983, Zilles and Wree 1985). All these areas do not contain an inner granular layer. This is a laminar pattern quite different from the appearance of the prefrontal cortex in primates, which shows an inner granular layer. The connectivity between the prefrontal cortex and the dorsomedial thalamic nucleus, however, is the same both in primates and rats. The area IL (infralimbic area) cannot be included in the prefrontal cortex because its architecture and connectivity are quite different compared with Cg1 through Cg3. IL receives afferents from the hippocampus, subiculum, thalamic midline nuclei, and the ventral tegmental area (Berger et al. 1976, Lindvall et al. 1978, Powell and Cowan 1954, Swanson 1981) and projects to the reuniens nucleus, the lateral hypothalamic area, and the nucleus of the solitary tract (Herkenham 1978, Shiosaka et al. 1980, van der Kooy et al. 1982). The cortical thickness is much less in IL than in the adjacent Cg3 area, and the laminar pattern shows a reduced number of layers. Therefore IL represents a part of the periallocortex, whereas

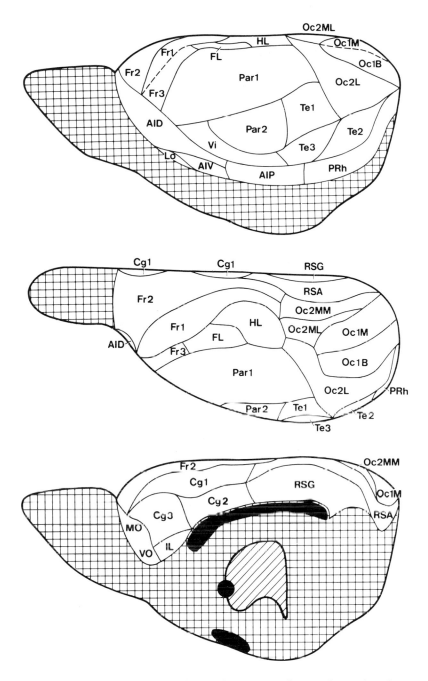

Figure 4.3 Map of the neocortical and adjoining periallocortical areas based on quantitative cyto- and myeloarchitectonical studies (Zilles et al. 1980, Zilles 1985, Zilles and Wree 1985) in (from top to bottom) lateral, dorsal, and medial views. Fr1–Fr3-frontal areas; Par1–Par2, FL, HL-parietal areas; Te1–Te3-temporal areas; Oc1B, Oc1M, Oc2L, Oc2MM, Oc2ML-occipital areas; Cg–Cg3-medial prefrontal cortex; IL-infralimbic area; MO, LO, VO-orbital corex; AID, AIP, AIV-insular cortex; PRh-perirhinal cortex; RSA, RSG-retrosplenial cortex. The allocortex and parts of the periallocortex are cross-hatched; the diencephalic-telencephalic transition is hatched.

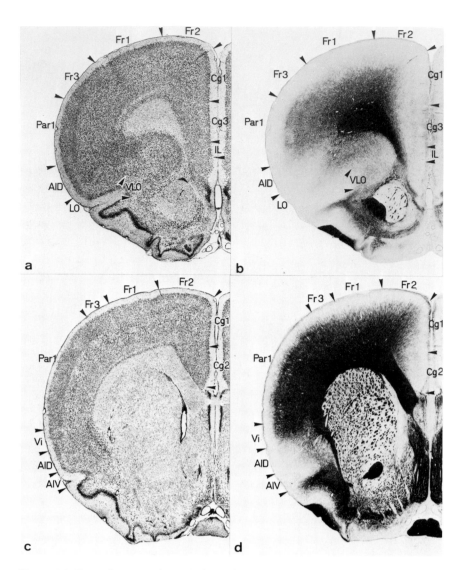

Figure 4.4 Coronal sections through the rat forebain from rostral to caudal levels. Sections in a, c, e, g, and i are stained for cell bodies; b, d, f, h, and j are stained for myelinated nerve fibers with a modification of Gallyas's silver method (for details, see Zilles 1985). The different neocortical and some of the adjoining periallocortical areas are delineated.

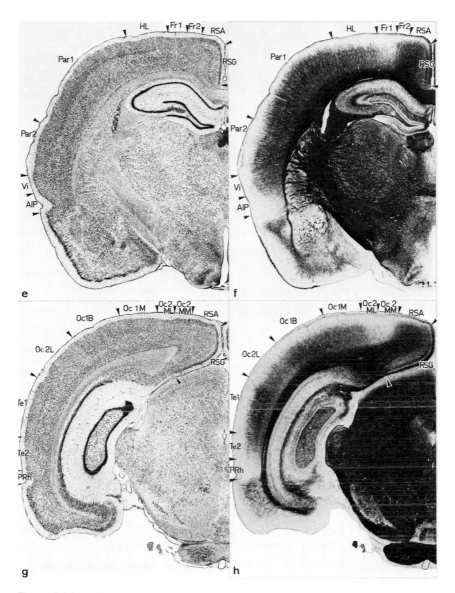

Figure 4.4 (cont.)

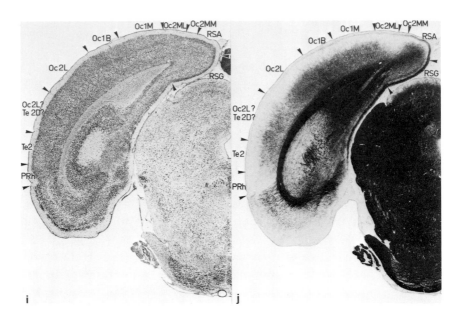

Figure 4.4 (cont.)

Cg1 through Cg3 can be classified as iso- to proisocortical areas. The mean cell density of the Cg areas is somewhat higher than that of the laterally adjacent frontal neocortical region. IL again has a higher mean cell density than do the dorsally bordering Cg areas. This results in a continuous decrease of the neuropil proportion from the classical neocortex (frontal areas) to the periallocortex (IL). The areal differences are also visible in myelin-stained sections, with the frontal areas showing the highest density of myelinated fibers, the Cg areas having a lower density, and the IL area having the lowest density (Zilles, Divac, Wree, and Schleicher, unpublished observations, 1989). A description of the structural and functional aspects of the medial prefrontal cortex as a frontal association area is given in chapter 18 by Kolb.

4.5 Insular Cortex

The insular cortex is located in the lateral transitional region from the frontal, parietal, and temporal (partly) neocortical areas dorsally to the paleocortex (anterior olfactory nucleus, piriform cortex) basally (figures 4.3 and 4.4). An anterior region with the dorsal and ventral parts of the agranular insular cortex (AID, AIV) and a posterior region with the posterior part of the agranular insular cortex (AIP) were delineated in Nissl- and myelin-stained sections (Zilles 1985, Zilles and Wree 1985). These areas do not show a clear isocortical structure and must be classified as proiso- and periallocortical areas. Because the claustrum can be found immediately below most of the rostrocaudal extent of the insular cortex, these areas have been named *claustrocortex* in an earlier cytoarchitectonical study (Zilles et al. 1980). According to Krettek and Price (1977), the rostrally and basally adjoining cortex, which extends to the medial hemispherical surface and borders the Cg cortex, is called *orbital cortex*. The orbital cortex has a periallocortical laminar structure and therefore is not discussed here. The same holds for the perirhinal cortex, which caudally abuts the insular cortex.

The insular cortex is connected with the cingulate, piriform, rostrosplenial, perirhinal, and entorhinal cortices, presubiculum, amygdala, claustrum, the caudate-putamen, pallidum, mediodorsal, and lateroposterior thalamic nuclei, and some other thalamic and rhombencephalic nuclei (Beckstead 1976, 1979, Divac et al. 1978a,b, Leonard 1969, 1972, Reep and Winans 1982, Zilles and Wree 1985). The insular cortex is architectonically characterized by the lack of an inner granular layer and by an extremely low myelin density (figure 4.4).

4.6 Gustatory Cortex

The gustatory cortex (figures 4.3 and 4.4) has tentatively been delineated as area Gu in a cytoarchitectonical study (Zilles 1985). In the approximate position of Gu, a taste area was described in a series of functional studies (Benjamin and Akert 1959, Benjamin and Pfaffmann 1955, Braun et al. 1982, Guldin and Markowitsch 1983, Lasiter and Glanzmann 1983, Lasiter et al. 1982, van der Kooy et al. 1982, Wolf, 1968). Gu shows an isocortical structure with a layer IV and can be differentiated from the agranular insular cortex. More recently the functional identification of Gu as a cortical area with a function in taste perception has been questioned (Cechetto and Saper 1987, Kosar et al. 1986a,b). The electrophysiological analysis has shown that only a part of AID represents the gustatory neocortex, whereas the granular area is a general visceral sensory cortex. Kosar and associates (1986a,b) have emphasized that the gustatory cortex is located in an agranular area, whereas Cechetto and Saper (1987) have characterized this region as dysgranular. Whether this contradiction is only a semantic problem or reflects a real disagreement in identification cannot be decided presently (cf. chapter 16 by Braun). Therefore the former area Gu has been renamed Vi (visceral sensory cortex) (figures 4.3 and 4.4).

4.7 Perirhinal and Retrosplenial Cortex

The perirhinal cortex (PRh) is found in the posterior part of the rhinal sulcus (figures 4.3 and 4.4). PRh is bordered by the entorhinal cortex and auditory belt regions. Because the laminar structure of PRh permits a classification as part of the periallocortex, no further discussion is necessary. More information about the perirhinal cortex is given by Deacon and colleagues (1983), Kosel and colleagues (1983), Krettek and Price (1977), and Zilles and Wree (1985).

The retrosplenial cortex (figures 4.3 and 4.4) comprises the areas RSA and RSG (Zilles et al. 1980, Zilles 1985, Zilles and Wree 1985), which can be classified as periallocortical regions. Therefore the reader is referred to Krettek and Price 1977 and Vogt et al. 1981 for further information.

4.8 Frontal Cortex

The frontal neocortical region of the rat comprises the agranular isocortical areas Fr1, Fr2, and Fr3 (Zilles 1985, Zilles and Wree 1985) (figures 4.3 and 4.4). This parcellation was recently corroborated by Schober (1986). These areas are surrounded by the cingulate cortex medially and by the insular and orbital cortices laterally and rostrobasally (Kolb 1984, Krettek and Price 1977). The agranular cytoarchitectonical structure of the frontal cortex suggests a motor function. This was corroborated by numerous electrophysiological studies (Donoghue and Parham 1983, Donoghue and Wise 1982, Gioanni and Lamarche 1985, Hall and Lindholm 1974, Neafsey et al. 1986, Sanderson et al. 1984, Sapienza et al. 1981). The lack of a clearly visible inner granular layer and the predominant inner pyramidal layer with large and densely packed pyramidal cells separates the Fr areas from the laterally and caudally adjoining parietal cortex in Nissl-stained preparations (figure 4.4). Myelin-stained sections add further supporting evidence for a fundamental borderline between frontal and parietal cortices because Fr1 through Fr3 have the lowest myelin content in layers I through III, compared with parietal, occipital, and temporal neocortical areas (figure 4.5a). Fr1 and Fr3 correspond to the lateral agranular frontal cortex (Ag_l) and Fr2 to the medial agranular frontal cortex (Ag_m) of Donoghue and Wise (1982). Whereas Fr1 and the rostral part of Fr2 contain many neurons in layer V projecting to the spinal cord (Miller 1987), Fr3 and the larger caudal part of Fr2 contain only a few or none of these neurons.

The representation of the head in these latter regions was demonstrated by Gioanni and Lamarche (1985), Neafsay and coworkers (1986), and Sanderson and coworkers (1984). Fr3 can probably be identified as a motor projection of the jaw by comparing the stereotaxic coordinates of this area in Zilles (1985) with the data given by Neafsey and coworkers (1986). The caudal part of Fr2 (rostrocaudal extent from +3 mm to −3 mm, with bregma as zero point) contains the motor representation of vibrissae and eye muscles (Hall and Lindholm 1974, Neafsey et al. 1986, Sanderson et al. 1984). A second forelimb motor area was described by Neafsey and Sievert (1982) in the rostromedial part of their AgL field. This suggests multiple representations to be an organizational principle in the rat cortex. A second hindlimb motor area, which abuts the second forelimb area at the medial side in the rostral part of AgM, was described more recently by Neafsey and coworkers (1986). Both areas together constitute a rostral motor area (RMA), which is said to be represented by parts of Fr1 and Fr2 (Neafsey et al. 1986). RMA contains corticospinal neurons and is less responsive to peripheral sensory input than are the other Fr1 areas. These characteristics support an interpretation of RMA as supplementary motor cortex. A comparison of the illustrations given by Neafsey and colleagues (1986) for the Fr1/Fr2 (AgL/AgM) borderline with the delineations, maps, and description of these two areas by Donoghue and Wise (1982), Zilles (1985), and Zilles and Wree (1985) reveals clear discrepancies. Whereas the latter authors describe a more lateral extent of Fr2 (3 mm rostral to bregma) up to 2.5 to 3 mm from the midline, Neafsey and coworkers (1986) show the lateral extent of AgM to be approximately 1 mm at this level. Moreover a relatively dense layer II and a conspicuously light layer III was described as architectonical criteria by Donoghue and Wise (1982), Zilles and colleagues (1980), Zilles (1985), and Zilles and Wree (1985) for Fr2 compared with Fr1. In figure 4a of Neafsey et al. 1986, the AgM/AgL border is clearly shown within Fr2 when defined according to these criteria. Therefore the presumed supplementary motor cortex containing the rostral forelimb and hindlimb areas is well within the limits of Fr2 constituting its rostral part. The frontal area Fr1 therefore represents the primary motor cortex (Donoghue and Wise 1982) with Fr3 as a somatotopical subfield.

Fr1 is delineated from Fr2 by cyto- and myeloarchitectonic features. Fr2 represents the supplementary motor cortex in its rostral part and the frontal eye field (Hall and Lindholm 1974, Leichnetz and Gonzalo-Ruiz 1987, Leichnetz et al. 1987, Neafsey et al. 1986, Reep et al. 1987) in its caudal part. Table 4.2 gives a comparison of the nomenclature used by different observers. The map of the rat frontal cortex proposed by Krieg (1946) differs in so many aspects from all the other anatomical and physiological studies that its areal pattern cannot be accepted as a basis for further studies.

An interesting problem for morphofunctional correlations was raised by the fact that the cortical motor functions are not restricted to the Fr areas. Donoghue and colleagues (1979), Hall and Lindholm (1974), Neafsey and coworkers (1986), Sanderson and coworkers (1984) and Sapienza and coworkers (1981) described a motor-sensory overlap for various somatotopic subfields. Motor reactions could also be elicited in highly granular regions (Donoghue and Wise 1982, Hummelsheim and Wiesendanger 1985). This led to the statement that parts of the granular cortex of Par1 can be considered as motor cortex (cf. Neafsey et al. 1986). On the other hand different levels of excitability and differences in connectivity (Afsharpour 1985, Collins et al. 1986, Leong 1983, McGeorge and Faull 1987) between granular and agranular cortical fields point to distinctions with correlates in architectonical pecularities. Cyto-

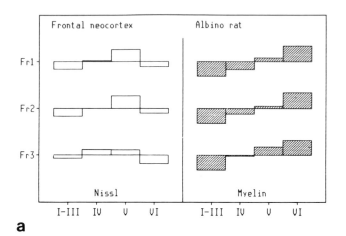

a

b

Organization of the Neocortex

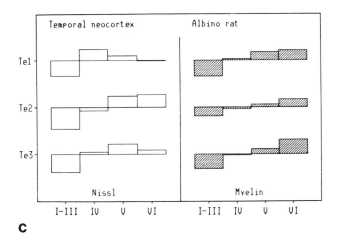

c

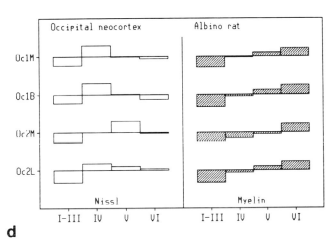

d

Figure 4.5 Relative densities of cell bodies and myelinated nerve fibers in layers I through III, IV, and VI, (a) of the frontal neocortical areas Fr1, Fr2, and Fr3, (b) of the parietal neocortical areas Par1, Par2, FL, and HL, (c) of the temporal neocortical areas Te1, Te2, and Te3, and (d) of the occipital neocortical areas Oc1M, Oc1B, Oc2M (O2MM + Oc2ML), and Oc2L. The mean density of each of the two variables over all layers is defined as 100 percent, and the actual values for each layer are expressed as a relative value on this basis.

Table 4.2 Nomenclature of the Frontal and Parietal Isocortical Areas of the Rat Used by Different Observers

Donoghue and Wise 1982, Donoghue and Parham 1983	Krettek and Price 1977, Kolb 1984	Neafsey et al. 1986	Zilles et al. 1980	Zilles 1985, Zilles and Wree 1985, Zilles (this chapter)
AG$_m$	Pr Cm	AgM, rostrodorsal part of AgL (RHL)	Prc$_m$, Prc3	Fr2
AG$_l$	Pr CI	AgL	Prc1-2	Fr1, Fr3
S I	—	EL, LI, NK, TI, Tr, Tt, r, d, Vc, Vi, ?; Df, Se, ab, Sup; Ae, Af, Ke, T5f	SM 1	Par1; FL; HL
S II	—	?	SM II	Par2

and myeloarchitectonical features therefore reflect much more projectional and intracortical than somatotopical characteristics. A detailed description of the function and organization of the frontal neocortex is given in chapter 8 by Neafsey.

The laminar pattern of the Fr1 through Fr3 areas shows an indistinct layer IV (inner granular layer). This permits the use of the term *agranular cortex* for the whole frontal region. Nevertheless some very small perikarya (*Körnerzellen*) comparable with the neurons in layer IV of Par1 can also be found immediately above layer V. This finding permits the delineation of a layer IV, although the general agranular character of the Fr areas should be emphasized. A quantitative analysis of the laminar pattern of the frontal cortical fields in Nissl- and myelin-stained material with an image analyzer (Schleicher et al. 1986, Zilles 1985, Zilles and Wree 1985, Zilles et al. 1980) is shown in figure 4.5a. The relatively largest gray-level index (GLI), which is a measure for the number of cell bodies per volume, is found in layer V of Fr1 through Fr3. The supragranular layers (I through III) and layer VI have the lowest GLIs in all three areas. Only Fr3 shows an increase in GLI of layer IV, which permits the delineation of this frontal area from the adjoining Fr1. Compared with the parietal areas (figure 4.5b), the GLI of layer IV in Fr3 is relatively and absolutely much lower and demarcates Fr3 from the adjacent Par1 (cf. also figure 4.6). The delineation of Fr2 from Fr1 is founded on the larger density of cell bodies in layer II and the lower density in layers III and IV of Fr2.

The quantitative evaluation of the myelin-stained sections gives a very similar picture not only for all frontal but also for all neocortical areas, when relative myelin densities are compared (figures 4.4 and 4.5a). The lowest values are consistently found in the supragranular

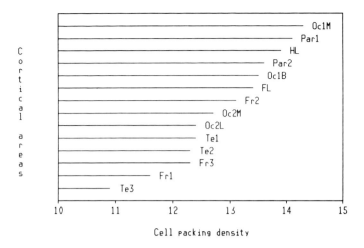

Figure 4.6 Mean cell-packing densities over all layers of the respective neocortical areas measured as gray level indices in Nissl-stained sections (proportion of the projection profiles of neuronal cell bodies, glial, and endothelial cell nuclei in percent per area; cf. Schleicher et al. 1986) of albino rats.

layers increasing stepwise from layer IV to layer VI, where the highest densities of myelinated axons can be seen. A clear distinction between frontal and parietal areas, however, can be made by a comparison of the absolute densities. There is an increase in myelination of only 5 percent in layer I to upper layer III and layer VI in the parietal compared with the frontal areas, but a very pronounced increase of 17 percent to 26 percent in the lower layer III to layer V. The myeloarchitecture reveals the frontal areas as absolutely lower myelinated parts of the cortex compared with the parietal areas (figure 4.7). At the same time the frontal areas retain the general laminar pattern of all neocortical regions with a monotonous increase of myelination from supragranular layers to the cortex/white matter border.

4.9 Parietal Cortex

The parietal neocortical region comprises four areas: Par1, Par2, FL (forelimb area), and HL (hindlimb area) (Zilles 1985, Zilles and Wree 1985). These areas are surrounded by the primary motor cortex (Fr1, Fr3) medially and rostrally, by the secondary visual cortex (Oc2ML, Oc2L), the auditory cortex (Te areas) caudally, and by the insular cortex basally (figure 4.3). All these areas have a clearly visible inner granular layer (*granular* or *dysgranular* cortex) and represent the somatosensory cortex. Par1, FL, and HL constitute the primary area, and Par2 the supplementary area (Welker 1971, 1976, Welker and Sinha 1972, Woolsey and LeMessurier 1948). The parietal areas receive input from cutaneous mechanoreceptors (Welker 1971, 1976) and are connected with

Zilles: Anatomy: Cyto- and Myeloarchitecture

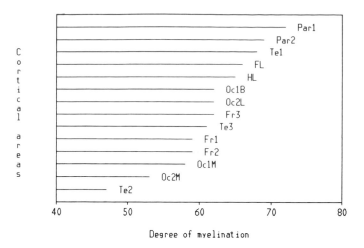

Figure 4.7 Mean densities of myelinated nerve fibers (degree of myelination) over all layers of the respective neocortical areas measured as gray level indices in myelin-stained sections of albino rats.

the primary motor cortex and the contralateral primary and supplementary somatosensory areas (Akers and Killackey 1978, Ivy and Killackey 1981, Jacobson 1970, Wise 1975). Many corticospinal neurons are found in layer V of the parietal neocortex (Miller 1987, Bates and Killackey 1984). This and electrophysiological studies lead to the conclusion that the whole frontal and parietal cortex is a motor cortex (Neafsey et al. 1986). Because the parietal cortex has a cytoarchitecture (see below) and connectivity (see chapter 14 by Chapin and Lin) different from that of the Fr areas, it seems justifiable to make a clear distinction between these regions.

The major part of the primary somatosensory cortex is represented by Par1. The laminar structure of this area expresses most clearly the typical features of a sensory cortex. As shown in figures 4.4 and 4.5b, the highest relative neuronal density is found in layer IV. The GLI of this layer and area is the largest compared with the patterns in all the other neocortical areas. Next to it are the GLIs in layer IV of FL and HL. The whole primary somatosensory area in the rat therefore takes a position regarding the laminar distribution of cell density, which is comparable with the primary visual cortex in most of the primates. The second largest relative cell density is found in layer V, followed by layer VI. The lowest GLIs in Par1 are visible in the supragranular layers. This sequence in cell densities is also principally the same in FL, HL, and Par2. This last area shows the lowest differences in GLIs between the granular and infragranular layers, which quantifies the impression of a less differentiated area by visual inspection of Nissl-stained specimens (figures 4.5 and 4.5b). A comparison of the mean absolute cell densities for all layers of neocortical areas demonstrates (figure 4.6), that four of the six areas with the largest GLIs are Par1, FL, HL, and Par2. Only the primary visual cortex (Oc1M + Oc1B) has comparably high cell densities.

The measurement of the densities of myelinated axons reveals the same layer sequence as already described for the frontal region (see above). In contrast to the frontal areas, layer IV of the parietal areas shows a relatively higher degree of myelination, whereas layer VI shows a lower degree of myelination. A comparison of the somatosensory cortex with the other neocortical areas demonstrates a uniquely high absolute level of myelination, which is about 13 percent lower in the latter regions. Par1 has the absolutely best-developed myelination of all neocortical areas (figure 4.7), followed by Par2.

Within the parietal areas somatotopic subdivisions have been described with electrophysiological methods (Chapin and Lin 1984, Chapin et al. 1987, Donoghue and Wise 1982, Donoghue and Parham 1983, Gioanni 1987, Neafsey et al. 1986), which are partially visible in cyto- or myeloarchitectonical specimens. The delineation of subareas within Par1 containing a conspicuous layer IV (granular zones), surrounded by less granular regions (perigranular zones) and areas with a low granularity (dysgranular zones), is the architectural basis for further parcellations. All zones together represent a single body map, but the dysgranular zones exhibit multimodal convergence (cutaneous and joint movements, directional specificity, bilateral representation), whereas the granular zones show a finely detailed map of cutaneous representation (Chapin and Lin 1984, Welker et al. 1984). The dysgranular zones are therefore transitional both in structure and function. Within Par1 the representation of the mystacial vibrissae is found most caudally and basally. It can be recognized as a granular zone by cell-dense vertical columns in coronal sections, which are surrounded by small dysgranular zones (figure 4.4). These dysgranular zones are the terminal areas of callosal projections (Olavarría et al. 1984). Because the thalamocortical projections are localized in the granular zones, a complementary organization of callosal and thalamic connections can be found.

At the mediodorsal border of Par1, two areas with a peculiar cytoarchitectonic organization can be found: FL and HL (figures 4.4 and 4.5b). These areas combine features of the frontal and parietal areas. A prominent, highly granular layer IV occurs together with large pyramidal cells in layer V (*sensorimotor amalgam*). Donoghue and Wise (1982) and Neafsey and coworkers (1986) have shown that motor responses can be elicited within the typical granular cortex of HL. Hummelsheim and Wiesendanger (1985) demonstrated that within the HL area, motor and proprioceptive zones overlap only to a small extent. The sensory zone is located more caudally. Thus the architectonically defined amalgam does not completely match with a functional amalgam. Afsharpour (1985) showed that the projections to the subthalamic nucleus originate in the frontal areas, are present to a lesser degree in FL and HL, and are absent in Par1. This corroborates the architectural aspect of FL and HL as regions with both motor and sensory traits.

A major problem is raised by the search for a rodent analog of the posterior parietal cortex in primates. Krieg (1946) described an area 7, which has a topology comparable with areas 5 and 7 in primates (Hyvärinen 1982). This parcellation could not be reproduced by quantitative cytoarchitectural studies (Zilles 1985, Zilles and Wree 1985, Zilles et al. 1980, 1984). Schober's (1986) cortical map does not contain a field comparable with Krieg's area 7. The position of Krieg's area 7 is represented by parts of Oc2ML and Oc2L in these studies. All these areas are classified here as secondary visual cortices. Experimental studies (Miller and Vogt 1984, Montero et al. 1973a,b, Olavarria and Montero 1981, Schober et al. 1976) have demonstrated strong reciprocal connections of these areas with the primary visual cortex. On the other hand the parcellation into Oc2MM, Oc2ML, and Oc2L does not imply that each of these areas represents a cytoarchitectonically homogeneous field (Zilles and Wree 1985). Further studies, especially with quantitative methods, are needed to exhaust the advantages of this approach for a more refined subdivision of this cortical region. Kolb and Walkey (1987) and Miller and Vogt (1984) have summarized and considerably extended findings arguing for a multimodal association cortex in the range between the primary somatosensory, auditory, and visual areas of the rat.

The supplementary somatosensory cortex (Par2) can be easily delineated from Par1 by its absolutely lower mean cell density (figure 4.6). The laminar pattern of this parameter on a relative scale (figure 4.5b) objectifies the impression of a less distinctive laminar differentiation gained by visual inspection.

Layers I through IV of Par2 have lower absolute and relative GLIs than those of Par1. The infragranular layers show a reversed relation. Myelin-stained sections do not give distinctive criteria for a delineation of Par2 from Par1, but the border between Par2 and the insular cortex can easily be demonstrated (figure 4.4). The somatotopical subdivisions of the supplementary somatosensory cortex shown in physiological studies are not reflected by recognizable architectural subdivisions. Histochemical methods are more effective in this respect (Wallace 1987). Par1 and Par2 receive afferent fibers from different thalamic sources (Donoghue et al. 1979, Ivy and Killackey 1981, Spreafico et al. 1987, Welker and Sinha 1972) and can therefore be distinguished also on the basis of differential connectivity. Despite these differences in connectivity, the parietal areas Par1, FL, HL, and Par2 form a family of cortical fields similar in cyto- and myeloarchitecture. The simultaneous presentation of the mean cell body and myelin densities (figure 4.8) demonstrates that all parietal areas form a cluster completely separated from the other sensory regions. There is no overlap between the frontal and parietal areas on a quantitative morphological basis.

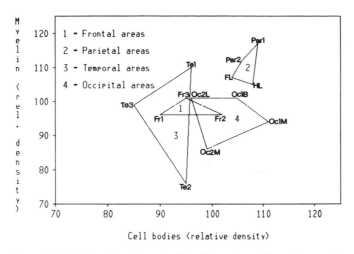

Figure 4.8 Relative densities of cell bodies and myelinated nerve fibers over all layers of the respective neocortical areas define clusters separating the parietal, temporal, and occipital areas. The frontal areas overlap the temporal and occipital clusters. The mean value of each of the two variables over all neocortical areas and layers is defined as 100 percent, and the mean value for each area is expressed as a relative value on this basis.

4.10 Temporal Cortex

The temporal neocortical region comprises three areas—Te1, Te2, and Te3 (Zilles 1985, Zilles and Wree 1985)—based on Nissl-stained specimens. Schober (1986) proposed the same parcellation in a cytoarchitectural study. These areas are surrounded by the parietal areas (Par1, Par2) dorsally and rostrally, the perirhinal area (PRh) basally, and the secondary visual area (Oc2I) dorsally and caudally (figure 4.3). The temporal areas have an inner granular layer that is most prominent in Te1. This anatomical feature assigns Te1 a position comparable with those of other primary sensory areas (Par1, Oc2). Te1 was therefore identified as primary auditory cortex (Zilles 1985, Zilles and Wree 1985). This cytoarchitectural identification must remain tentative pending corroboration by tracing and electrophysiological experiments. Ryugo and Killackey (1974) described a projection to layers IV and III of the temporal cortex from the ventral nucleus of the medial geniculate body (MGB) and a less dense projection to all layers of this cortex from the medial nucleus. This study was based on the Fink-Heimer procedure. Unfortunately no description of the position and extent of the respective cortical area was given. In an unpublished doctoral thesis Patterson (1977) described a subdivision of the auditory cortex into a granular area ("core") and less granular areas ("belts") on the basal and caudal margins of the core. The laminar structure of these areas permit a comparison of the core region with Te1 and the belt region with Te2 and Te3. Moreover Patterson (1977) showed a projection of the dorsal, caudal, ventrolateral, and marginal divisions of MGB to the belt areas with the Fink-Heimer technique and retrograde axonal transport. The ventral nucleus projects to the core and the medial nucleus to the core and areas dorsal and rostral to it. The afferent fibers from the medial nucleus of MGB terminate in a diffuse pattern not restricted to layer IV, whereas the axon terminals from the other nuclei of MGB are found in layers III and IV. The belt areas have therefore been classified by Scheel (1988) as a *specific* auditory belt area, which can be compared with Te2 and Te3, and an *unspecific* belt area, which is most probably located within Oc2L, Te1, and Par2. Scheel (1988) revealed this detailed pattern of connectivity with the iontophoretical injection of wheat-germ-agglutinin horseradish perioxidase into various cortical regions. The main results of this latter study with the observations of LeDoux and colleagues (1985), who used the same technique, but focused their study mainly on the subcortical projections of MGB. Summarizing these experiments, we can state that at least the major part of Te1 resemble the auditory core (primary auditory cortex) and Te2 and Te3 can be compared with the specific belt (secondary auditory cortex).

A recent reevaluation of the temporal cortex in Timm-stained sections (cf. chapter 5 by Zilles, Wree, and Dausch) gives architectural evidence for the rostral part of the unspecific belt region of Scheel (1988) as an area delineated from Par2. A comparison of myelin-stained and Timm-stained sections with adjacent Nissl-stained sections shows that a reliable delineation of the unspecific belt region is extremely difficult on the basis of the Nissl-stained sections, but an area with a lower myelin content can be found between the more dorsal part of Oc2L and Te1 (figures 4.4i,j) that may represent the dorsal part of the unspecific belt (Te2D). This dorsal part of the unspecific belt region is still included in the Oc2L area in this chapter. This situation emphasizes the multimodal associational character of Oc2L (see below). For further details on the connectivity of the temporal cortex, see Cipolloni and Peters 1979, Coleman and Clerici 1987, Herkenham 1980, Miller and Vogt 1984, Vaughan 1983, Vogt and Miller 1983, Webster 1985, and Winer and Larue 1987.

A quantitative analysis of the laminar pattern of temporal areas in Nissl- and myelin-stained sections shows that Te1 has (together with Par1 and Par2) the highest mean absolute myelin density (figure 4.7), whereas (together with the other temporal areas and the primary motor cortex) it has the lowest mean absolute cell density (figure 4.6). The overall degree of myelination alone separates the primary area Te1 from the secondary areas Te2 and Te3, with Te2 having the lowest degree (figure 4.7). If the relative densities (based on the mean value of the total neocortex) of myelin and cell bodies are taken into consideration, the temporal areas are found within a cluster separate from the other sensory regions and only partially overlapped by the frontal cortical areas (figure 4.8). The auditory cortex is therefore characterized by very low to very high myelin densities together with low cell-packing densities. Te1 has a laminar distribution of cell densities with the relatively highest values in layer IV, followed by layer V (figure 4.5c). This pattern permits the delineation from Te2 and Te3, which have much lower values in layer IV. Te1 differs most clearly from the adjoining Par1 in Nissl-stained sections because Te1 has relatively and absolutely lower cell densities in layer IV. The delineation of Te1 and Oc2L is mainly based on the much higher absolute and relative cell density in layer IV of Te1. The laminar patterns between Te1 and the adjoining Par2 are very similar both in cyto- and myeloarchitectural preparations, indicating that this border needs further analysis with other staining methods (cf. chapter 5 by Zilles, Wree, and Dausch). Te3 can be distinguished from Par2 by its absolutely and relatively lower cell densities in layer IV and Te3. The borderline between Te2 and Oc2L is also based on layer IV, which has absolutely and relatively lower cell densities in Te2. Summarizing these data, at least three different temporal areas can be identified in Nissl- and myelin-stained material. At the rostral border of Te1 to Par2, these preparations do not deliver criteria clear enough for a definite areal pattern. Additional techniques are necessary to decide the question of whether the unspecific belt region of Scheel (1988) can be delineated here as an anatomical entity.

4.11 Occipital Cortex

The occipital neocortical region comprises four areas: Oc1, Oc2MM, Oc2ML, and Oc2L (Zilles 1985, Zilles and Wree 1985). Schober (1986) corroborated this areal pattern in an independent cytoarchitectural study. These areas are surrounded by the retrosplenial agranular cortex (RSA) medially, by the frontal areas (Fr1, Fr2), the hindlimb area (HL), the primary somatosensory cortex (Par1), and the primary auditory cortex (Te1) rostrally, and by the temporal area Te2 and the perirhinal cortex (PRh) basally (figure 4.3). The occipital areas have an inner granular layer (for review, see Peters 1985) that is less prominent than the respective layer in the somatosensory region. Oc1 constitutes the primary visual cortex. Cc2MM, Oc2ML, and Oc2L represent the secondary visual and parieto-temporo-occipital association cortex. Although these latter areas show local differences in their cyto- and myeloarchitecture within each area, it was not possible until now to consistently delineate subareas in a larger sample of rat brains, even with computerized image analysis of Nissl- and myelin-stained sections (Zilles et al. 1980, Zilles and Wree 1985). Histochemical (cf. chapter 5), electrophysiological, and tracing methods (Espinoza and Thomas 1983, Montero 1973, 1981) seem more helpful, if the elaboration of a more detailed areal pattern is intended.

The primary visual cortex (Oc1) receives its main afferents from the dorsal nucleus of the lateral geniculate body and several other cortical and subcortical regions (cf. Peters 1985, Zilles and Wree 1985, chapter 13 by Goodale and Carey, chapter 12 by Dean) and projects to the secondary visual areas (e.g., Montero 1981), the superior colliculus (Schoffield et al. 1987), the lateral geniculate body, and a variety of other subcortical nuclei (for review, see Sefton and Dreher 1985, Zilles and Wree 1985). Oc1 of one side is the cortical target for input from both eyes. Zilles and associates (1984) have shown that Oc1 can be further subdivided into a monocular (Oc1M) and binocular (Oc1B) part. Oc1B is located as a rostrocaudally oriented strip lateral to Oc1M (figure 4.3). Oc1M receives input from the contralateral eye and Oc1B from both eyes, as demonstrated by transneuronal transport of a tritiated amino acid injected into the contralateral eye. Both subareas can also be recognized in Nissl- and myelin-stained sections by a higher cell density in combination with a lower myelin density in Oc1M compared with Oc1B. Oc1 reaches the occipital pole of the hemisphere (Ribak and Peters 1975, Tsang 1937, Winkelmann et al. 1972, Zilles et al. 1980, Zilles 1985, Zilles and Wree 1985). The expansion of Oc1 shows striking similarities with maps based on neurophysiological studies (Adams and Forrester 1968, Montero 1973, 1981) and differs from that displayed in Krieg's (1946) map.

The primary visual area Oc1 is surrounded medially, rostrally, and laterally by Oc2M (subdivided into Oc2MM and Oc2ML) and Oc2L. Layer IV of these areas has a much lower cell density, whereas the cell density is much higher in layer V, both on absolute and relative (figures 4.5d and 4.6) scales. The laminar distribution pattern of myelinated fibers is very similar between Oc1 and Oc2L, but Oc2M has a relatively lower density in layer V (figure 4.5d). Oc2M is also absolutely less myelinated than are the other occipital areas (figure 4.7). These cyto- and myeloarchitectural data together exhibit a clustering of the occipital areas that does not overlap with the other sensory or motor areas (figure 4.8). The primary visual cortex also shows a much higher mean cell density over all layers and both subfields (Oc1M, Oc1B) than do the other occipital areas (figure 4.7). The comparison of the mean myelin density through the whole cortical thickness of the respective areas demonstrates an increase in myelin density from medial to lateral; Oc1B and Oc2L as laterally located areas have a higher myelin content than do Oc1M and Oc2M (figure 4.7). Recently (Zilles 1985) Oc2M was subdivided into a more lateral and rostral field, Oc2ML, and a more medial and further caudally extending field, Oc2MM, on the basis of Nissl-stained sections and image analysis. Oc2MM has a higher cell density in layer II, a lower cell density in layers III and VI, and a lower degree of granularization of layer IV compared with O2cML. The adjoining agranular retrosplenial cortex (RSA) also has a cell-dense layer II, but all the other layers exhibit a density lower than in Oc2MM.

The primary visual cortex Oc1 has the smallest receptive field sizes (10° to 20°), whereas the visual responses in Oc2M and Oc2L are characterized by larger receptive fields (40° to 60°) (Montero et al. 1973a). Multiple representations of the visual field were found in Oc2 areas

(Espinoza and Thomas 1983, Miller and Vogt 1984, Montero 1981, Montero et al. 1973a,b, Olavarria and Montero 1984), which receive input from Oc1 by cortico-cortical connections. These findings corroborate the identification of Oc2M and Oc2L as secondary visual cortex. The multiple retinotopic arrangements may be reflected by the inhomogeneities in cytoarchitecture in the secondary visual areas. Miller and Vogt (1984) and Sukekawa (1988) have shown connections between nonvisual regions and the Oc2 areas. Because motor auditory and somatosensory functions were found in the rostrally and laterally surrounding areas, connections between these areas and Oc2M and Oc2L are of major interest for the identification of the secondary "visual" areas as multimodal association cortex.

References

Adams, A. D., and Forrester, J. M. (1968). The projection of the rat's visual field on the cerebral cortex. *Quart. J. Exp. Physiol.* 53:327–336.

Akers, R. M., and Killackey, H. P. (1978). Organization of corticocortical connections in the parietal cortex of the rat. *J. Comp. Neurol.* 181:513–538.

Afsharpour, S. (1985). Topographical projections of the cerebral cortex to the subthalamic nucleus. *J. Comp. Neurol.* 236:14–28.

Bates, C. A., and Killackey, H. P. (1984). The emergence of a discretely distributed pattern of corticospinal projection neurons. *Develop. Brain Res.* 13:265–273.

Beckstead, R. M. (1976). Convergent thalamic and mesencephalic projections to the anterior medial cortex in the rat. *J. Comp. Neurol.* 166:403–416.

Beckstead, R. M. (1979). An autoradiographic examination of cortico-cortical and subcortical projections of the mediodorsal-projection (prefrontal) cortex of the rat. *J. Comp. Neurol.* 184:43–62.

Benjamin, R. M., and Akert, K. (1959). Cortical and thalamic areas involved in taste discrimination in the albino rat. *J. Comp. Neurol.* 111:231–259.

Benjamin, R. M., and Pfaffmann, C. (1955). Cortical localization of taste in albino rat. *J. Physiol.* 28:56–64.

Berger, B., Thierry, A. M., Tassin, J. P., and Moyne, M. A. (1976). Dopaminergic innervation of the rat prefrontal cortex. A fluorescence histochemical study. *Brain Res.* 106:133–145.

Braun, J. J., Lasiter, P. S., and Kiefer, S. W. (1982). The gustatory neocortex of the rat. *Physiol. Psychol.* 10:13–45.

Brodmann, K. (1909). *Vergleichende Lokalisationslehre der Grosshirnrinde in ihren Prinzipien dargestellt auf Grund des Zellenbaus.* Leipzig: J. A. Barth.

Carey, R. G., and Neal, T. L. (1985). The rat claustrum: Afferent and efferent connections with visual cortex. *Brain Res.* 329:185–193.

Cechetto, D. F., and Saper, C. B. (1987). Evidence for a viscerotopic sensory representation in the cortex and thalamus in the rat. *J. Comp. Neurol.* 262:27–45.

Chapin, J. K., and Lin, C.-S. (1984). Mapping the body representation in the SI cortex of anesthetized and awake rats. *J. Comp. Neurol.* 229:199–213.

Chapin, J. K., Sadeq, M., and Guise, L. U. (1987). Corticocortical connections within the primary somatosensory cortex of the rat. *J. Comp. Neurol.* 263:326–346.

Cipolloni, P. B., and Peters, A. (1979). The bilaminar and banded distribution of the callosal terminals in the posterior neocortex of the rat. *Brain Res.* 176:33–47.

Coleman, J. R., and Clerici, W. J. (1987). Sources of projections to subdivisions of the inferior colliculus in the rat. *J. Comp. Neurol.* 262:215–226.

Collis, R. C., Santori, E. M., Der, T., Toga, A. W., and Lothman, E. W. (1986). Functional metabolic mapping during forelimb movement in rat. I. Stimulation of motor cortex. *J. Neurosci.* 6:448–462.

Cusick, C. G., and Lund, R. D. (1981). The distribution of callosal projection to the occipital-cortex in rats and mice. *Brain Res.* 214:239–259.

Deacon, T. W., Eichenbaum, H., Rosenberg, P., and Eckmann, K. W. (1983). Afferent connections of the perirhinal cortex in the rat. *J. Comp. Neurol.* 220:168–190.

Divac, I., Bjorklund, A., Lindvall, O., and Passingham, R. E. (1978a). Converging projections from the mediodorsal thalamic nucleus and mesencephalic dopaminergic neurons to the neocortex in three species. *J. Comp. Neurol.* 180:59–72.

Divac, I., Kosmal, A., Björklund, A., and Lindvall, O. (1978b). Subcortical projections to the prefrontal cortex in the rat as revealed by the horseradish peroxidase technique. *Neurosci.* 3:785–796.

Domesick, V. B. (1969). Projections from the cingulate cortex in the rat. *Brain Res.* 12:296–320.

Domesick, V. B. (1972). Thalamic relationship of the medial cortex in the rat. *Brain Behav. Evol.* 6:457–483.

Donoghue, J. P., and Parham, C. (1983). Afferent connections of the lateral agranular field of the rat motor cortex. *J. Comp. Neurol.* 217:390–404.

Donoghue, J. P., and Wise, S. P. (1982). The motor cortex of the rat: Cytoarchitecture and microstimulation mapping. *J. Comp. Neurol.* 212:76–88.

Donoghue, J. P., Kerman, K. L., and Ebner, F. F. (1979). Evidence for two organizational plans within the somatic sensory-motor of the rat. *J. Comp. Neurol.* 183:647–664.

Droogleever Fortuyn, A. B. (1914). Cortical cell-lamination of the hemispheres of some rodents. *Arch. Neurol. Psychol.* 6:221–354.

Espinoza, S. G., and Thomas, H. C. (1983). Retinotopic organization of striate and extrastriate visual cortex in the hooded rat. *Brain Res.* 272:137–144.

Farén, A., DeFelipe, J., and Regidor, J. (1984). Nonpyramidal neurons: General account. In A. Peters and E. G. Jones (eds.), *Ceebral Cortex.* Vol. 1 (pp. 201–253). New York and London: Plenum Press.

Feldman, M. L., and Peters, A. (1978). The forms of non-pyramidal neurons in the visual cortex of the rat. *J. Comp. Neurol.* 179:761–798.

Gioanni, Y. (1987). Cortical mapping and laminar analysis of the cutaneous and proprioceptive inputs from the rat foreleg: an extra- and intra-cellular study. *Exp. Brain Res.* 67:510 522.

Gioanni, Y., and Lamarche, M. (1985). A reappraisal of rat motor cortex organization by intracortical microstimulation. *Brain Res.* 344:49–61.

Guldin, W. O., and Markowitsch, H. J. (1983). Cortical and thalamic afferent connections of the insular and adjacent cortex of the rat. *J. Comp. Neurol.* 215:135–153.

Hajós, F., Zilles, K., Gallatz, K., Schleicher, A., Kaplan, I., and Werner, L., (1988a). Ramification patterns of vasoactive intestinal polypeptide (VIP)-cells in the rat primary visual cortex. An immunohistochemical study. *Anat. Embryol.* 178:197–206.

Hajós, F., Zilles, K., Schleicher, A., and Kalman, M. (1988b). Types and spatial distribution of vasoactive intestinal polypeptide (VIP) containing synapses in the rat visual cortex. *Anat. Embryol.* 178:207–217.

Hall, R. D., and Lindholm, E. P. (1974). Organization of motor and somatosensory neocortex in the albino rat. *Brain Res.* 66:23–38.

Hedlich, A., and Werner, L. (1988). Neuroglioforme Zellen im visuellen Cortex der Ratte. *J. Hirnforsch.* 29:107–116.

Hedlich, A., and Winkelmann, E. (1982). Neuronentypen des visuellen Cortex der adulten und juvenilen Ratte. *J. Hirnforsch.* 23:353–373.

Herkenham, M. (1980). The connections of the nucleus reuniens thalami: Evidence for a direct thalamo-hippocampal pathway in the rat. *J. Comp. Neurol.* 177:580–610.

Herkenham, M. (1978). Laminar organization of thalamic projections to the rat neocortex. *Science* 207:532–535.

Hummelsheim, H., and Wisendanger, M. (1985). Is the hindlimb representation of the rat's cortex a sensorimotor amalgam? *Brain Res.* 346:75–81.

Hyvärinen, J. (1982). *The Parietal Cortex of Memory and Man.* Berlin, Heidelberg, New York: Springer-Verlag.

Isseroff, A., Schwartz, M. L., Dekker, J. J., and Goldman-Rakic, P. S. (1984). Columnar organization of callosal and associational projections from rat frontal cortex. *Brain Res.* 293:213–223.

Ivy, G. O., and Killackey, H. P. (1981). The ontogeny of the distribution of callosal projection neurons in the rat parietal cortex. *J. Comp. Neurol.* 195:367–389.

Ivy, G. O., Gould, H. J., and Killackey, H. P. (1984). Variability in the distribution of callosal projection neurons in the adult rat parietal cortex. *Brain Res.* 306:53–61.

Jacobson, S. (1970). Distribution of commissural axon terminals in the rat neocortex. *Exp. Neurol.* 28:193–205.

Jones, E. G. (1984). Neurogliaform or spiderweb cells. In A. Peters and E. G. Jones (eds.), *Cerebral Cortex*. Vol. 1 (pp. 409–418). New York, London: Plenum Press.

Jones, E. G., and Hendry, S. H. C. (1984). Basket cells. In A. Peters and E. G. Jones (eds.), *Cerebral Cortex*. Vol. I (pp. 309–336). New York, London: Plenum Press.

Kolb, B. (1984). Functions of the frontal cortex of the rat: A comparative review. *Brain Res. Rev.* 8:65–98.

Kolb, B., and Walkey, J. (1987). Behavioural and anatomical studies of the posterior parietal cortex in the rat. *Behav. Brain Res.* 23:127–145.

Kosar, E., Grill, H. J., and Norgren, R. (1986a). Gustatory cortex in the rat. I. Physiological properties and cytoarchitecture. *Brain Res.* 379:329–341.

Kosar, E., Grill, H. J., and Norgren, R. (1986b). Gustatory cortex in the rat. II. Thalamocortical projection. *Brain Res.* 379:342–352.

Kosel, K. C., van Hoesen, G. W., and Rosene, D. L. (1983). A direct projection from the perirhinal cortex (area 35) to the subiculum in the rat. *Brain Res.* 269:347–351.

Krettek, J. E., and Price, J. L. (1977). The cortical projections of the mediodorsal nucleus and adjacent thalamic nuclei in the rat. *J. Comp. Neurol.* 171:157–192.

Krieg, W. J. S. (1946). Connections of the cerebral cortex. I. The albino rat. A topography of the cortical areas. *J. Comp. Neurol.* 84:221–275.

Krieg, W. J. S. (1947). Connections of the cerebral cortex. I. The albino rat. C. Extrinsic connections. *J. Comp. Neurol.* 86:267–394.

Lasiter, P. S., and Glanzmann, D. L. (1983). Axon collaterals of pontine taste area neurons project to the posterior ventromedial thalamic nucleus and to the gustatory neocortex. *Brain Res.* 258:299–304.

Lasiter, P. S., Glanzmann, D. L., and Mensah, P. A. (1982). Direct connectivity between pontine taste areas and gustatory neocortex in rat. *Brain Res.* 234:111–121.

LeDoux, J. E., Ruggiero, D. A., and Reis, D. J. (1985). Projections to the subcortical forebrain from anatomically defined regions of the medial geniculate body in the rat. *J. Comp. Neurol.* 242:182–213.

Leichnetz, G. R., and Gonzalo-Ruiz, A. (1987). Collateralization of frontal eye field (medial precentral/anterior cingulate) neurons projecting to the paraoculomotor region, superior colliculus, and medial pontine reticular formation in the rat: a fluorescent double-labeling study. *Exp. Brain Res.* 68:355–364.

Leichnetz, G. R., Hardy, S. G. P., and Carruth, M. K. (1987). Frontal projections to the region of the oculomotor complex in the rat: A retrograde and anterograde HRP study. *J. Comp. Neurol.* 263:387–399.

Leonard, C. M. (1969). The prefrontal cortex of the rat. I. Cortical projection of the mediodorsal nucleus. II Efferent connections. *Brain Res.* 12:321–343.

Leonard, C. M. (1972). The connections of the dorsomedial nucleus. *Brain Res.* 6:524–541.

Leong, S. K. (1983). Localizing the corticospinal neurons in neonatal, developing and mature albino rat. *Brain Res.* 265:1–9.

Leong, S. K., Shieh, J. Y., and Wong, W. C. (1984). Localizing spinal-cord-projecting neurons in adult albino rat. *J. Comp. Neurol.* 228:1–17.

Lindvall, O., Björklund, A., and Divac, I. (1978). Organization of catecholamine neurons projecting to the frontal cortex in the rat. *Brain Res.* 142:1–24.

Lund, J. S. (1984). Spiny stellate neurons. In A. Peters and E. G. Jones (eds.), *Cerebral Cortex*. Vol. 1 (pp. 255–308). New York, London: Plenum Press.

Marin-Padilla, M. (1984). Neurons of layer I: A developmental analysis. In A Peters and E. G. Jones (eds.), *Cerebral Cortex*. Vol. 1, (pp. 447–478). New York, London: Plenum Press.

Marin-Padilla, M., and Marin-Padilla, M. T (1982) Origin, prenatal development and structural organization of layer I of the human cerebral (motor) cortex: A Golgi study. *Anat. Embryol.* 164:161–206.

Markowitsch, H. J., and Guldin, W. O. (1983). Heterotopic interhemispheric cortical connections in the rat. *Brain Res. Bull.* 10:805–810.

McGeorge, A. J., and Faull, R. L. M. (1987). The organization and collaterization of corticostriate neurons in the motor and sensory cortex of the rat brain. *Brain Res.* 423:318–324.

Miller, M. W. (1987). The origin of corticospinal projection neurons in rat. *Exp. Brain Res.* 67:339–351.

Miller, M. W., and Vogt, B. A. (1984). Direct connections of rat visual cortex with sensory, motor, and association cortices. *J. Comp. Neurol.* 226:184–202.

Montero, V. M. (1973). Evoked responses in the rat's visual cortex to contralateral, ipsilateral and restricted photic stimulation. *Brain Res.* 53:192–196.

Montero, V. M. (1981). Comparative studies on the visual cortex. In C. N. Woolsey (ed.), *Cortical Sensory Organization*. Vol. 2 (pp. 33–81). Clifton: Humana Press.

Montero, V. M., Rojas, A., and Torrealba, F. (1973a). Retinotopic organization of striate and peristriate visual cortex in the albino rat. *Brain Res.* 53:197–201.

Montero, V. M., Bravo, H., and Fernandez, V. (1973b). Striate-peristriate cortico-cortical connections in the albino and gray rat. *Brain Res.* 53:202–207.

Morrison, J. H., Magistretti, P. J., Benoit, R., and Bloom, F. E. (1984). The distribution and morphological characteristics of the intracortical VIP-cell: an immunohistochemical analysis. *Brain Res.* 292:269–282.

Neafsey, E. J., and Sievert, C. (1982). A second forelimb motor area exists in rat frontal cortex. *Brain Res.* 232:151–156.

Neafsey, E. J., Bold, E. L., Haas, G., Hurley-Guis, K. M., Quirk, G., Sievert, C. F., and Terreberry, R. R. (1986). The organization of the rat motor cortex: A microstimulation mapping study. *Brain Res. Rev.* II:77–96.

Olavarria, J., and Montero, V. M. (1981). Reciprocal connections between the striate cortex and extrastriate cortical visual areas in the rat. *Brain Res.* 217:358–363.

Olavarria, J., and Montero, V. M. (1984). Relation of callosal and striate-extrastriate cortical connections in the rat: Morphological definition of extrastriate visual areas. *Exp. Brain Res.* 54:240–252.

Olavarria, J., and van Sluyters, R. C. (1983). Widespread callosal connections in infragranular visual cortex of the rat. *Brain Res.* 279:223–237.

Olavarria, J., and van Sluyters, R. C. (1985). Organization and postnatal development of callosal connections in the visual cortex of the rat. *J. Comp. Neurol.* 239:1–26.

Olavarria, J., van Sluyters, R. C. and Killackey, H. P. (1984). Evidence for the complementary organization of callosal and thalamic connections within rat somatosensory cortex. *Brain Res.* 291:364–368.

Patterson, H. A. (1977). An anterograde degeneration and retrograde axonal transport study of the cortical projections of rat geniculate body. Doctoral dissertation, Boston University.

Peters, A. (1984a). Chandelier cells. In A. Peters and E. G. Jones (eds.). *Cerebral Cortex.* Vol. 1 (pp. 361–380). New York, London: Plenum Pres.

Peters, A. (1984b). Bipolar cells. In A. Peters and E. G. Jones (eds.), *Cerebral Cortex.* Vol 1 (pp. 381–407). New York, London: Plenum Press.

Peters, A. (1985). The visual cortex of the rat. In A. Peters and E. G. Jones (eds.), *Cerebral Cortex.* Vol. 3 (pp. 19–80). New York, London: Plenum Press.

Peters, A., and Feldman, M. L. (1976). The projection of the lateral geniculate nucleus to area 17 of the rat cerebral cortex. I. General description. *J. Neurocytol.* 5:63–84.

Peters, A., and Kara, D. A. (1985a). The neuronal composition of area 17 of rat visual cortex. I. The pyramidal cells. *J. Comp. Neurol.* 234:218–241.

Peters, A., and Kara, D. A. (1985b). The neuronal composition of area 17 of rat visual cortex. II. The nonpyramidal cells. *J. Comp. Neurol.* 234:242–263.

Peters, A., and Kara, D. A. (1987). The neuronal composition of area 17 of rat visual cortex. IV. The organization of pyramidal cells. *J. Comp. Neurol.* 260:573–590.

Peters, A., and Kimerer, L. M. (1981). Bipolar neurons in rat visual cortex: A combined Golgi-electron microscope study. *J. Neurocytol.* 10:921–946.

Peters, A., and Proskauer, C. C. (1980). Smooth and sparsely-spined cells with myelinated axons in rat visual cortex. *Neuroscience* 5:2079–2092.

Peters, A., and Saldanha, J. (1976). The projection of the lateral geniculate nucleus to area 17 of the rat cerebral cortex. III. Layer VI. *Brain Res.* 105:533–537.

Peters, A., Kara, D. A., and Harriman, K. M. (1985). The neuronal composition of area 17 of rat visual cortex. III. Numerical considerations. *J. Comp. Neurol.* 238:263–274.

Peters, A., Meinecke, D. L., and Karamanlidis, A. N. (1987). Vasoactive intestinal polypeptide immunoreactive neurons in cat primary visual cortex. *J. Neurocytol.* 16:23–38.

Peters, A., Proskauer, C. C., Feldman, M. L., and Kimerer, L. (1979). The projection of the lateral geniculate nucleus to area 17 of the rat cerebral cortex. V. Degenerating axon terminal synapsing with Golgi impregnated neurons. *J. Neurocytol.* 8:331–357.

Peters, A., Proskauer, C. C., and Ribak, C. E. (1982). Chandelier cells in rat visual cortex. *J. Comp. Neurol.* 206:397–416.

Powell, T. P. S., and Cowan, W. M. (1954). The connections of the midline and intralaminar nuclei of the thalamus of the rat. *J. Anat.* 88:307–319.

Reep, R. L., Corwin, J. V., Hashimoto, A., and Watson, R. T. (1987). Efferent connections of the rostral portion of medial agranular cortex in rats. *Brain Res. Bull.* 19:203–221.

Reep, R. L., and Winans, S. S. (1982). Efferent connection of dorsal and ventral agranular insular cortex in the hamster, *Mesocricetus auratus.*, *Neurosci.* 7:2609–2635.

Ribak, C. E., and Peters, A. (1975). An autoradiographic study of the projections from the lateral geniculate body of the rat. *Brain Res.* 92:341–368.

Rieck, R., and Carey, R. G. (1984). Evidence for a laminar organization of basal forebrain afferents to the visual cortex. *Brain Res.* 297:374–380.

Ryugo, D. K., and Killackey, H. P. (1974). Differential telencephalic projections of the medial and ventral divisions of the medial geniculate body of the rat. *Brain Res.* 82:173–177.

Sanderson, K. J., Welker, W., and Shambes, G. M. (1984). Reevaluation of motor cortex and of sensorimotor overlap in cerebral cortex of albino rats. *Brain Res.* 292:251–260.

Sapienza, S., Talbi, B., Jacquemin, J., and Albe-Fessart, D. (1981). Relationship between input and output of cell in motor and somatosensory cortices of the chronic awake rat. *Exp. Brain Res.* 43:47–56.

Sarter, M. and Markowitsch, H. J. (1985). Convergence of intra- and interhemispheric cortical afferents: Lack of collateralization and evidence for a subrhinal cell group projecting heterotopically. *J. Comp. Neurol.* 236:283–296.

Scheel, M. (1988). Topographic organization of the auditory thalamocortical system in the albino rat. *Anat. Embryol.* 179:181–190.

Schleicher, A., Zilles, K., and Wree, A. (1986). A quantitative approach to cytoarchitectonics: software and hardware aspects of a system for the evaluation and analysis of structural inhomogeneities in nervous tissue. *J. Neuro. Sci. Meth*. 18:221–235.

Schober, W. (1986). The rat cortex in stereotaxic coodinates. *J. Hirnforsch*., 27:121–143.

Schober, W., and Winkelmann, E. (1977). Die geniculo-corticale Projektion bei Albinoratte. *J. Hirnforsch*. 18:1–20.

Schober, W., Luth, H.-J., and Gruschka, H. (1976). Die Herkunft afferenter Axone im striaren Kortex der Albinoratte: Eine Studie mit Meerrettich-Peroxidase. *Z. mikrosk.-anat. Forsch*. 90:300–415.

Schofield, B. R., Hallman, L. E., and Lin, C.-S. (1987). Morphology of corticotectal cells in the primary visual cortex of hooded rats. *J. Comp. Neurol*. 261:85–97.

Sefton, A. J., and Dreher, B. (1985). Visual system. In G. Paxinos (ed.), *The Rat Nervous System*. Vol. 1 (pp. 169–221). Sydney: Academic Press.

Shiosaka, S., Tohyama, M., Takagi, H., Takahshi, Y., Saitoh, Y., Sakumoto, T., Nakagawa, H., and Shimizu, N. (1980). Ascending and descending components of the medial forebrain bundle in the rat as demonstrated by the horseradish peroxidase blue reaction. *Exp. Brain Res*. 39:377–388.

Somogyi, P. (1977). A specific "axo-axonal" interneuron in the visual cortex of the rat. *Brain Res*. 136:345–350.

Somogyi, P., and Cowey, A. (1984). Double bouquet cells. In A. Peters and E. G. Jones (eds.). *Double Bouquet Cells*. (pp. 337–360). New York, London: Plenum Press.

Somogyi, P., Freund, T. F., and Kisvárday, Z. F. (1984). Different types of ^{3}H-GABA accumulating neurons in the visual cortex of the rat. Characterizing by combined autoradiography and Golgi impregnation. *Exp. Brain Res*. 54:45–56.

Spreafico, R., Barbaresi, P., Weinberg, R. J., and Rustioni, A. (1987). SII-projecting neurons in the rat thalamus: A single- and double-retrograde-trading study. *Somatosensory Res*. 4:359–375.

Stephan, H. (1963). Vergleichend-anatomische Untersuchungen am Uncus bei Insectivoren und Primaten. *Progr. Brain Res*. 3:111–121.

Stephan, H. (1975). Allocortex. In W. Bargmann (ed.), *Handbuch der mikroskopischen Anatomie des Menschen. Vol. 4, Nervensystem. Part 9*. Berlin, Heidelberg, New York: Springer—Verlag.

Sukekawa, K. (1988). Interconnections of the visual cortex with the frontal cortex in he rat. *J. Hirnforsch* 29:83–93.

Svetukhina, V. M. (1962). Cytoarchitectonics of cerebral neocortex in rodents (albino rat). *Arch. Anat. Gistol. Embryol*. 42:31–45.

Swanson, L. W. (1981). A direct projection from Ammon's horn to prefrontal cortex in the rat. *Brain Res*. 217:150–154.

Szentágothai, J. (1975). The "module-concept" in cerebral cortex architecture. *Brain Res.* 95:475–496.

Szentágothai, J. (1978). The neuron network of the cerebral cortex: A functional interpretation. *Proc. R. Soc. London Ser. B* 201:219–248.

Tsang, Y.-C. (1937). Visual centers in blinded rats. *J. Comp. Neurol.* 66:211–261.

van de Kooy, D., McGinty, J. F., Koda, L. Y., Gerfen, C. R., and Bloom, F. E. (1982). Visceral cortex: A direct connection from prefrontal cortex to the solitary nucleus in rat. *Neurosci. Lett.* 33:123–127.

Vaughan, D. W. (1983). Thalamic and callosal connections of the rat auditory cortex. *Brain Res.* 260:181–189.

Vogt, C., and Vogt, O. (1919). Allgemeinere Ergebnisse unserer Hirnforschung. *J. Psychol. Neurol.* 25:279–462.

Vogt, B. A., and Miller, M. W. (1983). Cortical connections between rat cingulate and visual, motor, and postsubicular cortices. *J. Comp. Neurol.* 216:192–210.

Vogt, B. A., Rosene, D. L., and Peters, A. (1981). Synaptic termination of thalamic and callosal afferents in cingulate cortex of the rat. *J. Comp. Neurol.* 201:265–283.

Wallace, M. N. (1987). Histochemical demonstration of sensory maps in the rat and mouse cerebral cortex. *Brain Res.* 418:178–182.

Webster, W. R. (1985). Auditory system. In G. Paxinos (ed.), *The Rat Nervous System.* Vol. 2 (pp. 153–184). Sydney: Academic Press.

Welker, C. (1971). Microelectrode delineation of fine grain somatotopic organization of SmI cerebral cortex in albino rat. *Brain Res.* 26:259–275.

Welker, C. (1976). Receptive fields of barrels in the somatosensory neocortex of the rat. *J. Comp. Neurol.* 166:173–190.

Welker, C., and Sinha, M. (1972). Somatotopic organization of SmII cerebral neocortex in albino rat. *Brain Res.* 37:132–136.

Welker, W., Sanderson, K. J., and Shambes, G. M. (1984). Patterns of afferent projections to transitional zones in the somatic sensorimotor cerebal cortex of albino rats. *Brain Res.* 292:261–267.

Werner, L. (1981). Klassifizierung von Nervenzellen verschiedener Altersstadien im visuellen Cortex der Ratte nach Darstellung im Nissl-Praparat. *Z. mikrosk.-anat. Forsch* 95:183–190.

Werner, L., Hedlich, A. Winkelmann, E., and Brauer, K. (1979). Versuch einer Identifizierung von Nervenzellen des visuellen Kortex der Ratte nach Nissl- und Golgi-Kopsch-Darstellung. *J. Hirnforsch.* 20:121–139.

Werner, L. Wilke, A., Blodner, R., Winkelmann, E., and Brauer, K. (1982). Topographical distribution of neuronal types in the albino rat's area 17. A qualitative and quantitative Nissl study. *Z. mikrosk.-anat. Forsch.* 96:433–453.

Werner, L., Hedlich, A., and Winkelmann, E. (1985). Neuronentypen im visuellen Kortex der Ratte, identifiziert in Nissl- und deimpragnierten Golgi-Präparaten. *J. Hirnforsch.* 26:173–186.

Winer, J. A., and Larue, D. T. (1987). Patterns of reciprocity in auditory thalamocortical and corticothalamic connections: Study with horseradish perioxidase and autoradiographic methods in the rat medial geniculate body. *J. Comp. Neurol.* 257:282–315.

Winkelmann, E., Kunz, G., and Winkelmann, A. (1972). Untersuchungen zur laminaren Organisation des Cortex cerebri der Ratte unter besonderer Berucksichtigung der Sehrinde (Area 17). *Z. mikrosk.-anat. Forsch.* 85:353–364.

Wise, S. P. (1975). The laminar organization of certain afferent and efferent fiber systems in the rat somatosensory cortex. *Brain Res.* 90:139–142.

Wolf, G. (1968). Projections of thalamic and cortical gustatory areas in the rat. *J. Comp. Neurol.* 132:519–530.

Woolsey, C. N., and LeMessurier, D. H. (1984). The pattern of cutaneous representation in the rat's cerebral corex. *Fed. Proc.* 7:137–138.

Wree, A., Kulig, G., Gutmann, P., and Zilles, K. (1985). Modification of callosal afferents of the primary visual cortex ipsilateral to the remaining eye in rats monocularly enucleated at different stages of ontogeny. *Cell Tissue Res.* 242:433–436.

Wree, A., Angenendt, H.-W., and Zilles, K. (1986). The size of the zone of origin of callosal afferents projecting to the primary visual cortex contralateral to the remaining eye in rats monocularly enucleated at different postnatal ages. *Anat. Embryol.* 174:91–96.

Zaborsky, L., and Wolff, J. R. (1982). Distribution patterns and individual variations of callosal connections in the albino rat. *Anat. Embryol.* 165:213–232.

Zilles, K. (1985). *The Cortex of the Rat. A Stereotaxic Atlas.* Berlin, Heidelberg, New York, Tokyo: Springer-Verlag.

Zilles, K., and Wree, A. (1985). Cortex: Areal and laminar structure. In G. Paxinos (ed.), *The Rat Nervous System.* Vol. 1, (pp. 375–415). Sydney: Academic Press.

Zilles, K., Zilles, B., and Schleicher, A. (1980). A quantitative approach to cytoarchitectonics. VI. The areal pattern of the cortex of the albino rat. *Anat. Embryol.* 159:335–360.

Zilles, K., Wree, A. Schleicher, A., and Divac, I. (1984). The monocular and binocular subfields of the rat's primary visual cortex. A quantitative morphological approach. *J. Comp. Neurol.* 226:391–402.

5 Anatomy of the Neocortex: Neurochemical Organization

Karl Zilles, Andreas Wree, and Nadja-Dorothee Dausch

The neurochemistry of the central nervous system is one of the most rapidly growing fields in modern neuroscience. It is impossible to cover all aspects of the neurochemical structure of the cortex in this chapter because the diversity of the methodical approaches and the tremendous amount of published results require selection. We have restricted our chapter to results derived from studies with the Timm stain, the 2-deoxyglucose method, and the immunohistochemistry and receptor autoradiography of some of the cortical transmitter systems. The Timm stain was selected because observations with this method have revealed valuable neurochemical aspects in the hippocampal region, which are of great importance for the understanding of structural-functional interrelations. This method, however, has been used only sporadically for the histochemical analysis of the neocortex, but valuable insights into the distribution of zinc-containing synaptic vesicles may be received also in this region of the forebrain. The local cerebral glucose utilization was chosen because this approach has opened wide perspectives for an interpretation of metabolically dependent cortical activities on an anatomical level. Finally, immunohistochemical and receptor autoradiographical observations represent a major battlefield of modern morphological research of the cortex, which is important also for neurophysiology, biochemistry, pharmacology, and neurology.

All these neurochemical techniques have revealed a considerable heterogeneity of the neocortex. The areal or laminar distributions found with one method, however, may not necessarily match the results based on a different method. Therefore a structural basis must be defined that gives a frame for the identification of cortical areas or layers independent from the actual neurochemical question and technique. The cytoarchitecture of the neocortex based on Nissl-stained sections was used by us as such a frame because this parcellation has reached a considerable degree of differentiation (cf. chapter 4 by Zilles), is corroborated by neurophysiological data, and can easily be reproduced also in laboratories without specialized histochemical equipment. Therefore we used adjacent Nissl-stained sections in Timm, 2-deoxyglucose, and receptor autoradiographical studies for the identification of cortical areas or layers. We found a good correlation between the position of areal and laminar borders in cytoarchitectural preparations and neurochemical observations in many cases. In other cases, however, the actual neurochemical technique can reveal subdivisions not visible in Nissl-stained sections, or cytoarchitectonically defined borders cannot be found in the neurochemical material. Apparently none of these different approaches alone can give a complete picture of the neocortical structure, but the cytoarchitecture delivers an independent relational system that allows a structurally meaningful and well-defined comparison between the different neurochemical aspects. Detailed descriptions of the histochemical methods can be found in Boast et al. 1986, Danscher 1981, Sokoloff et al. 1977, and Zilles et al. 1988.

5.1 The Neocortex of the Rat in Timm Stain

The sulphide-silver staining method by Timm (1958), modified by Danscher (1981), visualizes a transition metal (presumably zinc) inside the synaptic vesicles of asymmetric synapses. Approximately 10 percent of the clear round vesicles are stained (Pérez-Clausell and Danscher 1985). Axonal terminals containing these vesicles are visualized with the Timm stain with the light microscope. Although many attempts have been made to establish correlations between zinc-containing synaptic vesicles and various transmitters (e.g., glutamate, enkephalin), it remains unclear whether histochemically active zinc is associated with a certain transmitter system. Despite these uncertainties the method has revealed detailed areal and laminar (especially mossy fibers) patterns in the hippocampus, which can be correlated with functionally identified projections. Therefore this histochemical procedure may be useful also for the demonstration of axonal terminal fields in the neocortex, which are defined by zinc-containing synaptic vesicles. The Timm stain reveals an areal pattern, which further refines the parcellation found in cyto- or myeloarchitectural observations, and can classify sensory, motor, and associational areas by the characteristic laminar distribution of stained particles in these groups of neocortical areas. The following description is based on a densitometric analysis of Timm-stained serial sections with an image analyzer.

The medial prefrontal cortex (areas Cg1 through Cg3) and the frontal cortex (areas Fr1 through Fr3) show a nearly identical laminar pattern in Timm-stained sections (figure 5.1a,b). These areas have a first density maximum over layers I and II, a minimum in layer III, and a second maximum in the upper layer V. Minute differences permit a delineation of Cg1 from Cg3 and Cg2; Cg1 has a lower density than Cg3 in layer III and a somewhat higher density than Cg2 in layer V. The orbital cortex (Krettek and Price 1977), which is difficult to delineate both from cingulate and insular areas in Nissl-stained sections, is easily recognizable in Timm material by its much lower staining intensity. The parietal areas (Par1, Par2, FL, HL) are delineated from the frontal areas by a lower density of Timm-positive particles (figure 5.1c,d). Additionally the laminar pattern differs between the motor cortex with two maxima in density and the parietal cortex with three maxima in density (figure 5.2). The trilaminar pattern is caused by maxima in layers I and II, in upper layer V, and in layer VI, which are separated by minima in layer IV and at the border between layers V and VI. The minimum in layer IV is most conspicuous by its extremely low density, indicating that the synaptic terminals from the specific thalamic nuclei may be devoid of zinc-containing terminals. The cytoarchitectonical and functional sensorimotor amalgam (areas FL, HL; cf. chapter 4 by Zilles) shows a mixture between the characteristic features of the motor cortex (high overall density) and the somatosensory cortex (trilaminar pattern) in Timm preparation (figure 5.2). The mean density over all layers is somewhat higher in Par2 compared with Par1. The first maximum in Par2 extending over layers I through III is broader than in the other parietal areas.

The temporal areas (Te1 through Te3) have a trilaminar distribution, with the highest value in the lower layer I and a marked minimum in layer IV (figures 5.1e–h and 5.2). The primary auditory cortex (Te1) shows the lowest mean density of all temporal areas. Te1 is surrounded by areas with a higher density over all cortical layers. Additionally the minimum within layer IV is smaller in these nonprimary areas compared with the primary auditory cortex. The rostral part of the nonprimary temporal areas (Te3R) shows a higher density in all layers except for layer VI compared with Par2. This permits the delineation of Te3R from the caudal part of the supplementary somatosensory cortex. This border is barely visible in Nissl-stained sections. Te3V adjoins Te3R at the basal border of the latter area and shows a much higher overall density. Te3V resembles the cytoarchitectonically defined area Te3 (see chapter 4 by Zilles). In contrast to observations in Nissl-stained material, the border between Te3 and the caudally adjoining Te2 cannot be found in Timm-stained sections. Nevertheless, the approximate location of Te2 is indicated as Te2V in the cortical map constructed on the basis of densitometric measurements of Timm material (figure 5.3). Summarizing these findings about the temporal nonprimary areas, a ring of cortical areas displaying a high density of Timm-positive structures in a trilaminar distribution pattern surrounds the primary auditory cortex. This ring is comparable with the belt region described by Scheel (1988) for the auditory cortex of the rat in tracing studies. Te3R, Te3V, and Te2C constitute the larger part of this belt, whereas the rest may be included in Oc2L. This region surrounds the primary visual cortex (together with Oc2M; see chapter 4 by Zilles) and has a laminar pattern very similar to the nonprimary auditory cortex in Timm-stained sections. Nissl- and myelin-stained sections reveal an architectural inhomogeneity within Oc2L. Therefore it is possible that the rostrobasal part of Oc2L represents a nonprimary auditory area, tentatively named Te2D (figure 5.3).

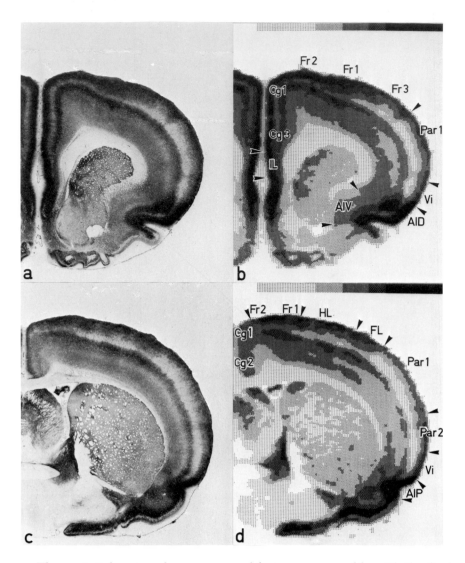

The occipital region shows a general feature comparable with the findings in other two sensory regions; i.e., the occipital areas have the lowest densities in the primary visual cortex and higher densities in the surrounding nonprimary areas (figure 5.1g,h). The trilaminar pattern of the parietal and temporal areas is not clearly visible in the occipital areas (figure 5.2), but measurements of distributional profiles reveal a third maximum in these areas. The areas Oc2MM and Oc2ML, delineated in Nissl-stained sections, cannot be separated in Timm material. Oc2L is difficult to delineate from Oc2M in Timm sections, although Oc2M has a somewhat higher density in layers II and III compared with Oc2L.

The Timm stain reveals a detailed areal pattern in the region of the putative gustatory cortex and the agranular insular region not visible in Nissl material. A region at the basal border of Par1 and Par2 is found that is characterized by a granular to dysgranular appearance in Nissl-stained sections. This area was classified as gustatory cortex (Gu) in

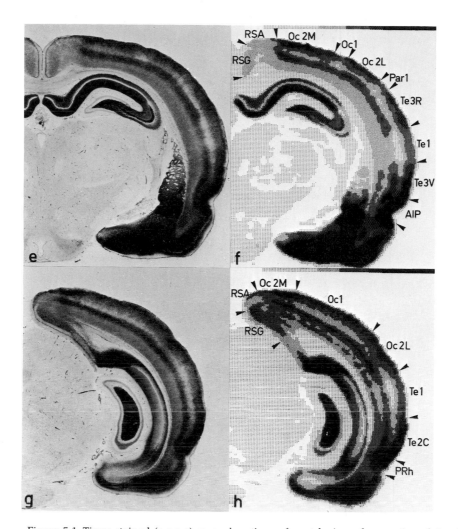

Figure 5.1 Timm-stained (a,c,e,g) coronal sections of a rat brain and respective plots of gray value distributions (b,d,f,h) after densitometry. The whole range of gray values is subdivided into five classes represented by the scales in b, d, f, and h. These scales indicate an increasing density of Timm-stained particles; for abbreviations, see table 5.1.

Zilles et al.: Anatomy: Neurochemical Organization

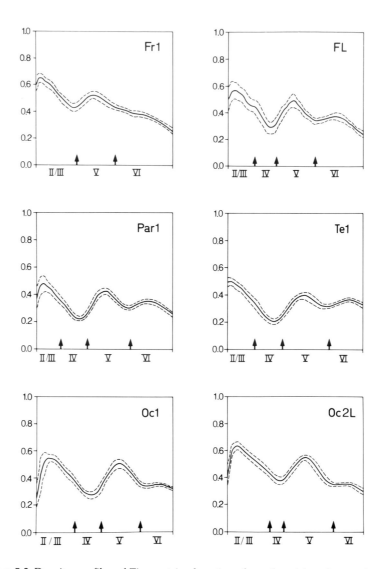

Figure 5.2 Density profiles of Timm-stained sections from the pial surface to the cortex/white-matter boundary of the cortical areas Fr1, FL, Par1, Te1, Oc1, and Oc2L. The different cortical thicknesses were standardized and the densitometric readings (y axis) are given between 0.0 (white) and 1.0 (black). Roman numerals indicate the cortical layers.

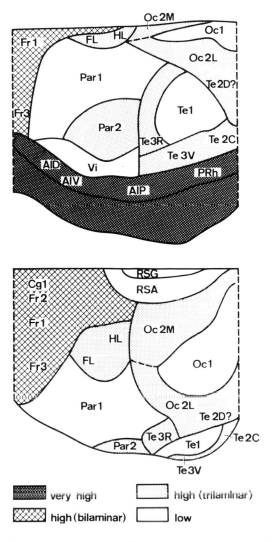

very high

high (bilaminar)

high (trilaminar)

low

Figure 5.3 Map of the cortical areas (for abbreviations, see table 5.1) of the central part of a hemisphere in lateral (top) and dorsal (bottom) views. The areas show different mean densities and laminar patterns with Timm stain.

cytoarchitectonical studies (Zilles 1985a). As discussed by Zilles in chapter 4, more recent findings (Cechetto and Saper 1987, Kosar et al. 1986a,b) have questioned the functional identification of this region. According to Cechetto and Saper (1987), the former Gu is a general visceral sensoric area and is therefore renamed area Vi. This area can be distinguished from Par1 and Par2 by its higher density in layer VI of Timm-stained sections. The basally adjoining insular cortex shows a much higher density (figure 5.1a,b and 5.3) and most probably contains the gustatory cortex.

Timm staining is an excellent method to delineate motor (bilaminar pattern) from sensory (trilaminar pattern) and primary areas (low density) from surrounding association cortex (high density).

5.2 Local Cerebral Glucose Utilization

In the adult mammalian brain energy metabolism depends almost entirely on glucose. Furthermore there exists a close relationship between energy metabolism and functional brain activity (Sokoloff 1981). The functional activity of the whole brain or of brain areas and nuclei can be visualized by the measurement of the local cerebral glucose utilization (LCGU). Studying in vitro the fate of a radioactively labeled analog of glucose (2-deoxy-D-[1-^{14}C]glucose) and subsequently using quantitative autoradiographic techniques, it is possible to measure the LCGU of practically every discrete brain region (for theoretical and technical details, see Sokoloff 1982, Sokoloff et al. 1977, Wree et al. 1988). The resulting LCGU map can be viewed as representing a "metabolic encephalography" (Sokoloff 1982). This map is therefore different from all the other approaches because the functional, mainly synaptical activity is the pertinent parameter. Because the activity is monitored in sections through the neocortex, the architectural relation is maintained. This method therefore allows the interpretation of cytoarchitectural parcellations in terms of function-related activity.

The LCGU of the auditory, parietal, sensory motor, frontal, retrosplenial, sulcal, and suprarhinal cortices (e.g., Bryan et al. 1983, Hungerbühler et al. 1981, McCulloch and Kelly 1983, Savaki et al. 1983, Sokoloff et al. 1977) has been determined. The exact position of these measurements, however, often remains unclear. In some tables it is mentioned that the measurements have been performed in layer IV, although this layer does not exist or is difficult to identify in all areas measured (e.g., in the frontal cortex; McCulloch et al. 1983). The difference in the range of the LCGU values found in the isocortex (65 μmol to 90 μmol glucose/100 g · min) is lower than the respective range covered by the various gray matters of all the other noncortical brain regions (35 μmol to 100 μmol glucose/100 g · min; Wree et al., in press).

In layer IV of a single barrel in the primary somatosensory area (Par1), stimulation of the respective vibrissa results in a glucose consumption of about 150 μmol glucose/100 g · min, whereas supragranular and infragranular layers show lower values (Durham and Woolsey 1977, Hand 1981). Another example for layer-specific LCGU measurements are the visual cortical areas (Batipps et al. 1981, Toga and Collins 1981).

To our knowledge no study exists in which all the neocortical areas of the rat brain were completely delineated according to architectonic criteria (Nissl stain, Burck 1973; myelin stain, Zilles 1985a; distribution of acetylcholinesterase, Karnovsky and Roots 1964, Zilles 1985a, Zilles and Wree 1985, Zilles et al. 1985b) and the respective LCGU was measured in corresponding autoradiographs (for technical details of the method used, see Wree et al. 1988). The LCGU values listed in table 5.1 represent the mean LCGU of the *whole* cortical area, excluding layer I. Layer I was omitted because it is partly lost in the cryostat sections. The following description of the cortical areas refers to figure 5.4 and to table 5.1.

Area Cg1 shows the highest LCGU, especially in the upper layers, and by this Cg1 can be separated from Cg2 and Cg3, which both have lower values. The orbital cortex shows a high LCGU, and the adjoining insular cortex shows a very low LCGU. The border visible in the LCGU plot (figure 5.4) fits perfectly with the architectonical border.

The areas Fr1 and Fr3 differ in LCGU distribution. Fr2 exhibits a higher glucose consumption, especially in layers II through V, compared with the laterally adjoining Fr1. Fr3 shows higher values than Fr1 in the supragranular layers. Furthermore Fr3 has the highest values in layer IV and in this respect resembles Par1.

All parietal areas have a characteristic appearance in the LCGU plots. HL and FL show high values not only in the inner granular layer but also in the supragranular layers and in layer V. FL has a higher LCGU than does HL. This difference may be caused by functional differences: The hindlimbs of the rats used for the 2-deoxyglucose experiments were restrained by plaster casts, whereas the forelimbs were freely movable. This is the usual method in nearly all deoxyglucose studies reported in the literature. It is necessary because many minute blood samples must be taken during the experiment, and for that a completely free, moving animal would greatly inhibit the strictly timed sampling. Comparisons with a few experiments on completely free, moving rats (own unpublished observations, 1988) have shown that the LCGU pattern is not changed in the neocortical areas, with the exception of HL. The LCGU of HL seems slightly increased in the completely free, moving rats. Within Par1 layer IV shows the highest LCGU values. Granular and dysgranular parts of Par1 are characterized by high LCGU values in layer IV. Par2 is separated from Par1 by a sharp border. Par2 shows a conspicuously higher LCGU in the range of the granular and supragranular layers than does Par1. The Vi area, which laterobasally follows Par2, again shows a lower LCGU and can thus be separated from Par2.

Te1, Te2, and Te3 can be separated from each other by their different

Table 5.1 Local Cerebral Glucose Utilization (μmol glucose/100g · min) in the Cortical Areas of the Rat Brain

Area	Abbreviation	LCGU	±	SD
Orbital cortex	O	85.5	±	4.6
Agranular insular cortex	A1	64.2	±	3.4
Perirhinal cortex	RRh	60.7	±	4.4
Cingulate cortex, area 1	Cg1	75.9	±	3.8
Cingulate cortex, area 2	Cg2	71.8	±	3.7
Cingulate cortex, area 3	Cg3	74.2	±	3.9
Frontal cortex, area 1	Fr1	69.3	±	2.8
Frontal cortex, area 2	Fr2	71.9	±	2.8
Frontal cortex, area 3	Fr3	69.9	±	2.6
Parietal cortex, area 1	Par1	70.4	±	2.9
Parietal cortex, area 2	Par2	71.4	±	5.2
Forelimb area	FL	72.7	±	5.5
Hindlimb area	HL	69.8	±	4.3
Visceral cortex	Vi	70.9	±	4.0
Temporal cortex, area 1	Te1	89.5	±	12.6
Temporal cortex, area 2	Te2	70.7	±	7.1
Temporal cortex, area 3	Te3	76.9	±	7.8
Occipital cortex, area 1, monocular part	Oc1M	71.9	±	5.5
Occipital cortex, area 1, binocular part	Oc1B	70.9	±	6.9
Occipital cortex, area 2, lateral part	Oc2L	70.8	±	6.9
Occipital cortex, area 2, mediolateral part	Oc2ML	71.1	±	5.3
Occipital cortex, area 2, mediomedial part	Oc2MM	66.8	±	4.8
Agranular retrosplenial cortex	RSA	69.7	±	3.2
Granular retrosplenial cortex	RSG	70.4	±	2.7

Mean LCGU values ± SD are given ($n = 7$).

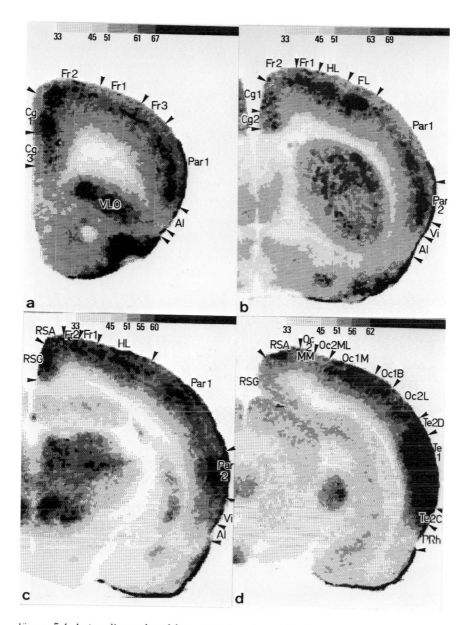

Figure 5.4 Autoradiographs of four coronal sections taken from one rat at (a) about 2.2 mm anterior to bregma, (b) about −0.3 mm posterior to bregma, (c) about −2.8 mm posterior to bregma, and (d) about −5.8 mm posterior to bregma (according to Zilles 1985a). The autoradiographs are transformed into local cerebral glucose utilization (μmol/ 100g · min) and different ranges are plotted in different print modes according to the scale. The areal borders are marked by arrow heads; for abbreviations see table 5.1.

Zilles et al.: Anatomy: Neurochemical Organization

LCGUs. Te1 exhibits the highest values of the whole cortex. On auto-radiographs it can easily be delineated with the naked eye. Mean LCGU values in the range of 100 μmol glucose/100 g · min are measured in this area. The laterobasally following area Te3 can be separated from Te1 by its lower LCGU values (table 5.1). LCGUs even lower are measured in Te2 (the only isocortical area not shown in figure 5.4), which follows Te3 caudally.

The primary visual areas Oc1M and Oc1B are characterized by high LCGUs mainly in the range of layer IV. In the lateral and especially in the medial direction, areas with lower values follow the Oc1 region. The medial secondary visual cortex, Oc2M, can be subdivided due to the low LCGUs in Oc2MM and higher values in Oc2ML. The lateral secondary visual areas Oc2L has lower LCGUs in layer IV compared with the neighboring Oc1B. The border between Oc2L and the laterally adjoining Te1 is easily recognizable by a high LCGU in Te1.

Although the retrosplenial areas (RSA, RSG) and the perirhinal area (PRh) should not be included into the isocortical areas, the respective LCGU data are given in table 5.1. The perirhinal area shows low LCGU values, which permit a delineation from Te3. RSA and RSG can be separated clearly in their rostral extent; RSG shows a higher LCGU than does RSA. More caudally the differences diminish. The border between RSA and the laterally adjoining Oc2MM is always clear-cut by higher values in RSA.

With respect to the LCGU distribution, the isocortex of the rat can clearly be subdivided into regions of different glucose consumption (figure 5.4). Borders in the LCGU picture match the respective borders seen in architectonical specimens. Nearly all architectonically founded borders are visible in the LCGU picture. Furthermore in the LCGU picture some areal borders are more clearly seen than in the adjacent Nissl-stained sections.

5.3 Transmitters and Receptors

This section is a short survey of the distribution of transmitters and transmitter receptors in the rat neocortex. The classical neurotransmitters are described in greater detail than the neuropeptides.

Acetylcholine

The cholinergic innervation of the rat neocortex originates from neurons in the basal forebrain. This region includes the medial septum with the horizontal and vertical limbs of the diagonal band, the ventral pallidum with scattered large neurons resembling the magnocellular basal "nucleus," the substantia innominata, the magnocellular preoptic nucleus, and the lateral hypothalamic area. The cholinergic nature of these neurons has been demonstrated with acetylcholinesterase (AChE) histochemistry after injection of the irreversible AChE-inhibitor diisopropylfluorophosphate (DFP), which indicates their ability to synthesize AChE (Bigl et al. 1982, Butcher and Woolf 1984, Woolf et al. 1983, Zilles 1985b). Nearly all of the neurons in this localization are also labeled with choline-acetyltransferase (ChAT) immunohistochemistry (Butcher and Woolf 1984, Eckenstein and Thoenen 1983, Satoh et al. 1983), corroborating their cholinergic nature. The frontal areas receive cholinergic afferents mainly from the ventral pallidum; the cingulate areas from the horizontal limb of the diagonal band; the parietal areas from the ventral pallidum, substantia innominata, lateral hypothalamus, and lateral preoptic area; and the occipital areas from these latter regions and the horizontal limb of the diagonal band (Bigl et al. 1982, Ichikawa and Hirata 1986, Luiten et al. 1985, Mayo et al. 1984, McKinney et al. 1983, Woolf et al. 1983, 1986). Within the magnocellular basal "nucleus," the anterior parts project to dorsomedial cortical regions and the posterior parts to ventrolateral cortical regions (Luiten et al. 1987).

The laminar pattern of cholinergic axons and terminals within the neocortex shows the highest densities in layers I, II, and VI of the frontal and cingulate areas, and in layers I to III and V to VI of parietal, temporal, and most (Oc2M, Oc2L) of the occipital areas (Eckenstein et al. 1988, Luiten et al. 1985, Parnavelas et al. 1986, Rieck and Carey 1984). The primary visual cortex (Oc1) has higher densities in layers I to III and IV to V with peak values in layer IV (Eckenstein et al. 1988). In addition to this extrinsic innervation, which determines the laminar pattern of ChAT-positive axons and terminals, an intrinsic cholinergic system of the rat neocortex has been described (Eckenstein and Thoenen 1983, Eckenstein et al. 1988, Houser et al. 1985, Johnston et al. 1981, Parnavelas et al. 1986), consisting of neurons distributed throughout layers II through VI, but concentrated in layers II and III. These ChAT-labeled cells are nonpyramidal neurons, and most of them can be identified as bipolar cells. The intrinsic cholinergic neurons form symmetric and asymmetric synapses with dendrites and somata of mostly ChAT-negative cells (Parnavelas et al. 1986). Recently ChAT-containing pyramidal neurons have been described in the frontal cortex of the rat (Nishimura et al. 1988).

Acetylcholine binds to nicotinic and muscarinic receptors in the rat neocortex. The muscarinic receptor can be subdivided further into M1 and M2 subtypes by labeling with tritiated pirenzepine or oxotremorine-M (Spencer et al. 1986). Tritiated N-methyl-scopolamine (NMS) reveals both M1 and M2 binding sites. The neocortical layers I, III, and IV contain the relatively highest densities of nicotinic receptors demonstrated with [^{3}H]-nicotine or [^{3}H]-acetylcholine with the muscarinic receptor blocker atropine (Clarke et al. 1985, Schwartz 1986). The immunocytochemical demonstration of nicotinic receptors with monoclonal antibodies reveals the cellular and subcellular distribution (Deutch et al. 1987, Schröder et al., in press a, Swanson et al. 1987). Immunoreactive perikarya were mainly seen in layers II, III, and V.

Stained dendrites were found in all layers. Immunocytochemical observations show immunoreactive products in the perinuclear zone of the cytoplasm, in the Golgi apparatus, along microtubules in the dendrites, and in postsynaptic densities.

M1 receptors are most densely packed in layers II and III of the motor, sensory (figures 5.5 to 5.8), and association cortices. M2 receptors show the highest densities in layer V of the primary (figure 5.5) and supplementary motor cortices; layer IV of the parietal, occipital, and primary auditory areas (figures 5.6 to 5.8); and layer VI of the visceral and secondary auditory cortices. The highest densities of NMS binding sites (M1 + M2) are found in layers II and III of the whole neocortex (Cortés and Palacios 1986, Wamsley et al. 1980, own unpublished observations, 1988). The laminar distribution pattern of NMS receptors is more similar to the M1 pattern than to the M2 pattern. This can be explained by the higher absolute density of M1 compared with M2 receptors in the cortex (Spencer et al. 1986). Vogt and colleagues (1987) have demonstrated muscarinic (mostly M1) receptors on smooth surfaces of pyramidal and multipolar cingulate neurons associated with postsynaptic densities of symmetric cholinergic synapses. Muscarinic cortical receptors show a decreasing density after lesions of the substantia innominata (de Belleroche et al. 1985). The pre- and postsynaptic localization of muscarinic receptors in the rat cortex was already stated by Aguilar and coworkers (1979). Immunocytochemical observations with a monoclonal antibody against muscarinic receptors (Matsuyama et al. 1988, Schröder et al., in press b,c) revealed reactive neuronal cell bodies in layers II, III, and V. Immunopositive apical dendrites, probably of pyramidal cells, are mainly present in layers III to V, and reactive postsynaptic membrane

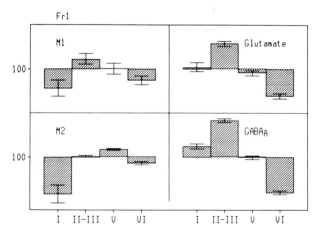

Figure 5.5 Laminar distribution of muscarinic M1 and M2 receptors, glutamate binding sites, and GABA$_A$ receptors in the primary motor cortex (Fr1) of the rat. The mean receptor density over all layers of the respective area is expressed as 100 percent, and the different layers are scaled in percentage on this basis. Five animals were used for these measurements.

Organization of the Neocortex

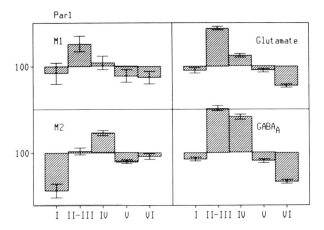

Figure 5.6 Laminar distribution of muscarinic M1 and M2 receptors, glutamate binding sites, and GABA$_A$ receptors in the primary somatosensory cortex (Par1) of the rat. The mean receptor density over all layers of the respective area is expressed as 100 percent, and the different layers are scaled in percentage on this basis. Five animals were used for these measurements.

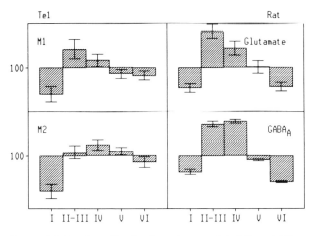

Figure 5.7 Laminar distribution of muscarinic M1 and M2 receptors, glutamate binding sites, and GABA$_A$ receptors in the primary auditory cortex (Te1) of the rat. The mean receptor density over all layers of the respective area is expressed as 100 percent and the different layers are scaled in percentage on this basis. Five animals were used for these measurements.

Zilles et al.: Anatomy: Neurochemical Organization

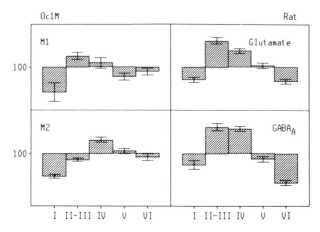

Figure 5.8 Laminar distribution of muscarinic M1 and M2 receptors, glutamate binding sites, and GABA$_A$ receptors in the primary visual cortex (Oc1) of the rat. The mean receptor density over all layers of the respective area is expressed as 100 percent, and the different layers are scaled in percentage on this basis. Five animals were used for these measurements.

densities are predominantly found in layers I to III. The subcellular distribution of immunopositive material is the same as in the cells reacting with antibodies against nicotinic receptors (see above). The laminar distributions of muscarinic receptors revealed by autoradiography agree well with these immunocytochemical results.

Glutamate
Although glutamate and aspartate have long been discussed as transmitter candidates in the neocortex, it is difficult to fulfill all rigorous criteria for transmitters (cf. Streit 1984). Because glutamate and aspartate are also used in the general metabolism, the demonstration of these amino acids alone cannot prove the transmitter-related pool. Electrophysiological evidence, studies of high-affinity uptake sites after lesions, and glutamate release after stimulation (Emson and Lindvall 1979, Mayer and Westbrook 1987, Takeuchi 1987) have supported the transmitter role of these compounds. Corticofugal systems to the amygdala, striatum, thalamus, tectum, substantia nigra, pons, and cuneate nucleus and the cortico-cortical and callosal systems seem to use glutamate and/ or aspartate as neurotransmitters (Baughman and Gilbert 1981, Fonnum and Malthe-Sørenssen 1981, Fosse and Fonnum 1987, Peinado and Mora 1986, Streit 1984). Further evidence for this role can be derived from the demonstration of glutamate receptors (see below) involved in neurotransmission.

Glutamate-containing neurons were demonstrated with immunohistochemical methods in all layers of the rat neocortex by using immunohistochemical methods including antibodies against glutamate (Ottersen and Storm-Mathisen 1984) or the glutamate-synthesizing enzyme glutaminase (Kaneko and Mizumo 1988). Neurons with intense immunoreactivity are visible in layer V and the deep part of layer VI, whereas the neurons in layers II through V show a light reaction. The majority of glutamate-containing cells are pyramidal cells. The glutamate-containing axon terminals show the highest density in layers I through IV, with peak values in layer IV of primary sensory areas.

The sodium-independent L-glutamate binding sites can be labeled with [^{3}H]-glutamate and give a first insight into the distribution of the places where glutamate can act as an excitatory transmitter. These binding sites show the highest densities in layers II and III of all neocortical areas, followed by layer IV in the primary sensory areas (figures 5.5 to 5.8). A higher density of glutamate-binding sites in layers I and II compared with layers V and VI was described also by Greenamyre and colleagues (1984). The glutamate-binding sites are further subdivided into N-methyl-D-aspartate (NMDA), quisqualate, and kainate receptors. The laminar distribution of NMDA receptors shows the highest values in the outer layers and declines toward the deeper neocortical layers (Maragos et al. 1988, Monaghan and Cotman 1985). Artola and Singer (1987) reported NMDA receptors in the rat visual cortex as a prerequisite for the induction of long-term potentiation. The quisqualate receptors show a similar laminar pattern, with the highest densities in the superficial and the lowest in the deeper neocortical layers (Monaghan et al. 1984, Rainbow et al. 1984b). The kainate receptors display a trilaminar distribution, with the highest densities in the superficial (I through III) and deep (V and VI) layers and lower densities in layer IV (Monaghan and Cotman 1982, Patel et al. 1986). This laminar pattern corresponds with the distribution of zinc-containing vesicles revealed by the Timm stain (see above). A further correspondence between Timm stain and kainate receptor distribution is visible in the hippocampus. The stratum lucidum, which contains the mossy fiber terminals, shows the highest densities both in Timm stain and kainate receptors. Therefore it can be hypothesized that the zinc-containing vesicles shown with Timm stain represent a subset of glutamate-containing vesicles acting at kainate receptors.

GABA The inhibitory neurotransmitter GABA (γ-aminobutyric acid) can be found exclusively in intrinsic neurons (Emson and Lindvall 1979, Lin et al. 1986, Meinecke and Peters 1987, Ribak 1978). Immunohistochemical observations based on the use of antibodies against the GABA-synthetizing enzyme glutamic acid decarboxylase (GAD) or GABA itself (Mugnaini and Oertel 1985, Ottersen and Storm-Mathisen 1984) and autoradiographic studies (Chronwall and Wolff 1978) permit a detailed analysis of the cortical cell types containing GABA or GAD and their laminar distribution. All layers show immunopositive neurons (10 percent to 15 percent of all neurons; Lin et al. 1986, Penny et al. 1986, but these neurons are more numerous in layers II and VI of the frontal and prefrontal cortices and in layers IV through VI of the parietal cortex than in the other layers (Esclapez et al. 1987). In contrast to these findings, Chmielowska and coworkers (1988) described the highest density in the supragranular layers of the parietal cortex. Meinecke and Peters (1987) and Ottersen and Storm-Mathisen (1984) described a uniform distribution through all layers (except in layer I, which had a lower number) of the neocortex, and Lin and associates (1986) found a slightly higher density of GAD-positive neurons in layer IV of the same cortical region. All multipolar and bitufted interneurons and 80 percent of the bipolar neurons are immunopositive (Meinecke and Peters 1987). Eighty-five percent of the neurons of layer I are GAD immunoreactive (Lin et al. 1986). Retzius-Cajal, basket, neuroglioform, bipolar, and bitufted cells were found to be GABAergic neurons (Chmielowska et al. 1988, Lin et al. 1986, Peters and Harriman 1988, Peters et al. 1982). GAD immunoreactive puncta, which are interpreted to represent GABA-containing presynaptic terminals, are observed with the greatest density in layer IV of the somatosensory and visual cortices (Chmielowska et al. 1988, Lin et al. 1986, Ribak 1978), followed by layers I and VI. The lowest density occurs in layer V. The GAD puncta are arranged around the cell bodies and proximal parts of apical and basal dendrites of pyramidal cells (Ribak 1978). Linkage of GAD axonal processes on large GAD puncta and immunoreactive cell bodies was observed by Lin and associates (1986) and Ottersen and Storm-Mathisen (1984), which could indicate a presynaptic disinhibition. The highest concentration of GABA is found in layer IV of the rat visual cortex (Ishikawa et al. 1983), which is in agreement with the densities of immunoreactive cell bodies and puncta. Colocalization of GABA with somatostatin (Lin et al. 1986, Schmechel et al. 1984), substance P (Penny et al. 1986), and vasoactive intestinal polypeptide (Peters and Harriman 1988) also has been demonstrated in the rat.

GABA acts on at least two different receptor sites—the $GABA_A$ and $GABA_B$ receptors (Johnston 1986). The $GABA_A$ sites are sensitive to the antagonist bicuculline and activate chloride ion channels, which leads to a hyperpolarization of the cell. The $GABA_B$ sites are sensitive to the agonist baclofen and influence calcium ion fluxes. $GABA_A$ sites are located synaptically (both pre- and postsynaptically) and extrasynaptically. The laminar distribution of $GABA_B$ receptors in the rat neocortex remains to be clarified. Palacios and colleagues (1981) have described a high concentration of $GABA_A$ receptors in layers I through IV, lower values in layer V, and still lower concentrations in layer VI. Studies with $[^3H]$-muscimol binding (5-8nM) in defined cortical areas show the highest $GABA_A$ densities in layers II and III, followed by layer I in the primary motor cortex of the rat. Layer V has even lower densities, but the lowest $GABA_A$ concentration is found in layer VI (figure 5.5). This laminar pattern is generally the same in the primary sensory areas (Par1, Te1, Oc1; see figures 5.6 to 5.8); here an inner granular layer can be delineated that shows the highest GABA$_A$-receptor densities together with layer III.

The laminar distributions of GABAergic terminals (see above) and GABA$_A$ receptors both show a maximum in layer IV. The distribution of GABA, enzymatically determined by Ishikawa and coworkers (1983) in the occipital cortex, matches perfectly the GABA$_A$-receptor distribution shown in figure 5.8. All these results argue for a preferential localization of GABAergic inhibitory processes in layers II through IV of the neocortex.

Serotonin (5-HT)

The serotoninergic innervation of the rat neocortex originates in the dorsal and median raphe nuclei. The axons ascend through the medial forebrain bundle to the frontal and cingulate areas and through the dorsal raphe cortical tract to most of the neocortical areas (Azmitia and Segal 1978). The axons from the median raphe nucleus show large spherical varicosities, and axons from the dorsal raphe nucleus show smaller pleomorphic (granular to fusiform) varicosities (Kosofsky and Molliver 1987). The latter axons predominate in the frontal and prefrontal areas, whereas the other cortical regions contain both axonal types. Axons with large spherical varicosities are mainly found in layers I through III of the parietal cortex, but are absent in the deeper layers. Serotoninergic axons are relatively uniformly distributed through all cortical layers (Lidov et al. 1980). In contrast to these findings, counting of 5-HT–containing varicosities (Beaudet and Descarries 1976, Descarries et al. 1975, Doucet et al. 1987, 1988), by in vivo differential pulse voltammetry (Lamour et al. 1983) and high-pressure liquid chromatography (Parnavelas et al. 1985) have clearly demonstrated a decrease in 5-HT and 5-HT terminals from superficial to deeper layers. These terminals form typical synaptic contacts (both symmetric and asymmetric) with spines, dendritic shafts, and rarely with somata of pyramidal and nonpyramidal neurons (Papadopoulos et al. 1987a,b, Parnavelas et al. 1985). Measurements of cortical 5-HT content reveal also an areal inhomogeneity, with the prefrontal areas having the highest 5-HT concentration (Reader 1981).

The 5-HT–binding sites of the rat neocortex can be subdivided into 5-HT$_1$ (with the subtypes 5-HT$_{1A}$, 5-HT$_{1B}$, and 5-HT$_{1C}$), 5-HT$_2$, and 5-HT$_3$ receptors. The 5-HT$_1$ receptors show highest densities in the frontal areas, decreasing values rostrocaudally, with the lowest densities in the occipital areas (Pazos and Palacios 1985, Zilles et al. 1985a). This areal distribution agrees with the distribution of 5-HT (see above). The laminar pattern of 5-HT$_1$ receptors is similar in all neocortical areas, with high values over layers I through III, low values over layer IV, very high values over layer V, and low values over layer VI (own unpublished observations, 1988). A considerable amount of the cortical 5-HT$_1$ receptors comprises the subtype 5-HT$_{1B}$ (especially in the frontal cortex),

5-HT$_{1A}$ receptors are intermediate, and 5-HT$_{1C}$ receptors represent the minority (Pazos and Palacios 1985). 5-HT$_2$ receptors are found in the rat neocortex in lower densities than are 5-HT$_1$ receptors. They reach a maximal density in layer IV and show an areal distribution similar to that of 5-HT$_1$ receptors (Pazos et al. 1985). 5-HT$_3$ receptors have the lowest density of all 5-HT–binding sites, with the highest values in the frontal and the lowest in the parietal areas (Kilpatrick et al. 1987). Conflicting results are found regarding the relation between 5-HT receptors and cholinergic innervation in the cortex. Cross and Deakin (1985) described a loss in 5-HT$_1$, but not 5-HT$_2$ receptors in the cortex after lesion-induced degeneration of cholinergic terminals, whereas Quirion and colleagues (1985) revealed a loss in 5-HT$_2$ receptors in the same model.

Noradrenaline (NE)
Noradrenaline-containing axons of the rat neocortex originate in the locus coeruleus and ascend via the dorsal tegmental bundle through the medial forebrain bundle, anterior septal region, and internal and external capsule (Tohyama et al. 1974; for review, see Emson and Lindvall 1979). More rostrally located areas seem to have a denser NE innervation than do more caudally located areas (Doucet et al. 1987, 1988), a finding that is also described above for 5-HT innervation. Measurements of NE concentrations in the frontal, parietal, temporal, and occipital areas (Palkovits et al. 1979) corroborate these findings by a decrease of NE concentrations along this rostrocaudal sequence. Within the neocortex the NE-containing axons show a layer-specific orientation with horizontal fibers in layer I, radially oriented fibers in layers II and III, short oblique or tortuous axon segments in layers IV and V, and strictly rostrocaudally oriented fibers in layer VI (Morrison et al. 1978). The highest density of NE-containing terminals is found in the superficial layers of frontal and parietal areas, with a continuous decrease down to layer VI (Doucet et al. 1987, 1988). The laminar-specific concentration of NE in the visual cortex differs from the density of terminals because the NE concentration in layer VI increases to values found in layers II and III (Parnavelas et al. 1985). The NE-containing varicosities form conventional synapses in the same manner as described for 5-HT terminals (see above; Papadopoulos et al. 1987b, Parnavelas et al. 1985).

Some studies have shown that the spontaneous activity of cortical neurons may be inhibited by β-adrenergic receptors and excited by α-adrenergic receptors (Olpe et al. 1980, Bevan et al. 1977). NE increases the response of neurons to excitatory or inhibitory input (Waterhouse et al. 1981, 1982) and the concentration of adenosine cyclic-3',5'-monophosphate (cAMP) in the brain by activation of adrenergic receptors. It has been shown that NE and vasoactive intestinal polypeptide (VIP) interact synaptically to increase the cortical cAMP levels (Schaad et al. 1987). Moreover both NE and VIP can promote glycogenolysis in astrocytes. Finally, NE and VIP may influence vasodilation of cortical blood vessels (for review, see Magistretti and Morrison 1988). Summarizing these aspects, NE can act on neurons (probably on the dendrites of pyramidal cells) by vertically ascending axonal branches of the longitudinally oriented NE-containing fibers in layer VI. VIP terminals are found on the same dendrites (see below). The horizontally oriented NE-containing axons in layer I may act on astrocytes and blood vessels together with VIP cell terminals.

NE acts on four types (α_1, α_2, β_1, β_2) of adrenergic receptors in the rat cortex (for review, see Gordon et al. 1988). The highest concentration of the postsynaptic α_1-receptors is located in the prefrontal cortex. The density decreases in the frontoparietal areas and reaches lowest values in the occipitotemporal region. The α_2-receptors show the highest concentration in the temporal areas, whereas the β-receptors are homogenously distributed over the whole neocortex (Diop et al. 1987).

The laminar distribution of α-receptors is quite uniform over all cortical layers (Young and Kuhar 1980), whereas the β-receptors (mainly β_1) show a higher density in layers I through III compared with the deeper layers (Palacios and Kuhar 1980, 1982, Rainbow et al. 1984a). β_1-receptors are highly concentrated in layers I and II, whereas β_2-receptors are most densely packed in layer IV and the deeper part of layer V (Rainbow et al. 1984a). Eighty percent of the β-adrenergic receptors in layers I and II are of the β_1 subtype. Equal proportions of both subtypes are found in layers IV and IVb. The distribution of β_1-receptors is therefore comparable with the laminar distribution of NE-containing terminals.

Aoki and colleagues (1987) reported a different laminar distribution for β-receptors using a polyclonal antibody and immunohistochemistry. According to this study, the supra- and intragranular layers have the same β-receptor densities, but the density in layer IV is lowered by about 15 percent. It is unclear whether the quantitation of optical densities in immunohistochemical specimens permits a comparison with autoradiographic results. The cellular localization of β-receptors in perikarya, dendrites, postsynaptic densities within spines, axons, and glial processes argues for both a neuronal and nonneuronal as well as pre- and postsynaptic localization.

Recently Jones and coworkers (1985) and Palacios and coworkers (1987) reported a conspicuously high density of the α_1-subtype in layer V. These receptors show a double band of very high densities on the superficial and lower borders of this layer. This double band fuses to a single layer in the cingulate cortex. Generally the α_1-receptor density is higher in the more rostral compared with the more caudal cortical regions. Palacios and Wamsley (1984) describe a high density of α_2-receptor in layers I and IV. This means that the α_1 and α_2-receptors display a different anatomical distribution. In the rat hippocampus α_2-receptors are found on GABA-containing axonal terminals, where they enhance GABA release (Pittaluga and Raiteri 1987). Presently it is unknown whether such a mechanism is also valid in the neocortex, but GABA$_A$ receptors on NE terminals increase NE release both in the hippocampus and cortex (Bonanno and Raiteri 1987).

Dopamine

The neocortical dopamine-containing fibers originate in the mesencephalon between the interpeduncular nucleus and the substantia nigra basally and the medial lemniscus dorsally (A9 cell group [substantia nigra pars compacta] and A10 cell group [ventral tegmental area]). They ascend through the medial forebrain bundle and terminate mainly in the frontal areas (Emson and Lindvall 1979, Oades and Halliday 1987). A convergence of dopaminergic afferents and fibers from the mediodorsal thalamic nucleus is found in a part of the frontal cortex, which can be identified as prefrontal cortex of the rat (Divac et al. 1978). This part comprises areas Cg1 through Cg3 (medial prefrontal cortex) and the dorsal part of the agranular insular cortex (cf. chapter 4 by Zilles). A lower degree of dopaminergic innervation was described also for the more caudally located cortical areas (Descarries et al. 1987, Doucet et al. 1988). The highest density of dopamine-containing terminals (varicosities) is found in layers II and III of the prefrontal cortex (Berger et al. 1988, Descarries et al. 1987, Doucet et al. 1988). The dopamine innervation displays the reversed laminar pattern of the 5-HT and NE innervation in the prefrontal cortex. The density of dopamine-containing varicosities is much lower in the frontal, parietal, temporal, and occipital areas. The terminals are mostly confined to the deeper layer VI in these regions (Descarries et al. 1987, Phillipson et al. 1987).

The dopamine receptors can be subdivided into D1 and D2 receptors. The D1 type is linked to and stimulates the adenylate cyclase system. D1 and D2 receptors interact in both opposing and synergistic fashions (for review, see Clark and White 1987). D1 receptors are found in much higher densities than are D2 receptors in the neocortex (Charuchinda et al. 1987, Dawson et al. 1986c, Palacios and Pazos 1987). Differing results have been reported regarding the areal and laminar distribution of both dopaminergic receptor subtypes (Boyson et al. 1986, Dawson et al. 1986a,b,c, Dawson et al. 1988, Martres et al. 1985a,b, Palacios and Pazos 1987). These differences may be caused, at least partially, by the use of different ligands and by the additional labeling of 5-HT$_2$ receptors to differing degrees, which again depends on the ligand and the brain region under observation. 5-HT$_2$ receptors can cause up to 50 percent of the activity in receptor autoradiography of the rat neocortex (Dawson et al. 1988). Despite these problems some general aspects of regional and laminar distributions can be revealed with the presently available techniques. D1 receptors show the highest concentrations in the prefrontal followed by the temporal and occipital areas (Dawson et al. 1986b, 1988). The frontoparietal areas (especially the motor cortex) have the lowest D1 receptor densities. The laminar distribution of the post-synaptic D1 receptor reaches the highest values in layers V and VI of the neocortex (Boysen et al. 1986, Dawson et al. 1986a,b,c, 1988). The lowest values are found in layers I through III. The D2 receptors seem to reach peak values also in layers V and VI (Martres et al. 1985a,b). The dopaminergic innervation density and the receptor density show a considerable mismatch when different areas are compared. For example, the occipital areas have a lower density of dopamine-containing afferents than do the frontal areas, but the receptors show an inverse relation. The laminar distribution of dopamine terminals (Descarries et al. 1987) and receptors, on the other hand, both have the highest values in layers V and VI.

Vasoactive Intestinal Polypeptide (VIP)

VIP and VIP receptors have particularly high concentrations in the rat neocortex (Lorén et al. 1979, Staun-Olsen et al. 1985). An extensive colocalization of VIP with classical transmitters (acetylcholine, Ecken-stein and Baughman 1984) and other peptides (somatostatin and cho-lecystokinin, Papadopoulos et al. 1987c) has been demonstrated. VIP is localized in nonpyramidal neurons (Connor and Peters 1984, Fuxe et al. 1977, Hajós et al. 1988a, McDonald et al. 1982a, Magistretti and Morrison 1985, Morrison et al. 1984, Sims et al. 1980). Most of these neurons are fusiform bipolar cells (Feldman and Peters 1978, Peters and Kimerer 1981). The VIP cells constitute 1.5 percent of the whole cortical neuronal population, with 76 percent bipolar cells and 24 percent mul-tipolar nonpyramidal cells (Hajós et al. 1988a). The majority of VIP is found in layers II and III of the rat visual cortex (figure 5.9). The fusiform bipolar cells (68 percent of the VIP cells) have dendrites spanning con-siderable distances from layer I to layer V. The ascending dendrite has a terminal tuft of roughly varicose branches in layer I. Oblique or

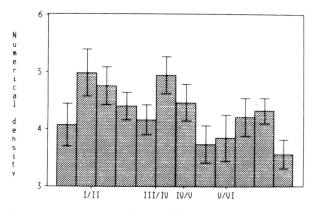

Figure 5.9 Laminar distribution of the VIP-positive varicosities in the primary visual cortex of the rat (from Hajós et al. 1988b). Three maxima can be recognized, which indicate the laminar distribution of these terminals.

Zilles et al.: Anatomy: Neurochemical Organization

transverse branches of the main dendrites are seen in layers II through VI. The axon originates from the proximal part of the descending dendrite. As with the dendrites the axonal branches are vertically oriented and descend to layer VI. They bear numerous en passant and terminal axonal varicosities. Dendrites and axons of these cells are confined to a small, vertically oriented cylinder. This type of spatial distribution leads to the hypothesis of the role of VIP cells as elements with a columnar regulatory function (Magistretti and Morrison 1985, Magistretti et al. 1981). Although this may be relevant for the fusiform cells, about 32 percent of the VIP cells show an irregular spatial distribution of their dendrites and axons. They are thought to give rise to a noncolumnar component of VIP innervation (Hajós et al. 1988a). This is corroborated by the laminar distribution of VIP axonal varicosities, which show three maxima, the first on the layers I/II border, the second within layer IV, and the third within the deeper layer VI (Hajós et al. 1988b). VIP axons form symmetrical synapses with dendritic shafts, spines, and cell bodies of pyramidal and nonpyramidal neurons. VIP dendrites and cell bodies form symmetrical and asymmetrical synapses with VIP-negative axons. Synaptic contacts between two VIP-positive structures are rarely found (Hajós et al. 1988b).

VIP receptors show a slightly higher concentration in the rostral compared with caudal neocortical areas (Besson et al. 1986, Staun-Olsen et al. 1985). Besson and associates (1986) described the highest density in layers IV and VI, where De Souza and colleagues (1985) revealed a preferential localization in layer I. On the other hand the illustrations of Besson and associates (1986) also show a high density of binding sites in layer I. This seems to permit a reconciliation of the controversy on the basis of a laminar distribution with peaks in layers I, IV, and VI. This pattern exactly reflects the distribution of VIP boutons (see above). Poulin and colleagues (1986) demonstrated additional VIP binding sites in vascular smooth muscles of cerebral arteries.

A variety of functions is claimed for VIP in the cortex, including cerebral vasodilation (Edvinsson 1982, Lee et al. 1984, Said 1982). Increased glycogenolysis (Magistretti et al. 1981), glucose utilization (McCulloch and Kelly 1983), and neuronal excitation (Phillis and Kirkpatrick 1980) are also found (for review, see Rostène 1984).

Somatostatin (SRIF)
SRIF-containing neurons of the rat neocortex belong to the group of bitufted and multipolar nonpyramidal cortical neurons (McDonald et al. 1982b, Meinecke and Peters 1986, Mizukawa et al. 1987). Laemle and Feldman (1985) have described also SRIF-containing pyramidal cells (for critical discussion, see McDonald et al. 1982b and Meinecke and Peters 1986). SRIF neurons are found in all areas and layers except layer I. A preferential localization of the cell bodies in layers II to III and V to VI is described. The SRIF-positive fibers are concentrated in layers I, V,

and VI, with maximal densities in layer I (Mizukawa et al. 1987, Naus et al. 1988). Colocalization of SRIF with VIP, neuropeptide Y, and GABA has been reported by Hendry and colleagues (1984), Lin and coworkers (1986), and Papadopoulos and coworkers (1987c).

Although a detailed analysis of the areal and laminar distribution of somatostatin receptors is lacking, a rough estimate given in the illustrations of Maurer and Reubi (1985) and McCarty and Plunkett (1987) shows a considerable inhomogeneity between the laminar patterns of different cortical areas. The upper cortical layers (I through III) contain very low densities, whereas the lower layers (IV through VI) display high densities with a bilaminar distribution in some areas or a decreasing density (from layers IV to VI) in other (frontoparietal) areas.

SRIF affects neurotransmission. Both excitatory and inhibitory effects on cortical neurons have been reported. The SRIF release can be increased by cholinergic stimulation and decreased by GABAergic stimulation (for review, see Parnavelas and McDonald 1983).

Cholecystokinin (CCK)

CCK-immunoreactive neurons of the bitufted and multipolar nonpyramidal varieties are found in the rat neocortex (Emson and Hunt 1981, McDonald et al. 1982c). They occur in all layers, including layer I, but are concentrated in layers II and III. Approximately 1 percent of the whole cortical neuronal population contains CCK. The axons of these cells form a particularly dense network in layers II and III.

CCK receptors are visualized in all areas and layers, with highest densities in layers IV and VI (Sekiguchi and Moroji 1986, Zarbin et al. 1983). Cortical neurons can be excited by iontophoretical application of CCK (Phillis and Kirkpatrick 1980).

Opioid Peptides

Bipolar and multipolar nonpyramidal cells as well as presumptive pyramidal neurons display immunoreactivity against dynorphin A and proenkephalin (McGinty et al. 1984). Proenkephalin immunoreactive cells are preferentially located in layers II to III and V to VI, whereas the density of dynorphin A cells is generally far below that of the proenkephalin cells. Dynorphin A is visualized mostly in pyramidal cells of layer V. More recently Fallon and Leslie (1986) have described a somewhat different distribution and cellular localization. They found dynorphin B immunoreactivity exclusively in nonpyramidal cells and preferentially located in layers II to III and V to VI. Proenkephalin-containing cells are rarely seen in the neocortex. The dynorphin B cells can be identified as part of the cortical local circuit system. Proopiomelanocortin cannot be found in significant amounts within the neocortex of the rat.

Three distinct types of opioid receptors (μ, δ, and κ) have been described in the rat brain (Mansour et al. 1987, 1988, McLean et al.

1986). The three receptor types show different densities within the neocortex. The μ receptors have the highest, the δ receptors a moderate, and the κ receptors the lowest density. The primary visual cortex (Oc1) shows the lowest concentration of all three receptors, whereas the frontal and parietal areas have the relatively highest densities. The receptors display bilaminar distributions in most of the neocortical regions. The highest densities are found for the μ receptors in layers I and IV and for the δ and κ receptors in layers II to III and V to VI. Significant amounts of κ receptors can be visualized only in layers V and VI of the primary visual cortex and the occipitotemporal region.

Presently a sufficient knowledge of the cortical function of the opioid system is lacking, although numerous functional aspects have been described for other brain regions (for review, see Mansour et al. 1988).

References

Aguilar, J. S., M. Criado, and E. de Robertis, 1979. Pre- and postsynaptic localization of central muscarinic receptors. *Eur. J. Pharmacol.* 57:227–230.

Aoki, C., T. H. Joh, and V. M. Pickel, 1987. Ultrastructural localization of β-adrenergic receptor-like immunoreactivity in the cortex and neostriatum of rat brain. *Brain Res.* 437:264–282.

Artola, A., and W. Singer, 1987. Long-term potentiation and NMDA receptors in rat visual cortex. *Nature* 330:649–652.

Azmitia, E. C., and M. Segal, 1978. An autoradiographic analysis of the differential ascending projections of the dorsal and median raphe nuclei in the rat. *J. Comp. Neurol.* 179:641–668.

Batipps, M., M. Miyaoka, M. Shinohara, L. Sokoloff, and C. Kennedy, 1981. Comparative rates of local cerebral glucose utilization in the visual system of conscious albino and pigmented rats. *Neurology* 31:58–62.

Baughman, R. W., and C. D. Gilbert, 1981. Aspartate and glutamate as possible neurotransmitters in the visual cortex. *J. Neurosci.* 1:427–439.

Beaudet, A., and L. Descarries, 1976. Quantitative data on serotonin nerve terminals in adult rat neocortex. *Brain Res.* 111:301–309.

Berger, B., G. Doucet, and L. Descarries, 1988. Density of the dopamine innervation in rat cerebral cortex after neonatal 6-hydroxydopamine or adult stage DSP-4 noradrenaline denervations: A quantitative autoradiographic study. *Brain Res.* 441:260–268.

Besson, J., A. Sarrieau, M. Vial, J.-C. de Marie, G. Rosselin, and W. Rostène, 1986. Characterization and autoradiographic distribution of vasoactive intestinal peptide binding sites in the rat central nervous system. *Brain Res.* 398:329–336.

Bevan, P., C. M. Bradshaw, and E. Szabadi, 1977. The pharmacology of adrenergic neuronal responses in the cerebral cortex: Evidence for excitatory α- and inhibitory β-receptors. *Br. J. Pharmac.* 59:635–641.

Bigl, V., N. J. Woolf, and L. L. Butcher, 1982. Cholinergic projection from the basal forebrain to frontal, parietal, temporal, occipital, and cingulate cortices: A combined fluorescent tracer and acetylcholinesterase analysis. *Brain Res. Bull.* 8:727–749.

Boast, C. A., E. W. Snowhill, and C. A. Alter, 1986. *Quantitative Receptor Autoradiography*. New York: Alan R. Liss.

Bonanno, G., and M. Raiteri, 1987. Release-regulating GABA$_A$ receptors are present on noradrenergic nerve terminals in selective areas of the rat brain. *Synapse* 1:254–257.

Boyson, S. J., P. McGonigle, and P. B. Molinoff, 1986. Quantitative autoradiographic localization of the D$_1$ and D$_2$ subtypes of dopamine receptors in rat brain. *J. Neurosci.* 6:3177–3188.

Bryan, R. M., R. A. Hawhins, A. M. Mans, D. W. Davis, and R. B. Page, 1983. Cerebral glucose utilization in awake unstressed rats. *Am. J. Physiol.* 244:C270–C275.

Burck, H. C., 1973. *Histologische Technik*. Stuttgart: Thieme Verlag.

Butcher, L. L., and N. J. Woolf, 1984. Histochemical distribution of acetylcholinesterase in the central nervous system: Clues to the localization of cholinergic neurons. In *Handbook of Chemical Neuroanatomy, Vol. 3: Classical Transmitters and Transmitter Receptors in the CNS, Part II*. A. Björklund, T. Hökfelt, and M. J. Kuhar (eds). Amsterdam: Elsevier Biomedical Press, pp. 1–50.

Cechetto, D. F., and C. B. Saper, 1987. Evidence for a viscerotopic sensory representation in the cortex and thalamus in the rat. *J. Comp. Neurol.* 262:27–45.

Charuchinda, C., P. Supavilai, M. Karobath, and J. M. Palacios, 1987. Dopamine D$_2$ receptors in the rat brain: Autoradiographic visualization using a high-affinity selective agonist ligand. *J. Neurosci.* 7:1352–1360.

Chmielowska, J., M. G. Stewart, and R. C. Bourne, 1988. γ-aminobutyric acid (GABA) immunoreactivity in mouse and rat first somatosensory (SI) cortex: Description and comparison. *Brain Res.* 439:155–168.

Chronwall, B., and J. R. Wolff, 1978. Classification and location of neurons taking up ^{3}H-GABA in the visual cortex of rats. In *Amino Acids as Chemical Transmitters*. F. Fonnum (ed). New York: Plenum Press, pp. 297–303.

Clark, D., and F. J. White, 1987. Review: D1 dopamine receptor—The search for a function: A critical evaluation of the D1/D2 dopamine receptor classification and its functional implications. *Synapse* 1:347–388.

Clarke, P. B. S., R. D. Schwartz, S. M. Paul, C. B. Pert, and A. Pert, 1985. Nicotinic binding in rat brain: Autoradiographic comparison of [3H]acetylcholine, [3H]nicotine, and [125I]-α-bungarotoxin. *J. Neurosci.* 5:1307–1315.

Connor, J. R., and A. Peters, 1984. Vasoactive intestinal polypeptide immunoreactive neurons in rat visual cortex. *Neuroscience* 12:1027–1044.

Cortés, R., and J. M. Palacios, 1986. Muscarinic cholinergic receptor subtypes in the rat brain. I. Quantitative autoradiographic studies. *Brain Res.* 362:227–238.

Cross, A. J., and J. F. W. Deakin, 1985. Cortical serotonin receptor subtypes after lesion of ascending cholinergic neurones in rat. *Neurosci. Lett.* 60:261–265.

Danscher, G., 1981. Histochemical demonstration of heavy metals. A revised version of the sulphide silver method suitable for both light and electronmicroscopy. *Histochemistry* 71:1–16.

Dawson, T. M., P. Barone, A. Sidhu, J. K. Wamsley, and T. N. Chase, 1986a. Quantitative autoradiographic localization of D-1 dopamine receptors in the rat brain: Use of the iodinated ligand [^{125}I] S C H 23982. *Neurosci. Lett.* 68:261–266.

Dawson, T. M., D. R. Gehlert, R. T. McCabe, A. Barnett, and J. K. Wamsley, 1986b. D-1 dopamine receptors in the rat brain: A quantitative autoradiographic analysis. *J. Neurosci.* 6:2352–2365.

Dawson, T. M., D. R. Gehlert, and J. K. Wamsley, 1986c. Quantitative autoradiographic localization of central dopamine D-1 and D-2 receptors. In *Neurobiology of Central D1-Dopamine Receptors*. G. R. Breese, J. Creese (eds). New York, London: Plenum Press, pp. 93–118.

Dawson, T. M., P. Barone, A. Sighu, J. K. Wamsley, and T. N. Chase, 1988. The D1 dopamine receptors in the rat brain: Quantitative autoradiographic localization using an iodinated ligand. *Neuroscience* 26:83–100.

de Belleroche, J., I. M. Gardiner, M. H. Hamilton, and N. J. M. Birdsall, 1985. Analysis of muscarinic receptor concentration and subtypes following lesion of rat substantia innominata. *Brain Res.* 340:201–209

Descarries, L., A. Beaudet, and K. C. Watkins, 1975. Serotonin nerve terminals in adult rat neocortex. *Brain Res.* 100:563–588.

Descarries, L., B. Lemay, G. Doucet, and B. Berger, 1987. Regional and laminar density of the dopamine innervation in adult rat cerebral cortex. *Neuroscience* 21:807–824.

De Souza, E. B., H. Seifert, and M. J. Kuhar, 1985. Vasoactive intestinal peptide receptor localization in rat forebrain by autoradiography. *Neurosci. Lett.* 56:113–120.

Deutch, A. Y., J. Holliday, R. H. Roth, L. L. Y. Chun, and E. Hawrot, 1987. Immuno-histochemical localization of a neuronal nicotinic acetychloline receptor in mammalian brain. *Pros. Natl. Acad. Sci. USA* 84:8697–8701.

Diop, L., R. Brière, L. Grondin, and T. A. Reader, 1987. Adrenergic receptor and catecholamine distribution in rat cerebral cortex: Binding studies with [^{3}H]prazosin, [^{3}H]idazoxan and [^{3}H]dihydroalprenolol. *Brain Res.* 402:403–408.

Divac, I., A. Björklund, O. Lindvall, and R. E. Passingham, 1978. Converging projections from the mediodorsal thalamic nucleus and mesencephalic dopaminergic neurons to the neocortex in three species. *J. Comp. Neurol.* 180:59–72.

Doucet, G., M. A. Audet, and L. Descarries, 1987. Numbered density of monoamine innervations in two regions of adult neocortex. *Neuroscience* 22 (suppl.):S114.

Doucet, G., L. Descarries, M. A. Audet, S. Garcia, and B. Berger, 1988. Autoradiographic method for quantifying regional monoamine innervations in the rat brain. Application to the cerebral cortex. *Brain Res*. 441:233–259.

Durham, D., and T. A. Woolsey, 1977. Barrels and columnar cortical organization: Evidence from 2-deoxyglucose (2-DG) experiments. *Brain Res*. 137:169–174.

Eckenstein, F., and R. W. Baughman, 1984. Two types of cholinergic innervation in cortex, one co-localized with vasoactive intestinal polypeptide. *Nature* 309:153–155.

Eckenstein, F., and H. Thoenen, 1983. Cholinergic neurons in the rat cerebral cortex demonstrated by immunohistochemical localization of choline acetyltransferase. *Neurosci. Lett*. 36:211–215.

Eckenstein, F. P., R. W. Baughman, and J. Quinn, 1988. An anatomical study of cholinergic innervation in rat cerebral cortex. *Neuroscience* 26:457–474.

Edvinson, L., 1982. Vasoactive intestinal polypeptide and the cerebral circulation. In *Vasoactive Intestinal Peptide*. S. I. Said, (ed). New York: Raven Press, pp. 149–159.

Emson, P. C., and S. P. Hunt, 1981. Anatomical chemistry of the cerebral cortex. In *The Organization of the Cerebral Cortex*. F. O. Schmitt, F. C. Worden, G. Adelman, and S. G. Dennis (eds.). Cambridge, Mass: MIT Press, pp. 325–345.

Emson, P. C., and O. Lindvall, 1979. Distribution of putative neurotransmitters in the neocortex. *Neuroscience* 4:1–30.

Esclapez, M., G. Campistron, and S. Trottier, 1987. Immunocytochemical localization and morphology of GABA-containing neurons in the prefrontal and frontoparietal cortex of the rat. *Neurosci. Lett*. 77:131–136.

Fallon, J. H., and F. M. Leslie, 1986. Distribution of dynorphin and enkephalin peptides in the rat brain. *J. Comp. Neurol*. 249:293–336.

Feldman, M. L., and A. Peters, 1978. The forms of non-pyramidal neuron in the visual cortex of the rat. *J. Comp. Neurol*. 179:761–794.

Fonnum, F., and D. Malthe-Sørenssen, 1981. Localization of glutamate neurons. In *Glutamate: Transmitter in the Central Nervous System*. P. J. Roberts, J. Storm-Mathisen, and G. A. R. Johnston eds. London: John Wiley & Sons Ltd., pp. 205–222.

Fosse, V. M., and Fonnum, F., 1987. Biochemical evidence for glutamate and/or aspartate as neurotransmitters in fibers from the visual cortex to the lateral posterior nucleus (pulvinar) in rats. *Brain Res*. 400:219–224.

Fuxe, K., T. Hökfelt, S. I. Said, and V. Mutt, 1977. VIP and the nervous system: Immunohistochemical evidence for localization in central and periphal nerves, particularly intracortical neurons of the cerebral cortex. *Neurosci. Lett*. 5:241–246.

Gordon, B., E. E. Allen, and P. Q. Trombley, 1988. The role of norepinephrine in plasticity of visual cortex. *Progr. Neurobiol*. 30:171–191.

Greenamyre, J. T., A. B. Young, and J. B. Penney, 1984. Quantitative autoradiographic distribution of L-[$_3$H]glutamate-binding sites in rat central nervous system. *J. Neurosci*. 4:2133–2144.

Hajós, F., K. Zilles, K. Gallatz, A. Schleicher, I. Kaplan, and L. Werner, 1988a. Ramification patterns of vasoactive intestinal polypeptide (VIP)-cells in the rat primary visual cortex. *Anat. Embryol.* 178:197–206.

Hajós, F., K. Zilles, A. Schleicher, and M. Kálmán, 1988b. Types and spatial distibution of vasoactive intestinal polypeptide (VIP)-containing synapses in the rat visual cortex. *Anat. Embryol.* 178:207–217.

Hand, P., 1981. The 2-deoxyglucose method. In *Neuroanatomical Tract Tracing Methods*. L. Heimer and M. J. Robards (eds). New York and London: Plenum Press, pp. 511–538.

Hendry, S. H. C., E. G. Jones, and P. C. Emson, 1984. Morphology, distribution, and synaptic relations of somatostatin and neuropeptide Y-immunoreactive neurons in rat and monkey neocortex. *J. Neurosci.* 4:2497–2517.

Houser, C. R., G. D. Crawford, P. M. Salvaterra, and J. E. Vaughn, 1985. Immunocytochemical localization of choline acetyltransferase in rat cerebral cortex: A study of cholinergic neurons and synapses. *J. Comp. Neurol.* 234:17–34.

Hungerbühler, J. P., J. C. Saunders, J. H. Greenberg, and M. Reivich, 1981. Functional neuroanatomy of the auditory cortex studied with (2-^{14}C)deoxyglucose. *Exp. Neurol.* 71:104–121.

Ichikawa, T., and Y. Hirata, 1986. Organization of choline acetyltransferase-containing structures in the forebrain of the rat *J. Neurosci.* 6:281–292.

Ishikawa, K., Watabe, S., and Goto, N., 1983. Laminal distribution of γ-aminobutyric acid (GABA) in the occipital cortex of rats: Evidence as a neurotransmitter. *Brain Res.* 277:362–364.

Johnston, G. A. R., 1986. Multiplicity of GABA receptors. In *Benzodiazepine/GABA Receptors and Choline Channels: Structural and Functional Properties*. New York: Alan R. Liss, pp: 57–71.

Johnston, M. V., M. McKinney, and J. T. Coyle, 1981. Neocortical cholinergic innervation: A description of extrinsic and intrinsic components in the rat. *Exp. Brain Res.* 43:159–172.

Jones, L. S., L. L. Gauger, and J. N. Davis, 1985. Anatomy of brain alpha₁-adrenergic receptors: In vitro autoradiography with [^{125}I]-HEAT. *J. Comp. Neurol.* 231:190–08.

Kaneko, T., and N. Mizumo, 1988. Immunohistochemical study of glutaminase-containing neurons in the cerebral cortex and thalamus of the rat. *J. Comp. Neurol.* 267:590–602.

Karnovsky, M. L., and L. Roots, 1964. A "direct-coloring" thiocholin method for choline esterase. *J. Histochem. Cytochem.* 12:219–221.

Kilpatrick, G. J., B. J. Jones, and M. B. Tyers, 1987. Identification and distribution of 5-HT₃ receptors in rat brain using radioligand binding. *Nature* 330:746–748.

Kosar, E., H. J. Grill, and R. Norgren, 1986a. Gustatory cortex in the rat. I. Physiological properties and cytoarchitecture. *Brain Res.* 379:329–341.

Kosar, E., H. J. Grill, and R. Norgren, 1986b. Gustatory cortex in the rat. II. Thalamocortical projection. *Brain Res.* 379:342–352.

Kosofsky, B. E., and M. E. Molliver, 1987. The serotoninergic innervation of cerebral cortex: Different classes of axon terminals arise from dorsal and median raphe nuclei. *Synapse* 1: 153–168.

Krettek, J. E., and J. L. Price, 1977. The cortical projections of the mediodorsal nucleus and adjacent thalamic nuclei in the rat. *J. Comp. Neurol.* 171:157–192.

Laemle, L. K., and S. C. Feldman, 1985. Somatostatin (SRIF)-like immunoreactivity in subcortical and cortical visual centers of the rat. *J. Comp. Neurol.* 233:452–462.

Lamour, Y., J. P. Rivot, D. Pointis, and L. Ory-Lavollee, 1983. Laminar distribution of serotonergic innervation in rat somatosensory cortex, as determined by in vivo electrochemical detection. *Brain Res.* 259:163–166.

Lee, T. J.-F., A. Saito, and I. Berezin, 1984. Vasoactive intestinal polypeptide-like substance: The potential transmitter for cerebral vasodilation. *Science* 224:898–900.

Lidov, H. G. W., R. Grzanna, and M. E. Molliver, 1980. The serotonin innervation of the cerebral cortex in the rat—an immunohistochemical analysis. *Neuroscience* 5:207–227.

Lin, C.-S., S. M. Lu, and D. E. Schmechel, 1986. Glutamic acid decarboxylase and somatostatin immunoreactivities in rat visual cortex. *J. Comp. Neurol.* 244:369–383.

Lorén, I., P. C. Emson, J. Fahrenkrug, A. Björklund, I. Alumets, R. Håkanson, and F. Sundler, 1979. Distribution of vasoactive intestinal polypeptide in the rat and mouse brain. *Neuroscience* 4:1953–1976.

Luiten, P. G. M., R. P. A. Gaykema, J. Traber, and D. G. Spencer, 1987. Cortical projection patterns of magnocellular basal nucleus subdivisions as revealed by anterogradely transported *Phaseolus vulgaris* leucoagglutinin. *Brain Res.* 413:229–250.

Luiten, P. G. M., D. G. Spencer, J. Traber, and R. P. A Gaykema, 1985. The pattern of cortical projections from the intermediate parts of the magnocellular nucleus basalis in the rat demonstrated by tracing with *Phaseolus vulgaris*-leucoagglutinin. *Neurosci. Lett.* 57:137–142.

Magistretti, P. J., and H. J. Morrison, 1985. VIP-neurons in the neocortex. *TINS* 8:7–8.

Magistretti, P. J., and J. H. Morrison, 1988. Noradrenaline- and vasoactive intestinal peptide-containing neuronal systems in neocortex: Functional convergence with contrasting morphology. *Neuroscience* 24:367–378.

Magistretti, P. J., J. H. Morrison, W. J. Shoemaker, V. Sapin, and F. E. Bloom, 1981. Vasoactive intestinal polypeptide induced glycogenolysis in mouse cortical slices: A possible regulatory mechanism for the local control of energy metabolism. *Proc. Natl. Acad. Sci. USA* 78:6535–6539

Mansour, A., H. Khachaturian, M. E. Lewis, H. Akil, and S. J. Watson, 1987. Autoradiographic differentiation of mu, delta, and kappa opioid receptors in the rat forebrain and midbrain. *J. Neurosci.* 7:2445–2464.

Mansour, A., H. Khachaturian, M. E. Lewis, H. Akil, and S. J. Watson, 1988. Anatomy of CNS opioid receptors. *TINS* 11:308–314.

Maragos, W. F., J. B. Penney, and A. B. Young, 1988. Anatomic correlation of NMDA and ³H-TCP-labeled receptors in rat brain. *J. Neurosci.* 8:493–501.

Martres, M.-P., M.-L. Bouthenet, N. Sales, P. Sokoloff, and J.-C. Schwartz, 1985a. Widespread distribution of brain dopamine receptors evidenced with [¹²⁵I]iodosulpride, a highly selective ligand. *Science* 228:752–755.

Martres, M.-P., N. Sales, M.-L. Bouthenet, and J.-C. Schwartz, 1985b. Localization and pharmacological characterization of D-2 dopamine receptors in rat cerebral neocortex and cerebellum using [¹²⁵I]iodosulpride. *Eur. J. Pharmacol.* 11:211–219.

Matsuyama, T., P. G. M. Luiten, D. G. Spencer, and A. D. Strosberg, 1988. Ultrastructural localization of immunoreactive sites for muscarinic acetylcholine receptor proteins in the rat cerebral cortex. *Neurosci. Res. Communications* 2:69–76.

Maurer, R., and J. C. Reubi, 1985. Brain somatostatin receptor subpopulation visualized by autoradiography. *Brain Res.* 333:178–181.

Mayer, M. L., and G. L. Westbrook, 1987. The physiology of excitatory amino acids in the vertebrate central nervous system. *Progr. Neurobiol.* 28:197–276.

Mayo, W., B. Dubois, A. Ploska, F. Javoy-Agid, Y. Agid, M. Le Moal, and H. Simon, 1984. Cortical cholinergic projections from the basal forebrain of the rat, with special reference to the prefrontal cortex innervation. *Neurosci. Lett.* 47:149–154.

McCarty, R., and L. M. Plunkett, 1987. Quantitative autoradiographic analysis of somatostatin binding sites in discrete areas of rat forebrain. *Brain Res. Bull.* 18:29–34.

McCulloch, J., and P. A. T. Kelly, 1983. A functional role for vasoactive intestinal polypeptide in the anterior cingulate cortex. *Nature* 304:438–440.

McCulloch, J., P. A. T. Kelly, R. Uddman, and L. Edvinsson, 1983. Functional role for vasoactive intestinal polypeptide in the caudate nucleus: A 2-deoxy[¹⁴C]glucose investigation. *Proc. Natl. Acad. Sci. USA* 80:1472–1476.

McDonald, J. K., J. G. Parnavelas, A. N. Karamanlidis, and N. Brecha, 1982a. The morphology and distribution of peptide-containing neurons in adult and developing visual cortex of the rat. II. Vasoactive intestinal polypeptide. *J. Neurocytol.* 11:825–837.

McDonald, J. K., J. G. Parnavelas, A. N. Karamanlidis, N. Brecha, and J. I. Koenig, 1982b. The morphology and distribution of peptide-containing neurons in the adult and developing visual cortex of the rat. I. Somatostatin. *J. Neurocytol.* 11:809–824.

McDonald, J. K., J. G. Parnavelas, A. N. Karamanlidis, G. Rosenquist, and N. Brecha, 1982c. The morphology and distribution of peptide-containing neurons in the adult and developing visual cortex of the rat. III. Cholecystokinin. *J. Neurocytol.* 11:881–895.

McGinty, J. F., D. van der Kooy, and F. E. Bloom, 1984. The distribution and morphology of opioid peptide immunoreactive neurons in the cerebral cortex of rats. *J. Neurosci.* 4:1104–1117.

McKinney, M., J. T. Coyle, and J. C. Hedreen, 1983. Topographic analysis of the innervation of the rat neocortex and hippocampus by the basal forebrain cholinergic system. *J. Comp. Neurol.* 217:103–121.

McLean, S., R. B. Rothman, and M. Herkenham, 1986. Autoradiographic localization of μ- and δ-opiate receptors in the forebrain of the rat. *Brain Res.* 378:49–60.

Meinecke, D. L., and A. Peters, 1986. Somatostatin immunoreactive neurons in rat visual cortex: A light and electron microscopic study. *J. Neurocytol.* 15:121–136.

Meinecke, D. L., and A. Peters, 1987. GABA immunoreactive neurons in rat visual cortex. *J. Comp. Neurol.* 261:388–404.

Mizukawa, K., P. L. McGeer, S. R. Vincent, and E. G. McGeer, 1987. The distribution of somatostatin-immunoreactive neurons and fibers in the rat cerebral cortex: Light and electron microscopic studies. *Brain Res.* 426:28–36.

Monaghan, D. T., and C. W. Cotman, 1982. The distribution of [^{3}H]kainic acid binding sites in rat CNS as determined by autoradiography. *Brain Res.* 252:91–100.

Monaghan, D. T., and C. W. Cotman, 1985. Distribution of N-methyl-D-aspartate-sensitive L-[^{3}H]glutamate binding sites in rat brain. *J. Neurosci.* 5:2909–2919.

Monaghan, D. T., D. Yao, and C. W. Cotman, 1984. Distribution of [^{3}H]AMPA binding sites in rat brain as determined by quantitative autoradiography. *Brain Res.* 324:160–164.

Morrison, J. H., R. Grzanna, M. E. Molliver, and J. T. Coyle, 1978. The distribution and orientation of noradrenergic fibers in neocortex of the rat: An immunofluorescence study. *J. Comp. Neurol.* 181:17–40.

Morrison, J. H., P. J. Magistretti, R. Benoit, and F. E. Bloom, 1984. The distribution and morphological characteristics of the intracortical VIP-cell: An immunohistochemical analysis. *Brain Res.* 292:269–282.

Mugnaini, E., and W. H. Oertel, 1985. An atlas of the distribution of GABAergic neurons and terminals in the rat CNS as revealed by GAD immunohistochemistry. In *Handbook of Chemical Neuroanatomy, Vol. 4. GABA and Neuropeptides in the CNS, Part I.* A. Björklund and T. Hökfelt (eds). Amsterdam: Elsevier, pp. 436–608.

Naus, C. C. G., F. D. Miller, J. H. Morrison, and F. E. Bloom, 1988. Immunohistochemical and in situ hybridization analysis of the development of the rat somatostatin-containing neocortical neuronal system. *J. Comp. Neurol.* 269:448–463.

Nishimura, Y., M. Natori, and M. Mato, 1988. Choline acetyltransferase immunopositive pyramidal neurons in the rat frontal cortex. *Brain Res.* 440:144–148.

Oades, R. D., and G. M. Halliday, 1987. Ventral tegmental (A10) system: Neurobiology. I. Anatomy and connectivity. *Brain Res.Rev.* 12:117–165.

Olpe, H. R., A. Glatt, J. Laszlo, and A. Schellenberg, 1980. Some electrophysiological and pharmacological properties of the cortical noradrenergic projection of the locus coeruleus in the rat. *Brain Res. Rev.* 186:9–19.

Ottersen, O. P., and J. Storm-Mathisen, 1984. Glutamate- and GABA-containing neurons in the mouse and rat brain, as demonstrated with a new immunocytochemical technique. *J. Comp. Neurol.* 229:374–392.

Palacios, J. M., and M. J. Kuhar, 1980. Beta-adrenergic-receptor localization by light microscopic autoradiography. *Science* 208:1378–1380.

Palacios, J. M., and M. J. Kuhar, 1982. Beta adrenergic receptor localization in rat brain by light microscopic autoradiography. *Neurochem. Internat.* 4:473–490.

Palacios, J. M., and A. Pazos, 1987. Visualization of dopamine receptors: A progress review. In *Dopamine Receptors*. I. Creese and C. M. Frazer (eds). New York: A. Liss, pp. 175–197.

Palacios, J. M., and J. K. Wamsley, 1984. Catecholamine receptors. In *Handbook of Chemical Neuroanatomy, Vol. 3: Classical Transmitters and Transmitter Receptors in the CNS, Part II*. A. Björklund, T. Hökfelt, and M. J. Kuhar (eds). Amsterdam, New York, Oxford: Elsevier, pp. 325–351.

Palacios, J. M., D. Hoyer, and R. Cortés, 1987. α_1-adrenoreceptors in the mammalian brain: Similar pharmacology but different distribution in rodents and primates. *Brain Res.* 419:65–75.

Palacios, J. M. J. K. Wamsley, and M. J. Kuhar, 1981. High affinity GABA receptors— autoradiographic localization. *Brain Res.* 222:285–307.

Palkovits, M., L. Záborsky, M. J. Brownstein, M. I. K. Fekete, J. P. Herman, and B. Kanyicska, 1979. Distribution of norepinephrine and dopamine in cerebral cortical areas of the rat. *Brain Res. Bull.* 4:593–601.

Papadopoulos, G. C., J G. Parnavelas, and R. M. Buijs, 1987a. Monoaminergic fibers form conventional synapses in the cerebral cortex. *Neurosci. Lett.* 76:275–279.

Papadopoulos, G. C., J G. Parnavelas, and R. M. Buijs, 1987b. Light and electron microscopic immunocytochemical analysis of the serotonin innervation of the rat visual cortex. *J. Neurocytol.* 16:883–892.

Papadopoulos, G. C., J G. Parnavelas, and M. E. Cavanagh, 1987c. Extensive co-existence of neuropeptides in the rat visual cortex. *Brain Res.* 420:95–99

Parnavelas, G., and J. K. McDonald, 1983. The cerebral cortex. In *Chemical Neuroanatomy*. P. C. Emson (ed.) New York: Raven Press, pp. 505–549.

Parnavelas, J. G., H. C. Moises, and S. G. Speciale, 1985. The monoaminergic innervation of the rat visual cortex. *Proc. R. Soc. London B* 223:319–329.

Parnavelas, J. G., W. Kelly, E. Franke, and F. Eckenstein, 1986. Cholinergic neurons and fibres in the rat visual cortex. *J. Neurocytol.* 15:329–336.

Patel, S., B. S. Meldrum, and J. F. Collins, 1986. Distribution of [^{3}H]kainic acid and binding sites in the rat brain: In vivo and in vitro receptor autoradiography. *Neurosci. Lett.* 70:301–307.

Pazos, A., and J. M. Palacios, 1985. Quantitative autoradiographic mapping of serotonin receptors in the rat brain. I. Serotonin-1 receptors. *Brain Res.* 346:205–230.

Pazos, A., R. Cortés, and J. M. Palacios, 1985. Quantitative autoradiographic mapping of serotonin receptors in the rat brain. II. Serotonin-2 receptors. *Brain Res.* 346:231–249.

Peinado, J. M., and F. Mora, 1986. Glutamic acid as a putative transmitter of the inter-hemispheric corticocortical connections in the rat. *J. Neurochem.* 47:1598–1603.

Penny, G. R., S. Afsharpour, and S. T. Kitai, 1986. Substance P–immunoreactive neurons in the neocortex of the rat: A subset of the glutamic acid decarboxylase-immunoreactive neurons. *Neurosci. Lett.* 65:53–59.

Pérez-Clausell, J., and G. Danscher, 1985. Intravesicular localization of zinc in rat telencephalic boutons. A histochemical study. *Brain Res.* 337:91–98.

Peters, A, and L. M. Kimerer, 1981. Bipolar neurons in rat visual cortex. A combined Golgi-electron microscopic study. *J. Neurocytol.* 9:163–183.

Peers, A., and K. M. Harriman, 1988. Enigmatic bipolar cell of rat visual cortex. *J. Comp. Neurol.* 267:409–432.

Peters, A., C. C. Proskauer, and C. E. Ribak, 1982. Chandelier cells in rat visual cortex. *J. Comp. Neurol.* 206:397–416.

Phillipson, O. T., I. C. Kilpatrick, and M. W. Jones, 1987. Dopaminergic innervation of the primary visual cortex in the rat, and some correlations with human cortex. *Brain Res. Bull.* 18:621—633.

Phillis, J. W., and J. R. Kirkpatrick, 1980. The actions of motilin, luteinizing hormone releasing hormone, cholecystokinin, somatostatin, vasoactive intestinal peptide, and other peptides on rat cerebral cortical neurons. *Can. J. Physiol. Pharmacol.* 58.612–621.

Pittaluga, A., and M. Raiteri, 1987. GABAergic nerve terminals in rat hippocampus possess α_2-adrenoceptors regulating GABA release. *Neurosci. Lett.* 76:363–367.

Poulin, P., Y. Suzuki, K. Lederis, and O. P. Rorstadt, 1986. Autoradiographic localizaion of binding sites for vasoactive intestinal peptide (VIP) in bovine cerebral arteries. *Brain Res.* 381:382–384.

Quirion, R., J. Richard, and T. V. Dam, 1985. Evidence for the existence of serotonin tpe-2 receptors on cholinergic terminals in rat cortex. *Brain Res.* 333:345–349.

Rainbow, T. C., B. Parson, and B. B. Wolfe, 1984a. Quantitative autoradiography of β_1- and β_2-adrenergic receptors in rat brain. *Poc. Natl. Acad. Sci. USA* 81:1585–1589.

Rainbow, T. C., C. M. Wieczorek, and S. Halpain, 1984b. Quantitative autoradiography of binding sites for [^{3}H]AMPA, a structural analogue of glutamic acid. *Brain Res.* 309:173–177.

Reader, T. A. 1981. Distribution of catecholamines and serotonin in the rat cerebral cortex: Absolute levels and relative proportions. *J. Neural Transmission* 50: 13–27.

Ribak, C. E., 1978. Aspinous and sparsely-spinous stellate neurons in the visual cortex of rats contain glutamic acid decarboxylase. *J. Neurocytol.* 7:461–478.

Rieck, R., and R. G. Carey, 1984. Evidence of a laminar organization of basal forebrain afferents ot the visual cortex. *Brain Res.* 297:374–380.

Rostène, W. H., 1984. Neurobiological and neuroendocrine functions of the vasoactive intestinal peptide (VIP). *Progr. Neurobiol.* 22:103–129.

Said, S. I., 1982. Vasodilator action of VIP: Introduction and general considerations. In *Vasoactive Intestinal Peptide*. S. I. Said (ed), New York: Raven Press, pp. 145–148.

Satoh, K., D. M. Armstrong, and H. C. Fibiger, 1983. A comparison of the distribution of central cholinergic neurons as demonstrated by acetylcholinesterase pharmacohisto-chemistry and choline acetyltransferase immunohistochemistry. *Brain Res. Bull.* 11:693–720.

Savaki, H. E., M. Desban, J. Glowinski, and M. J. Besson, 1983. Local cerebral glucose consumption in the rat. II. Effects of unilateral substantia nigra stimulation in the conscious and in halothane-anesthetized animals. *J. Comp. Neurol.* 213:46–65.

Schaad, N. C., M. Schorderet, and P. J. Magistretti, 1987. Prostaglandins and the synergism between VIP and noradrenaline in the cerebral cortex. *Nature* 328:637–640.

Scheel, M., 1988. Topographic organization of the auditory thalamocortical system in the albino rat. *Anat. Embryol.* 179:181–190.

Schmechel, D. E., B. G. Vickrey, D. Fitzpatrick, and R. P. Elde, 1984. GABAergic neurons of mammalian cerebral cortex: Widespread subclass defined by somatostatin content. *Neurosci. Lett.* 47:227–232.

Schröder, H., K. Zilles, A. Maelicke, and F. Hajös, (in press a). Immunohistochemical localization of cortical nicotinic cholinreceptors in rat and man. *Brain Research*.

Schröder, H., K. Zilles, P. G. Luiten, and A. D. Strosberg, (in press b). Human cortical neurons contain both nicotinic and muscarinic acetylcholine receptors—an immunohistochemical double-labelling study. *Synapse*.

Schröder, H., K. Zilles, P. G. Luiten, and A. D. Strosberg, (in press c). Immunocyto-chemical visualization of muscarinic cholinoreceptors in the human cerebral cortex. *Brain Research*.

Schwartz, R. D., 1986. Autoradiographic distribution of high affinity muscarinic and and nicotinic cholinergic receptors labeled with [^{3}H]acetylcholine in rat brain. *Life Science* 38:2111–2119.

Sekiguchi, R., and T. Moroji, 1986. A comparative study on characterization and distribution of cholecystokinin binding sites among the rat, mouse and Guinea pig brain. *Brain Res.* 399:271–281.

Sims, K. B., D. L. Hoffman, S. I. Said, E. A. Zimmerman, 1980. Vasoactive intestinal polypeptide (VIP) in mouse and rat brain. An immunocytological study. *Brain Res.* 186:165–183.

Sokoloff, L., 1981. Relationship among local functional activity, energy metabolism, and blood flow in the central nervous system. *Fed. Proc.* 40:2311–2316.

Sokoloff, L., 1982. The radioactive deoxyglucose method: Theory, procedure, and application for the local cerebral glucose utilization in the central nervous system. *Adv. Neurochem.* 4:7–36.

Sokoloff, L., M. Reivich, C. Kennedy, M. H. DesRosiers, C. S. Patlak, K. D. Pettigrew, O. Sakurada, and M. Shinohara, 1977. The (^{14}C)deoxyglucose method for the measurement of local cerebral glucose utilization: Theory, procedure, and normal values in the conscious and anaesthetized albino rat. *J. Neurochem.* 28:897–917.

Spencer, D. G., E. Horváth, and J. Traber, 1986. Direct autoradiographic determination of M1 and M2 muscarinic acetylcholine receptor distribution in the rat brain; Relation to cholinergic nuclei and projections. *Brain Res.* 380:59–68.

Staun-Olsen, P., B. Ottesen, S. Gammeltoft, and J. Fahrenkrug, 1985. The regional distribution of receptors for vasoactive intestinal polypeptide (VIP) in the rat central nervous system. *Brain Res.* 330:317–321.

Streit, P., 1984. Glutamate and aspartate as transmitter candidates for systems of the cerebral cortex. In *Cerebral Cortex*, Vol. 2. A. Peters and E. G. Jones (eds). New York and London: Plenum Press, pp. 119–143.

Swanson, L. W., D. M. Simmons, P. J. Whiting, and J. Lindstrom, 1987. Immunohistochemical localization of neuronal nicotinic receptors in the rodent central nervous system. *J. Neurosci.* 7:3334–3342.

Takeuchi, A., 1987. The transmitter role of glutamate in nervous systems. *Japan. J. Physiol.* 37:559–572.

Timm, F., 1958. Zur Histochemie der Schwermetalle. Das Sulfid-Silberverfahren. *Dt. Zschr. gerichtl. Med.* 46:706–711.

Toga, A. W., and R. Collins, 1981. Metabolic response of optic centers to visual stimuli in the albino rat: Anatomical and physiological considerations. *J. Comp. Neurol.* 199:433–464.

Tohyama, M., T. Maeda, and N. Shimizu, 1974. Detailed noradrenaline pathways of locus coeruleus neuron to the cerebral cortex with use of 6-hydroxydopa. *Brain Res.* 79:139–144.

Vogt, B. A., B. Townes Anderson, and D. L. Burns, 1987. Dissociated cingulate cortical neurons: Morphology and muscarinic acetylcholine receptor binding properties. *J. Neurosci.* 7:959–971.

Wamsley, J. K., M. A. Zarbin, N. J. M. Birdsall, and M. J. Kuhar, 1980. Muscarinic cholinergic receptors: Autoradiographic localization of high and low affinity agonist binding sites. *Brain Res.* 200:1–12.

Waterhouse, B. D., H. C. Moises, and D. J. Woodward, 1981. Alpha-receptor-mediated facilitation of somatosensory cortical neuronal responses to excitatory synaptic inputs and iontophoretically applied acetylcholine. *Neuropharmacology* 20:907–920.

Waterhouse, B. D., H. C. Moises, H. H. Yeh, and D. C. Woodward, 1982. Norepinephrine enhancement of inhibitory synaptic mechanisms in cerebellum and cerebral cortex: Mediation by β-adrenergic receptors. *J. Pharmac. Exp. Ther.* 221:495–506.

Woolf, N. J., F. Eckenstein, and L. L. Butcher, 1983. Cholinergic projections from the basal forebrain to the frontal cortex: A combined fluorescent tracer and immunohistochemical analysis in the rat. *Neurosci. Lett.* 40:93–98.

Woolf, N. J., M. C. Hernit, and L. L. Butcher, 1986. Cholinergic and noncholinergic projections from the rat basal forebrain revealed by combined choline acetyltransferase and *Phaseolus vulgaris* leucoagglutinin immunohistochemistry. *Neurosci. Lett.* 66:281–286.

Wree, A., A. Schleicher, K. Zilles, and T. Beck, 1988. Local cerebral glucose utilization in the Ammon's horn and dentate gyrus of the rat brain. *Histochemistry* 88:415–426.

Wree, A., K. Zilles, and A. S. Schleicher, (in press). Local cerebral glucose utilization in the neocortical areas of the rat brain. *Anat. Embryol.*

Young, W. S., and M. J. Kuhar, 1980. Noradrenergic α1 and α2 receptors: Light microscopic autoradiographic localization. *Proc. Natl. Acad. Sci. USA* 77:1696–1700.

Zarbin, M. A., R. B. Innis, J. K. Wamsley, S. H. Snyder, and M. J. Kuhar, 1983. Autoradiographic localization of cholecystokinin receptors in rodent brain. *J. Neurosci.* 3:877–906.

Zilles, K., 1985a. *The Cerebral Cortex of the Rat. A Stereotaxic Atlas.* Berlin, Heidelberg, New York. Springer-Verlag.

Zilles, K., 1985b. Morphological studies on brain structures of the NZB mouse: An animal model for the aging human brain? In *Senile Dementia of the Alzheimer Type.* J. Traber and W. H. Gispen (eds). Berlin, Heidelberg: Springer-Verlag, pp. 355–365.

Zilles, K., and A. Wree, 1985. Cortex: Areal and laminar structure. In *The Rat Nervous System, Vol. 1.* G. Paxinos (ed). Sydney, New York, London: Academic Press, pp. 375–416.

Zilles, K., A. Schleicher, T. Glaser, J. Traber, and M. Rath, 1985a. The ontogenetic development of serotonin (5-HT$_1$) receptors in various cortical regions of the rat brain. *Anat. Embryol.* 172:255–264.

Zilles, K., A. Wree, A. Schleicher, and I. Divac, 1985b. The monocular and binocular subfields of the rat's primary visual cortex. A quantitative morphological approach. *J. Comp. Neurol.* 226:391–402.

Zilles, K., A. Schleicher, M. Rath, and A. Bauer, 1988. Quantitative receptor autoradiography in the human brain. Methodical aspects. *Histochemistry* 90:129–137.

6

An Introduction to the Electrical Activity of the Cerebral Cortex: Relations to Behavior and Control by Subcortical Inputs

Cornelius H. Vanderwolf

It is a capital mistake to theorize before one has data. Insensibly one begins to twist facts to suit theories instead of theories to suit facts. (Sherlock Holmes in *Scandal in Bohemia*)

6.1 Neural Basis of the Electrocorticogram

An electrode placed anywhere on or in the mammalian cerebral cortex reveals spontaneous variations in electrical potential occurring at relatively low frequencies (mostly in the range of 1 Hz to 50 Hz) and with an amplitude of no more than 3 mV to 4 mV (usually in range of 0.1 mV to 2.0 mV). Sensory stimuli may result in an electrical potential (evoked potential) that is similar to some of the components of the spontaneous electrocorticogram. Evidence accumulating over the past 50 years has indicated that these macropotentials are primarily due to slow potential changes that occur in neuronal dendrites and somata as a result of synaptic activity. Synaptic activity, however, does not necessarily give rise to macropotentials of the type seen in mammalian cerebral cortex. For example, the neural ganglia in invertebrates such as lobsters, crabs, or insects generally do not generate significant slow wave activity despite the presence of an abundance of spontaneous action potentials. Similarly the mammalian spinal cord and cerebellum generate very little spontaneous slow wave activity.

As a first step in understanding this, imagine that a synaptic input has opened ion channels in a limited region of the apical dendrite of an elongated neuron such as a cortical pyramidal cell. Positive current, entering the cell in the form of Na^+ or Ca^{++} ions, tends to be conducted throughout the interior of the cell because the cytoplasm has an electrical resistance much lower than that of the fatty cell membrane outside the active synaptic zone. Current also escapes through the cell membrane, however, partly as a resistive flow and partly as a capacitative flow, and returns to the active synaptic zone by an extracellular route. This extracellular current flows through multiple pathways in accordance with the electrical properties of the cells, membranes, and fluid spaces surrounding the active cell. As a result the extracellular current flow is very diffuse compared with the intracellular current flow, which is confined to a narrow channel. Current flowing through the resistance imposed by the extracellular elements results in a voltage that can be detected by an electrode placed at a considerable distance from the active cell. Because the current flow at any given point outside the active cell is only a fraction of the total current flow generated by the active synaptic zone, the extracellular potential is small compared with the potential recorded by an intracellular electrode.

The geometry of the active neuron is an important determinant of the extent of current flow in remote regions. Imagine a cell whose dendrites are arranged radially in a spherical configuration. Imagine further an active dendritic synaptic zone localized as a concentric shell about the cell soma. In such a situation current flows would tend to be confined to the region enclosed by the dendrites, and an electrode placed some distance away from the cell might fail to detect any potential change at all. These considerations suggest that elongated cells, such as the pyramidal cells of the neocortex or of the hippocampal formation, are more likely than the more spherical local circuit neurons to generate large field potentials.

If local synaptic activity (in an apical dendrite of a pyramidal cell, for example) results in the entry of positive charge into a cell, the affected region is termed an *active sink* because the cell membrane actively changes in conductance. The region in which current leaves the cell—probably mainly the soma, the initial segment of the axon, and the basal dendrites in this case—is referred to as a *passive source* of current because the properties of the membrane are not actively changed. A source-sink pair is often referred to as a *dipole*. An extracellular electrode placed near the active sink will record a negative potential (positive charges are moving away from the electrode and into the dendrite), whereas an extracellular electrode placed near the passive source will record a positive potential. Between the zone in which a negative potential can be recorded and the zone in which a positive potential can be recorded, there may be a narrow null zone in which no potential at all can be detected (figure 6.1). Immediately after an excitatory input to the apical dendrite, the cell in our example may receive an inhibitory input to the cell soma. In this case the cell soma might constitute an active source if local synaptic action results in an outflow of positive charge (local hyperpolarization). A nearby extracellular electrode would detect positivity, whereas an extracellular electrode near a remote dendrite region of the same cell might detect negativity due to the presence of a passive sink. These examples show that the mere presence of local negative or positive extracellular potentials does not constitute evidence for the existence of local zones of active depolarization of hyperpolarization. The situation is further complicated by evidence that both dendrites and cell somata can display either active depolarization or active hyperpolarization.

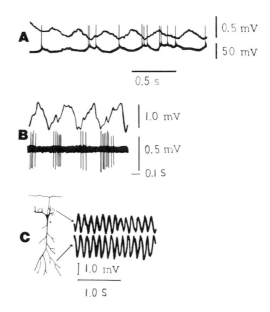

Figure 6.1 Various aspects of hippocampal electrophysiology. (A) Upper trace, extracellular slow wave activity recorded from the CA4 pyramidal cell layer; lower trace, intracellular record from a CA4 pyramidal cell. Positive potentials go upward. Note that both the extracellular potential and the membrane potential show spontaneous slow fluctuations. Hyperpolarization of the cell is synchronized with a positive extracellular potential, and depolarization of the cell (often sufficient to produce an action potential) is synchronized with a negative extracellular potential. (Redrawn from Fujita and Sato 1964.) (B) Upper trace, extracellular potential recorded from the molecular (dendritic) layer of the dentate gyrus; lower trace extracellular unitary action potentials recorded from the dentate cell layer. Note that unit spikes occur in bursts immediately afer maximum negativity in the molecular layer. This negativity is probably due, at least in part, to depolarization of granule cell dendrites. (Redrawn from Colom and Bland 1987.) (C) Sketch of a CA1 pyramidal cell together with records of RSA derived from the basal dendritic layer of CA1 (stratum oriens) and from near the terminal branches of the apical dendrites of CA1 (stratum moleculare). Note that the two records are 180° out of phase; positive potentials occur in stratum oriens in synchrony with negative potentials in stratum moleculare and vice versa. In a null zone, marked by a dot, no RSA is recorded. (Records are redrawn from Whishaw et al. 1976.) The extracellular RSA appears to be due to superimposed potentials originating from both hippocampal pyramidal cells and dentate granule cells.

Extracellular currents generated by synaptic potentials in a single neuron are rather small. Consequently significant extracellular potentials appear only if the currents from large numbers of cells can summate. This can happen if (1) elongated cells are arranged parallel to one another, like trees in a forest, and (2) if the same type of synaptic activity occurs synchronously in large numbers of cells. If cells have different types of synaptic activity at the same time, the extracellular currents might cancel one another. All the necessary conditions are met in the case of hippocampal and neocortical pyramidal cells, which are elongated, arranged in parallel, and often active in synchrony. Consequently the hippocampus and neocortex give rise to prominent extracellular slow wave activity. If cells are depolarized and hyperpolarized in a nonsynchronized manner, one might expect to see low-amplitude field potentials. This is the traditional explanation of the occurrence of low-voltage fast activity (LVFA) in the neocortex (figure 6.2), leading to the term *desynchronized activity* for this waveform. Similarly, irregular slow waves or spindles are sometimes referred to as *synchronized activity*. As mentioned, the mammalian cerebellar cortex does not generate a slow electrocorticogram despite the existence of large numbers of Purkinje cells, which are elongated, arranged in parallel, and have very extensive dendrites. One suggested explanation of this puzzle (and the related puzzle of the absence of slow waves in invertebrate ganglia) is that neighboring neurons in structures such as the cerebellum show little tendency toward synchronized activity. If this explanation is correct, another fundamental question presents itself. What advantage (if any) is there in having synchronized neural activity in the cerebral cortex?

In both the hippocampus and the neocortex, slow wave activity sometimes consists of rather irregular waves, whereas at other times highly rhythmical activity occurs (figures 6.1, 6.2, and 6.3). Thus in the hippocampus the rhythmical activity consists of a nearly sinusoidal waveform of about 4 Hz to 12 Hz (rhythmical slow activity, or RSA). This waveform has been accounted for on the basis of the properties of networks of neurons. It is assumed that the axons of pyramidal cells possess collaterals that excite interneurons (figure 6.4). Many of these interneurons have an inhibitory effect, probably mediated by γ-aminobutyric acid, which affects a number of pyramidal cells, including those that excited the interneuron in the first place. Thus if a pyramidal cell fires as a result of a dendritic excitatory postsynaptic potential, it will immediately afterward become hyperpolarized, and firing will cease. Nearby pyramidal cells that did not fire may also be hyperpolarized. Because the pyramidal cells have ceased firing, the inhibitory interneuron also becomes quiescent, allowing the entire cycle to be repeated. The result is that pyramidal cells alternately depolarize and hyperpolarize in synchrony, giving rise to prominent rhythmical extracellular slow waves.

LOW VOLTAGE
FAST ACTIVITY

SPINDLE

IRREGULAR
SLOW
ACTIVITY

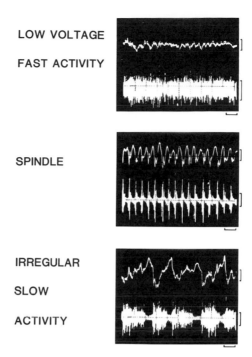

Figure 6.2 Slow waves and multiunit activity (MUA) recorded simultaneously from a bipolar surface-to-depth (layer V) electrode pair in parietal neocortex in a rat. Unit activity is derived from the deep electrode. Deep positivity (surface negativity) is indicated by an upward deflection. Note that during low-voltage fast activity (LVFA), MUA occurs as a continuous discharge. During spindle activity brief rhythmical bursts of MUA occur in phase with the deep negative component of the slow waves, presumably as a result of synchronized depolarization of neural dendrites and somata lying near the deep electrode. Long-lasting suppression of MUA occurs during the deep positive component of the slow waves. Presumably this component is due to synchronized hyperpolarization of local neural somata and dendrites. During large-amplitude irregular slow activity, long duration bursts of MUA are interrupted by arrhythmic periods of MUA suppression that correlate with deep positive waves (presumably arising from hyperpolarization of neural dendrites and somata). Note that spindle activity reliably recruits the largest units detected by the electrode. Calibration, 0.5 mV for slow waves, 0.050 mV for MUA, 200 ms. (From Vanderwolf 1988)

A
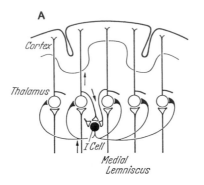

B
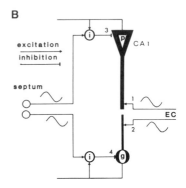

Figure 6.3 Neural models proposed to explain the origin of rhythmical slow waves. (A) A scheme suggesting that recurrent inhibition in the thalamus results in synchronized activity in thalamocortical fibers, which in turn produce synchronized rhythmical activity in neocortical cells. When thalamic cells fire in response to an excitatory input (from medial lemniscus) they are immediately silenced by inhibitory interneurons (I cell) that had been excited by an input from the thalamic cells. The I cells then fall silent because they no longer receive an excitatory input, allowing the entire cycle to be repeated. (From Andersen and Eccles 1962) Later research has shown that the hypothetical I cells may be located in the thalamic reticular nucleus (Steriade et al 1985). (B) A more complex model designed to account for hippocampal RSA, as proposed by Buzsáki and colleagues (1983). This model assumes four independent rhythmical inputs (1–4), each of which is capable of generating field RSA. Inputs to the same neurons are nearly synchronous (1–3 and 2–4), but inputs to the pyramidal cells (p) and granule cells (g) are phase shifted. i = inhibitory interneuron. Inputs from the septal nuclei are assumed to be cholinergic, whereas the entorhinal input may be glutaminergic. Evidence discussed in the text raises the possibility that the entorhinal input is strongly facilitated by a serotonergic input. Further improvements in this type of model have been proposed by Leung (1984).

There is evidence that such cyclical processes occur in the thalamus as well as in the neocortex and hippocampus. In the thalamus the result is a series of rhythmical bursts of action potentials in thalamocortical fibers that drive rhythmical activities in the neocortex such as spindle waves or the alpha rhythm (figure 6.2). Thus thalamic cells act as pacemakers for the rhythmical cortical potentials. Similarly there is evidence that rhythmical bursts in septohippocampal fibers drive the rhythmical waves of RSA in the hippocampus. Rhythmical firing in the perforant path input from the entorhinal cortex to the hippocampus and dentate gyrus also appears to contribute to RSA (figure 6.4). There may be additional collateral inhibitory circuits in both neocortex and hippocampus that contribute to the observed rhythms. A further possibility is that some cells in the thalamus (and perhaps in other sites)

Organization of the Neocortex

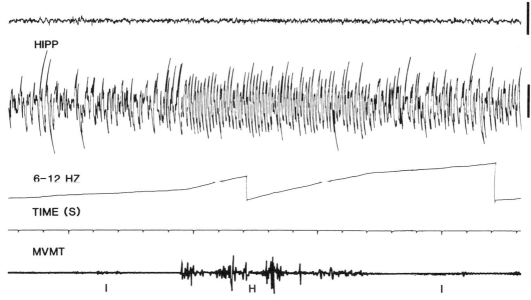

Figure 6.4 Hippocampal and neocortical activity in relation to behavior in a normal rat. CTX = sensorimotor neocortex; HIPP = dorsal hippocampus; 6-12 Hz = 6-Hz to 12-Hz activity from hippocampus integrated over 10-s periods, time in seconds; MVMT = output from a magnet-and-coil type of movement sensor; I = behavioral immobility; H = spontaneous head movement, calibration in millivolts. Note the presence of hippocampal rhythmical slow activity (RSA) and an increase in the slope of integrated 6-Hz to 12-Hz activity during head movement, while large-amplitude irregular activity (LIA) occurs during immobility. Low-voltage fast activity (LVFA) is present in the neocortex during both immobility and movement.

possess inherently rhythmical processes in the cell membrane. Such cells could act as pacemakers of cerebral rhythms, much as cells in the sinoatrial node pace the beating of the heart.

It is apparent that simple models of the type illustrated in figure 6.4 do not go very far in accounting for the origin of brain waves. The suggested circuits may account for rhythmical waveforms, but do not account for irregular waveforms or explain how the same tissue can generate quite different waveforms at different times.

6.2   Introduction to Cerebral Activity and Behavior

The following sections deal with the relations between behavior and the electrocorticogram, the cortical evoked potentials, and the unit activity that is correlated with these macropotentials. A central concept in the discussion is that many aspects of cerebral activity vary in close correlation with concurrent motor activity. Second, behavior-related variations in cerebral macropotentials are largely due to the joint action of ascending cholinergic and serotonergic projections, which exert a strong control over the activity of the cerebral cortex. As a result of this, blockade of central cholinergic and serotonergic neurotransmission produces severe generalized disturbances in the control of adaptive behavior.

The foregoing concepts depart sharply from the commonly held views in this field. For the past three decades, and longer, research on the electrocorticogram and the general physiology of the cerebral hemispheres has been dominated by two intertwined theories: (1) cerebral electrical activity is closely related to consciousness and the sleep-wake cycle, and (2) a reticulothalamocortical pathway, involving the intralaminar nuclei of the thalamus, plays the major role in the control of cortical electrical activity. The first of these theories is of special importance because it has exerted a wide influence on brain research. It is commonly stated that the appearance of LVFA in the neocortex is related to wakefulness or consciousness, whereas the appearance of large amplitude irregular slow waves is related to sleep or coma. However, serious investigators of cerebral physiology have long been well aware that this interpretation does not agree with the facts. In the words of N. Kleitman (1963, p. 30), a pioneer in sleep research, "It is clear that the EEG by itself not only fails to gauge the depth of sleep but the very presence of behavioral sleep." M. Jouvet (1967, p. 119), another eminent sleep researcher, corroborates this: "Yet in no case does the state of the corticogram allow us to presume whether an animal is asleep or awake." In a critical review of data and hypotheses relating to conventional concepts of the reticular activating system, the electrocorticogram, and behavioral arousal, Vanderwolf and Robinson (1981, p. 461) conclude "that neocortical slow wave activity is not well correlated with arousal level or consciousness and, further, that the states of sleep and waking are not dependent on the integrity of the cerebral cortex or the ascending reticulocortical projections."

The process of solving scientific problems is sometimes compared with the work of a detective. Bearing this in mind, let us follow the advice of the master sleuth quoted at the beginning of the chapter (Doyle 1981) and begin at the beginning. What are the facts concerning the relation of cerebral macropotentials to behavior, and how can these facts be accounted for in terms of modern findings in neuroanatomy, neuropharmacology, and electrophysiology? The following sections present a synopsis of a recent, more extensive review of this field (Vanderwolf 1988). References are organized according to topic in table 6.1.

Table 6.1 Selected References on Cerebral Electrical Activity and Behavior

1. Genesis of brain waves, general reviews
    Andersen and Andersson 1968, Bullock and Basar 1988, Elul 1972,
    Purpura 1959, Shepherd 1977, Spencer 1977

2. Anatomy, physiology, and pharmacology of the hippocampal formation
    a. Reviews and symposia
    Bland 1986, Buzsáki and Vanderwolf 1985, Ciba Foundation Symposium
    1978, Isaacson and Pribram 1975 (vol. 1), 1986, Lopes da Silva and
    Arnolds 1978, Seifert 1983, Stumpf 1965

    b. Selected experimental papers
    Bland et al. 1975, 1980, Bland and Whishaw 1976, Fujita and Sato 1964,
    Leung and Yim 1986, Núñez et al. 1987, Vinogradova et al. 1980,
    Winson 1974

3. Hippocampus: Electrophysiology, pharmacology, and role in behavior
    a. Reviews and symposia
    Black 1975, Buzsáki and Vanderwolf 1985, Ciba Foundation Symposium
    1978, Isaacson and Pribram 1975, 1986 (vols. 2, 3, 4), Lopes da Silva and
    Arnolds 1978, O'Keefe 1979, O'Keefe and Nadel 1978, Robinson 1980,
    Seifert 1983, Vanderwolf 1988

    b. Selected experimental papers
    Arnolds et al. 1984, Buzsáki 1986, Buzsáki et al. 1981, 1983, Dudar et al.
    1979, Feder and Ranck 1973, Fox and Ranck 1981, Green and Arduini
    1954, Kolb and Whishaw 1977, Konopacki et al. 1987, Kramis et al.
    1975, Leung 1980, 1982, 1984, Leung et al. 1982, Muller and Kubie 1987,
    Muller et al. 1987, O'Keefe 1976, Ranck 1973, Robinson and Green 1980,
    Robinson et al. 1977, Rose 1983, Rowntree and Bland 1986, Sainsbury
    1970, Sainsbury et al. 1987, Stewart and Vanderwolf 1987a,b,
    Vanderwolf 1969, Vanderwolf and Baker 1986, Vanderwolf et al. 1985,
    Welsh et al. 1985, Whishaw 1972, Whishaw and Vanderwolf 1973,
    Whishaw et al. 1986, Winson 1972

4   Cingulate cortex: Electrophysiology and behavior
    Borst et al. 1987, Leung and Borst 1987

5. Neocortical electrophysiology

    a. Reviews
    Andersen and Andersson 1968, Elul 1972, Spencer 1977

    b. Selected experimental papers
    Ball et al. 1977, Calvet et al. 1964, 1973, Fox and O'Brien 1965, Ingvar
    1955, Jasper and Stefanis 1965, Kellaway et al. 1966, Moruzzi and
    Magoun 1949, Schaul et al. 1978, Spencer and Brookhart 1961a,b

6. Neocortex: Electrophysiology and pharmacology in relation to behavior
    a. Reviews
    Vanderwolf 1988, Vanderwolf and Robinson 1981

    b. Selected experimental papers
    Beyer and Sawyer 1964, Fleming and Bigler, 1974, Leung et al. 1982,
    Pickenhain and Klingberg 1965, Rougeul et al. 1972, Schwartzbaum and
    Kreinick 1973, Schwartzbaum et al. 1971, Starr 1964, Stewart et al. 1984,
    Vanderwolf 1984, Vanderwolf and Baker 1986, Vanderwolf et al. 1987,
    Vanderwolf and Pappas 1980, Vanderwolf et al. 1980

Table 6.1 (continued)

7. Thalamic control of the electrocorticogram
Andersen and Andersson 1968, Angeleri et al. 1969, Belardetti et al. 1977, Jahnsen and Llinás 1984a,b, Schlag and Chaillet 1963, Semba et al. 1980, Steriade et al. 1985, Vanderwolf and Stewart 1988, Villablanca and Salinas-Zeballos 1972

8. Brain cholinergic systems: Electrophysiology, anatomy, and role in behavior

a. Reviews
Butcher and Woolf 1986, Pepeu 1973, Vanderwolf 1988

b. Selected experimental papers
Armstrong et al. 1983, Belardetti et al. 1977, Bigl et al. 1982, Cuculic et al. 1968, Detari and Vanderwolf 1987, Detari et al. 1984, Divac 1975, Jasper and Tessier 1971, Johnston et al. 1981, Kanai and Szerb 1965, Lamour et al. 1984, 1986, Lehmann et al. 1980, Lewis and Shute 1967, LoConte et al. 1982, Saper 1984, Satoh and Fibiger 1986, Shute and Lewis 1967, Szerb 1967, Whishaw et al. 1985, Woolf and Butcher 1986

9. Brain serotonergic systems: Electrophysiology, anatomy, and role in behavior

a. Reviews
Azmitia 1978, Steinbusch and Nieuwenhuys 1983, Trulson and Jacobs 1981, Vanderwolf 1988

b. Selected experimental papers
Andén et al. 1966, Dahlström and Fuxe 1964, Lidov et al. 1980, McGinty et al. 1973, McGinty and Harper 1976, Rasmussen et al. 1984, Trulson and Jacobs 1979

10. The electrocorticogram, brainstem, sleep, and related neuropharmacology
Reviews
Jouvet 1967, 1972, Kleitman 1963, Moruzzi 1972, Pompeiano 1967, Siegel 1979, Steriade and Hobson 1976

11. Dopaminergic control of serotonin-dependent cerebral activity
Balfour and Iyaniwura 1985, Horn et al. 1971, Vanderwolf 1975, Vanderwolf and Stewart 1986

12. Neuropathology: Possible role of brain cholinergic and serotonergic systems in dementia, depression, schizophrenia, and phencyclidine-induced psychosis

a. Reviews
Hutton and Kenny 1985, Schaffer et al. 1980, Schiebel et al. 1986, Snyder 1980, Stahl et al. 1982, Weil-Malherbe 1978, Whitford 1986

b. Selected experimental papers
Bennett et al. 1979, Bowen et al. 1983, Crow et al. 1979, Davies and Maloney 1976, Fauman et al. 1976, Luby et al. 1959, Luisada 1978, Palmer et al. 1987, Vanderwolf 1987a,b, Whitehouse et al. 1981

6.3 Hippocampal Activity in Relation to Behavior

The rat provides an excellent subject for work in behavioral electrophysiology. Rat neuroanatomy, neuropharmacology, and behavior have been well studied in comparison with other laboratory animals, thus providing useful background information for electrophysiological work. Further, rats are convenient in size and can be raised and maintained with minimal cost. For these reasons most recent work in the field has made use of the rat.

Let us suppose that we have prepared a rat with chronic recording electrodes placed at appropriate sites in the neocortex and the hippocampus. We connect the electrodes to an appropriate recording device by means of a light, flexible cable and place the rat on a small platform connected to a movement-sensing device. The rat moves about freely and can also be induced to eat, drink, or go to sleep if the appropriate conditions are arranged. Figure 6.3 illustrates some of the phenomena that are observed. If the rat stands motionless with its head held up and eyes fully open, hippocampal activity consists of an irregular pattern of slow waves punctuated at irregular intervals by large-amplitude sharp waves (hippocampal "spikes"). Let us refer to this pattern as a whole as *large-amplitude irregular activity* (LIA). If the rat turns its head or walks across the platform, hippocampal activity changes to a pattern of RSA, with a frequency of about 7 Hz to 9 Hz. Sharp waves are totally suppressed. If, instead of walking, the rat sits up (supported by the hind legs and tail) and begins to wash its face, RSA is observed during the act of sitting up, but LIA appears during the rhythmical rubbing movements of the forepaws. LIA also occurs during chewing food, licking water, or chattering the teeth together (a defensive behavior seen in many rodents) but RSA always occurs during any kind of locomotion, stepping, or change in posture. Any type of sensory stimulus, painful or not, that elicits the latter type of movements elicits also RSA. Sensory stimuli that do not elicit such movements do not in general elicit RSA, even though they may elicit such behaviors as blinking, ear movement, the startle response, or prolonged immobility (freezing). Let us refer to the behaviors that are consistently accompanied by RSA as *type 1 behaviors* and those with no consistent relation to RSA as *type 2 behaviors* (figure 6.5). Usually type 2 behaviors are accompanied by LIA, but sometimes they are accompanied by RSA, for example, when type 1 and type 2 movements occur simultaneously. Moving the head while drinking water is an example of this.

More extensive investigations have revealed that the change from LIA to RSA is merely one aspect of a general change in hippocampal activity that correlates with the occurrence of type 1 behavior. Other indications of this change are (1) increases in 20-Hz to 60-Hz fast wave activity, (2) changes in evoked potentials, (3) increases in firing rate of "theta cells" (putative interneurons) in Ammon's horn, (4) decreases in

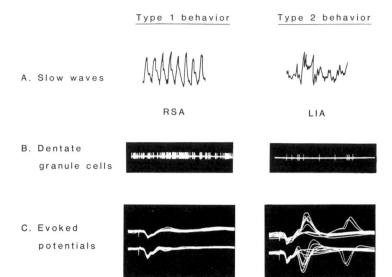

Figure 6.5 Hippocampal activity in relation to behavior in the rat. *Type 1 behavior* includes walking, running, jumping, swimming, rearing, digging, manipulation of objects with the forelimbs, isolated movements of the head or one limb, and shifts of posture. *Type 2 behavior* includes (1) alert immobility in any posture and (2) licking, chewing, chattering the teeth, sneezing, startle response, vocalization, shivering, tremor, face washing, scratching the fur, pelvic thrusting, ejaculation, defecation, urination, piloerection. (A) Walking is associated with rhythmical slow activity (RSA), and alert immobility is associated with large-amplitude irregular activity (LIA). (B) A dentate granule cell, identified by electrophysiological criteria, fires at a high rate during walking and a low rate during drinking. (C) Evoked potentials occurring in stratum pyramidale (upper trace) and stratum radiatum (lower trace) of field CA1 after stimulation of the angular bundle during walking (type 1 behavior) or drinking (type 2 behavior). Ten superimposed sweeps. The early in-phase potentials are volume conducted from the dentate gyrus. Note that phase-reversed evoked potentials often occur in CA1 during drinking, but never occur during walking. (From Vanderwolf 1988, redrawn from Vanderwolf et al. 1975 and Buzsaki et al. 1983.)

firing rate in many, but not all, complex spike cells (putative pyramidal cells) in Ammon's horn, and (5) increases in the firing rate of dentate granule cells. Theta cells and dentate granule cells often fire in bursts during a particular phase of the RSA cycle (figure 6.1). Pyramidal cells also tend to do this, but the relation is usually less obvious, in part because pyramidal cells fire at rather low rates. Figure 6.5 illustrates a number of these changes, whereas table 6.1 provides a list of references in the field of hippocampal electrical activity and behavior. Recent studies have also shown that the cingulate cortex generates a rhythmical electrical pattern that resembles hippocampal RSA both in morphology and in relations to behavior (table 6.1).

Although the relation between hippocampal slow wave activity and spontaneous behavior in the rat is well described by the concepts of type 1 and type 2 behavior, complications arise when a wider range of experimental situations are considered. Although dogs, mice, and Mongolian gerbils resemble rats insofar as they display RSA almost exclusively during type 1 behavior, rabbits, cats, and guinea pigs often generate clear RSA during such type 2 behaviors as waking immobility or face washing. Thus the latter animals may display either LIA or RSA during a type 2 behavior such as waking immobility. Even in the rat clear RSA can be induced during complete immobility by a variety of experimental manipulations including prolonged aversive conditioning, exposure to predator species, treatment with anesthetics, cholinomimetic or neuroleptic drugs, or surgical lesions of the hypothalamus or midbrain. These findings at first raised serious doubts about the validity of the type 1/type 2 behavior distinction.

Clarification of the field was achieved when it was found that cholinergic blocking drugs such as atropine, scopolamine, or hemicholinium generally eliminate all RSA occurring during type 2 behavior, regardless of how it is induced or of the species of animal studied, but do not eliminate the RSA occurring during type 1 behavior. Peripherally acting antimuscarinic drugs, such as atropine methylnitrate, are ineffective. Thus the natural RSA pattern evidently consists of an atropine-sensitive component and an atropine-resistant component. Figure 6.6 illustrates one of the many demonstrations of this. These data suggest that atropine-sensitive RSA may depend on the well-known cholinergic projections to the hippocampal formation from the medial septal nucleus and the nucleus of the diagonal band. This hypothesis is supported by many different experimental findings: (1) Release of acetylcholine in the hippocampus correlates with the occurrence of RSA. (2) Injection of cholinergic agonists systemically, or directly into the hippocampus, produces RSA. Isolated in vitro slices of hippocampus will generate an RSA-like waveform when exposed to cholinergic agonists. (3) Rhythmical firing of medial septal cells correlates with the occurrence of RSA. (4) Surgical ablation of the septal area abolishes all RSA, but a cell-specific neurotoxic lesion (ibotenic acid) of the septal nuclei produces a

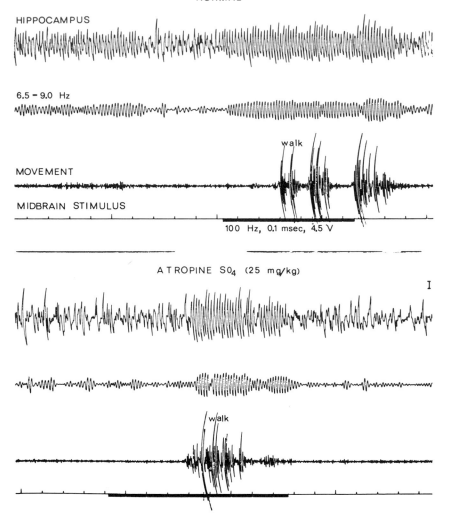

Figure 6.6 Effects of atropine on hippocampal rhythmical slow activity (RSA) and behavior elicited by stimulation of the midbrain reticular formation. Hippocampal activity is shown as an unfiltered record and also after passage through a bandpass filter system (6.5 Hz to 9.0 Hz). (Top four tracings) Undrugged rat. Note that (1) RSA accompanies small spontaneous movements (probably head movements); (2) RSA begins at onset of stimulation even though rat is motionless; walking begins only after a delay of about 3 s; (3) RSA persists during the centrally elicited walking. (Bottom four tracings) After treatment with atropine sulfate (50 mg/kg intraperitoneally). Note that (1) behavior is essentially unchanged; walking begins after a latent period of several seconds; (2) RSA still accompanies walking behavior; but (3) the RSA initially present during immobility appears to have been abolished. Reticular stimulation is constant throughout, 0.1-ms pulses at 100 Hz and 4.5 V. Calibration, time marks 1.0 s, 0.5 mV. (From Vanderwolf 1975)

partially selective loss of the RSA that can occur during type 2 behavior. This mimics the effect of atropine or scopolamine. Therefore it is safe to conclude that the atropine-sensitive type of RSA, which can occur during type 2 behavior, depends on a cholinergic input to the hippocampus from the medial septum and diagonal band.

The problem of the neurochemical basis of atropine-resistant RSA resisted analysis for several years. However, it now appears that atropine-resistant RSA depends on an input to the hippocampus from the serotonin-containing cells of the midbrain. This hypothesis is supported by the following observations: (1) Parachlorophenylalanine, which blocks the synthesis of serotonin, reduces or eliminates atropine-resistant RSA. Reserpine, which results in the enzymatic degradation of serotonin (as well as other monoamines) has a similar effect. (2) 5,7-Dihydroxytryptamine, which has a specific neurotoxic effect on serotonergic neurons (when combined with a systemic injection of desmethylimipramine to protect noradrenergic neurons), reduces or eliminates atropine-resistant RSA when it is injected locally among the serotonergic neurons of the midbrain. Thus a combination of specific serotonergic depletion (by parachlorophenylalanine or 5,7-dihydroxytryptamine) plus cholinergic blockade (by atropine or scopolamine) produces a rat that displays continuous LIA regardless of concurrent behavior. (3) Surgical lesions that interrupt known ascending serotonergic pathways abolish atropine-resistant RSA. (4) Blockade of dopaminergic and no radrenergic neurotransmission by means of surgical lesions, pharmacological depletion, or receptor blockade, or by treatment with 6-hydroxydopamine does not abolish atropine-resistant RSA. Therefore it is unlikely that catecholamines are directly involved in the generation of this waveform. (5) Electrical stimulation of the median raphe in freely moving rats produces atropine-resistant RSA in correlation with loco motion. (6) Although the details remain to be worked out, it appears that serotonergic cells of the dorsal and median raphe nuclei fire in correlation with gross motor activity.

Taken together, these data indicate that when a normal rat engages in a type 1 behavior, a combination of cholinergic and serotonergic inputs to the hippocampus generate RSA plus a variety of other electrophysiological changes that correlate with RSA. Under some circumstances the cholinergic input can act independently, resulting in an atropine-sensitive type of RSA occurring during type 2 behavior.

Atropine-resistant RSA is associated only with active type 1 movements and cannot be elicited by a purely passive movement imposed by the experimenter. Further, atropine-resistant RSA can be elicited in a curare-treated rat. Consequently this waveform does not occur as a result of feedback from moving body parts. This is also true of atropine-resistant neocortical LVFA, which is discussed in the next section.

How do these findings in awake or drug-treated rats relate to the activity seen during natural sleep? Our rat on the recording platform is unlikely to go to sleep, even though it would normally sleep during the daytime because it is in a very exposed position. However, if the rat is provided with some possibility of concealment, such as that afforded by a small cardboard box, it will usually fall asleep after a delay of several hours. During quiet sleep our rat lies motionless for long periods, with its head resting on the floor of the box and its eyes closed. The trunk and tail are often curled up in a C shape. During this behavior hippocampal slow wave activity is very irregular (LIA) and often has a higher amplitude than that seen during waking immobility. Complex cells in general fire at higher rates than in an awake rat, but theta cells fire sporadically at a low rate.

With the onset of active sleep, muscle tone disappears. This can be demonstrated electromyographically if the rat was previously prepared with flexible wire electrodes fixed in various muscle groups, but is also evident on visual inspection because the body slumps limply on the floor as muscle tone disappears. In the hippocampus clear RSA appears coincident with the disappearance of muscle tone and persists continuously for many seconds (average duration of about 2 min) until the active sleep episode ends. Then the rat usually awakens briefly and moves about before settling down to sleep again. Throughout an episode of active sleep, brief twitches of the muscles occur at irregular intervals. Almost any muscle group may be involved, but in rats limb and vibrissae movements appear to be especially common. The explanation of this curious state of affairs, in which phasic muscular activity appears on a background of hypotonia or atonia, is that spinal and cranial motor neurons are subjected to a strong descending inhibitory influence throughout an episode of active sleep. This accounts for the atonia. The muscular twitches arise as a result of powerful excitatory barrages descending via the reticulospinal, pyramidal, and rubrospinal tracts. There is evidence that if the descending inhibitory effect is eliminated (lesions in the region of the locus coeruleus appear to do this), the effects of the descending excitatory barrages are allowed full expression, resulting in vigorous coordinated motor activity. This can be regarded as an experimentally induced form of sleep-walking. (Sleep-walking in humans is said to occur during slow wave sleep.) Therefore active sleep appears to be a condition in which the brain generates patterns of neural activity similar to those that result in normal behavior in the waking state, but output is blocked at the level of the final common path. According to this view, the presence of RSA in the hippocampus during active sleep can be regarded as one of numerous signs of the activation of motor control programs. However, there is a difficulty: Hippocampal RSA is continuously present during active sleep, but muscular twitches occur only intermittently. A solution to this problem was provided by studies showing that in atropine-treated rats bursts of hippocampal RSA correlate closely with the occurrence of bursts of muscle activity during active sleep (figure 6.7). The RSA that

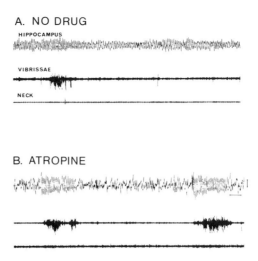

A. NO DRUG

HIPPOCAMPUS

VIBRISSAE

NECK

B. ATROPINE

Figure 6.7 Hippocampal slow wave activity during active sleep after deprivation of active sleep. (A) Undrugged rat. Note the higher-frequency RSA during electromyographic (EMG) burst in muscles under vibrissae and lower-frequency RSA in interval after the muscle twitch. (B) After atropine sulfate (40 mg/kg intraperitoneally). Note that RSA occurs only in relation to EMG bursts. Neck muscle activity is abolished during active sleep in the normal state, but persists in the atropinized rat. (From Vanderwolf et al. 1978).

is normally present in the intervals between the bursts of muscle activity is evidently of the atropine-sensitive type. Thus atropine-resistant RSA is correlated with motor activity sleep in much the same way as it is in the waking state.

6.4 Neocortical Activity in Relation to Behavior

Let us return to the rat on the movement-sensor platform (figure 6.3). It is apparent that spontaneous neocortical activity differs in appearance from spontaneous hippocampal activity. The pattern of unit firing seen in the two structures also differs. Neocortical LVFA is associated with an irregular continuous pattern of action potentials, whereas hippocampal RSA tends to be associated with a bursting pattern of action potentials (figures 6.1 and 6.2). In the neocortex LVFA is usually present for long periods of time, with no obvious relation to concurrent motor activity. A clear relation between neocortical activity and behavior, however, can be demonstrated readily by means of the evoked potential technique. The transcallosal evoked response provides a convenient means of studying cerebral evoked potentials without the complications introduced by the use of natural sensory stimuli. These complications include movement-related variations in receptor orientation, variation in receptor sensitivity and spontaneous variations in subcortical synaptic transmission. To study the transcallosal evoked potential, it is necessary to implant a stimulating electrode in one hemisphere and a

Vanderwolf: Introduction to Electrical Activity

recording electrode at the mirror-image point in the opposite hemisphere. Good results are obtained with electrodes placed in frontal or parietal neocortex (figure 6.8). Brief (0.1 ms to 1.0 ms) single current pulses presented to one hemisphere result in an evoked response on the other side. Stimulation of corpus callosum fibers in the midline evokes a similar response at a shorter latency, but section of the callosal fibers between stimulating and recording electrodes placed in opposite hemispheres causes the evoked response to disappear. Therefore the response completely depends on excitation of callosal fibers. Extensive work in anesthetized animals has shown that the initial effect of a callosal volley is usually excitatory, causing depolarizing postsynaptic potentials and cell discharge, and that few neurons are excited antidromically compared with the number excited orthodromically. After initial excitation, many neurons are hyperpolarized, and firing is inhibited. Therefore we are observing mainly the postsynaptic response of neocortical neurons that are first excited and then inhibited by a callosal volley. The latter effect may be due to recurrent inhibition (figure 6.4).

The transcallosal evoked response in a freely moving rat consists of an early component and late components (figure 6.8). The early component peaks in 5 ms to 10 ms, is usually negative both at the surface and in layer V of the neocortex, and is accompanied by unit discharges, indicating a widespread excitatory effect. It is probably due to summed excitatory postsynaptic potentials. The main late component peaks at

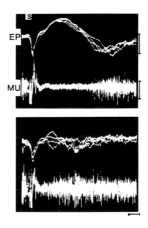

Figure 6.8 Effect of motor activity on the transcallosal response. EP = bipolar transcortical record of slow wave evoked response in left sensorimotor cortex, deep positivity up; MU = multiunit activity derived from the deep member of the same bipolar electrode pair; S = monopolar stimulation of right sensorimotor cortex at twice threshold (228 μA). (Top) Waking immobility. (Bottom) Walking elicited by pushing. Note the large late deep positive component of the evoked potential and associated multiunit suppression during immobility and the small late deep positive component and associated multiunit activity during elicited walking. The early deep negative component is only slightly altered. Four superimposed single sweeps in each behavioral condition. Calibration, EP = 0.5 mV and MU = 0.05 mV, 20 ms. (From Vanderwolf et al. 1987)

40 ms to 80 ms, is negative at the surface and positive in layer V, and is accompanied by a strong suppression of unit discharges. These effects are probably due to widespread synchronized inhibitory postsynaptic potentials occurring in pyramidal cells.

If the transcallosal evoked response is elicited during the course of spontaneous behavior, the development of the late components in particular varies strikingly in correlation with concurrent motor activity. Figure 6.8 shows that during waking immobility (rat standing still, head up, eyes wide open) the main late component is large and is associated with a long period of suppression of multiunit activity. During walking, the late component is strongly reduced in amplitude and duration, and the period of suppression of multiunit activity is shortened. The correlation between behavior and the development of the cortical evoked potentials is best demonstrated by a video technique in which a view of the oscilloscope used for recording and a view of the rat are combined on the same tape. Slow-motion playback of the tape can be used to generate data of the type shown in figure 6.9. In general it appears that the late component of the transcallosal evoked potential is well developed during waking immobility and other type 2 behavior, but is strongly reduced during type 1 behavior.

Although the relation between concurrent motor activity and the development of sensory evoked potentials has not been studied as extensively as the relation between concurrent motor activity and the transcallosal evoked potentials, there are indications that similar rules exist in both cases. For example, the late component of visual evoked

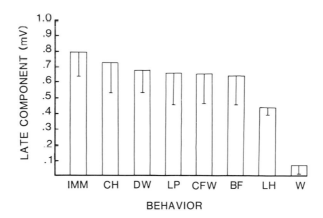

Figure 6.9 Peak amplitude of the late component of the transcallosal evoked response in relation to various spontaneous behaviors in the rat. Transcortical bipolar records; the stimuli were monopolar cathodal pulses (0.5 ms duration, 0.5 Hz, 2.5 times threshold). Means and standard deviations were derived from 40 single sweeps/condition/rat, 5 to 6 rats/condition. IMM = alert immobility; CH = chewing food pellet; DW = drinking water; LOP = licking forepaws; CFW = circular or rotary paw movements during face washing; BF = biting food; LH = lateral head movement; W = spontaneous walking. (From Vanderwolf et al. 1987)

potentials is smaller in freely moving rats when hippocampal RSA is present than it is when hippocampal RSA is absent. Therefore one can say that the development of at least some types of evoked potentials in the neocortex of the rat varies in relation to behavior in a manner suggestive of the relation beween behavior and hippocampal RSA.

Spontaneous neocortical activity does not correlate in any really obvious way with concurrent motor activity. Waking rats sometimes display spindle-shaped bursts of very rhythmical (6-Hz to 10-Hz waves associated with brief rhythmical bursts of unit activity (figure 6.2). These 6-Hz to 10-Hz spindles *never* occur during walking or other type 1 behavior, athough they do occur occasionally during immobility. Thus there is a hint of a relation to movement in the pattern of occurrence of this waveform, but the effect is not very clear. The relation to concurrent motor activity can be demonstrated in a more obvious manner by artificially triggering the spindles so that they occur more frequently. For example, a stroboscopic flash of light will trigger spindle activity in the visual projection areas quite reliably during waking immobility or face washing (type 2 behavior), but fails completely when the flashes are applied during a type 1 behavior such as walking.

Although variations in the pattern of the spontaneous neocorticogram do not display any compelling correlation with spontaneous motor activity, a very striking correlation appears after systemic injections of atropine, scopolamine, or other antimuscarinic drugs (figure 6.10). Large-amplitude irregular slow waves, associated with a burst-suppression pattern of unit activity (figure 6.2), occur during behavioral immobility even though the rats are in a normal waking posture with the head up and the eyes open. (Atropine, but not scopolamine, tends to cause some drooping of the eyelids, probably owing to a ganglionic blocking action.) The large-amplitude slow waves also occur during active type 2 behaviors such as chattering or gnashing of the teeth, tremor, and face washing (if it occurs for several seconds in the absence of postural shifts). During type 1 behaviors, however, such as walking, rearing, changes in posture, or lateral or vertical head movements, an LVFA pattern occurs. If the rat engages in head movement and walking *continuously*, i.e., no periods of immobility or other type 2 behavior, even of only 1-s to 2-s duration, large-amplitude slow waves will not occur at all. If the rat remains quiet for long periods, large-amplitude slow waves occur continuously throughout the period of immobility.

These observations suggest that the LVFA pattern of the normal rat is produced by two distinct inputs, much as hippocampal RSA is generated by two distinct inputs. One input, sensitive to atropine, can generate LVFA during type 2 behavior, whereas the other input, resistant to atropine, generates LVFA only in close correlation with the occurrence of type 1 behavior. Current evidence indicates that atropine-sensitive LVFA is produced by activity in the cholinergic projections

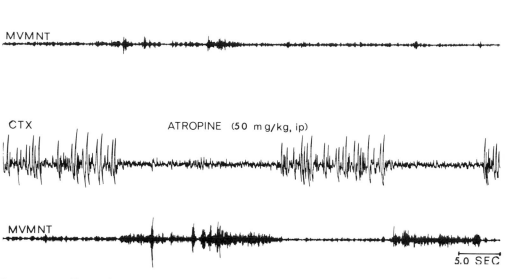

Figure 6.10 Effects of atropine sulfate on neocortical electrical activity in relation to behavior. CTX = neocortical wave activity; MVMNT = output of magnet-and-coil type of movement sensor. (Upper traces) Undrugged rat displays continuous low voltage fast activity (LVFA) with no relation to motor activity. (Lower traces) After atropine, large-amplitude slow waves occur during immobility, but LVFA persists during spontaneous motor activity (head movements and stepping). (From Vanderwolf 1984)

from the basal forebrain to the neocortex, whereas atropine-resistant LVFA depends on ascending serotonergic projections.

Evidence supporting the role of the basal forebrain cholinergic system in the genesis of atropine-sensitive LVFA includes the following points: (1) Release of acetylcholine from the surface of the neocortex is greater during periods of LVFA than during periods of large amplitude irregular slow waves, in both anesthetized and freely moving animals. (2) Treatment with acetylcholine or anticholinesterases (by systemic or intracarotid injection or by local application on the neocortex) produces LVFA. (3) Treatment with centrally acting antimuscarinic drugs (atropine, quinuclidinyl benzilate, scopolamine) blocks one type of LVFA, but antimuscarinic drugs that fail to penetrate the blood-brain barrier (atropine methylnitrate) are ineffective. (4) Destruction of basal forebrain cells by local injection of kainic acid (a cell-specific neurotoxin) also abolishes one type of LVFA, mimicking the effect of centrally acting antimuscarinic drugs. (5) Basal forebrain neurons that can be driven antidromically by electrical stimulation of the neocortex fire at much higher rates during periods of LVFA than during periods of large irregular slow activity or 6-Hz to 10-Hz spindle activity. Anatomical evidence indicates that such cells are likely to contain the cholinergic marker enzymes choline acetyltransferase and acetylcholinesterase.

Evidence supporting the role of ascending serotonergic projections in the genesis of atropine-resistant LVFA includes the following points: (1) The serotonin-depleting drugs reserpine and parachlorophenylalanine eliminate atropine-resistant LVFA. Therefore a combination of either of these drugs with either atropine or scopolamine abolishes all LVFA, producing an awake animal that displays continuous large-amplitude irregular activity in its cortex, regardless of ongoing behavior (figure 6.11). Painful stimuli or strong electrical stimulation of the midbrain reticular formation, hypothalamus, or medial thalamus fails to produce LVFA in these preparations. (2) Local injections of 5,7-dihydroxytryptamine into the serotonergic cell groups in the midbrain (in combination with a systemic injection of desmethylimipramine to protect noradrenergic neurons) result in a chronic loss of atropine-resistant LVFA, mimicking the effect of reserpine or parachlorophenylalanine. (3) Blockade of dopaminergic and noradrenergic neurotransmission by means of surgical lesions, pharmacological depletion, or receptor blockade or by

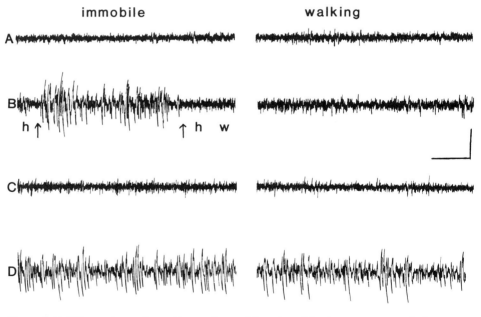

Figure 6.11 Effects of atropine sulfate and parachlorophenylalanine on neocortical electrical activity in relation to behavior in a rat. (A) Normal rat displays LVFA during both waking immobility and spontaneous walking. (B) After treatment with atropine (50mg/kg intraperitoneally), large irregular slow waves occur during immobility (between arrows), but LVFA occurs during head movements (h) and walking (w). (C) A day after completion of treatment with parachlorophenylalanine (500 mg/kg/day intraperitoneally for 3 days), the neocortex displays LVFA during both waking immobility and spontaneous walking. (D) After treatment with atropine in addition to parachlorophenylalanine, all LVFA disappears, and large irregular slow waves occur during both immobility and walking. Calibration, 5 s, 1 mV.

treatment with a neurotoxin (6-hydroxydopamine) does not abolish atropine-resistant LVFA. (4) In rats pretreated with reserpine, 5-hydroxytryptophan (the immediate precursor of serotonin) restores atropine-resistant LVFA. A similar (and better) restoration is produced by monoamine oxidase inhibitors (pargyline, tranylcypromine) that produce rapid increases in brain serotonin levels in reserpine-treated rats. Serotonin agonists such as 5-methoxy-N, N-dimethyltryptamine or β-phenylethylamine also restore atropine-resistant LVFA in reserpine-treated rats, but catecholamine precursors and agonists, such as L-DOPA, amphetamine, or apomorphine, are ineffective. (5) Electrical stimulation of the median raphé in freely moving rats produces atropine-resistant LVFA in correlation with locomotion. These findings indicate that brain serotonin is necessary for the occurrence of atropine-resistant LVFA but that brain catecholamines are not directly involved in it.

It should also be mentioned that the form of the transcallosal evoked potential is no longer correlated with concurrent motor activity in rats that are treated with a combination of reserpine plus scopolamine or parachlorophenylalanine plus scopolamine. In such preparations the late component of the transcallosal evoked potential is always of large amplitude and long duration, as it is in type 2 behavior in the normal state. Thus it appears that behavior-related modulation of evoked potentials, as well as the occurrence of LVFA, are controlled by cholinergic and serotonergic inputs to the neocortex. Whether the many findings of behavior-related variations in human sensory evoked potentials are all fundamentally due to variations in ascending cholinergic and serotonergic activity remains to be determined.

How does the theory of dual cholinergic-serotonergic control of neocortical activation apply to sleep? Returning again to our rat on the movement sensor platform, we observe that quiet sleep is associated with the development of large-amplitude irregular slow waves in the neocortex. Brief episodes of rhythmical waves of 10-Hz to 16-Hz (sleep spindles) appear as well. The overall pattern is very similar to the one occurring during waking immobility in an atropine-treated rat. Current evidence indicates that the onset of irregular slow waves during quiet sleep is associated with reduced activity in basal forebrain cholinergic neurons and also in ascending serotonergic projections. An earlier view that ascending serotonergic activity is actually increased during slow-wave sleep no longer is tenable.

With the onset of active sleep, long trains of continuous LVFA occur in the neocortex. Experiments with atropinized rats indicate that the LVFA accompanying phasic muscular twitches is of the atropine-resistant type, whereas the LVFA occurring during the intertwitch intervals is of the atropine-sensitive type. Thus the situation in the neocortex is very similar to the situation observed in the hippocampus. Whether the atropine-resistant waveforms occurring in both the neocortex and hippocampus during active sleep depend on ascending serotonergic activity has not been definitely established. In cats the firing rate of dorsal raphé neurons falls to a very low level during an active sleep episode, but bursts of activity tend to occur in correlation with the phasic muscular twitches. Thus it may be that ascending serotonergic activity is responsible for atropine-resistant RSA and LVFA during sleep as well as in the waking state.

The theory that neocortical LVFA is controlled jointly by a cholinergic input from the basal forebrain and a serotonergic input from the brainstem stands in opposition to an older view that neocortical activation is controlled by a reticulothalamocortical pathway, involving especially the intralaminar nuclei of the thalamus. There are many findings that indicate that the thalamus is of minor importance in the genesis of neocortical LVFA: (1) Near-total destruction of thalamic neurons by a surgical lesion or by local injection of kainic acid does not abolish LVFA. (2) Partial or total transection of the brainstem just caudal to the thalamus abolishes the neocortical LVFA normally produced by stimulation of some sites in the intralaminar nuclei, but does not abolish thalamocortical transmission, as indicated by the persistence of cortical evoked potentials elicited by thalamic stimulation. (3) Combined treatment with reserpine plus scopolamine or atropine abolishes all neocortical LVFA, but does not abolish thalamocortical transmission, as indicated by cortical evoked potentials elicited by thalamic stimulation. The first of these observations shows that thalamocortical transmission is unnecessary for the genesis of neocortical LVFA, whereas the second and third observations show that it is not sufficient to produce LVFA. Consequently it is unlikely that the thalamus plays any essential role in activation of the neocortex.

References to neocortical electrophysiology, pharmacology, and relations to behavior and sleep are given in table 6.1.

6.5 Does Dopamine Regulate Serotonergic Control of Cerebral Activity?

Rats treated with antimuscarinic drugs, such as scopolamine or atropine, tend to be hyperactive, moving the head and walking about (type 1 behavior) more than normal. The basis of this effect is uknown, but may be due to a blockade of dopamine reuptake by these drugs. Atropine-resistant hippocampal RSA and atropine-resistant neocortical LVFA are very frequently present in rats treated with antimuscarinic drugs because these wave patterns occur in close correlation with the occurrence of type 1 movements. If an adequate dose of a neuroleptic drug is given subsequent to the antimuscarinic drug, a dramatic effect occurs. The previously hyperactive rat soon becomes quite immobile, usually sitting in a hunched posture, and only occasionally moving the head or changing posture. During the periods of immobility, large-amplitude irregular patterns of activity occurs continuously in both the neocortex and hippocampus, just as before the administration of the neuroleptic. Similarly whenever a type 1 movement occurs (spontaneous head turns, stepping, postural change, or struggling when handled), atropine-resistant RSA and atropine-resistant LVFA occur in association with it. Thus the neuroleptic decreases the probability of occurrence of the atropine-resistant cerebral waveforms, as well as the associated type 1 behavior, but does not alter the waveforms themselves. Different neuroleptics (chlorpromazine, haloperidol, pimozide, spiroperidol, trifluoperazine) have much the same effect, differing only in potency.

Because atropine-resistant hippocampal RSA and atropine-resistant neocortical LVFA depend on the presence of serotonin, and because the major common effect of the various neuroleptic drugs is blockade of dopamine receptors, the foregoing observations suggest that ascending serotonergic activity may be controlled by dopamine receptors. The action of dopamine agonists appears to be consistent with this hypothesis. If an atropine- or scopolamine-pretreated rat is given D-amphetamine (which releases dopamine from presynaptic terminals) or apomorphine (a direct acting dopamine agonist) in adequate doses, type 1 behavior (walking, rearing, head movement) occurs continuously for nearly an hour. In correlation with this, atropine-resistant RSA and atropine-resistant LVFA also occur continuously. Thus the atropine-resistant cerebral waveforms occur in normal relation to behavior after the administration of dopamine agonists, but the probability of their occurrence, and the occurrence of the associated type 1 behavior, is greatly increased.

Although these phenomena are very clear cut, they are not easily interpreted. Neuroanatomical demonstrations of serotonergic inputs to dopaminergic neurons suggest that serotonergic neurons control the activity of dopaminergic neurons rather than the other way around. There is also evidence, however, that dopamine can modulate the release of serotonin from axon termninals in the cerebral cortex. Perhaps this is the mechanism by which dopaminergic agonists and antagonists exert their effect on atropine-resistant (serotonin-dependent) cerebral activity.

6.6 Behavior-Related Cerebral Activity: What Does it Mean?

The electrical activity of the neocortex of the rat appears to consist of three principal patterns, as shown in figure 6.2. Large-amplitude irregular slow activity appears to be a fundamental pattern because it occurs spontaneously in large slabs of cortex that have been surgically isolated from the remainder of the nervous system. Therefore, even in intact animals, this waveform may be generated by circuits confined to the neocortex. The remaining patterns—LVFA and rhythmical spindle activity—do not occur in isolated cerebral cortex and presumably are not endogenous to the neocortex. The LVFA pattern appears in the neocortex as a result of cholinergic and serotonergic inputs, as we have seen. Rhythmical spindle activity, both the 10-Hz to 16-Hz spindles that occur during slow-wave sleep or after treatment with anticholinergic drugs, and the 6-Hz to 10-Hz spindles that occur in the undrugged waking state, appear to depend on an input from the thalamus. Thus large thalamic lesions abolish neocortical spindles without abolishing either LVFA or large irregular slow waves.

Hippocampal activity appears to be somewhat simpler than neocortical activity. The LIA pattern and its associated sharp waves may be analogous to the large irregular slow waves of the neocortex, whereas the RSA pattern is analogous to LVFA. Like LVFA, RSA appears to be generated in response to cholinergic and serotonergic inputs (figure 6.12), and the two waveforms have similar relations to behavior. However, the hippocampus does not seem to possess any prominent waveform that is analogous to neocortical spindle activity in terms of function (i.e., relation to behavior) even though hippocampal RSA has a superficial morphological similarity to neocortical spindle activity.

A classical approach to the significance of these different waveforms would be to prevent them from occurring and to observe the effect of this on physiology and behavior. Treatment with either parachlorophenylalanine or intracerebral 5,7-dihydroxytryptamine plus a central cholinergic blocking drug provides a means of eliminating all cerebral activation (hippocampal RSA as well as neocortical LVFA) without suppressing all cerebral activity and without eliminating all active behavior.

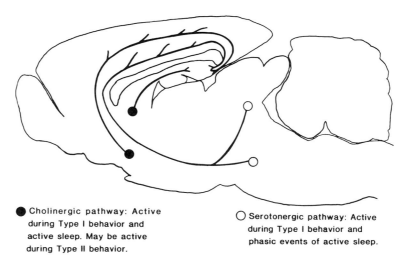

● Cholinergic pathway: Active during Type I behavior and active sleep. May be active during Type II behavior.

○ Serotonergic pathway: Active during Type I behavior and phasic events of active sleep.

Figure 6.12 Diagram illustrating part of the proposed pathways that determine the occurrence of low-voltage fast activity in the neocortex and rhythmical slow activity in the hippocampus.

Organization of the Neocortex

Previously the only available means of eliminating all cerebral activation were deep anesthesia or gross surgical lesions of the brainstem, procedures that are incompatible with any spontaneous behavior at all.

Rats subjected to simultaneous selective blockade of central cholinergic and serotonergic function display an interesting pattern of behavioral deficits and surviving behavioral capacities. They walk about and rear up on the hind legs as normal rats do, swim very well, readily climb up a vertical wire screen, and sit up to wash the face in a normal manner. However, the surviving motor patterns do not occur in normal sequence or in normal relation to environmental stimuli. The rats will walk off the edge of a table without the slightest hesitation. They are incapable of swimming reliably to a large visible platform in the center of a water-filled tank, a task that normal rats master in one or two trials. They are also incapable of avoiding (or even escaping) an electric shock by jumping out of a box, a task that normal rats master in two to six trials. The deficits are not restricted to learned behavior because the normal sequential pattern of grooming, generally regarded as an unlearned taxon-specific behavior, is also severely disrupted. It appears that combined central cholinergic and serotonergic blockade, which eliminates neocortical LVFA and hippocampal RSA, produces a severe generalized impairment of behavioral organization without producing any clear paralysis or akinesia. Because somewhat similar effects are produced by surgical decortication in rats, the facts suggest that many normal cortical functions are abolished when LVFA and RSA are abolished.

Why should the loss of LVFA and RSA produce such devastating effects on behavior? At one time, it was widely accepted that LVFA and RSA were indications of consciousness or arousal. On this basis it would be said presumably that blockade of central cholinergic and serotonergic function produce a lack of consciousness or of arousal. However, the fact that the experimental subjects walk about actively with the head held up in a normal posture and the eyes open make such suggestions meaningless. The rats might be described as demented or psychotic, but, in terms of ordinary English usage, they are certainly not unconscious. It is also unlikely that the behavioral deficits are due to any simple loss of sensory input to the neocortex. Visual, somesthetic, and auditory evoked potentials can be readily demonstrated in the appropriate neocortical areas after central cholinergic and serotonergic blockade.

A reasonable interpretation of the behavioral deficits produced by combined central cholinergic and serotonergic blockade is suggested by the electrophysiological data. As concluded previously (Vanderwolf 1988), "it is probably impossible for the neocortex to carry out its normal function in the presence of continuous large-amplitude irregular slow wave activity, a condition in which the activity of vast numbers of its output neurons is cut short for 100 ms or more, two or three times per second. Similarly, in the hippocampus deprived of cholinergic and serotonergic inputs, the continued irregular occurrence of sharp waves, associated with undifferentiated bursts of large numbers of cells of different types, may be incompatible with normal function. As a result the analysis of sensory input, the organization of motor output, the long-term storage of information, or whatever else the cerebal cortex does, cannot proceed normally in the absence of cholinergic and serotonergic inputs."

In may seem puzzling that although many aspects of cerebral electric activity correlate strongly with motor activity in a normal rat, experimental treatments that abolish this type of cerebral activity do not abolish motor activity. Instead such treatments produce rather complex deficits in the overall organization of behavior. A similar effect is produced by surgical removal of the cerebral cortex (see chapter 10 by Whishaw). The role of the cerebrum evidently is to guide, control, or organize the occurrence of various motor patterns such as walking, rearing, or standing motionless, which the details of muscular coordination are managed largely by the brainstem, spinal cord, and cerebellum.

The electrophysiological data discussed here suggest that the cerebral cortex may be particularly involved in the control of type 1 behaviors such as locomotion or the manipulation of objects. The behavior-related variations in hippocampal, neocortical, and cingulate activity all suggest this. Type 1 behaviors play a very general role in many functional systems including food getting, reproduction, avoidance of predators, and behavioral thermoregulation. Consequently, if cholinergic and serotonergic inputs constitute essential components of the neural machinery that controls type 1 behavior, one might expect to see a broad spectrum of behavioral deficits when central cholinergic and serotonergic transmission are interfered with. This corresponds to what is observed.

It is probable that central cholinergic and serotonergic dysfunction play significant roles in human neurological and psychiatric disorders. It is now clear that Alzheimer's disease is associated with a reduction in cholinergic and serotonergic input to the cerebral cortex. It has long been believed that serotonin plays a role in depression, and there have been suggestions of a role in schizophrenia as well. Recent work on rats has shown that phencyclidine suppresses atropine-resistant (serotonergic-dependent) activation of the neocortex and hippocampus. Because phencyclidine produces a schizophrenialike behavioral syndrome in humans, this finding, though indirect, tends to support the hypothesis of a serotonergic deficit in schizophrenia. Conceivably the beneficial effects of dopamine antagonists (neuroleptics) in schizophrenia are related to an indirect modulation of serotonin-dependent cerebral activity. Clearly much work remains to be done.

Acknowledgments

Research described in this chapter was supported by a grant from the Natural Sciences and Engineering Research Council. I thank R. K. Cooley for technical assistance, L. Mitchell for typing, and B. Kolb, L.-W. S. Leung, and B. Robertson for their comments on an early draft of the manuscript.

References

Andén, N. E., Dahlström, A., Fuxe, K., et al. (1966). Ascending monoamine neurons to the telencephalon and diencephalon. *Acta Physiologica Scandinavica* 67:313–326.

Andersen, P., and Andersson, S. A. (1968). *Physiological Basis of the Alpha Rhythm*. New York: Appleton-Century-Cofts.

Andersen, P., and Eccles, J. C. (1962). Inhibitory phasing of neuronal discharge. *Nature (London)* 1976:645–647.

Angeleri, F., Marchesi, G. F., and Quattrini, A. (1969). Effects of chronic thalamic lesions on the electrical activity of the neocortex and on sleep. *Archives Italiennes de Biologie* 107:633–667.

Armstrong, D. M., Saper, C. B., Levey, A. I., et al. (1983). Distribution of cholinergic neurons in rat brain: Demonstrated by the immunocytochemical localization of choline acetyltransferase. *Journal of Comparative Neurology* 216:53–68.

Arnolds, D. E. A. T., Lopes da Silva, F. H., Boeijinga, P., et al. (1984). Hippocampal EEG and motor activity in the cat: The role of eye movements and body acceleration. *Behavioral Brain Research* 12:121–135.

Azmitia, E. C. (1978). The serotonin-producing neurons of the midbrain median and dorsal raphé nuclei. In L. L. Iverson, S. D. Iverson and S. H. Snyder (eds.), *Handbook of Psychopharmacology, V. 9, Chemical Pathways in the Brain* (pp. 233–314). New York: Plenum Press.

Balfour, D. J. K., and Iyaniwura, T. T. (1985). An investigation of amphetamine-induced release of 5-HT from rat hippocampal slices. *European Journal of Pharmacology* 109:395–399.

Ball, G., Gloor, P., and Schaul, N. (1977). The cortical electromicrophysiology of pathological delta waves in the EEG of cats. *Electroencephalography and Clinical Neurophysiology* 43:346–361.

Belardetti, F., Borgia, R., and Mancia, M. (1977). Prosencephalic mechanisms of ECoG desynchronization in cerveau isolé cats. *Electroencephalography and Clinical Neurophysiology* 42:213–225.

Bennett, J. P., Enna, S. J., Bylund, D. B., et al. (1979). Neurotransmitter receptors in frontal cortex of schizophrenics. *Archives of General Psychiatry* 36:927–934.

Beyer, C., and Sawyer, C. H. (1964). Effects of vigilance and other factors on nonspecific acoustic responses in the rabbit. *Experimental Neurology* 10:156–169.

Bigl, V., Woolf, N. J., and Butcher, L. L. (1982). Cholinergic projections from the basal forebrain to frontal, parietal, temporal, occipital, and cingulate cortices: A combined fluorescent tracer and acetylcholinesterase analysis. *Brain Research Bulletin* 8:727–749.

Black, A. H. (1975). Hippocampal electricity activity and behavior. In R. L. Isaacson and K. H. Pribram (eds.), *The Hippocampus, Vol. 2, Neurophysiology and Behavior* (pp. 129–167). New York: Plenum Press.

Bland, B. H. (1986). The physiology and pharmacology of hippocampal formation theta rhythms. *Progress in Neurobiology* 26:1–54.

Bland, B. H. Andersen, P., and Ganes, T. (1975). Two generators of hippocampal theta activity in rabbits. *Brain Research* 94:199–218.

Bland, B. H. Anderson, P., Gaines, T., and Sveen, O. (1980). Automated analysis of rhythmicity of physiologically identified hippocampal formation neurons. *Experimental Brain Research* 38:205–219.

Bland, B. H., and Whishaw, I. Q. (1976). Generators and topography of hippocampal theta (RSA) in the anesthetized and freely moving rat. *Brain Research* 118:259–280.

Borst, J. G. G., Leung, L.-W. S., and MacFabe, D. F. (1987). Electrical activity of the cingulate cortex. II. Cholinergic modulation. *Brain Research* 407:81–93.

Bowen, D. M., Allen, S. J., Benton, S. J., et al. (1983) Biochemical assessment of serotonergic and cholinergic dysfunction and cerebral atrophy in Alzheimer's disease. *Journal of Neurochemistry* 41:266–272.

Bullock, T. H., and Basar, E. (1988). Comparison of ongoing compound field potentials in the brains of invertebrates and vertebrates. *Brain Research Reviews* 13:57–75.

Butcher, L. L., and Woolf, N. J. (1986). Central cholinergic systems: Synopsis of anatomy and overview of physiology and pathology. In A. B. Scheibel and A. F. Wechsler (eds.), *The Biological Substrates of Alzheimer's Disease* (pp. 73–86). New York: Academic Press.

Buzsáki, G. (1986). Hippocampal sharp waves: Their origin and significance. *Brain Research* 398:242–252.

Buzsáki, G., Grastyan, E., Czopf, J., et al. (1981). Changes in neuronal transmission in the rat hippocampus during behavior. *Brain Research* 225:235–247.

Buzsáki, G., Leung, L.-W. S., and Vanderwolf, C. H. (1983). Cellular bases of hippocampal EEG in the behaving rat. *Brain Research Reviews* 6:139–171.

Buzsáki, G., and Vanderwolf, C. H. (eds.). (1985). *Electrical Activity of the Archicortex*. Budapest: Akademiai Kiado.

Calvet, J., Calvet, M. C., and Scherrer, J. (1964). Etude stratigraphique corticale de l'activité EEG spontanneé. *Electroencephalography and Clinical Neuophysiology* 17:109–125.

Calvet, J., Fourment, A., and Thieffry, M. (1973). Electrical activity in neocortical projection and association areas during slow wave sleep. *Brain Research* 52:173–187.

Ciba Foundation Symposium 58. (1978). *Functions of the Septo-Hippocampal System*. Amsterdam: Elsevier.

Colom, L. V., and Bland, B. H. (1987). State-dependent spike train dynamics of hippocampal formation neurons: Evidence for theta-on and theta-off cells. *Brain Research* 422:277–286.

Crow, T. J., Baker, H. F., Cross, A. J., et al. (1979). Monoamine mechanisms in chronic schizophrenia: Post mortem neurochemical findings. *British Journal of Psychiatry.* 134:249–256.

Cuculic, Z., Bost, K., and Himwich, H. E. (1968). An examination of a possible cortical cholinergic link in the EEG arousal reaction. *Progress in Brain Research* 28:27–39.

Dahlström, A., and Fuxe, K. (1964). Evidence for the existence of monoamine-containing neurons in the central nervous system. I. Demonstration of monoamines in the cell bodies of brain stem neurons. *Acta Physiologica Scandinavica* 62 (Suppl. 232):1–55.

Davies, P., and Maloney, A. J. F. (1976). Selective loss of central cholinergic neurons in Alzheimer's disease. *Lancet* 2:1403.

Detari, L., and Vanderwolf, C. H. (1987). Activity of identified cortically projecting and other basal forebrain neurones during large slow waves and cortical activation in anaesthetized rats. *Brain Research* 437:1–8.

Detari, L., Juhasz, G., and Kukorelli, T. (1984). Firing properties of cat basal forebrain neurones during sleep-wakefulness cycles. *Electroencephalography and Clinical Neurophysiology* 58:362–368.

Divac, I. (1975). Magnocellular nuclei of the basal forebrain project to the neocortex, brainstem and olfactory bulb. Review of some functional correlates. *Brain Research* 93:385–398.

Doyle, A. C. (1981). A scandal in Bohemia. In *The Celebrated Cases of Sherlock Holmes* (pp. 15–30). London: Octopus Books. (First published in 1891–92)

Dudar, J. D., Whishaw, I. Q., and Szerb, J. C. (1979). Release of acetylcholine from the hippocampus of freely moving rats during sensory stimulation and running. *Neuropharmacology* 18:673–678.

Elul, R. (1972). The genesis of the EEG. *International Review of Neurobiology* 15:228–272.

Fauman, B., Aldinger, G., Fauman, M., and Rosen, P. (1976). Psychiatric sequelae of phencyclidine abuse. *Clinical Toxicology* 9:529–538.

Feder, R., and Ranck, J. B. Jr. (1973). Studies on single neurons in dorsal hippocampal formation and septum in unrestrained rats. Part II. Hippocampal slow waves and theta cell firing during bar pressing and other behaviors. *Experimental Neurology* 41:532–555.

Fleming, D. E., and Bigler, E. D. (1974). Relationship between photically evoked afterdischarge occurrence and hippocampal EEG rhythms in restrained and unrestrained albino rats. *Physiology and Behavior* 13:757–761.

Fox, S. E., and Ranck, J. B., Jr. (1981). Electrophysiological characteristics of hippocampal complex-spike cells and theta cells. *Experimental Brain Research* 41:399–410.

Fox, S. S., and O'Brien, J. H. (1965). Duplication of evoked potential waveform by curve of probability of firing of a single cell. *Science*. 147:888–890.

Fujita, Y., and Sato, T. (1964). Intracellular records from hippocampal pyramidal cells in rabbit during theta rhythm activity. *Journal of Neurophysiology* 27:1011–1025.

Green, J. D., and Arduini, A. A. (1954). Hippocampal electrical activity in arousal. *Journal of Neurophysiology* 17:533–557.

Horn, A. S., Coyle, J. T., and Snyder, S. H. (1971). Catecholamine uptake by synaptosomes from rat brain: Structure-activity relationships of drugs with differential effects on dopamine and norepinephrine neurons. *Molecular Pharmacology* 7:66–80.

Hutton, J. T., and Kenny, A. D. (1985). *Senile Dementia of the Alzheimer Type*. New York: A. R. Liss, Inc.

Ingvar, D. (1955). Electrical activity of isolated cortex in the unanesthetized cat with intact brain stem. *Acta Physiologica Scandinavica* 33:151–168.

Isaacson, R. L., and Pribram, K. H. (1975). *The Hippocampus, Vols. 1 and 2*. New York: Plenum Press.

Isaacson, R. L., and Pribram, K. H. (1986). *The Hippocampus, Vols 3 and 4*. New York, Plenum Press.

Jahnsen, H., and Llinás, R. (1984a). Electrophysiological properties of guinea-pig thalamic neurones: An *in vitro* study. *Journal of Physiology (London)* 349:205–226.

Jahnsen, H., and Llinás, R. (1984b). Ionic basis for the electroresponsiveness and oscillatory properties of guinea-pig thalamic neurones *in vitro*. *Journal of Physiology (London)* 349:227–247.

Jasper, H., and Stefanis, C. (1965). Intracellular oscillatory rhythms in pyramidal tract neurones in the cat. *Electroencephalography and Clinical Neurophysiology* 18:541–553.

Jasper, H. H., and Tessier, J. (1971). Acetylcholine liberation from cerebral cortex during paradoxical (REM) sleep. *Science* 172:601–602.

Johnston, M. V., McKinney, M., and Coyle, J. T. (1981). Neocortical-cholinergic innervation: A description of extrinsic and intrinsic components in the rat. *Experimental Brain Research* 43:159–172.

Jouvet, M. (1967). Neurophysiology of the states of sleep. *Physiological Reviews* 47:117–177.

Jouvet, M. (1972). The role of monoamines and acetylcholine containing neurons in the regulation of the sleep waking cycle. *Ergebnisse der Physiologie* 64:166–307.

Kanai, T., and Szerb, J. C. (1965). Mesencephalic reticular activating system and cortical acetylcholine output. *Nature (London)* 205:80–82.

Kellaway, P., Gol, A., and Proler, M. (1966). Electrical activity of the isolated cerebral hemisphere and isolated thalamus. *Experimental Neurology* 14:281–304.

Kleitman, N. (1963). *Sleep and Wakefulness*. Chicago: University of Chicago Press.

Kolb, B., and Whishaw, I. Q. (1977). Effects of brain lesions and atropine on hippocampal and neocortical electroencephalograms in the rat. *Experimental Neurology* 56:1–22.

Konopacki, J., MacIver, M. B., Bland, B. H., and Roth, S. H. (1987). Carbachol-induced EEG "theta" activity in hippocampal brain slices. *Brain Research* 405:196–198.

Kramis, R., Vanderwolf, C. H., and Bland, B. H. (1975). Two types of hippocampal rhythmical slow activity in both the rabbit and the rat: Relations to behavior and effects of atropine, diethyl ether, urethane and pentobarbital. *Experimental Neurology* 49:58–85.

Lamour, Y., Dutar, P., and Jobert, A. (1984). Septo-hippocampal and other medial-septum diagonal band neurons: Electrophysiological and pharmacological properties. *Brain Research* 309:227–239.

Lamour, Y., Dutar, P., Rascol, O., and Jobert, A. (1986). Basal forebrain neurons projecting to the rat frontoparietal cortex: Electrophysiological and pharmacological properties. *Brain Research* 362:122–131.

Lehmann, J., Nagy, J. I., Atmadja, S., and Fibiger, H. C. (1980). The nucleus basalis magnocellularis: The origin of a cholinergic projection to the neocortex of the rat. *Neuroscience* 5:1161–1174.

Leung, L. S. (1980). Behavior-dependent evoked potentials in the hippocampal CA1 region of the rat. I. Correlation with behavior and EEG. *Brain Research* 198.95–117.

Leung, L.-W. S. (1982). Nonlinear feedback model of neuronal populations in hippocampal CA1 region. *Journal of Neurophysiology* 47:845–868.

Leung, L.-W. S. (1984). Model of gradual phase shift of theta rhythm in the rat. *Journal of Neurophysiology* 52:1051–1065.

Leung, L.-W. S., and Borst, J. G. G. (1987). Electrical activity of the cingulate cortex. I. Generating mechanisms and relations to behavior. *Brain Research* 407:68–80.

Leung, L.-W. S., Harvey. G. C., and Vanderwolf, C. H. (1982). Combined video and computer analysis of the relation between the interhemispheric response and behavior. *Behavioral Brain Research* 6:195–200.

Leung, L. S., Lopes da Silva, F. H., and Wadman, W. J. (1982). Spectral characteristics of the hippocampal EEG in the freely moving rat. *Electroencephalography and Clinical Neurophysiology* 54:203–219.

Leung, L.-W. S., and Yim, C. Y. (1986). Intracellular records of theta rhythm in hippocampal CA1 cells of the rat. *Brain Research* 367:323–327.

Lewis, P. R., and Shute, C. C. D. (1967). The cholinergic limbic system: Projection to hippocampal formation, medial cortex, nuclei of the ascending cholinergic reticular system, and the subfornical organ and supra-optic crest. *Brain* 90:521–540.

Lidov, H. G. W., Grzanna, R., and Molliver, M. E. (1980). The serotonin innervation of the cerebral cortex in the rat: An immunohistochemical analysis. *Neuroscience* 5:207–227.

Lo Conte, G., Casamenti, F., Bigl, V., et al. (1982). Effects of magnocellular forebrain nuclei lesions on acetylcholine output from the cerebral cortex, electrocorticogram and behaviour. *Archives Italiennes de Biologie* 120:176–188.

Lopes da Silva, F. H., and Arnolds, D. E. A. T. (1978). Physiology of the hippocampus and related structures. *Annual Review of Physiology* 40:185–216.

Luby, E. D., Cohen, B. D., Rosenbaum, G., et al. (1959). Study of a new schizophrenomimetic drug—Sernyl. *American Medical Association Archives of Neurology and Psychiatry* 81:363–369.

Luisada, P. V. (1978). The phencyclidine psychosis: Phenomenology and treatment. In R. C. Petersen and R. C. Stillman (eds.), *Phencyclidine (PCP) Abuse: An Appraisal. U.S. National Institute of Drug Abuse Research Monograph* 21:241–253.

McGinty, D. J., Harper, R. M., and Fairbanks, M. K. (1973). 5-HT-containing neurons: Unit activity in behaving cats. In J. Barchas and E. Usdin (eds.), *Serotonin and Behavior* (pp. 267–279). New York: Academic Press.

McGinty, D. J., and Harper, R. M. (1976). Dorsal raphé neurons: Depression of firing during sleep in cats. *Brain Research* 101:569–575.

Moruzzi, G. (1972). The sleep-waking cycle. *Ergebnisse der Physiologie* 64:1–165.

Moruzzi, G., and Magoun, H. W. (1949). Brainstem reticular formation and activation of the EEG. *Electroencephalography and Clinical Neurophysiology* 1:455–473.

Muller, R. U., and Kubie, J. L. (1987). The effect of changes in the environment on the spatial firing of hippocampal complex-spike cells. *Journal of Neuroscience* 7:1951–1968.

Muller, R. U., Kubie, J. L., and Ranck, J. B. Jr. (1987). Spatial firing patterns of hippocampal complex-spike cells in a fixed environment. *Journal of Neuroscience* 7:1935–1950.

Núñez, A., Garcia-Austt, E., and Buño, W., Jr. (1987). Intracellular Θ-rhythm generation in identified hippocampal pyramids. *Brain Research* 416:289–300.

O'Keefe, J. (1976). Place units in the hippocampus of the freely moving rat. *Experimental Neurology* 51:78–109.

O'Keefe, J. (1979). A review of the hippocampal place cells. *Progress in Neurobiology* 13:419–439.

O'Keefe, J., and Nadel, L. (1978). *The Hippocampus as a Cognitive Map.* Oxford: Clarendon Press.

Palmer, A. M., Francis, P. T., Benton, J. S., et al. (1987). Presynaptic serotonergic dysfunction in patients with Alzheimer's disease. *Journal of Neurochemistry* 48:8–18.

Pepeu, G. (1973). The release of acetylcholine from the brain: An approach to the study of central cholinergic mechanisms. *Progress in Neurobiology* 2:257–288.

Pickenhain, L., and Klingberg, F. (1965). Behavioural and electrophysiological changes during avoidance conditioning to light flashes in the rat. *Electroencephalography and Clinical Neurophysiology* 18:464–476.

Pompeiano, O. (1967). The neurophysiological mechanisms of the postural and motor events during desynchronized sleep. *Research Publications of the Association for Nervous and Mental Disease* 45:351–423.

Purpura, D. P. (1959). Nature of electrocortical potentials and synaptic organizations in cerebral and cerebellar cortex. *International Review of Neurobiology* 1:47–163.

Ranck, J. B., Jr. (1973). Studies on single neurons in dorsal hippocampal formation and septum in unrestrained rats. Part 1. Behavioral correlates and firing repertoires. *Experimental Neurology* 41:461–531.

Rasmussen, K., Heym, J., and Jacobs, B. L. (1985). Activity of serotonin-containing neurons in nucleus centralis superior of freely moving cats. *Experimental Neurology* 83:302–317.

Robinson, T. E. (1980). Hippocampal rhythmic slow activity (RSA; theta): A critical analysis of selected studies and discussion of possible species-differences. *Brain Research Reviews* 2:69–101.

Robinson, T. E., and Green, D. G. (1980). Effects of hemicholinium-3 and choline on hippocampal electrical activity during immobility vs. movement. *Electroencephalography and Clinical Neurophysiology* 50:314–323.

Robinson, T. E., Kramis, R. C., and Vanderwolf, C. H. (1977). Two types of cerebral activation during active sleep: Relations to behavior. *Brain Research* 124:544–549.

Rose, G. (1983). Physiological and behavioral characteristics of dentate granule cells. In W. Seifert (ed.), *Neurobiology of the Hippocampus* (pp. 449–472). London: Academic Press.

Rougeul, A., Letalle, A., and Corvisier, J. (1972). Activite rhythmique du cortex somesthesique primaire en relation avec l'immobilite chez le chat libre eveille. *Electroencephalography and Clinical Neurophysiology* 33:23–39.

Rowntree, C. I., and Bland, B. H. (1986). An analysis of cholinoceptive neurons in the hippocampal formation by direct microinfusion. *Brain Research* 362:98–113.

Sainsbury, R. S. (1970). Hippocampal activity during natural behavior in the guinea pig. *Physiology and Behavior* 5:317–324.

Sainsbury, R. S., Heynen, A., and Montoya, C. P. (1987). Behavioral correlates of hippocampal type 2 theta in the rat. *Physiology and Behavior* 39:513–519.

Saper, C. B. (1984). Organization of cerebral cortical afferent systems in the rat. II. Magnocellular basal nucleus. *Journal of Comparative Neurology* 222:313–342.

Satoh, K., and Fibiger, H. C. (1986). Cholinergic neurons of the laterodorsal tegmental nucleus: Efferent and afferent connections. *Journal of Comparative Neurology* 253:277–302.

Schaffer, C. B., Pandey, G., Noll, K. M., et al. (1980). Introduction and theories of affective disorders. In G. C. Palmer (ed.), *Neuropharmacology of Central Nervous System and Behavioral Disorders* (pp. 1–35). New York: Academic Press.

Schaul, N., Gloor, P., Ball, G., and Gotman, J. (1978). The electromicrophysiology of delta waves induced by systemic atropine. *Brain Research* 143:475–486.

Scheibel, A. B., Wechsler, A. F., and Brazier, M. A. B. (1986). *The Biological Substrates of Alzheimer's Disease*. UCLA Forum in Medical Sciences. Orlando: Academic Press, no. 27.

Schlag, J. D., and Chaillet, F. (1963). Thalamic mechanisms involved in cortical desynchronization and recruiting responses. *Electroencephalography and Clinical Neurophysiology* 15:39–62.

Schwartzbaum, J. S., and Kreinick, C. J. (1973). Interrelationships of hippocampal electroencephalogram, visually evoked response, and behavioral reactivity to photic stimuli in rats. *Journal of Comparative and Physiological Psychology* 85:479–490.

Schwartzbaum, J. S., Kreinick, C. J., and Gustafson, J. W. (1971). Cortical evoked potentials and behavioral reactivity to photic stimuli in freely moving rats. *Brain Research* 27:295–307.

Seifert, W. (1983). *Neurobiology of the Hippocampus*. London: Academic Press.

Semba, K., Szechtman, H., and Komisaruk, B. R. (1980). Synchrony among rhythmical facial tremor, neocortical 'alpha' waves, and thalamic non-sensory neuronal bursts in intact awake rats. *Brain Research* 195:281–298.

Shepherd, G. M. (1977). The olfactory bulb: A simple system in the mammalian brain. In J. M. Brookhart, V. B. Mountcastle, E. R. Kandel, and S. R. Geiger (eds.), *Handbook of Physiology: Section 1: The Nervous System, Vol. 1, Cellular Biology of Neurons, Part 2* (pp. 945–968). Bethesda: American Physiological Society.

Shute, C. C. D., and Lewis, P. R. (1967). The ascending cholinergic reticular system: Neocortical, olfactory and subcortical projections. *Brain* 90:497–520.

Siegel, J. M. (1979). Behavioral functions of the reticular formation. *Brain Research Reviews* 1:69–105.

Snyder, S. H. (1980). Phencyclidine. *Nature* 285:355–356.

Spencer, W. A. (1977). The physiology of supraspinal neurons in mammals. In J. M. Brookhart, V. B. Mountcastle, E. R. Kandel, and S. R. Geiger (eds.), *Handbook of Physiology: Section 1: The Nervous System, Vol. 1, Cellular Biology of Neurons, Part 2* (pp. 969–1021). Bethesda: American Physiological Society.

Spencer, W. A., and Brookhart, J. M. (1961a). Electrical patterns of augmenting and recruiting waves in depths of sensorimotor cortex of cat. *Journal of Neurophysiology* 24:26–49.

Spencer, W. A., and Brookhart, J. M. (1961b). A study of spontaneous spindle waves in sensorimotor cortex of cat. *Journal of Neurophysiology* 24:50–65.

Stahl, S. M., Ciaranello, R. D., and Berger, P. A. (1982). Platelet serotonin in schizophrenia and depression. In B. T. Ho, J. C. Schoolar, and E. Usdin (eds.), *Serotonin in Biological Psychiatry. Advances in Biochemical Psychopharmacology, Vol. 34* (pp. 183–198). New York: Raven Press.

Starr, A. (1964). Influence of motor activity on click-evoked responses in the auditory pathway of waking cats. *Experimental Neurology* 10:191–204.

Steinbusch, H. W. M., and Nieuwenhuys, R. (1983). The raphe nuclei of the rat brainstem: A cytoarchitectonic and immunohistochemical study. In P. C. Emson (ed.), *Chemical Neuroanatomy* (pp. 131–207). New York: Raven Press.

Steriade, M., Deschenes, M., Domich, L., and Mulle, C. (1985). Abolition of spindle oscillations in thalamic neurons disconnected from nucleus reticularis thalami. *Journal of Neurophysiology* 54:1473–1497.

Steriade, M., and Hobson, J. A. (1976). Neuronal activity during the sleep-waking cycle. In G. A. Kerkut and J. W. Phillis (eds.), *Progress in Neurobiology, Vol. 6* (pp. 155–376). Oxford: Pergamon Press.

Stewart, D. J., MacFabe, D. F., and Vanderwolf, C. H. (1984). Cholinergic activation of the electrocorticogram: Role of the substantia innominata and effects of atropine and quinuclidinyl benzilate. *Brain Research* 322:219–232.

Stewart, D. J., and Vanderwolf, C. H. (1987a). Hippocampal rhythmical slow activity following ibotenic acid lesions of the septal region. I. Relations to behavior and effects of atropine and urethane. *Brain Research* 423:88–100.

Stewart, D. J., and Vanderwolf, C. H. (1987b). Hippocampal rhythmical slow activity following ibotenic acid lesions of the septal region. II. Changes in hippocampal activity during sleep. *Brain Research* 423:101–108.

Stumpf, Ch. (1965). Drug action on the electrical activity of the hippocampus. *International Review of Neurobiology* 8:77–138.

Szerb, J. C. (1967). Cortical acetylcholine release and electroencephalographic arousal. *Journal of Physiology (London)* 192:329–343.

Trulson, M. E., and Jacobs, B. L. (1979). Raphe unit activity in freely moving cats: Correlation with level of behavioral arousal. *Brain Research* 163:135–150.

Trulson, M. E., and Jacobs, B. L. (1981). Activity of serotonin-containing neurons in freely moving cats. In B. L. Jacobs and A. Gelperin (eds.), *Serotonin Neurotransmission and Behavior* (pp. 339–365). Cambridge, Mass.: MIT Press.

Vanderwolf, C. H. (1969). Hippocampal electrical activity and voluntary movement in the rat. *Electroencephalography and Clinical Neurophysiology* 26:407–418.

Vanderwolf, C. H. (1975). Neocortical and hippocampal activation in relation to behavior: Effects of atropine, eserine, phenothiazines, and amphetamine. *Journal of Comparative and Physiological Psychology* 88:300–323.

Vanderwolf, C. H. (1984). Aminergic control of the electrocorticogram: A progress report. In A. A. Boulton, G. B. Baker, W. Dewhurst, and M. Sandler (eds.), *Neurobiology of the Trace Amines* (pp. 163–183). Clifton, N.J.: Humana Press.

Vanderwolf, C. H. (1987a). Suppression of serotonin-dependent cerebral activation: A possible mechanism of action of some psychotomimetic drugs. *Brain Research* 414:109–118.

Vanderwolf, C. H. (1987b). Near-total loss of "learning" and "memory" as a result of combined cholinergic and serotonergic blockade in the rat. *Behavioral Brain Research* 23:43–57.

Vanderwolf, C. H. (1988). Cerebral activity and behavior: Control by central cholinergic and serotonergic systems. *International Review of Neurobiology* 30:225–340.

Vanderwolf, C. H., and Baker, G. B. (1986). Evidence that serotonin mediates non-cholinergic neocortical low voltage fast activity, non-cholinergic hippocampal rhythmical slow activity and contributes to intelligent behavior. *Brain Research* 374:342–356.

Vanderwolf, C. H., Kramis, R., Gillespie, L. A., et al. (1975). Hippocampal rhythmic slow activity and neocortical low voltage fast activity: Relations to behavior. In R. L. Isaacson and K. H. Pribram (eds.), *The Hippocampus, Volume 2: Neurophysiology and Behavior* (pp. 101–128) New York: Plenum Press.

Vanderwolf, C. H., Harvey, G. C., and Leung, L.-W. S. (1987). Transcallosal evoked potentials in relation to behavior in the rat: Effects of atropine, *p*-chlorophenylalanine, reserpine, scopolamine and trifluoperazine. *Behavioral Brain Research* 25:31–48.

Vanderwolf, C. H., Kramis, R., and Robinson, T. E. (1978). Hippocampal electrical activity during waking behaviour and sleep: Analyses using centrally acting drugs. *Functions of the Septo-Hippocampal System* (pp. 199–226). Ciba Foundation Symposium 58 (new series). Amsterdam: Elsevier, Excerpta Medica, North-Holland.

Vanderwolf, C. H., Leung, L.-W. S., and Cooley, R. K. (1985). Pathways through cingulate, neo- and entorhinal cortices mediate atropine-resistant hippocampal rhythmical slow activity. *Brain Research* 347:58–73.

Vanderwolf, C. H., and Pappas, B. A. (1980). Reserpine abolishes movement-correlated atropine-resistant neocortical low voltage fast activity. *Brain Research* 202:79–94.

Vanderwolf, C. H., and Robinson, T. E. (1981). Reticulo-cortical activity and behavior: A critique of the arousal theory and a new synthesis. *Behavioral and Brain Sciences* 4:459–514.

Vanderwolf, C. H., Robinson, T. E., and Pappas, B. A. (1980). Monoamine replacement after reserpine: Catecholaminergic agonists restore motor activity but phenylethylamine restores atropine-resistant neocortical low-voltage fast activity. *Brain Research* 202:65–77.

Vanderwolf, C. H., and Stewart, D. J. (1986). Joint cholinergic-serotonergic control of neocortical and hippocampal electrical activity in relation to behavior: Effects of scopolamine, Ditran, trifluoperazine, and amphetamine. *Physiology and Behavior* 38:57–65.

Vanderwolf, C. H., and Stewart, D. J. (1988). Thalamic control of neocortical activation: A critical re-evaluation. *Brain Research Bulletin* 20:529–538.

Villablanca, J., and Salinas-Zeballos, M. E. (1972). Sleep-wakefulness, EEG, and behavioral studies of chronic cats without the thalamus: The "athalamic cat." *Archives Italiennes de Biologie* 110:383–411.

Vinogradova, O. S., Brazhnik, E. S., Karanov, A. M., and Zhadina, S. D. (1980). Neuronal activity of the septum following various types of deafferentation. *Brain Research* 187:353–368.

Weil-Malherbe, H. (1978). Serotonin and schizophrenia. In W. B. Essman (ed.), *Serotonin in Health and Disease, Vol. 3, The Central Nervous System* (pp. 231–291). New York: Spectrum Publications.

Welsh, D. K., Richardson, G. S., and Dement, W. C. (1985). A circadian rhythm of hippocampal theta activity in the mouse. *Physiology and Behavior* 35:533–538.

Whishaw, I. Q. (1972). Hippocampal electroencephalographic activity in the Mongolian gerbil during natural behaviours and wheel running and in the rat during wheel running and conditioned immobility. *Canadian Journal of Psychology* 26:219–239.

Whishaw, I. Q., Bland, B. H., Robinson, T. E., and Vanderwolf, C. H. (1976). Neuromuscular blockade: The effects of two hippocampal RSA (theta) systems and neocortical desynchronization. *Brain Research Bulletin* 1:573–581.

Whishaw, I. Q., O'Connor, W. T., and Dunnett, S. B. (1985). Disruption of central cholinergic systems in the rat by basal forebrain lesions or atropine: Effects on feeding, sensorimotor behaviour, locomotor activity, and spatial navigation. *Behavioral Brain Research* 17:103–115.

Whishaw, I. Q., and Vanderwolf, C. H. (1973). Hippocampal EEG and behavior: Changes in amplitude and frequency of RSA (theta rhythm) associated with spontaneous and learned movement patterns in rats and cats. *Behavioral Biology* 8:461–484.

Whitehouse, P. J., Price, D. L., Clark, A. W., et al. (1981). Alzheimer's disease: Evidence for selective loss of cholinergic neurons in the nucleus basalis. *Annals of Neurology* 10:122–126.

Whitford, G. M. (1986). Alzheimer's disease and serotonin: A review. *Neuropsychobiology* 15:133–142.

Winson, J. (1972). Interspecies differences in the occurrence of theta. *Behavioral Biology* 7:479–487.

Winson, J. (1974). Patterns of hippocampal theta rhythm in the freely moving rat. *Electroencephalography and Clinical Neurophysiology* 36:291–301.

Woolf, N. J., and Butcher, L. L. (1986). Cholinergic systems in the rat brain. III. Projections from the pontomesencephalic tegmentum to the thalamus, tectum, basal ganglia, and basal forebrain. *Brain Research Bulletin* 16:603–637.

III Motor Systems

7 Motor Functions of the Neocortex

Bryan Kolb

Since the time of Hughlings-Jackson, we have known that impairments of movement arise from cortical damage to the classical motor region (Brodmann's area 4 in the primate) as well from damage to much of the rest of the cortex. Although it is accepted that the motor contributions of the different cortical regions are dissociable, little is known about the nature of their relative contributions. It has proved difficult to dissociate different regions in humans because of (1) an absence of patients with lesions restricted to the appropriate (anatomically and electrophysiologically defined) regions of neocortex, and (2) the impossibility of making any controlled anatomical manipulations. Thus the study of nonhuman animals must provide the analogs in which the relative contributions of these areas are uncovered. Although studies with monkeys have demonstrated various motor impairments after lesions to the primary motor, parietal, and prefrontal cortices, only modest progress has been made in dissociating the contributions of different cortical areas to the control of movement. One reason for this is that studies with nonhuman primates have focused on a specific kind of movement, namely, reaching, and have ignored the other kinds of movements that monkeys make in their natural world. This problem is not easily solved, however, because it is usually impractical to study free-ranging monkeys with the degree of precision necessary in studies of motor control. The advantage of the rat is that it can be studied in a wider range of behavioral situations, and such investigations may shed light on the role of the cortex in motor control.

A significant hindrance to the study of cortical control of movement in nonprimates in general and in rodents in particular has been the widely held conviction that monkeys and apes are the only animals whose movements are really analogous to those of humans. About thirty years ago the belief developed that the effects of motor cortex damage became progressively more serious as one compared rodents to carnivores to primates. For example, Lassek (1954, pp. 65–66) concluded that removal of Brodmann's area 4 in primates causes "an enduring paralysis of isolated movements, especially in the digits. A flaccid type of paralysis occurs in the proximal joints, whereas the wrists and fingers pass through a period of moderate spasticity." In contrast "the motor cortex appears to be largely dispensable in mammals ranking below primates. [Ablation of motor cortex in the rat or cat] is attended by only negligible transitory deficits" (Lassek 1954, p. 67). If indeed Lassek's observations were valid, it is hardly surprising that investigators of motor function would want to focus on the primate cortex. In fact, however, the conclusion drawn from the comparison of deficits in reaching in monkeys and walking in rats or cats is not valid. Whereas only posture and locomotion were observed in early studies of rodents with motor decortications, more recent work has shown that the movement of the wrist, hand, and fingers is impaired in rodents as well as in primates after motor cortex lesions. Indeed chapter 9 by Bures and Bracha shows striking parallels not only between the behavioral changes after motor decortication in rats and monkeys but also in the electrophysiological correlates of movements in the two orders.

To determine the nature of the involvement of the neocortex in the execution of different movements and behaviors in the rat, it is reasonable to begin by carefully studying the behavior of rats with complete neodecortications. When Whishaw and I (1984) began to reexamine the behavior of the decorticate preparation, we were surprised to discover that the animals appeared remarkably normal when observed in a laboratory cage and that it was possible to virtually eliminate the feeding deficits with appropriate preoperative and postoperative experiences. Furthermore, although the study of more complex behaviors such as learning, sexual, and maternal behaviors in the 1920s, 1930s, and 1940s by both Lashley and Beach had emphasized the behavioral losses of these animals, Whishaw and I (1984) as well as Oakley (1983) found that the animals were capable of many learned and species-typical behaviors, although the details of behavior were often quite clumsy and sometimes even peculiar. It is now clear that the role of the cortex has been poorly understood for many behaviors. Whishaw's chapter 10 summarizes what is known about the behavior of the decorticate rat and provides us with an important reference point as we try to unravel the role of discrete cortical regions in the control of movement.

Having identified the changes in the control of movement after decortication, it is now possible to begin to look at the localization of motor control functions in the cortex. First Neafsey reviews in chapter 8 the anatomical and electrophysiological organization of the motor cortex, which can be defined as the cortex forming the motor ratunculus. In the next chapter Bures and Bracha review the effects of cortical lesions of the ratunculus on skilled movements in the rat, especially reaching. Detailed discussions of other types of movement changes, especially those of placing responses, can be found in a review by Bures and colleagues (1983).

A comparison of the motor losses of complete neodecorticate (Whishaw, chapter 10) and motor decorticate (Bures and Bracha, chapter 9) rats reveals that there is a lot we do not know. The decorticate rat has far more severe behavioral loss than can be accounted for by the loss of the motor and sensory ratunculus. There must be significant contributions of the other sensory systems in the guidance of movement as well as from the frontal regions forming the prefrontal cortex. The contribution of the visual input to motor control is reviewed by Goodale and Carey (chapter 10), and that of the prefrontal region is alluded to in chapter 18 and in a review by Kolb and Whishaw (1983).

References

Beach, F. (1940). Effects of cortical lesions upon the copulatory behavior of male rats. *Journal of Comparative Psychology* 29:193–244.

Bures, J., Buresova, O., and Huston, J. P. (1983). *Techniques and Basic Experiments for the Study of Brain and Behavior*. 2nd ed. Amsterdam: Elsevier.

Kolb, B., and Whishaw, I. Q. (1983). Dissociation of the contributions of the prefrontal, motor, and parietal cortex to the control of movement in the rat: An experimental review. *Canadian Journal of Psychology* 37:211–232.

Lassek, A. M. (1954). *The Pyramidal Tract*. Springfield, IL: Charles C. Thomas.

Lashley, K. S. (1921). Studies of cerebral function in learning. III. The motor areas. *Brain* 44:255–285.

Oakley, D. A. (1983). Learning capacity outside neocortex in animals and man: Implications for therapy after brain-injury. In G. C. L. Davey (ed.), *Animal Models of Human Behavior*. New York: John Wiley & Sons, 247–266.

Whishaw, I. Q., and Kolb, B. (1984). Behavioral and anatomical studies of rats with complete or partial decortication in infancy: Functional sparing, crowding, or loss and cerebral growth or shrinkage. In R. Almli and S. Finger (eds.), *Early Brain Damage: Neurobiology and Behavior*. New York: Academic Press, 117–138.

8 The Complete Ratunculus: Output Organization of Layer V of the Cerebral Cortex

Edward J. Neafsey

[E]very area of the cortex can be viewed as a motor area, or layer V itself could be termed the "motor cortex." (Diamond 1979)

This chapter describes the motor output organization of the sensorimotor cortex of the rat; in addition it proposes a scheme for the overall motor output organization of the entire cortex, including the hippocampus and piriform cortex. This latter task becomes feasible when all cortical output is considered to be directed at only three major targets: body, eyes-head, and viscera (Diamond 1979, Neafsey et al. 1986b). Just as Lawrence and Kuypers (1968a, b) provided insight into the functions of the various descending motor pathways by focusing on the motor neurons they controlled, important insights into the organization of the cerebral cortex can be achieved by focusing on the motor or effector targets of its output.

8.1 Somatic Motor Cortex

Cytoarchitecture

The topography of the major cytoarchitectonic fields in the rat frontal and parietal cortex has been agreed upon (Donoghue and Wise 1982) and provides a convenient terminology to designate various subdivisions in this rather large expanse of cortex. In addition, in a number of instances cytoarchitectonic borders correspond with functional borders (see below). Figure 8.1 depicts a dorsolateral view of the left cerebral cortical surface of the rat, with the midline at the top of the figure and the frontal pole at the left. Proceeding from medial to lateral at the level of bregma (B), five major cytoarchitectonic regions are indicated by the heavy lines: AGM, medial agranular; AGL, lateral agranular; S-I, granular primary somatosensory (barrelfield); S-II, granular secondary somatosensory; and INS, insular cortex. AGM, the rat's frontal eye field, can be distinguished from AGL, the primary motor cortex, on the basis of the denser layer II in AGM. The border between AGL and S-I may be thought of as the rat's "central sulcus," which separates the primary somatic motor cortex from the primary somatic sensory cortex. (Some of these regions may be subdivided further. For example, Chapin and

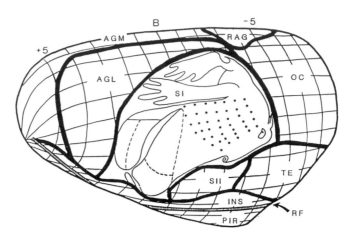

Figure 8.1 Dorsolateral view of rat left hemisphere with 1-mm^2 grid (boxes) and cytoarchitectonic borders (heavy lines) indicated. Frontal pole is at left, midline is at top, and numbers (+5, −5) denote distance in millimeters rostral and caudal to bregma. B = bregma; RF = rhinal fissure; AGM = agranular medial; AGL = agranular lateral; S-I = granular primary somatosensory; S-II = granular secondary somatosensory; INS = insular; PIR = piriform; RAG = retrosplenial agranular; OC = occipital visual; TE = temporal auditory. A ratunculus has been superimposed on S-I after Chapin and Lin (1984). (Modified from figure 2 of Neafsey et al. 1986a. Used with the publisher's permission.)

Lin (1984) have subdivided S-I into granular, perigranular, and dysgranular zones; and Krettek and Price (1977) and Kosar and colleagues (1986) have subdivided INS into agranular and granular portions. For completeness the visual (OC), auditory (TE), retrosplenial agranular (RAG), and piriform (PIR) cortical areas are also labeled. An overall, detailed description of rat cortical cytoarchitecture has been provided by Zilles (1985).

Microstimulation Mapping

In a recent review (Neafsey et al. 1986a) my coworkers and I described in detail our experiments investigating the organization of the rat somatic motor cortex using intracortical microstimulation (300-ms trains of 0.25-ms pulses at 350 Hz, currents less than 50 μA) in rats anesthetized with ketamine HCl (100 mg/kg). One of the major findings of these experiments was the discovery of a second motor representation near the frontal pole. Figure 8.2 illustrates the results of two typical mapping experiments in which two forelimb motor areas were delineated, one just rostral and lateral to bregma, corresponding to the "traditional" primary forelimb motor area (Hall and Lindholm 1974, Woolsey 1958), and another located far rostrally, with an intervening zone where neck or vibrissae movements were elicited at the lowest thresholds (also cf. Sanderson et al. 1984). This rostral forelimb motor area overlaps the separate rostral patch of corticospinal neurons near

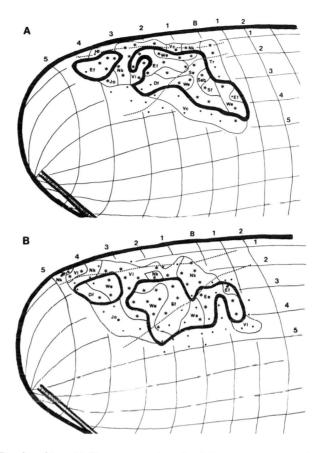

Figure 8.2 Results of two (A,B) separate microstimulation mapping experiments. Numbers indicate millimeters rostral or caudal to bregma (B). Each square on grid represents 1 mm². Asterisks denote stimulation points where the threshold current was below 25 μA, small dots denote points where threshold current was below 50 μA, and large dots denote points where threshold current was below 100 μA. Small dots outside areas enclosed by lines indicate points where no response was seen below maximum current used in that experiment. Dashed lines indicate cytoarchitectonic borders between AGM and AGL (medial line) and between AGL and S-I (lateral line). Df = digit flexion; Ee = elbow extension; Ef = elbow flexion; Hf = hip flexion; Jo = jaw open; Nk = neck muscle twitch; Sab = shoulder abduction; Se = shoulder extension; Sf = shoulder flexion; Tr = trunk; Vc = vibrissae contralateral; Vi = vibrissae ipsilateral; We = wrist extension. (From figure 3 of Neafsey et al. 1986a. Used with the publisher's permission.)

the frontal pole, first described by Hicks and D'Amato (1977) and subsequently confirmed by others (Neafsey and Sievert 1982, Wise et al. 1979). Detailed mapping experiments of the rostral motor area revealed in some animals a small, medially located hindlimb area (figure 8.2A), indicating that a "complete" body representation may exist here and suggesting that this rostral motor area may be the rat's homolog of the primate's supplementary motor area (Neafsey and Sievert 1982, Wise et al. 1979). Medial to the caudal forelimb motor area, a long, narrow vibrissae-neck (Vc, Vi, Nk) movement zone was found, in agreement with other studies (Hall and Lindholm 1974, Sanderson et al. 1984). Note also that in general movements were elicited from small, irregularly shaped patches of cortex, each including several adjacent stimulation points, thereby creating a mosaic pattern of organization for the somatic motor cortex. (It must be mentioned, however, that on the borders between two movement zones, it was not unusual for both movements to be evoked at low-current intensities. This "overlap," which is *not* shown on the maps, may at least in part account for the variability among different published rat motor cortical maps (Gioanni and Lamarche 1985, Hall and Lindholm 1974, Neafsey et al. 1986a, Sanderson et al. 1984, Woolsey 1958). Other sources of variability between studies include different stimulation parameters, electrodes, and anesthetics.

Histological analysis located the rostral motor area in AGL, with the rostral hindlimb subdivision extending slightly into AGM. With this one exception the border between AGM and AGL corresponded to the functional border between the vibrissae-eyes-neck movement cortex (AGM) and the limb-jaw-tongue movement cortex (AGL). The caudal forelimb motor area was located in both AGL and S-I, with low-threshold responses (<25 μA) seen in both regions, although in any particular experiment thresholds were usually lower in AGL than in S-I.

The detailed internal organization of the hindlimb, jaw-lips-tongue, and vibrissae motor areas was also studied (Neafsey et al. 1986a), and a composite map summarizing the low-current intensity (<50 μA) responses from all of the mapping experiments is illustrated in figure 8.3. This map is a highly idealized picture because there was significant variability from animal to animal in the detailed internal organization of each major motor region. Nonetheless the map does depict typical features. The thin solid lines superimpose a 1-mm^2 grid in perspective on the cortical surface. The heavy dotted lines outline the major functional subdivisions in the motor cortex such as the forelimb or hindlimb areas; the light dotted lines indicate the typical internal organization within each of these regions. Both the rostral and caudal motor regions exhibit a somatotopic organization, as described by all other studies (Gioanni and Lamarche 1985, Hall and Lindholm 1974, Sanderson et al. 1984, Woolsey 1958). There are a number of examples, however, where adjacent cortical movement zones do *not* represent adjacent body parts,

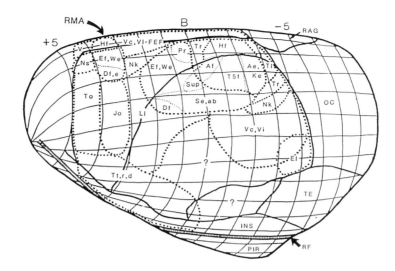

Figure 8.3 Idealized summary map of responses evoked with currents below 50 μA. The light lines superimpose a 1-mm² grid, and the heavier solid lines indicate the cytoarchitectonic borders as described in figure 8.1. The heavy dotted lines surround the major subdivisions of the motor cortex, and the light dotted lines indicate the typical internal organization within the forelimb and hindlimb areas. The arrow at top left indicates the rostral motor area (RMA). Most abbreviations are defined in captions to figures 8.1 and 8.2. Ae = ankle extension; Af = ankle flexion; E1 = eyelid; FEF = frontal eye field; Ke = knee extension; Lf − lower lip; Ns − nose twitch; Pr = pronation; Sup = supination; T1 = tail; To = tongue out; Tt, r, d = tongue tip twitch, tongue right side twitch (contralateral), or tongue dorsum twitch; T5f = toe 5 flexion. Question marks are found in unmapped parts of S-I and S-II that may also be motor regions. (Adapted from figure 13 of Neafsey et al. 1986a. Used with the publisher's permission.)

such as the border between the caudal hind limb area and the more medial vibrassae area.

Overlap

One striking feature that distinguishes this map from most previous maps is the large amount of S-I "sensory" cortex that yielded motor responses at currents less than 50 μA. For example, note the large expanse of S-I (and INS) cortex where microstimulation elicits tongue (Tt, r, d) or lower lip (Ll) movements. This "extension" of motor cortex into S-I was particularly well demonstrated by Gioanni and Lamarche (1985), who evoked vibrissae and eyelid movements from S-I barrelfield granular cortex, the results of which are included on the map in figure 8.3 (portions of S-I labeled Vc, Vi, and E1). Parts of S-I (and S-II) labeled with a question mark in figure 8.3 have not yet been mapped but may be "motor" as well.

This overlap of "motor" cortex with "sensory" cortex does not of course mean that no distinction can be made between these cortical regions. For example, a number of investigators have demonstrated qualitative and quantitative differences in the peripheral sensory inputs to these regions. S-I's granular zone forelimb representation receives primarily cutaneous inputs, while S-I's dysgranular zone forelimb area receives primarily deep (joint and muscle) inputs (Chapin and Lin 1984, Welker et al. 1984). By comparison AGL's caudal forelimb area also receives primarily deep inputs, whereas AGL's rostral forelimb area receives virtually no peripheral sensory input from the contralateral forelimb (Sievert and Neafsey 1983, Welker et al. 1984). These differences are much more significant than some slight difference in microstimulation threshold current.

The common feature of cortex where low-threshold movement responses to electrical stimulation are elicited is that this cortex gives rise to direct, descending corticospinal and corticobulbar projections (Wise et al. 1979), supporting Diamond's observation, quoted at the beginning of the chapter, that layer V of the cerebral cortex (even in "sensory cortex") should be considered as motor cortex. Wise and Donoghue (1986) have proposed a differential overlap scheme for the rat sensorimotor cortex, with complete overlap for the hindlimb sensory and motor regions, partial overlap between the forelimb sensory and motor regions, and absence of overlap between vibrissae sensory and motor regions. As noted, however, Gioanni and Lamarche (1985) have clearly demonstrated that vibrissae movements can be elicited at low currents (<50 μA) from the vibrissae, barrelfield somatic sensory cortex, a finding that calls into question the basic premise of the differential overlap scheme and suggests that the simpler, complete overlap theory presented above is more correct.

Frontal Eye Field

The border between AGM and AGL also represents the lateral border of the vibrissae motor cortex. In several studies (Hall and Lindholm 1974, Sanderson et al. 1984), the AGM cortex has also been associated with eye, eyelid, and pupillary motor responses, and we also have elicited such responses from this cortex (Neafsey et al. 1986a). Such a combination of responses may appear puzzling, but can likely be explained by two observations: (1) AGM has strong direct projections to the superior colliculus (Leichnetz and Gonzalo-Ruiz 1987, Neafsey et al. 1986b, Reep et al. 1987), and (2) electrical stimulation of the superior colliculus in the rat evokes coordinated eye, eyelid, and vibrissae movements (McHaffie and Stein 1982). Thus the border between AGM and AGL is a watershed, separating medial, eyes-head cortex in AGM from lateral, limb-jaw-tongue cortex in AGL. AGM and the medially adjacent anterior cingulate (AC) and prelimbic (PL) cortices have been termed the frontal eye field in the rat and other species, due not only to the eyes-head movements evoked here by electrical stimulation (Hall and Lindholm 1974, Hess 1969, Kaada 1960, Sinnamon and Galer 1984) but also to the significant, reciprocal connections between this cortex and the visual cortex (Miller and Vogt 1984). Also consistent with this view are the results of lesion studies that have concluded that this antero-medial cortex functions as part of a "spatial mapping system" that "includes the superior colliculus and serves attentional orienting functions" (Kolb 1984; cf. also Crowne and Pathria 1982, Foreman 1983). Rats with lesions of this cortex are unable to learn the Morris water maze task and are impaired in learning the location of reward in the radial maze task, as well as showing significant contralateral neglect (Sutherland et al. 1982). Finally, single units in the anteromedial frontal cortex of the rat change their discharge rate during head-orienting movements (Kanki et al. 1983).

8.2 Overall Cortical Output Organization

Somatic Motor Cortex

The preceding discussion of the juxtaposition of sensorimotor cortex and frontal eye field cortex introduced two of the three major targets of cortical layer V output: body (somatic) and eyes-head. As just discussed, *somatic* output cortex corresponds to the entire sensorimotor cortex, anatomically defined as the source of direct descending corticobulbar and corticospinal projections and physiologically defined as the cortex where electrical stimulation produces limb-jaw-tongue movement.

Eyes-Head Motor Cortex

Eyes-head output cortex corresponds in part with the already described frontal eye field cortex located in AGM-AC-PL, but also includes other cortical regions with projections to the superior colliculus, including the visual cortex (OC, Diamond 1979 and Olavarria and Van Sluyters 1982), the auditory cortex (TE, Diamond 1979 and Faye-Lund 1985), the posterior cingulate retrosplenial cortex (RSA + RSG, Neafsey et al. 1986b, Sikes et al. 1988, and Vogt et al. 1986). The piriform (PIR) olfactory cortex is also included in this group because its deepest layers (termed the endopiriform nucleus) have recently been shown to project directly to the superior colliculus (Neafsey et al. 1986b). Of course many of these cortical regions project to other targets in addition to the tectum, but a tectal output is the common factor that allows these different cortical areas to be functionally linked. It is interesting to note that the hippocampal formation, although lacking direct projections to the superior colliculus, does project strongly to the medial frontal eyes-head cortex (Ferino et al. 1987, Sorensen 1985, Swanson and Kohler 1986). Identification of this target for hippocampal output as eyes-head orientation output cortex may help explain the deficits in spatial mapping and maze performance seen following hippocampal lesions (Morris et al. 1982, O'Keefe and Nadel 1978, Sutherland et al. 1982).

Visceral Motor Cortex

The third and last major target of cortical layer V output is the viscera, defined broadly as the respiratory musculature and the internal organs of the body controlled by the autonomic nervous system. *Visceral* output cortex is anatomically defined as cortex that gives rise to direct projections to either the solitary nucleus of vagus (NTS) or to the periaqueductal gray (PAG). The NTS is a major brainstem respiratory control region (the dorsal respiratory group; McCrimmon et al. 1987) and also receives visceral afferent inputs from cranial nerves VIII, IX, and X (Contreras et al. 1982). Direct cortical projections to the NTS arise from the insular (Neafsey et al. 1986b, Saper 1982, van der Kooy et al. 1984) and infralimbic (Terreberry and Neafsey 1983, 1987, van der Kooy et al. 1984) cortices of the rat, and stimulation in both evokes cardiovascular, respiratory, and gastric responses (Burns and Wyss 1985, Hurley-Gius and Neafsey 1986, Ruggiero et al. 1987, Terreberry and Neafsey 1984). The insular and infralimbic cortices also give rise to strong projections to the PAG, as does the intervening orbital (OR) cortex (Hardy and Leichnetz 1981, Neafsey et al. 1986b). The PAG has also been associated with visceral function, particularly with various autonomic components of the "defense response" (Yardley and Hilton 1986) and with control of reproductive behaviors (Fahrbach et al. 1986). In addition the PAG has been linked to respiratory control because it acts as key brain area in the production of vocalizations (Larson and Kistler 1986, Muller-Preuss and Jurgens 1976, Yajima et al. 1980). For these reasons the orbital cortex has been included in the realm of "visceral cortex," even though it lacks direct projections to the NTS. (It should also be pointed out that the orbital cortex is not the only cortex with a projection to the PAG; the insular, infralimbic, prelimbic, anterior cingulate, and retrosplenial cortices also project to the PAG (Neafsey et al. 1986b).

The hippocampal formation, whose relationship with eyes-head cortex has been discussed above, can also be considered to be in part a visceral output cortex for two reasons. First, although the hippocampal formation lacks direct projections to the NTS or PAG, hippocampal stimulation has recently been shown to evoke large heart rate and blood pressure responses (Ruit and Neafsey 1988) that appear to be mediated in part by the massive projection from the hippocampus to the infralimbic cortex (Swanson 1981). Second, if the notion of visceral is expanded to include hormonal regulation of bodily organs, then the hippocampal formation, with its well-documented projections to the hypothalamus (Swanson 1983) and its important role in feedback control of corticosterone levels (Dunn and Orr 1984, McEwen et al. 1979, Sapolsky et al. 1983a, b 1984, Stumpf and Sar 1981), clearly merits classification as a visceral output type of cortex and may even deserve the name "endocrine motor cortex."

Overall Topography of Cortical Output

The topographical relationships of these three types of cortical outputs are illustrated in figure 8.4, using the flattened but topologically correct map of the rat cerebral hemisphere originally provided by Swanson (1983). Figure 8.4A is a modified version of Swanson's map on which the major cortical cytoarchitectonic fields have been labeled. Note that the corpus callosum (CC) is found at the top of the figure, the frontal pole is to the left, the olfactory bulb–olfactory nucleus (OB-ON) and piriform cortex (PIR) are at the lower left, and the hippocampal formation occupies most of the right side of the figure. The neocortex is found primarily in the upper left quadrant of the figure.

In figure 8.4B the same map is reproduced with stippling over the *somatic* motor cortex in AGL, S-I, and S-II. This same region is the source of direct descending corticobulbar and corticospinal projections. In figure 8.4C the stippling indicates the *eyes-head* motor output cortex in AGM, PL, ACD, ACV, RSA, RSG, OC1 + OC2, and TE1 + TE1 + TE3. Note that this cortex almost completely surrounds the somatic motor cortex. In addition note the small stippled strip of this cortex in the upper part of the piriform (PIR) cortex, corresponding to projection from the endopiriform cortex to the superior colliculus (Neafsey et al. 1986b); in the intact brain this strip would be located just ventral to the rhinal fissure. Finally, in figure 8.4D the stippling indicates the *visceral* output cortex in INS, OR, and IL. This cortex appears to close the rostral gap in the ring of eyes-head cortex around the somatic output cortex. As discussed above, the medial frontal anterior cingulate (ACD, ACV), prelimbic (PL), and infralimbic (IL) cortices receive a strong input from the ventral CA1 and subicular subdivisions of the hippocampal formation and from the entorhinal (ENT) cortex, suggesting that these regions have both eyes-head and visceral output functions, especially when their other, neuroendocrine-related projections to the hypothalamus are also considered.

8.3 Discussion

The scheme described in this chapter classifies the entire cerebral cortex as "motor" cortex, implying that the primary function of cerebral cortical output is control over bodily movement or secretion. Such a statement inevitably raises several questions. What about the frontal lobes and their role in "higher" brain function? Where is the association cortex? Where in the cerebral cortex do learning and memory reside? There are no simple answers to these questions, but one recent study on the effects of frontal lobe lesions in humans (Guitton et al. 1985) suggests that such lesions do cause a *motor* deficit, which consists in an inability

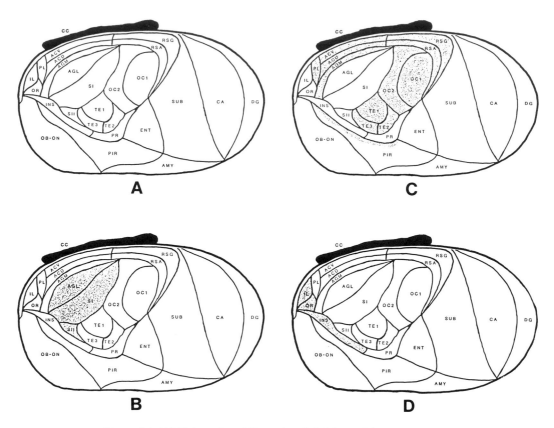

Figure 8.4 (A) Major cytoarchitectonic subdivisions of the rat cerebral cortex are depicted on a flattened map of the left cerebral hemisphere adapted from Swanson 1983. Frontal pole is at left, corpus callosum (CC) at top. ACD = anterior cingulate dorsal; ACV = anterior cingulate ventral; AGL = agranular lateral; AGM = agranular medial; AMY = amygdala; CA = CA1–CA4 fields of hippocampus; DG = dentate gyrus; ENT = entorhinal; IL = infralimbic; INS = insular; OB-ON = olfactory bulb–olfactory nucleus; OC1 = occipital visual (area 17); OC2 = occipital visual (area 18); OR = orbital; PL = prelimbic; PR = perirhinal; RSA = retrosplenial agranular; RSG = retrosplenial granular; S-I = granular primary somatosensory; S-II = granular secondary somatosensory; SUB = subiculum; TE1–TE3 = temporal auditory. (B) Same map with stippling over cortex that gives rise to corticospinal-corticobulbar projections. (C) Same map with stippling over cortex that gives rise to cortical projections to the tectum. (D) Same map with stippling over cortex that gives rise to cortical projections to the NTS; OR is included on basis of its projections to the PAG (see text).

to *suppress* eye movements to visual stimuli. Such a subtle loss of eyes-head motor control could have devastating behavioral effects that, if not carefully analyzed, could lead to the conclusion that frontal lobe lesions produce no motor symptoms but only deficits involved in higher-order attentional processes. As to the association cortex, Diamond's (1979) answer was simple: just as layer V is motor everywhere, layers II and III, the origins of cortico-cortical projections, are association cortex everywhere. Indeed the amount of cortex exclusively labeled as "association" has declined markedly in recent years as one after another of the traditional association areas has been reclassified as an area related to one of the primary sensory modalities (Diamond 1979, Kaas 1987). Learning and memory remain a mystery, but in humans the evidence from Alzheimer's disease and other memory disorders is overwhelming that alterations in brain structure and function produce profound memory deficits (Squire 1986, Zola-Morgan et al. 1986). The temporal lobe, including the hippocampal formation and amygdala, have been strongly indicated as brain areas where lesions or altered function can lead to memory deficits (Mahut et al. 1982, Murray and Mishkin 1984, Squire 1986, Zola-Morgan and Squire 1984). The insight that will seamlessly integrate these findings with the scheme for cortical motor output proposed in this chapter has yet to occur to me, but the basic observation that all cortical areas, including the hippocampus and piriform cortex, are "motor" and influence the body in some relatively direct way is important and should be kept in mind whenever the role of the cortex in psychological processes is discussed.

References

Burns, S. M., and Wyss, J. M. (1985). The involvement of the anterior cingulate cortex in blood pressure control. *Brain Res.* 340:71–77.

Chapin, J. K., and Lin, C.-S. (1984). Mapping the body representation in the SI cortex of anesthetized and awake rats. *J. Comp. Neurol.* 229:199–213.

Contreras, R. J., Beckstead, R. M., and Norgren, R. (1982). The central projections of the trigeminal, facial, glossopharyngeal and vagus nerves: an autoradiographic study in the rat. *J. Auton. Nerv. Syst.* 6:303–322.

Crowne, D. P., and Pathria, M. N. (1982). Some attentional effects of unilateral frontal lesions in the rat. *Behav. Brain Res.* 6:25–39.

Diamond, I. T. (1979). The subdivisions of neocortex: a proposal to revise the traditional view of sensory, motor, and association areas. In J. M. Sprague and A. N. Epstein (eds.), *Progress in Psychobiology and Physiological Psychology*. New York: Academic Press, 1–43.

Donoghue, J. P., and Wise, S. P. (1982). The motor cortex of the rat: cytoarchitecture and microstimulation mapping. *J. Comp. Neurol.* 212:76–88.

Dunn, J. D., and Orr, S. E. (1984). Differential plasma corticosterone responses to hippocampal stimulation. *Exp. Brain Res.* 54:1–6.

Fahrbach, S. E., Morrell, J. I., and Pfaff, D. W. (1986). Identification of medial preoptic neurons that concentrate estradiol and project to the midbrain in the rat. *J. Comp. Neurol.* 247:364–382.

Faye-Lund, H. (1985). The neocortical projection to the inferior colliculus in the albino rat. *Anat. Embryol.* 173:53–70.

Ferino, F., Thierry, A. M., and Glowinski, J. (1987). Anatomical and electrophysiological evidence for a direct projection from Ammon's horn to the medial prefrontal cortex in the rat. *Exp. Brain Res.* 65:421–426.

Foreman, N. (1983). Distractibility following simultaneous bilateral lesions of the superior colliculus or medial frontal cortex in the rat. *Behav. Brain Res.* 8:177–194.

Gioanni, Y., and Lamarche, M. (1985). A reappraisal of rat motor cortex organization by intracortical microstimulation. *Brain Res.* 344:49–61.

Guitton, D., Buchtel, H. A., and Douglas, R. M. (1985). Frontal lobe lesions in man cause difficulties in suppressing reflexive glances and in generating goal-directed saccades. *Exp. Brain Res.* 58:455–472.

Hall, R. D., and Lindholm, E. P. (1974). Organization of motor and somatosensory neocortex in the albino rat. *Brain Res.* 66:23–38.

Hardy, S. G. P., and Leichnetz, G. R. (1981). Frontal cortical projections to the periaqueductal gray in the rat: a retrograde and orthograde horseradish peroxidase study. *Neurosci. Lett.* 23:13–17.

Hess, W. R. (1969). *Hypothalamus and Thalamus. Experimental Observations.* Stuttgart: Georg Thieme Verlag.

Hicks, S. P., and D'Amato, C. J. (1977). Locating corticospinal neurons by retrograde axonal transport of HRP. *Exp. Neurol.* 56:410–420.

Hurley-Gius, K. M., and Neafsey, E. J. (1986). The medial frontal cortex and gastric motility: microstimulation results and their possible significance for the overall pattern of organization of rat frontal and parietal cortex. *Brain Res.* 365:241–248.

Kaada, B. R. (1960). Cingulate, posterior orbital, anterior insular and temporal pole cortex. In H. W. Magoun (ed.), *Handbook of Physiology-Neurophysiology II.* Washington, D.C.: American Physiological Society, 1345–1372.

Kaas, J. H. (1987). The organization of neocortex in mammals: implications for theories of brain function. *Ann. Rev. Psychol.* 38:129–151.

Kanki, J. P., Martin, T. L., and Sinnamon, H. M. (1983). Activity of neurons in the anteromedial cortex during rewarding brain stimulation, saccharin consumption and orienting behavior. *Behav. Brain Res.* 8:69–84.

Kolb, B. (1984). Functions of the frontal cortex of the rat: a comparative review. *Brain Res. Rev.* 8:65–98.

Kosar, E., Grill, H. J., and Norgren, R. (1986). Gustatory cortex in the rat. I. Physiological properties and cytoarchitecture. *Brain Res.* 379:329–341.

Krettek, J. E., and Price, J. L. (1977). The cortical projections of the mediodorsal nucleus nucleus and adjacent thalamic nuclei in the rat. *J. Comp. Neurol.* 171:157–192.

Larson, C. R., and Kistler, M. K. (1986). The relationship of periaqueductal gray neurons to vocalization and laryngeal EMG in the behaving monkey. *Exp. Brain Res.* 63:596–606.

Lawrence, D. G., and Kuypers, H. G. J. M. (1968a). The functional organization of the motor system in the monkey. I. The effects of bilateral pyramidal lesions. *Brain* 91:1–14.

Lawrence, D. G., and Kuypers, H. G. J. M. (1968b). The functional organization of the motor system in the monkey. II. The effects of lesions of the descending brain-stem pathways. *Brain* 91:15–33.

Leichnetz, G. R., and Gonzalo-Ruiz, A. (1987). Collateralization of frontal eye field (medial precentral/anterior cingulate) neurons projecting to the paraoculomotor region, superior colliculus, and medial pontine reticular formation in the rat: a fluorescent double-labeling study. *Exp. Brain Res.* 68:355–364.

Mahut, H., Zola-Morgan, S., and Moss, M. (1982). Hippocampal resections impair associative learning and recognition memory in the monkey. *J. Neurosci.* 2:1214–1229.

McCrimmon, D. R., Speck, D. F., and Feldman, J. L. (1987). Role of the ventrolateral region of the nucleus of the tractus solitarius in processing respiratory afferent input from vagus and superior laryngeal nerves. *Exp. Brain Res.* 67:449–459.

McEwen, B. S., Davis, P. G., Parsons, B., and Pfaff, D. W. (1979). The brain as a target for steroid hormone action. *Annual Review of Neuroscience* 2:65–112.

McHaffie, J. G., and Stein, B. E. (1982). Eye movements evoked by electrical stimulation in the superior colliculus of rats and hamsters. *Brain Res.* 247:243–253.

Miller, M. W., and Vogt, B. A. (1984). Direct connections of rat visual cortex with sensory, motor, and association cortices. *J. Comp. Neurol.* 226:184–202.

Morris, R. G. M., Garrud, P., Rawlins, J. N. P., and O'Keefe, J. (1982). Place navigation impaired in rats with hippocampal lesions. *Nature* 297:681–683.

Muller-Preuss, P., and Jurgens, U. (1976). Projections from the 'cingular' vocalization area in the squirrel monkey. *Brain Res.* 103:29–43.

Murray, E. A., and Mishkin, M. (1984). Severe tactual as well as visual memory deficits follow combined removal of the amygdala and hippocampus in monkeys. *J. Neurosci.* 4:2565–2580.

Neafsey, E. J., Bold, E. L., Haas, G., Hurley-Gius, K. M., Quirk, G., Sievert, C. F., and Terreberry, R. R. (1986a). The organization of the rat motor cortex: a microstimulation mapping study. *Brain Res. Rev.* 11:77–96.

Neafsey, E. J., Hurley-Gius, K., and Dimitrios, A. (1986b). The topographical organization of neurons in the rat medial frontal, insular and olfactory cortex projecting to the solitary nucleus, olfactory bulb, periaqueductal gray and superior colliculus. *Brain Res.* 377:261–270.

Neafsey, E. J., and Sievert, C. (1982). A second forelimb motor area exists in rat frontal cortex. *Brain Res.* 232:151–156.

O'Keefe, J., and Nadel, L. (1978). *The Hippocampus as a Cognitive Map.* New York: Oxford University Press.

Olavarria, J., and Van Sluyters, R. C. (1982). The projection from striate and extrastriate cortical areas to the superior colliculus in the rat. *Brain Res.* 242:332–336.

Reep, R. L., Corwin, J. V., Hashimoto, A., and Watson, R. T. (1987). Efferent connections of the rostral portion of medial agranular cortex in rats. *Brain Res. Bull.* 19:203–221.

Ruggiero, D. A., Mraovitch, S., Granata, A. R., Anwar, M., and Reis, D. J. (1987). A role of the insular cortex in cardiovascular function. *J. Comp. Neurol.* 257:189–207.

Ruit, K. G., and Neafsey, E. J. (1988). Cardiovascular and respiratory responses to electrical and chemical stimulation of the hippocampus in anesthetized and awake rats. *Brain Res.* 457:310–321.

Sanderson, K. J., Welker, W., and Shambes, G. M. (1984). Reevaluation of motor cortex and of sensorimotor overlap in cerebral cortex of albino rats. *Brain Res.* 292:251–260.

Saper, C. B. (1982). Convergence of autonomic and limbic connections in the insular cortex of the rat. *J. Comp. Neurol.* 210:163–173.

Sapolsky, R. M., Krey, L. C., and McEwen, B. S. (1983a). Corticosterone receptors decline in a site-specific manner in the aged rat brain. *Brain Res.* 289:235–240.

Sapolsky, R. M., Krey, L. C., and McEwen, B. S. (1983b). The adrenocortical stress-response in the aged male rat: impairment of recovery from stress. *Exp. Geront.* 18:55–64.

Sapolsky, R. M., Krey, L. C., and McEwen, B. S. (1984). Glucocorticoid-sensitive hippocampal neurons are involved in terminating the adrenocortical stress response. *Proc. Natl. Acad. Sci. USA* 81:6174–6177.

Sievert, C. F., and Neafsey, E. J. (1983). A chronic unit study of the sensory properties of neurons in the forelimb areas of rat sensorimotor cortex. *Neurosci. Abst.* 9:310.

Sikes, R. W., Vogt, B. A., and Swadlow, H. A. (1988). Neuronal responses in rabbit cingulate cortex linked to quick-phase eye movements during nystagmus. *J. Neurophysiol.* 59:922–936.

Sinnamon, H. M., and Galer, B. S. (1984). Head movements elicited by electrical stimulation of the anteromedial cortex of the rat. *Physiol. Behav.* 33:185–190.

Sorensen, K. E. (1985). Projection of the entorhinal area to the striatum, nucleus accumbens, and cerebral cortex in the guinea pig. *J. Comp. Neurol.* 238:308–322.

Squire, L. R. (1986). Mechanisms of memory. *Science* 232:1612–1619.

Stumpf, W. E., and Sar, M. (1981). Steroid hormone sites of action in the brain. In K.

Fuxe, J. A. Gustafsson, and L. Wetterberg (eds.), *Steroid Hormone Regulation of the Brain*. New York: Pergamon Press, 41–50.

Sutherland, R. J., Kolb, B., and Whishaw, I. Q. (1982). Spatial mapping: definitive disruption by hippocampal or medial frontal cortical damage in the rat. *Neurosci. Lett.* 31:271–276.

Swanson, L. W. (1981). A direct projection from Ammon's horn to prefrontal cortex in the rat. *Brain Res.* 217:150–154.

Swanson, L. W. (1983). The hippocampus and the concept of the limbic system. In W. Seifert (ed.), *Neurobiology of the Hippocampus*. New York: Academic Press, 3–19.

Swanson, L. W., and Kohler, C. (1986). Anatomical evidence for direct projections from the entorhinal area to the entire cortical mantle in the rat. *J. Neurosci.* 6:3010–3023.

Terreberry, R. R., and Neafsey, E. J. (1983). Rat medial frontal cortex: a visceral motor region with a direct projection to the solitary nucleus. *Brain Res.* 278:245–249.

Terreberry, R. R., and Neafsey, E. J. (1984). The effects of medial prefrontal cortex stimulation on heart rate in the awake rat. *Neurosci. Abstr.* 10:614.

Terreberry, R. R., and Neafsey, E. J. (1987). The rat medial frontal cortex projects directly to autonomic regions of the brainstem. *Brain Res. Bull.* 19:639–649.

van der Kooy, D., Koda, L. Y., McGinty, J. F., Gerfen, C. R., and Bloom, F. E. (1984). The organization of projections from the cortex, amygdala, and hypothalamus to the nucleus of the solitary tract in rat. *J. Comp. Neurol.* 224:1–24.

Vogt, B. A., Sikes, R. W., Swadlow, H. A., & Weyand, T. G. (1986). Rabbit cingulate cortex: cytoarchitecture, physiological border with visual cortex, and afferent cortical connections of visual, motor, postsubicular, and intracingulate origin. *J. Comp. Neurol.* 248:74–94.

Welker, W., Sanderson, K. J., and Shambes, G. M. (1984). Patterns of afferent projections to transitional zones in the somatic sensorimotor cerebral cortex of albino rats. *Brain Res.* 292:261–267.

Wise, S. P., and Donoghue, J. P. (1986). Motor cortex of rodents. In E. G. Jones and A. Peters (eds.), *Cerebral Cortex. Sensorimotor Areas and Aspects of Cortical Connectivity*. New York: Plenum Press, 243–270.

Wise, S. P., Murray, E. A., and Coulter, J. D. (1979). Somatotopic organization of corticospinal and corticotrigeminal neurons in the rat. *Neuroscience* 4:65–78.

Woolsey, C. N. (1958). Organization of somatic sensory and motor areas of the cerebral cortex. In H. F. Harlow and C. N. Woolsey (eds.), *Biological and Biochemical Bases of Behavior*. Madison: University of Wisconsin Press, 63–82.

Yajima, Y., Hayashi, Y., and Yoshii, N. (1980). The midbrain central gray substance as a highly sensitive neural structure for the production of ultrasonic vocalization in the rat. *Brain Res.* 198:446–452.

Yardley, C. P., and Hilton, S. M. (1986). The hypothalamic and brainstem areas from which the cardiovascular and behavioural components of the defence reaction are elicited in the rat. *J. Auton. Nerv. Syst.* 15:227–244.

Zilles, K. (1985). *The Cortex of the Rat. A Stereotaxic Atlas.* New York: Springer Verlag.

Zola-Morgan, S., and Squire, L. R. (1984). Preserved learning in monkeys with medial temporal lesions: sparing of motor and cognitive skills, *J. Neurosci.* 4:1072–1085.

Zola-Morgan, S., Squire, L. R., and Amaral, D. G. (1986). Human amnesia and the medial temporal region: enduring memory impairment following a bilateral lesion limited to field CA1 of the hippocampus. *J. Neurosci.* 6:2950–2967.

9 The Control of Movements by the Motor Cortex

Jan Bures and Vlastimil Bracha

From gross locomotion to discrete skills, movement represents the main output of the animal brain. Although the evolution of vertebrates has resulted in the gradual addition of several hierarchically organized levels of supraspinal motor control to the spinal mechanisms, the appearance of the motor cortex and the pyramidal tract in mammals was a major development in the functional organization of the brain (Ariens Kappers et al. 1960, Nauta and Karten 1970, Armand 1982). It meant that the growing mass of mammalian telencephalon was not entirely devoted to analysis and representation of environment, but a part of it was reserved for direct regulation of the activity of spinal motoneurons. This arrangement made it possible to exert independent control over individual muscles and muscle groups. Because it formed a parallel connection of the cortex to lower centers, the presence of the motor cortex complicates the answer to the question of which behaviors are primarily dependent on cortical versus subcortical mechanisms. The cortical contribution may range from a slight modification of movements emitted by the lower centers (changes of amplitude and timing of individual components) to completely new movement sequences that have never been a part of the innate repertoire of the animal. The motor cortex can be expected to play a particularly important role in the elaboration of discrete voluntary movements, the acquisition of new motor skills, and in the instrumentation of already existing unconditioned reflexes.

This chapter reviews the two principal ways of exploring the role of the motor cortex in skilled movement: The first is to remove the motor cortex and to examine changes in movements and movement patterns. The second is to correlate movements with electrical, biochemical, or morphological measures of cortical activity. The review is selective, focusing on the most studied movement pattern in rats, namely, reaching for food or objects.

9.1 Reaching

Rats use their forepaws for a wide range of behaviors. Thus they typically hold small pieces of food with both forepaws and display impressive dexterity when manipulating them in close coordination with the movements of jaw, lips, and tongue. Highly coordinated use of forepaws and orofacial musculature also occurs during grooming as animals hold fur, the tail, or a hindlimb with one or both forepaws. These fine movements of forepaws are part of a highly prepared stereotypical behavior integrated at subcortical levels and are therefore not much impaired by the ablation of the motor cortex. In fact efficient grooming is preserved in chronically decerebrate rats (Grill and Norgren 1978b). On the other hand the motor cortex is required for independent limb control during reaching for objects that cannot be accessed simultaneously by both paws. Tests of skilled forelimb movements in rats were introduced in the 1930s (Tsai and Maurer 1930, Yoshioka 1930, Peterson 1931, Peterson 1934). When rats are forced to reach for food through a narrow opening, they learn to reach through this opening with one paw, grasp the piece of food, and carry it to the mouth. In doing so, most rats show a clear preference for using one forepaw. This general procedure has proved very useful in the study of skilled forelimb use in rats.

Spontaneous Forepaw Preference

When determining forepaw preference, it is essential to eliminate possible biasing influence of the experimental situation. In a typical arrangement food is placed into a 6-cm–long tubular feeder (11-mm inside diameter) mounted outside the experimental cage and accessible through a hole in the center of the front wall, 5 cm above the floor. The position of food in the feeder can be adjusted with a closely fitting piston to different distances from the cage orifice of the tube. Photoelectric sensors monitor the presence of the food in the feeder as well as the insertion of the forepaw into the tube (figure 9.1A). The animal is required to produce an axial extension of the forelimb to grasp the food and carry it to the mouth or to remove it from the feeder by a raking movement and recover it by mouth at the feeder entrance or from the cage floor. The latter possibility is excluded in cages with a grid floor through which falling pellets are lost. The raking movements can be suppressed more efficiently when using a tubular feeder separated from the cage wall by a 5-mm to 10-mm gap through which pellets that are not firmly grasped disappear.

   A simpler reaching movement is produced in an apparatus equipped with an open tray feeder placed outside the experimental cage, the front wall of which consists of vertical bars. Only one limb can be extended through the vertical slits between the bars to reach for food. The movement is less constrained than in the case of the tubular feeder: it is not necessarily axial because the reaching forelimb can approach the food from above and/or from the side. The difficulty of the task can be controlled by changing the dimensions of the tray (width, rim) or pellet, by introducing a gap between the tray and the grid wall, by preventing

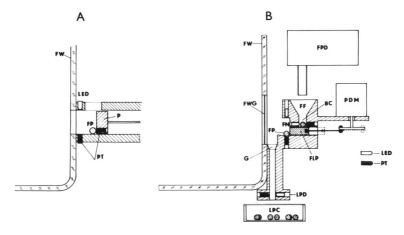

Figure 9.1 Examples of two types of feeders used in the reaching experiments. (A) Manually baited tubular feeder. FW = front wall of the experimental box; PT = photo-transistors; LED = light-emitting diode; FP = food pellet; P = piston forming the feeder bottom. PT_1 and PT_2 monitor insertion of the forepaw into the feeder and removal of the food pellet, respectively. (B) An automated open tray feeder. FN = feeder niche; FF = food funnel; FPD = food pellet dispenser; BC = buffer chamber; PDM = piston drive mechanisms; FLP = feeder loading piston; G = adjustable gap; LPD = lost pellet detector; LPC = lost pellet collector. The photoelectrically detected removal of the pellet from the feeder activates the loading mechanism. The piston moves to the backward position (interrupted contours), and the pellet prepared in the buffer chamber falls into the loading channel and is pushed into the feeder. A new pellet is delivered from the pellet dispenser into the buffer chamber. Pellets not firmly grasped fall into the gap and are counted and collected.

raking by a horizontal ledge above the tray (Whishaw et al. 1986), or by putting the pellet on a moving conveyor belt (Evenden and Robbins 1984). When the tray is accessible from the center of the cage wall, the animal can freely choose the posture suited to reaching with the preferred forepaw. Figure 9.1B shows an automatized version of this type of feeder.

Forced Use of Left or Right Forepaws

The rat's choice of the forepaw used for reaching can be influenced in various ways:

1. *Apparatus bias* The feeder or the access to the feeder is arranged in a way that facilitates reaching with one forepaw and constrains reaching with the other. Thus placing the entrance to the tubular feeder close to the right-hand corner of the cage facilities reaching with the right forepaw. It is worth noting, however, that even these constraints may not prevent rats with strong biases from adopting postures that allow the use of the left paw. More efficient restriction of a paw can be achieved when an additional narrow (15-mm) vertical plate is mounted to the left of the feeder entrance (Schwarting et al. 1987).

2. *Effector bias* The use of one forepaw can be prevented by mechanical means. Immobilization by bandaging is not very efficient because

the rat soon removes the bandage by gnawing. A better solution is to fit one forepaw with a bracelet (Whishaw et al. 1986), the size of which prevents the animal from either introducing the forepaw into the feeder or between the bars of the cage. A metal bracelet, which can be rapidly assembled from two separate parts, is shown in figure 9.2. Reaching with a forepaw also can be prevented by denervation (compression of the brachial plexus in the axilla) or by injecting the wrist and elbow with novocaine. Various degrees of forelimb paralysis preclude performance of fine movements.

3. *Training bias* Even in the absence of apparatus and effector bias, forepaw preference can be induced by shaping, i.e., by making the reward available to reaches performed with one but not the other forepaw (Gonzales et al. 1986). Because the reaches are too rapid to allow reliable manual control of food presentation, Wetzel and Bures (unpublished data, 1989) used an automatic device for this purpose. A miniature magnet was implanted under the skin of the wrist of the left paw, and a similar piece of nonmagnetic material was implanted into the right paw. An induction coil placed around the feeder entrance (figure 9.3) signaled the approach of the left but not right paw. Penetration of either paw into the feeder was monitored by the photoelectric sensor. Coincidence of the inductive and photoelectric signals indicating movement of the left paw activated a solenoid that moved the pellet out of the reach of the animal. Thus the feeder was always empty for the left paw and baited for the right paw. The conditions could be reversed by a simple change of the program.

Effect of Brain Lesions on Forepaw Preference

When all external or peripheral biasing influences are eliminated, the preferential use of the left or right forepaw is probably due to minor asymmetries of brain morphology or metabolism. Such asymmetry can be accentuated deliberately or created by lateralized brain lesions interfering with the putative neural substrate of reaching. If the lesion is made in naive animals, training reveals its effect by preference established in subsequent reaching tests. Siegfried and Bures (1980) showed in this way that rats with a unilateral 6-OHDA (6-hydroxydopamine)

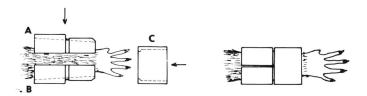

Figure 9.2 Scheme of the aluminum bracelet used to prevent rats from reaching with the selected forepaw. The inner half segments A and B are joined by the outer ring C.

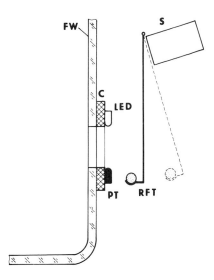

Figure 9.3 Apparatus for combined inductive and photoelectric detection of reaching. C = inductive coil around the feeder entrance; LED = light-emitting diode; PT = phototransistor; RFT = retractable food tray; S = solenoid. Reaching with the magnet-carrying forepaw generates overlapping inductive and photoelectric signals, the coincidence of which prevents access to food by activation of the feeder-retracting solenoid.

lesion of the substantia nigra reach consistently with the forepaw ipsilateral to the lesion. Castro (1977) trained rats with a unilateral lesion of the motor cortex in an apparatus biasing the use of the contralateral forepaw and found clear preference of the ipsilateral limb. Similar results were obtained after unilateral sectioning of the medullary pyramid (Kartje-Tillotson and Castro 1980).

A more common approach establishes the forepaw preference in intact animals and attempts to change it by unilateral lesions, interfering with the movement of the preferred forepaw. There are two basic versions of this procedure: (1) *free testing*, in which the animal is allowed to reach with either paw, and the effect of the lesion is assessed by overall change of performance (e.g., number of pellets retrieved per minute) and by change of preference (e.g., from 90 percent right to 85 percent left); and (2) *forced testing*, in which the animal is forced to use the paw contralateral to the lesion while the use of the ipsilateral limb is prevented (e.g., by a bracelet; Whishaw et al. 1986). This makes it possible to assess the limits of the animal's reaching abilities under conditions when only the affected limb can provide access to food.

The limits of postlesion recovery can also be established with bilateral lesions. Castro (1972a) trained rats to reach across a gap and then removed the frontal cortex of both hemispheres. The lesion caused a large drop in performance persisting during 30 daily sessions. In the early postlesion tests the rats were unable to extend the paw into the feeder. Extension amplitude gradually increased, and toward the end of training the rats succeeded in touching the pellets, but still failed to grasp them properly and carry them to the mouth. A similar but weaker deficit was observed under the same conditions after bilateral sectioning of the medullary pyramids (Castro 1972b), perhaps because some motor cortex output was mediated through the corticorubrospinal system.

Cortical Lesions Interfering with Reaching

Attempts to establish the cortical substrate of reaching have produced results that vary with the character of the movement (grasping versus raking), testing conditions (free or forced use of the impaired paw), and duration of the postlesion recovery and/or training. Despite the various sources of variability, all experimental evidence available confirms the early reports by Peterson (1934) and Peterson and Fracarol (1938) showing that reaching is controlled by a highly localized area of the contralateral motor cortex. According to Peterson and Devine (1963), extirpation of about 2 mm^2 of motor cortex, 1.6 mm rostral and 2.7 mm lateral from bregma in the hemicortex, contralateral to the preferred forepaw, induces transfer of reaching to the nonpreferred forelimb. The critical area corresponds reasonably well to the region from which forelimb movements can be elicited by low-threshold intracortical stimulation (Hall and Lindholm 1974). Larger lesions have been used by other authors (Castro 1972a,b, 1977, Price and Fowler 1981), who generally have found that the impairment in forelimb use is proportional to the volume of the ablated motor cortex. Whishaw and colleagues (1986) used lesions limited to the forepaw motor area (small), encompassing the major part of the sensorimotor cortex (medium), or additionally including the adjacent neocortex (large) of one hemisphere. Under free-testing conditions lesions produced a size-dependent increase of preference for the limb contralateral to the intact hemisphere, and this asymmetry increased with practice. When the use of the forelimb ipsilateral to the lesion was prevented by a bracelet, rats with small or medium lesions were able to reach with the paw contralateral to the lesion, and their performance greatly improved with practice. Only large lesions prevented improvement with forced practice, probably because they disrupted postural mechanisms, the presence of which is a prerequisite for independent limb use. The difference between the results of free and forced tests in rats with medium lesions may be at least partly due to sensory neglect, which may be overcome by the forced use of the neglected paw.

Although motor cortex lesions interfere with reaching, impairment of reaching does not necessarily imply cortical damage. Lateralized reaching is disrupted by contralateral caudate-globus pallidus lesions (Siegfried et al. 1980, Schneider and Olazabal 1984, Hamilton et al. 1985, Pisa 1988) or by dopamine depletion of neostriatum after 6-OHDA lesions of the substantia nigra (Siegfried and Bures 1980, Uguru-Okorie and Arbuthnott 1981, Evenden and Robbins 1984, Sabol 1985). Reaching is supported by complex cortico-subcortical circuits and cannot be implemented by pyramidal control of the performing limb alone.

Functional Blockade of Motor Cortex

The effects of motor cortex lesions described above have been confirmed by experiments in which the function of the critical areas is blocked. Attempts to influence reaching by cooling or local drug treatment (Jasper and Bonvallet 1934, Peterson and Carter 1936, Peterson 1949) of the exposed motor cortex date back to the 1930s, more recently reaching with the contralateral forepaw has been disrupted by focal epileptic discharge (Islam and Bures 1975).

The effect of unilateral cortical spreading depression (CSD) on lateralized reaching has been examined by Buresova and colleagues (1958). A CSD wave elicited by the application of a 2 percent KCl solution to the occipital cortex of the hemisphere contralateral to the preferred paw stopped reaching after 1 to 2 minutes (i.e., at a time when the slowly propagating wave of neural depolarization had entered the frontal cortex). On average the impairment lasted for 40 minutes and was sometimes accompanied by a shift of forepaw preference, which did not outlast the termination of the interfering condition. Martin and Webster (1974) used more protracted CSD to induce a persistent change of paw preference. CSD was elicited by application of 25 percent KCl on the hemisphere contralateral to the preferred forepaw on two consecutive days, and 200 reaches were elicited with the nonpreferred paw under these conditions. The enforced shift persisted in tests performed several days later in the absence of CSD. The handedness shift induced by reversible central blockade was comparable to that caused by transient immobilization of the preferred forepaw during the 200 forced practice trials.

CSD waves do not penetrate into a cortical area treated with 0.1-M or 0.2-M $MgCl_2$ (Bures 1960). Buresova and Bures (1960) and Bures and Buresova (1960) applied a filter paper soaked with 1.7 percent $MgCl_2$ onto the exposed sensorimotor cortex contralateral to the preferred forepaw. This treatment did not interfere with reaching. CSD elicited 20 to 30 minutes later from the occipital cortex did not penetrate into the frontal cortex and caused only a very short-lasting (4.7 minutes on average) impairment of reaching. This protective effect of a single $MgCl_2$ application lasted several hours. The combination of a functional decortication procedure with a treatment preserving function in a circumscribed cortical area is an analog of the cortical island technique employed for demonstrating that a definite cortical area can sustain the examined function alone, without the participation of the rest of the neocortex.

9.2 Orofacial Activities

Movements of jaws, tongue, vibrissae, and rhinarium can be obtained from stimulation of large parts of the motor cortex, but few studies have examined the effects of cortical lesions on these movements. Castro (1972c) reported that lesions of the sensorimotor cortex impaired the capability of rats to lap small food pellets from the compartments of a testing tray placed outside the experimental box and accessible through a horizontal slit in the wall. The failure was due to inadequate tongue protrusion. The same rats, however, had no apparent difficulties when drinking from a drinking spout. In a follow-up study (Castro 1975) essentially similar results were obtained with smaller lesions aimed at the tongue area of the motor cortex. The deficit was decreased when the lesions were placed in two stages with a 30- to 40-day interoperative delay.

Whishaw and Kolb (1983) used a simple method to measure the amplitude of tongue protrusion. One end of a plastic ruler was smeared with a mash of chocolate cookies and placed perpendicularly against the wire mesh wall of the cage. The animal was allowed to lick the sweet mixture through the wires of the cage. The cleared area of the ruler indicated the maximum amplitude of tongue protrusion, which decreased from 11 mm in intact rats to 4.4 mm, 1.3 mm, and 2.0 mm in rats with bilateral ablation of the motor cortex, orbital frontal cortex, and complete decortication, respectively. Ablation of the medial frontal or parietal cortex did not interfere with tongue use. The impaired rats failed to extend the tongue when lapping water spilled on a horizontal surface and nibbled rather than licked the drinking spouts. On the other hand, during grooming episodes decorticate rats were able to use the tongue for licking the back, hindquarters, abdomen, and genitalia (Whishaw et al. 1981). Normal grooming was also observed in decerebrate rats (Grill and Norgren 1978b), who failed to protrude their tongue beyond the upper incisors when stimulated by intraoral infusion of sapid fluids (Grill and Norgren 1978a).

An interesting finding pointing to impaired fine control of biting and chewing after motor cortex lesions reported by Whishaw and colleagues (1983), who observed that claws on the hindpaws of decorticate or hemidecorticate rats and rats with bilateral ablation of the motor cortex are about twice as long (5 mm) as those in control rats (2.6 mm). This is a manifestation of abolished claw cutting, a part of normal grooming behavior of intact rats. The lesioned rats were unable to remove plastic claws attached to their digits, although they oriented to them as normal animals. Inefficient biting and chewing thus seemed to account for the disruption of claw cutting.

Tongue control can be disrupted by lesions of lateral, but not medial, striatum (Pisa 1988), as has also been found for reaching (see above). Such findings support the view that the motor cortex and basal ganglia are parts of a corticosubcortical loop that is essential for normal motor performance (Alexander et al. 1986).

9.3 Latch Box Problems

The motor cortex can be expected to be important for efficient control of coordinated movements used for solving latch box problems. The role of the cerebral cortex in this type of manipulative task was examined first by Lashley (1935), who concluded that impairment of their acquisition is influenced more by the size of the lesion than by its locus. In a more recent study Spiliotis and Thompson (1973) used latches that required selective movements of the head, forepaws, and/or jaw. A rat could get access to food in the goal box by opening a one-way door locked by (1) a butterfly button, which had to be rotated clockwise from horizontal (locked) to vertical (open) position; (2) a barrel bolt, which had to be slid to the right; and (3) a hook, which had to be pulled out from an eyelet. Rats trained in all three problems sustained bilateral cortical or subcortical lesions and were tested for retention after recovery. Rats with anterior cortex lesions showed poor skill retention on all three problems whereas rats with posterior cortex ablation exhibited normal retention. Subsequently Thompson and colleagues (1984) examined the influence of various cortical lesions on the acquisition of problems 2 and 3 in rats preoperatively trained on problem 1. The errors to criterion ranged from 8.3 in sham operated animals to 45.2 and 23.4 in rats with frontal and frontocingulate ablations, respectively. Lesions of the parietal, occipital, and posterior cingulate cortex did not affect performance.

The effect of frontal and lateral parietal lesions on the retention of preoperatively acquired problems 1 and 2 was examined also by Gentile and coworkers (1978). The results were essentially similar to those of Spiliotis and Thompson (1973). The impairment caused by frontal lesions was attributed not to the failure to perform individual partial movements constituting the correct response but rather to an inability to organize them into an effective spatiotemporal pattern (i.e., to apraxia). This conclusion was questioned by Kolb and Whishaw (1983), who found that problem 1 was disrupted by orbital frontal and motor cortex lesions, problem 2 by orbital frontal lesion, and problem 3 (latch 1 covered by a plexiglas window, making only one end of the latch accessible to manipulation with one forepaw) by medial frontal lesion. Decorticated animals were unable to master any of the problems when motivated by food reward, but eventually succeeded in opening them when escaping from ice water. The authors argued that the differential effect of cortical lesions on the three latches reflects the type of movement used for manipulating the particular latch (snout, snout and paws, and paws only for latches 1, 2, and 3, respectively).

9.4 Instrumental Modification of Reaching

The motor cortex plays a key role in motor learning such as in the acquisition of movements or movement sequences that are not a part of the usual repertoire of the animal's behavior. Motor learning leads to establishment of new motor programs that can be viewed as equivalent to new memory engrams. The latter probably are contained within the motor system and are as amenable to experimental analysis as are the memories forming the basis of other types of learning. A disadvantage of this approach, however, is the difficulty in deciding what is a new movement and how it differs from the innate movements (Adams 1984). According to Grillner and Wallen (1985), most movements of vertebrates can be derived from tetrapod locomotion. Thus the movement repertoire evolves from whole-limb synergies through the activation of separate joints and finally to the fine control of individual digits. It is not easy to decide, however, whether lateralized reaching of rats is derived independently or from a modification of other movements, such as grasping, scratching, digging, or walking. This question may be answered by detailed quantitative description and direct comparison of the acquired and related innate movements. The major flaw of this approach is the dubious completeness of the list of innate reactions and the somewhat arbitrary criteria used for such comparisons. A more straightforward approach that avoids the dichotomy between acquired and innate behaviors uses conditioning of selected movements and movement sequences. Exact quantification of the movement before and after learning is again a prerequisite of such analysis.

Quantification of Reaching
The highly constrained reaching into a tubular feeder is well suited for quantitative description because it reduces the degrees of freedom of the actual movement (axial forelimb extension and flexion), stabilizes the position of the animal in front of the feeder, and allows reliable recording of the fundamental parameters of the movement. Videorecording analysis (Moroz and Bures 1983) showed that reaching movement of an overtrained rat consists of three successive and partly overlapping phases: (1) a simultaneous shoulder, elbow, and wrist extension that propels the paw into the feeder so that the digits and palm are above the pellet; (2) grasping the pellet by flexion of the fingers and wrist; and (3) extraction of the pellet from the feeder by simultaneous flexion of wrist, elbow, and shoulder. As shown in figure 9.4, extension, which is measured from the appearance of the fingers at the feeder entrance to their maximum protrusion, lasts for 60 ms. Finger flexion then lasts for 40 ms and is accompanied by relatively slow forelimb flexion. Retraction is complete after 300 ms as the pellet-holding paw disappears from the feeder. Retraction is more rapid (160 ms) after unsuccessful reaches because it is not slowed down by manipulation of

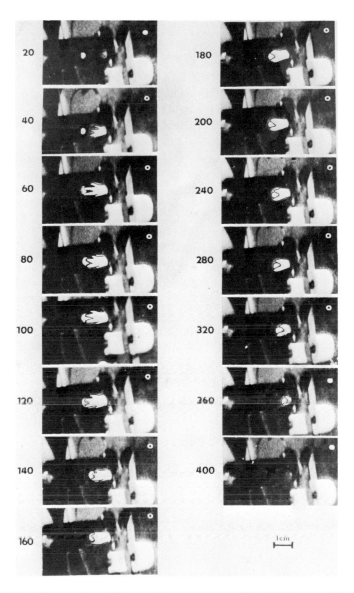

Figure 9.4 A videorecording of the reaching movement of the right forepaw. The numbers indicate time in milliseconds. Activation of the photoelectric sensor at the feeder entrance is signaled in frame 40 by the change of the white dot in the right upper corner to a circle. Note that the paw contacts the pellet in frame 60 and manipulates it with the fingers during frames 80 and 100. Retraction starting in frame 120 overlaps with grasping of the pellet and continues to frame 400. The photoelectric sensor signal changes again between frames 320 and 360. (From Moroz and Bures 1983)

the pellet. Statistical analysis of these components of reaching indicated high reproducibility of the rapid extension and finger flexion to retraction onset, which lasted 58 ± 10 ms (SD) and 49 ± 10 ms (SD) on average, respectively. The high velocity (up to 0.40 m/s) of extension suggests that this component represents a relatively inflexible ballistic movement (Brooks and Thach 1981). This is supported by the observation that the forepaw does not explore the inside of the feeder, but rather moves in abrupt isolated thrusts. Similarly the failure to contact and grasp the pellet does not initiate an immediate correction, but the flexion is completed and a correction attempted during the next reach. It seems that the extension and grasping are quasi-ballistic preprogrammed movements with limited feedback control, whereas the subsequent flexion is more influenced by the tactile and proprioceptive signals generated by contact with the target.

Reaching monitored by photoelectrical or mechanical sensors inside the feeder forms only the last portion of a more complex movement that involves the body and head as well as the nonpreferred forepaw and the hindlimbs. Using a videorecording technique, Bracha (1987) demonstrated that the entire sequence starts about 300 ms before the forepaw enters the feeder (zero time). The animal leans toward the feeder and inserts its nose into the entrance while the preferred forelimb is held in a semiflected position 10 mm to 20 mm below and 20 mm away from the lower edge of the feeder (zero of the coordinate system, figure 9.5). The head movement serves a double purpose: It ascertains the presence of food inside the feeder and provides a stable starting point for movement onset. The actual reaching begins about 200 ms later; the forepaw moves rapidly along the ipsilateral side of the snout into the feeder, where it decelerates over the last 5 mm to 10 mm from the target. After an unsuccessful reach the paw is retracted to a point 10 mm to 15 mm outside the feeder, from which a correction movement can reach the feeder during 40 ms. Correction movements are repeated with a frequency of 3 Hz and 4 Hz until the pellet is retrieved.

Rewarding Specified Movement Properties

In most attempts to modify the form of a limb movement by operant conditioning, the food pellet is substituted by an operandum. Displacement of the operandum by the forepaw is rewarded by the delivery of reinforcement. The following parameters of the reaching response have been examined with this procedure:

1. *Slowing of the retraction phase of reaching* (Hernandez-Mesa and Bures 1985)   Rats were rewarded by intracerebral self-stimulation for reaching into the tubular feeder in which the food was replaced by a ball-shaped plastic operandum. The movement of the operandum toward the feeder entrance was monitored by mechanical contacts. Reward was delivered only when the forepaw retraction time (movement of the operandum from the bottom to the entrance to the feeder) exceeded a predetermined

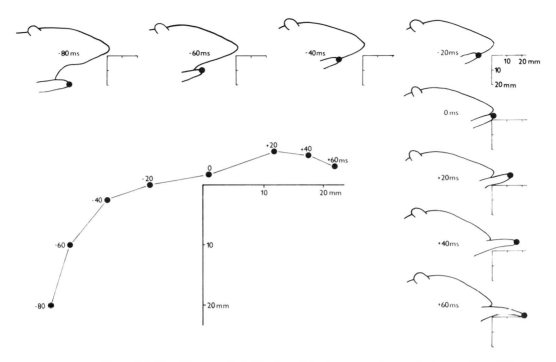

Figure 9.5 The videorecorded side view of the forepaw trajectory during reaching. (Above and at right) Schemes indicating the position of the head and of the right forepaw with respect to the lower edge of the tubular feeder entrance at 20-ms intervals before (−) and after (+) forepaw appearance at the feeder entrance (zero time). The curve represents the positions of the forepaw fingertips at the indicated times, with the lower edge of the feeder orifice corresponding to the origin of the coordinate system.

threshold value (e.g., 512 ms), which was never encountered during a normal reaching. Most rats were able to prolong retraction beyond 512 ms within a single session.

2. *Decreasing the velocity of the ballistic extension* (Zhuravin and Bures 1986) Rats were trained to reach into a horizontal tube containing an axially moving piston operandum, the movement of which was monitored by three photoelectric sensors between the points 13.0 mm, 15.1 mm, and 17.3 mm from the tube entrance. The movement was monitored with a computer that also controlled an electromechanical device that delivered a food pellet whenever the velocity of the operandum remained below a preset threshold value during the preceding extension. More than 20 sessions of 512 reaches were needed to reduce the extension velocity from the initial 0.32 m/s to 0.145 m/s.

3. *Increasing the duration of extension* (Bracha et al. 1987) Rats were trained to reach through a circular opening in the wall of the cage and push a hinged vertical panel across a 10-mm gap. The displacement of the panel delivered a pellet into a receptacle on the cage floor. The panel could be locked by a computer-operated solenoid for 20 ms to 120 ms after extension onset. The animal was rewarded when contin-

uously pushing against the locked panel during this interval and displacing it as soon as it was released. Whereas during standard reaching flexion starts about 100 ms after the forepaw is introduced into the feeder, the modified reaching was characterized by prolonged extension (during the isometric pressure against the locked panel and during the subsequent isotonic push) and by a corresponding delay of flexion onset (up to 300 ms). Most rats mastered the 20-ms prolongation of extension in a single 15-minute session, but required 5 to 10 sessions to overcome the 120-ms block.

4. *Increasing the demands on the visuomotor control of reaching* (Evenden and Robbins 1984)   Rats were trained to reach through a horizontal slit in the cage wall (1.5 cm wide and 12 cm above the cage floor) and remove small food pellets from a conveyor belt moving with a velocity of up to 3 cm/s. Pellets were presented at 5-s intervals and came either from left or right. The behavior was scored as percentage of correct retrievals, percentage of omissions (i.e., failures to reach to a presented pellet), and paw preference (i.e., the number of correct retrievals made with the left and right paw, respectively). Well-trained animals correctly retrieved 66 percent of the pellets, made 2.4 percent omissions, and displayed 85 percent paw preference.

5. *Changing self-paced reaching into signaled reaching* (Moroz and Bures 1983)   Rats were trained to reach into a tubular feeder in which the entrance was equipped with a solenoid-operated guillotine shutter. Solid-state programming equipment opened the shutter for 1024 ms and simultaneously presented an acoustic signal. Reaching accomplished during this interval prolonged the shutter opening time to 2.5 s, thus permitting the animal to complete the reach. In a discriminated version of this task (Storozhuk et al. 1984), a low tone and a high tone (600 Hz and 3000 Hz, respectively) were used as the CS^+ and CS^- to signal the presence and absence of food in the feeder. The behavior was evaluated by scoring the latency of the first reach, the percentage of omissions, and the percentage of errors of commission (reaching triggered by CS^-). The median reach latencies were 184 ms for nondiscriminated and 385 ms for discriminated reaching, respectively.

The forelimb movements made in various bar-pressing tasks closely resemble those made in reaching (Glick and Jerussi 1974, Church et al. 1986, Schwarting et al. 1987). Such tasks can be used to evaluate the behavioral effects of motor cortex lesions. Price and Fowler (1981) trained rats to press two horizontal disks for which the access was limited to either right or left forepaws. The bar-press force was monitored by force transducers, and responses exceeding a 16-g threshold were reinforced by access to water on a fixed ratio 5 schedule. Intact rats used both paws with approximately equal efficiency and emitted responses with about a 30-g mean peak force. In a later study Fowler and colleagues (1986) also used a pull-type operandum consisting of a 1-mm wire bail that formed a horizontal triangle, the apex of which was connected to the force transducer. The 18-mm base of the triangle could be grasped and pulled across a 25-mm distance toward the cage with a maximum force approaching 200 g. After unilateral ablation of the sensorimotor cortex, contralateral paw responses decreased by 95 percent in rate and by 60 percent in peak force. The impairment was less severe and recovery was faster in the forelimb ipsilateral to the lesion, but the performance never returned to the prelesion level. The longer duration of the emitted movements was attributed to a shift from preprogrammed to feedback-controlled movements. Gonzales and co-workers (1986) trained rats to rapidly press two adjacent levers separated by a vertical glass partition. The rat first had to use the left forepaw to press the right lever once and then the right lever twice. Response sequences in which the duration exceeded the most rapid presses by 20 percent were not rewarded. After three weeks of training, interresponse times ranged from 650 ms to 800 ms between the two levers and from 200 ms to 250 ms on the same lever. One week after bilateral ablation of the motor cortex, the interresponse time between levers increased to 900 ms to 1580 ms, and it remained increased in 3 of 4 rats for more than six weeks. The same-lever interresponse time was increased slightly one week after the lesion, but returned to the preoperative value within three weeks. The authors suggested that the prolongation of the between-lever interreponse time reflects the slowed motor function after damage of the pyramidal tract. This impairment is expressed more when joining two different movements than when repeating the same movement.

9.5 Electrophysiological Correlates of Reaching

The application of electrophysiological methods to study the activation of the motor cortex of rats during skilled movements is relatively recent. These studies take three forms: gross potential studies, unit activity studies, and measures of excitability changes. Most of these studies have focused almost exclusively on the electrical correlates of reaching.

Gross Potentials
Megirian and colleagues (1974) implanted a row of parasagittal electrodes over the frontoparietal cortex of rats and recorded EEGs in animals performing the lateralized reaching task. Averaged event-related potentials, which were synchronized by forepaw extension into the feeder, consisted of negative slow potential (20 μV to 50 μV) culminating 28 ms after reach detection. This main component was preceded and followed by less pronounced positive waves, corresponding to preparatory neural activity and to forepaw retraction, respectively. The reach-related potentials attained the maximum amplitude over the cortical forepaw area, but could be recorded over the entire parietal cortex of the hemisphere contralateral to the reaching paw as well as in the

ipsilateral hemisphere, although at a lower amplitude. The findings in rats closely resemble the potentials accompanying similar forelimb movements in cats (Rosenfield and Fox 1972) and monkeys (Gemba et al. 1981).

Unit Activity

Plastic unit activity changes corresponding to gross event-related potentials were recorded in the forepaw area of the sensorimotor cortex contralateral to the preferred forepaw by Dolbakyan and colleagues (1977), Stashkevich and Bures (1981), Moroz and Bures (1984), Storozhuk and colleagues (1984), and Zhuravin and Bures (1988). Typical perireach histograms (figure 9.6) showed clear excitatory peaks starting 50 ms to 100 ms before reach detection and culminating during maximum extension. Other units displayed more prolonged tonic excitation, phasic inhibition, or complex excitation-inhibition sequences. Similar histograms were also obtained by Wise and Donoghue (1986) in rats trained to generate an isometric force with their forelimbs. Electrolytic marking of electrode position showed that the recorded cells were located in the lateral agranular cortex, corresponding to the primary motor cortex.

Perireach histograms of individual neurons can be subsumed by a population response (Dolbakyan et al. 1977), which is expressed by the percentage of neurons excited or inhibited (with respect to the prereach background activity) at various intervals before and after reach detection. A typical population response in the contralateral motor cortex (figure 9.7) was characterized by prominent excitation starting about 150 ms before and culminating about 40 ms after reach detection and exponentially decaying over the subsequent 0.5 s. Inhibitory reactions were less frequent, started earlier, and synchronized less clearly with the movement. The population response in the ipsilateral cortex had a similar inhibitory component, but excitation was almost absent. The population responses of motor cortex neurons characteristically differed

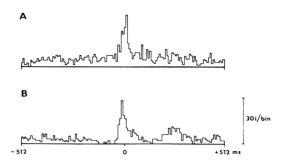

Figure 9.6 Characteristic perireach histograms obtained from single neurons in the forepaw region of the sensorimotor cortex of rats reaching into the tubular feeder. Abscissa shows time (ms) before (−) of after (+) reach detection (zero). Each histogram consists of 64 bins of 16 ms and is based on 30 to 40 reaches. Calibration, 30 spikes/bin.

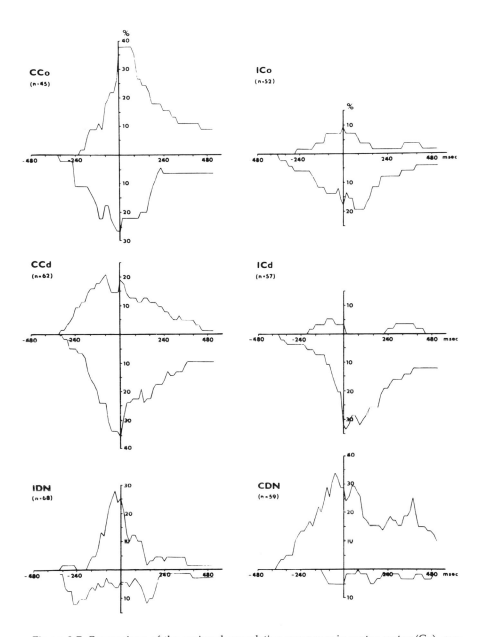

Figure 9.7 Comparison of the perireach population responses in motor cortex (Co), caudate nucleus (Cd), and dentate nucleus (DN) contralateral (C) or ipsilateral (I) to the reaching forepaw. The numbers indicate the sample size. Ordinate shows percentage of neurons in the respective sample showing at the given time in statistically significant excitatory (upward) or inhibitory (downward) reactions. Abscissa shows time (ms) before (−) or after (+) reaching. Note the similarity of the excitatory population response in the ipsilateral dentate nucleus and contralateral motor cortex. (From Hernandez-Mesa and Bures 1978)

from population responses in the head of the caudate nucleus and in the dentate nucleus. The activity of all three structures was modified during reaching in a way consonant with the view (Brooks et al. 1981) that preprogrammed ballistic movements are elaborated in the cerebellum and transmitted through the motor thalamus to task-specific assemblies of pyramidal cells in the motor cortex, whereas the caudate nucleus controls the postural adjustments indispensable for successful reaching. When one of these centers is eliminated, modified movement can still be performed by the remaining centers. Thus reach-synchronized single-pulse stimulation of the ipsilateral dentate nucleus prevents successful completion of the movement because it not only disrupts the patterned activity of the stimulated center but also interferes with the activity of the motor cortex. The changes were not limited to the post-stimulus part of the cortical perireach histograms, but could also be seen in the premotor activity, which started considerably earlier (300 ms before reach detection), when the interfering stimulus was on. Such modification of the perireach activity is probably an anticipatory change reflecting the attempts of the animal to cope with the blockage of the cortico-cerebello-cortical loop by changing the preprogrammed movement to a feedback-controlled movement. Modification of perireach histograms of motor cortex neurons has been reported in rats trained to slow down the ballistic component of reaching (Zhuravin and Bures 1988). As pointed out by Wise and Donoghue (1986), the motor cortex activity not only controls movement production but probably also engages in generation of the corollary discharge addressed to somatosensory centers, which will receive the movement-induced signals. Mismatch between the anticipated input and real input may be used to improve adjustment of the movement to changing environmental influences.

Some motor cortex neurons are activated during movement preparation. Preparatory activity overlaps with the early phase of movement execution, but can be separated from the latter during discriminated signaled reaching. Motor cortex units showed increased activity in the first 120 ms after CS^+ onset, which is about 200 ms before the second peak corresponding to the actual forepaw movement (Storozhuk et al. 1984). Pure preparatory activity uncontaminated by movement was also present during correct reactions to CS^- and during errors of omission (no reaction to CS^+). The presence of preparatory activity can be best demonstrated when a warning signal precedes the actual "go" signal. Tanji and Evarts (1979) and Kubota and Hamada (1979) showed in monkeys that activity of the motor cortex is changed during presentation of the warning signal alone, in the absence of any EEG activity. Experiments of this type, which are also feasible in rats, support the "response set" concept (Neafsey et al. 1978) that the performance of discrete movements requires preliminary priming of the mechanisms controlling their integration with the rest of the body.

Excitability Changes

Activation of the motor cortex during reaching is also reflected by excitability changes, which can be examined by monitoring the threshold or amplitude of responses to reach-triggered stimulation. This approach cannot be used, however, for examination of excitability in the premovement interval. In an attempt to assess perireach excitability changes, Islam and Bures (1975) recorded interictal activity of an epileptic focus elicited by application of 1-percent picrotoxin on the forepaw area of the motor cortex. Computer-plotted perireach histograms of epileptic spikes showed an inhibitory trough 300 ms to 100 ms before reach onset, an excitatory peak corresponding to extension, and a less pronounced postreach inhibition. Although the cross-correlation of the interictal activity with reaching was highly significant, the interpretation of results is not simple. The decreased incidence of spikes in the prereach interval can either reflect prevailing cortical inhibition in the phase of postural preparation of the forepaw movement or express the decreased probability of reaching in the interval after an interictal spike. In fact reaching was blocked during ictal episodes in the contralateral but not the ipsilateral motor cortex. Various forms of focal epileptic activity probably account for the disruption of reaching caused by the local application of drugs to the critical cortical area.

The excitability of the motor cortex not only changes in the course of individual movements, but its more prolonged modulation may influence the selection of the reaching paw. This was demonstrated by Hernandez-Mesa and Bures (1985), who trained rats to reach for a ball-shaped operandum in a horizontal tube. Successful movements were reinforced by a rewarding brain stimulation applied either to the left or right medial forebrain bundle at the level of the lateral hypothalamus. The stimulation side did not influence forepaw preference in strongly lateralized animals, but in a group of eight latently ambidextrous rats, stimulation of the lateral hypothalamus ipsilateral to the preferred forepaw increased reaching with the normally nonpreferred forepaw from 15 percent to 60 percent. Similar results were obtained in monkeys (Hopkins and Kuypers 1976), who showed a strong preference for operating the microswitch that delivered rewarding brain stimulation by using the hand contralateral to the hypothalamic electrode. A possible explanation for these observations was recently offered by Aou and colleagues (1988), who demonstrated the facilitating influence of rewarding hypothalamic stimulation on the ipsilateral motor cortex in monkeys. Because connections between the lateral hypothalamus and the motor cortex have been demonstrated in rats (Kita and Oomura 1981), it is conceivable that the shift of forepaw preference observed in the experiments of Hernandez-Mesa and Bures (1985) is due to the facilitation of the ipsilateral motor system at the cortical level, although the participation of subcortical centers (caudate nucleus) must also be taken into account (Zimmerberg and Glick 1975). In fact asymmetric excitability of motor nerves in the preferred and nonpreferred forelimbs was reported in one of the first studies of handedness (Jasper 1932).

9.6 Biochemical and Morphological Correlates of Reaching

The well-established lateralization of the cortical representation of reaching makes handedness a suitable model for biochemical studies. Hyden and Egyhazi (1964) examined the RNA content and base composition of the frontal area of the motor cortex in rats and reported changes elicited by the forced transfer of handedness. A more recent study (Fuchs et al. 1983) did not detect any asymmetries of [^{3}H]-leucine uptake in the sensorimotor forelimb cortex of trained rats. Krivanek and Buresova (1972) measured the acetylcholinesterase activity of the motor cortex of rats with spontaneous, forced, reversed, and overtrained (4 days) handedness and found it to be 10 percent higher in the contralateral than in the ipsilateral hemisphere in the overtrained group. Similar results were obtained after 6 and 14 days of training by Aleksidze and Balavadze (1971). Greenough (1985) found, however, no reaching-induced regional difference in binding of nicotinic and muscarinic ligands in the rat motor cortex.

Clear movement-related metabolic changes were obtained with (^{14}C-labeled) 2-deoxyglucose (2-dg) uptake (Fuchs et al. 1983, Greenough 1984). Well-trained rats were injected with the radiolabeled 2-dg, allowed to reach for 45 minutes, and killed immediately afterward. Heavy labeling was found in the forepaw region of the sensorimotor cortex and caudate-putamen contralateral to the active limb. Greater 2-dg uptake was also found in the ipsilateral cerebellar hemisphere and superior and inferior colliculi. Sharp (1984) used the 2-dg technique to trace the metabolic changes caused by 45 minutes of intermittent stimulation of the sensorimotor cortex, eliciting repetitive discrete forelimb movements (50-ms–long trains of 300 Hz, 0.5-ms pulses applied five times per second) in rats under ketamine anesthesia. The 2-dg uptake showed the greatest increase in the stimulated area and an increase in the somatosensory cortex, the second motor cortex (M-II), caudate-putamen, and in a number of subcortical structures of the stimulated hemisphere. Comparison of 2-dg autoradiograms after either 45 minutes of motor cortex stimulation or reaching shows similar metabolic patterns and indicates that the increased 2-dg is a manifestation of increased activity rather than of the plastic changes underlying learning.

Conversely overtrained reaching is accompanied by morphological changes outlasting the actual motor activity. Greenough and colleagues (1985) showed that after 16 days of training the apical dendritic fields of layer V pyramidal cells in the forelimb area of the sensorimotor cortex are larger in the hemisphere contralateral to the trained forepaw. Furthermore Withers and Greenough (1987) found increased total dendritic length in a specific type of pyramidal cells in cortical layers II and III of the sensorimotor cortex contralateral to the reaching forepaw.

9.7 Conclusions

The experimental evidence reviewed in this chapter shows that although most research into the neural mechanisms of skilled movements has been studied almost exclusively in primates (Brooks and Thach 1981), similar studies of skilled forelimb use can also be conducted on rats. Lesions of comparable areas of the motor cortex cause similar deficits of motor function in rats and monkeys, characterized by an inability to generate independent manipulatory movements with small muscle groups (digits, wrists, tongue), to organize them into precisely timed sequences, and to perform them rapidly and with the usual force. Electrophysiological evidence indicates that the phasic activation of the motor cortex precedes the movement by a time interval similar to that found in monkeys. Furthermore local metabolic changes point toward participation of the motor cortex in the skilled movements of rats. At the same time these studies show that the motor cortex does not implement the movements alone but instead in close cooperation with a number of cortical and subcortical structures, particularly the basal ganglia and cerebellum. The task of future investigations is not to examine the motor cortex in isolation but rather to provide a better understanding of its integration with the complex neural circuits subserving movement control in general and the acquisition of motor skills in particular.

References

Adams, J. A. (1984). Learning of movement sequences. *Psychol. Bull.* 96:3–28.

Aleksidze, N. G., and Balavadze, M. B. (1971). Changes of acetylcholinesterase activity in specific regions of rat cerebral cortex during learning (in Russian). *Doklady Ak. Nauk SSSR* 198:1455–1456.

Alexander, G. E., DeLong, M. R., and Strick, P. L. (1986). Parallel organization of functionally segregated circuits linking basal ganglia and cortex. *Ann. Rev. Neurosci.* 9:357–381.

Aou, S., Oomura, Y., Woody, C. D., and Nishino, H. (1988). Effects of behaviorally rewarding electrical stimulation on intracellularly recorded neuronal activity in the motor cortex of awake monkeys. *Brain Res.* 439:31–38.

Ariens Kappers, C. U., Huber, G. C., and Crosby, E. C. (1960). *The Comparative Anatomy of the Nervous System of Vertebrates, Including Man.* New York: Hafner.

Armand, J. (1982). The origin, course and termination of corticospinal fibers in various mammals. *Progr. Brain Res.* 57:329–360.

Bracha, V. (1987). Videorecording analysis of reaching for food in rats. *Physiol. Bohemoslov.* 36:366.

Bracha, V., Zhuravin, I. Q., and Bures, J. (1987). Instrumental prolongation of the extension phase of reaching. *Physiol. Bohemoslov.* 36:522.

Brooks, V. B., and Thach, W. T. (1981). Cerebellar control of posture and movement. In V. B. Brooks (ed.), *Handbook of Physiology. The Nervous System II.* Washington, D.C.: American Physiological Society, 847–946.

Bures, J. (1960). Block of Leao's spreading cortical depression by bivalent cations. *Physiol. Bohemoslov.* 9:202–209.

Bures, J., and Buresova, O. (1960). The use of Leao's spreading cortical depression in research on conditioned reflexes. In H. H. Jasper and G. D. Smirnov (eds.), *Moscow Colloquium on EEG of Higher Nervous Activity, EEG Clin. Neurophysiol. Suppl.* 13:359–376.

Buresova, O., and Bures, J. (1960). The use of partial functional decortication in study of the localization of condition reflexes. *Physiol. Bohemoslov.* 9:210–218.

Buresova, O., Bures, J., and Beran, V. (1958). A contribution to the problem of dominant hemisphere in rats. *Physiol. Bohemoslov.* 7:29–37.

Castro, A. J. (1972a). The effects of cortical ablations on digital usage in the rat. *Brain Res.* 37:173–185.

Castro, A. J. (1972b). Motor performance in rats: The effects of pyramidal tract section. *Brain Res.* 44:313–323.

Castro, A. J. (1972c). The effects of cortical ablations on tongue usage in the rat. *Brain Res.* 45:251–253.

Castro, A. J. (1975). Tongue usage as a measure of cerebral cortical localization in the rat. *Exp. Neurol.* 47:343–352.

Castro, A. J. (1977). Limb preference after lesions of the cerebral hemisphere in adult and neonatal rats. *Physiol. Behav.* 18:605–608.

Church, W. H., Sabol, K. E., Justice, J. B., Jr., and Neill, D. B. (1986). Striatal dopamine activity and unilateral bar pressing in rats. *Pharmacol. Biochem. Behav.* 25:865–871.

Dolbakyan, E., Hernandez-Mesa, N., and Bures, J. (1977). Skilled forelimb movements and unit activity in the motor cortex and caudate nucleus of rats. *Neuroscience* 2:73–80.

Evenden, J. L., and Robbins, T. W. (1984). Effects of unilateral 6-hydroxydopamine lesions of the caudate putamen on skilled forepaw use in the rat. *Behav. Brain Res.* 14:61–68.

Fowler, S. C., Gramling, S. E., and Liao, R.-M. (1986). Effects of pimozide on emitted force, duration and rate of operant response maintained at low and high levels of required force. *Pharmacol. Biochem. Behav.* 25:615–622.

Fuchs, J. L., Bajjalieh, S. M., Hoffman, C. A., and Greenough, W. T. (1983). Regional brain 2-deoxyglucose uptake during performance of a learned reaching task. *Soc. Neurosci. Abstr.* 9:54.

Gemba, H., Hashimoto, S., and Sasaki, K. (1981). Cortical field potentials preceding visually initiated hand movement in the monkey. *Exp. Brain Res.* 42:435–441.

Gentile, A. M., Green, S., Nieburgs, A., Schmelzer, W., and Stein, D. G. (1978). Disruption and recovery of locomotor and manipulatory behavior following cortical lesions in rats. *Behav. Biol.* 22:417–455.

Glick, S. D., and Jerussi, T. P. (1974). Spatial and paw preferences in rats: their relationship to rate-dependent effects of D-amphetamine. *J. Pharmacol. Exp. Therap.* 188:714–725.

Gonzalez, M. F., Poncelet, A., Loken, J. A., and Sharp, F. R. (1986). Quantitative measurement of interresponse times to assess forelimb motor function in rats. *Behav. Brain Res.* 22:75–84.

Greenough, W. T. (1984). Structural correlates of information storage in the mammalian brain: A review and hypothesis. *Trends Neurosci.* 7:229–233.

Greenough, W. T. (1985). The possible role of experience-dependent synaptogenesis, or synapses on demand, in the memory process. In N. M. Weinberger, J. L. McGaugh, and G. Lynch (eds.), *Memory Systems of the Brain*. New York: Guilford Press, 77–103.

Greenough, W. T., Larson, J. L., and Withers, G. S. (1985). Effects of unilateral and bilateral training in a reaching task on dendritic branching of neurons in the rat motor-sensory forelimb cortex. *Behav. Neural Biol.* 44:301–314.

Grill, H. J., and Norgren, R. (1978a). The taste reactivity test. II. Mimetic responses to gustatory stimuli in chronic thalamic and chronic decerebrate rats. *Brain Res.* 143.281–297.

Grill, H. J., and Norgren, R. (1978b). Neurological tests and behavioral deficits in chronic thalamic and chronic decerebrate rats. *Brain Res.* 143:299–312.

Grillner, S., and Wallen, P. (1985). Central pattern generators for locomotion, with special reference to vertebrates. *Ann. Rev. Neurosci.* 8:233–261.

Hall, R. D., and Lindholm, E. P. (1974). Organization of motor and somatosensory neocortex in the albino rat. *Brain Res.* 66:23–38.

Hamilton, M. H., Garcia-Munoz, M., and Arbuthnott, G. W. (1985). Separation of the motor consequences from other actions of unilateral 6-hydroxydopamine lesions in the nigrostriatal neurones of rat brain. *Brain Res.* 348:220–228.

Hernandez-Mesa, N., and Bureš, J. (1978). Skilled forelimb movements and unit activity of cerebellar cortex and dentate nucleus in rats. *Physiol. Bohemoslov.* 27:199–208.

Hernandez-Mesa, N., and Bures, J. (1985). Lateralized rewarding brain stimulation affects forepaw preference in rats. *Physiol. Behav.* 34:495–499.

Hopkins, D. A., and Kuypers, H. G. J. M. (1976). Response lateralization and self-stimulation in normal and split brain monkeys. In A. Wauquier and E. T. Rolls (eds.), *Brain Stimulation Reward*. Amsterdam: North Holland Publishers, 557–579.

Hyden, H., and Egyhazi, E. (1964). Changes in RNA content and base composition in cortical neurons of rats in a learning experiment involving transfer of handedness. *Proc. Nat. Acad. Sci. USA* 52:1030–1035.

Islam, S., and Bures, J. (1975). Interaction between the activity of an epileptic focus and discrete skilled movements in rats. *EEG Clin. Neurophysiol.* 39:651–656.

Jasper, H. H. (1932). L'action asymétrique des centres sur la chronaxie des nerfs symétrique droit et gauche chez les Mammifères. *C. R. Soc. Biol.* 110:702–705.

Jasper, H. H., and Bonvallet, M. (1934). Rôle de l'écorce dans l'organisation asymétrique des chronaxies des nerfs symétriques chez les rats droiters et gauchers. *C. R. Soc. Biol.* 116:991–994.

Kartje-Tillotson, G., and Castro, A. J. (1980). Limb preference after unilateral pyramidotomy in adult and neonatal rats. *Physiol. Behav.* 24:293–296.

Kartje-Tillotson, G., Neafsey, E. J., and Castro, A. J. (1985). Electrophysiological analysis of motor cortical plasticity after cortical lesions in newborn rats. *Brain Res.* 332:103–111.

Kita, H., and Oomura, Y. (1981). Reciprocal connections between the lateral hypothalamus and the frontal cortex in the rat: electrophysiological and anatomical observations. *Brain Res.* 213:1–16.

Kolb, B., and Whishaw, I. Q. (1983). Dissociation of the contributions of the prefrontal, motor, and parietal cortex to the control of movement in the rat: an experimental review. *Can. J. Psychol.* 37:211–232.

Krivanek, J., and Buresova, O. (1972). Cortical acetylcholinesterase and "handedness" in rats. *Experientia* 28:291–292.

Kubota, H., and Hamada, Y. (1979). Preparatory activity of monkey pyramidal tract neurons related to quick movement onset during visual tracking performance. *Brain Res.* 168:435–439.

Lashley, K. S. (1935). Studies of cerebral function in learning. XI. The behavior of the rat in latch box situations. *Comp. Psychology Monographs* 11:1–42.

Martin, D., and Webster, W. G. (1974). Paw preference shifts in the rat following forced practice. *Physiol. Behav.* 13:745–748.

Megirian, D., Buresova, O., Bures, J., and Dimond, S. (1974). Electrophysiological correlates of discrete forelimb movements in rats. *EEG Clin. Neurophysiol.* 36:131–139.

Moroz, V. M., and Bures, J. (1983). A telerecording analysis of reaching disruptions of rats after stimulation or lesion. *Physiol. Behav.* 31:255–257.

Moroz, V. M., and Bures, J. (1984). Effects of lateralized reaching and cerebellar stimulation on unit activity of motor cortex and caudate nucleus in rats. *Exp. Neurol.* 84:47–57.

Nauta, W. J. H., and Karten, H. J. (1970). A general profile of the vertebrate brain, with sidelights on the ancestry of cerebral cortex. In F. O. Schmitt (ed.), *The Neurosciences.* New York: Rockefeller University Press, 7–26.

Neafsey, E. J., Hull, C. D., and Buchwald, N. A. (1978). Preparation for movement in the cat. II. Unit activity in the basal ganglia and thalamus. *EEG Clin. Neurophysiol.* 44:714–723.

Peterson, G. M. (1931). A preliminary report on right- and left-handedness in the rat. *J. Comp. Psychol.* 12:243–250.

Peterson, G. M. (1934). Mechanisms of handedness in the rat. *Comp. Psychology Monographs* 9:1–67.

Peterson, G. M. (1949). Changes of handedness in the rat by local application of acetylcholine to the cerebral cortex. *J. Comp. Physiol. Psychol.* 42:404–412.

Peterson, G. M., and Carter, G. W. (1936). The local application of drugs to the motor cortex of the rat. *J. Comp. Psychol.* 212:123–129.

Peterson, G. M., and Devine, J. V. (1963). Transfers in handedness in the rat resulting from small cortical lesions after limited forced practice. *J. Comp. Physiol. Psychol.* 56:752–756.

Peterson, G. M., and Fracarol, C. (1938). The relative influence of the locus and mass of destruction upon the control of handedness by the cerebral cortex. *J. Comp. Neurol.* 68:173–190.

Pisa, M. (1988). Motor functions of the striatum in the rat: critical role of the lateral region in tongue and forelimb reaching. *Neuroscience* 24:453–463.

Price, A. W., and Fowler, S. C. (1981). Deficits in contralateral and ipsilateral forepaw motor control following unilateral cortical ablations in rats. *Brain Res.* 205:81–90.

Rosenfeld, J. P., and Fox, S. S. (1972). Movement related macropotentials in cat cortex. *EEG Clin. Neurophysiol.* 32:75–80.

Sabol, K. E., Neill, D. B., Wages, S. A., Church, W. H., and Justice, J. B. (1985). Dopamine depletion in a stiatal subregion disrupts performance of a skilled motor task in the rat. *Brain Res.* 335:33–34.

Schneider, J. S., and Olazabal, U. E. (1984). Behaviorally specific limb use deficits following globus pallidus lesions in rats. *Brain Res.* 308:341–346.

Schwarting, R., Nagel, J. A., and Huston, J. P. (1987). Asymmetries of brain dopamine metabolism related to conditioned paw usage in the rat. *Brain Res.* 417:75–84.

Sharp, F. R. (1984). Regional (^{14}C) 2-deoxyglucose uptake during forelimb movements evoked by rat motor cortex stimulation: cortex, diencephalon, midbrain. *J. Comp. Neurol.* 224:259–285.

Siegfried, B., and Bures, J. (1980). Handedness in rats: blockade of reaching behavior by unilateral 6-OHDA injections into substantia nigra and caudate nucleus. *J. Physiol. Psychol.* 8:360–368.

Siegfried, B., Fischer, J., and Bures, J. (1980). Intracranial colchicine impairs lateralized reaching in rats. *Neuroscience* 5:529–541.

Spiliotis, P. H., and Thompson, R. (1973). The "manipulative response memory system" in the white rat. *Physiol. Psychol.* 1:101–114.

Stashkevich, I. S., and Bures, J. (1981). Correlation analysis of neuronal interaction in the motor cortex of rats during performance of a discrete instrumental reaction. *Int. J. Neurosci.* 12:1–6.

Storozhuk, V. M., Bracha, V., Brozek, G., and Bures, J. (1984). Unit activity of motor cortex during acoustically signalled reaching in rats. *Behav. Brain Res.* 12:317–326.

Tanji, J., and Evarts, E. V. (1979). Anticipatory activity of motor cortex neurons in relation to direction of an intended movement. *J. Neurophysiol.* 31:785–797.

Thompson, R., Gallardo, K., and Yu, J. (1984). Cortical mechanisms underlying acquisition of latch box problems in the white rat. *Physiol. Behav.* 32:809–817.

Tsai, L. S., and Maurer, S. (1930). "Right handedness" in white rats. *Science* 72:436–438.

Uguru-Okorie, D. C., and Arbuthnott, G. W. (1981). Altered paw preference after unilateral 6-hydroxydopamine injections into lateral hypothalamus. *Neuropsychologia* 19:463–467.

Whishaw, I. Q., and Kolb, B. (1983). "Stick out your tongue": Tongue protrusion in neocortex and hypothalamic damaged rats. *Physiol. Behav.* 30:471:480.

Whishaw, I. Q., Kolb, B., Sutherland, R. J., and Becker, J. B. (1983). Cortical control of claw cutting. *Behav. Neuroscience* 97:370–380.

Whishaw, I. Q., Nonneman, A. J., and Kolb, B. (1981). Environmental constraints on motor abilities used in grooming, swimming, and eating by decorticate rats. *J. Comp. Physiol. Psychol.* 95:792–804.

Whishaw, I. Q., O'Connor, W. T., and Dunnett, S. T. (1986). The contributions of motor cortex, nigrostriatal dopamine and caudate-putamen to skilled forelimb use in the rat. *Brain* 109:805–843.

Wise, S. P., and Donoghue, J. P. (1986). Motor cortex of rodents. In E. G. Jones and A. Peters (eds.), *Cerebral Cortex, Vol. 5. Sensory-Motor Areas and Aspects of Cortical Connectivity.* New York: Plenum Press, 243–270.

Withers, G. S., and Greenough, W. T. (1987). Differential plasticity between two subtypes of pyramidal cells in the motor-sensory forelimb cortex as a consequence of reach training. *Soc. Neurosci. Abstr.* 13:1596.

Yoshioka, J. G. (1930). Handedness in rats. *J. Genet. Psychol.* 38:471–474.

Zhuravin, I. A., and Bures, J. (1986) Operant slowing of the extension phase of the reaching movement in rats. *Physiol. Behav.* 36:611–617.

Zhuravin, I. A., and Bures, J. (1988). Changes of cortical and caudatal unit activity accompanying operant slowing of the extension phase of reaching in rats. *Int. J. Neuroscience* 39: 147–152.

Zimmerberg, B., and Glick, S. D. (1975). Changes in side preference during unilateral electrical stimulation of the caudate nucleus in rats. *Brain Res.* 86:335–338.

10 The Decorticate Rat

Ian Q. Whishaw

If the centers are so tiny and well defined that moving an electrode on the surface of the brain by just a few millimeters is sufficient to distinguish them, then it cannot be difficult to destroy them. Nevertheless, again and again the remains of centers are discovered that have to crowd together as uncomfortably as fish in a pond that is drying out. What happens to the centers if one has removed a hemisphere? They flee before the cutting knife with astounding speed, into the other hemisphere. And still the "wanderlust" of these marvelous centers is not exhausted. They are still encountered even after the mantle is destroyed. (Goltz 1892, p. 603)

The idea that the cortex might have a general function, or at least that the operations that are performed in its different areas might have something in common, is implicit in a great deal of theoretical and experimental brain literature. To Gall and Spurzheim (1810–1819) the cortex housed the faculties listed on their phrenological maps, e.g., mirthfulness, acquisitiveness, amativeness, etc. To Flourens (1824) the cortex was the interface with the mind and so must have mental attributes such as intelligence and will. To Loeb (1900) and Pavlov (1927) the cortex was the organ of associative learning. To Goltz (1892) the cortex was the seat of understanding, reasoning power, and intelligence. C. Judson Herrick (1926) felt much the same way, but stated his position if not as clearly at least more prosaically. To Lashley (1950) the cortex was the organ of learning and memory. More recently Oakley (1981a) has made the cortex the organ of representational and abstract memory. To MacLean (1982) the cortex is the organ of emotion and expression. Phillips and colleagues (1984) speculate that the cortex is the Sherlock Holmes of the brain, sensitive to suspicious coincidence. The feature of these theories is that they do little more than substitute the neocortex for a facsimile of Descartes's (1664) mind. Perhaps the absence of more definitive statements has left fertile ground for the unabashed claim that normal human development and superior intellectual performance can be achieved in the absence of the neocortex (Lorber 1968).

If the theoretical approaches illustrated in the collage above have been unproductive, the findings of the occasional empirical sorties have often been misleading. Accordingly it has been suggested at various times that species-typical behaviors are subcortical. It has also been suggested that the cortex suppresses strong response tendencies, is largely inhibitory in function, is a source of arousal, suppresses exaggerated defensive reactions, matures behavior, contributes to body weight set-point, and is involved more in sexual behavior than in learning (see Oakley 1979a for a review). There is even a strong philosophical bias in some schools that the cortex is more important to higher animals like primates than to lower animals like rats (Lassek 1954).

What has been missing in approaches to cortical function is a strong commitment to naturalistic studies that emphasize careful description of motor patterns of animals in variegated natural environments or analogs of such environments. As has been pointed out by others (see Robinson 1983), this important phase of research has been neglected in laboratory studies of brain and behavior. Even when behavior is adequately described it is often treated as an epiphenomenon and not a primary objective of the research. Thus it must be stated apologetically that we still have no complete catalog of effects of cortex lesions on rat behavior and no satisfying theories of cortical function.

A major objective of this chapter is to describe the behavioral capacities of animals without cortex. This description is a necessary first step toward determining what aspects of behavior should be assigned properly to subcortical structures and what aspects of behavior depend on the cortex. It is noteworthy that since this research approach was initiated by Flourens (1824), the behavioral capacities accorded to subcortical structures have been steadily revised upward. Consequently many aspects of complex behavior and learning once referred to cortical structures are now recognized to importantly depend on subcortical portions of the forebrain and the brainstem.

10.1 Decortication

The term *neodecortication* refers to a preparation in which only neocortex has been removed. With the additional removal of midline limbic cortex and hippocampus, the preparation is referred to as *decorticate*. There has been no careful comparison of the behavior of neodecorticate and decorticate animals, but it should be expected that they be similar because the neocortex and limbic areas are major targets for reciprocal connections. Furthermore, when preparations involving neocortex and midline cortex removal have been compared with preparations involving the additional removal of the hippocampal formation, no obvious behavioral differences have been seen (Vanderwolf et al. 1978; Whishaw and Kolb 1983a). *Decorticate* is therefore used here to refer to all of these preparations. If removals include the caudate-putamen, i.e., complete *telencephalic* removal, behavioral capacities are reduced further as compared with decortication. In proportion to the extent of the additional removals, animals lost the ability to eat, drink, groom, and maintain themselves in laboratory environments (Grill and Norgren 1978; Sorenson and Ellison 1970). These preparations have been referred to as *thalamic*, but most of the thalamus proper undergoes complete secondary degeneration.

Removals are usually made by aspiration after removal of the frontal and parietal bones and retraction of the meninges (Whishaw 1974). Removal of the meninges and blood vessels can also produce a complete lesion (Oakley and Russell 1979, 1980), but there is no evidence of significant differences in the end points of the two techniques. Leao's spreading depression can be used for acute decortication (Bures and Buresova 1969). Techniques for removal in the neonatal animal are similar to those for adults, except that hypothermic anesthesia is preferred over barbiturate anesthesia (Kolb and Whishaw 1981). Excellent survival follows operations performed between 1 and 8 days after birth and later than 25 days after birth. With operations performed between 8 and 25 days, most animals experience respiratory failure (Kolb and Whishaw 1981). An attempt at pharmacological removal has been made, but the lesions are incomplete (Pereira and Russell 1981), as are lesions produced by heat applied to the neonate's skull (Murphy et al. 1981).

10.2 Anatomical Changes

Cortical removals do not directly injure subcortical structures, but subcortical structures undergo secondary changes, which become more apparent as survival time is extended (figure 10.1) Brain weighing at removal indicates a decline in weight to about 1.3 g, compared with control values of about 2.2 g in male rats. This represents a loss of between 36 percent (Vanderwolf et al. 1978) to 39 percent (Whishaw et al. 1981b) of total brain weight. The caudate-putamen, hippocampus, and thalamus appear intact one week postoperation. By one year postoperation, the caudate-putamen and globus pallidus have shrunk by 30 percent by area, and the hippocampus has shrunk by about 4 percent by area (Whishaw et al. 1981b). Shrinkage of the anterior thalamus is about 50 percent and of the posterior thalamus about 40 percent, and for the brainstem shrinkage is about 26 percent of control area (Kolb et al. 1983a). With time the lateral ventricles enlarge. The hippocampus shifts, and its movement occurs partly as a result of shrinkage of the underlying thalamus, which allows the fornix to sag. Nissl-stained coronal sections show that with time the anterior and ventral nuclei of the thalamus, the geniculate bodies, the globus pallidus, and portions of the caudate-putamen undergo retrograde degeneration. Darkly stained spherical globs appear within the necrotic tissue of these structures. Stains for calcium using von Kossa's technique (Braun 1975) or with alazarin red S for calcium—with or without pretreating tissue with ethylenediaminetetraacetic acid (EDTA) to chelate calcium and prevent

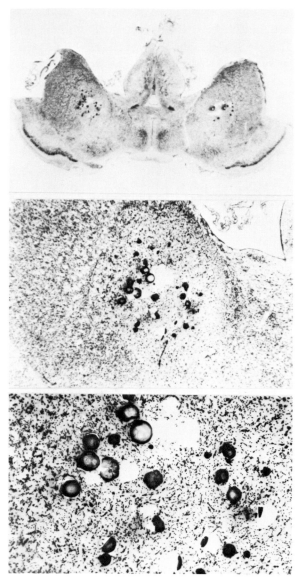

Figure 10.1 Coronal sections through the brain of a rat killed one year postoperation, illustrating the typical extent of cortical removal with an example of subcortical change illustrated by the histological appearance of the globus pallidus. The dark substance comprises deposits of calcium. (Adapted from Whishaw et al. 1981.)

staining (Whishaw et al. 1981b)—indicate that the globs are indeed calcium, which apparently accumulates over time (Whishaw and Kolb 1984a).

Neonatal decortication performed on rats less than 5 days of age produces a different pattern of subcortical change than occurs after adult damage. Progressively earlier damage produces comparatively greater decreases in adult brain weight such that brain weight may be reduced by as much as 50 percent (brain weight as low as 1 g) if lesions are made at birth (Whishaw and Kolb 1984b). Measurements of subcortical structures show that there is more shrinkage than occurs after adult operation, but the gliosis and calcification typical after adult operation is not present. The nuclei that degenerate after adult operation are gone, and the remaining nuclei of the thalamus appear to have undergone a topographic reorganization and are hard to identify. The hippocampus shrinks relatively less than do other structures, but Ammon's horn and the dentate gyrus are characterized by peculiarly shaped gyri (Kolb et al. 1983a). The subiculum also undergoes changes marked by peculiar cytoarchitectonics (Kolb et al. 1986).

Injections of retrograde tracers true blue or nuclear yellow into the striatum, hippocampus, or subiculum of adult or neonate decorticate rats indicate that most expected afferents are present. In neonates label is not found in the ventral tegmental area or thalamus after true blue injection into the striatum and hippocampus, respectively. Acetylcholinesterase staining shows that the normal striatal patchy organization is present. In sum, within the changes that take place subcortically after neonatal decortication, there is little evidence for the development of new pathways or the reorganization of expected pathways (Kolb et al. 1986, Lanca et al. 1986).

10.3   Recovery

The most incapacitating impairment after adult decortication is an inability to eat and drink. At the descriptive level there are discrepancies in reports on the extent of these deficits. Braun (1975) found that decorticate rats were aphagic and adipsic (ate no food and drank no water) for a median of 3 days, were anorexic and adipsic for an additional 2 to 3 days, ate dry food and were adipsic for an additional 9 days, and maintained themselves on food and water only after 35 days. He argued that this paralleled the recovery of lateral hypothalamic-lesioned rats (Teitelbaum and Epstein 1962), suggesting a communality between these areas in the orchestration of consummatory behavior. More severe deficits were reported by Vanderwolf and colleagues (1978). Their rats were completely aphagic for 10 to 19 days and required tube feeding for 14 to 45 days to stay alive; only 1 of 18 ever drank water from a metal tube.

A reexamination of the feeding abilities of decorticate rats shows that recovery is rapid, the deficits only superficially resemble those of lateral hypothalamic-damaged rats, and that initial and enduring feeding impairments are related to impairments in motor acts of food ingestion (Whishaw et al. 1981b). The differences between this study and those described above relate to variations in feeding procedure. Briefly the rats have difficulty with mouth movements and so require easy access to food and water. By using remedial feeding procedures that help compensate for the animals' motor impairments, it is possible to have an animal spontaneously maintaining weight on dry food and water as early as 5 days postoperation, and all rats can recover to this point by 10 days. The rats' initial deficits are marked by very weak biting (e.g., rats cannot chew through the paint on a pencil) and difficulty in manipulating pieces of food into the mouth for swallowing. Also they are deficient in the ability to protrude their tongue to lick (Whishaw and Kolb 1983b).

By presenting various types of food on a spatula, the following features of early feeding capacities were revealed: Within 24 hours postoperation the rats ate mash, unfamiliar foods, dry chow, and tap and sugar water from a spatula. They sampled nonnutritive substances such as petrolatum, but did not persist in ingestive attempts for as long as they did with nutritive substances, and they rejected noxious substances. Although initially anorexic, when given mash in a low-rimmed dish in their cage, they chewed on the edge of the dish and ingested enough food to arrest weight loss as early as 2 to 4 days postoperation. At about this time they also began to chew on hard food pellets. If given a little practice drinking by having a water spout presented directly to the mouth, they quickly resumed spontaneous drinking.

As recovery proceeds to the point where animals can maintain themselves, biting strength increases until they grind up large quantities of food. Dexterity must remain a problem because much of this food is dropped. Normal tongue protrusion ability never recovers fully, but with time the rats are able to lick from a surface (Whishaw and Kolb 1989). Perseverative locomotion initially interrupts sustained eating or drinking, but major aspects of this problem dissipate as rats become efficient enough to maintain body weight. As a result of feeding difficulties the rats undergo an initial decline in body weight to about 70 percent of control levels and then recover to about 90 percent of control weight.

Neonatal decortication produces no interruption in suckling as pups are seen to have food in their stomach within 24 hours postoperation. They show a decline in body weight of about 30 percent early in postoperation, and they have a chronic body weight loss of about 10 percent in adulthood (Kolb and Whishaw 1981). As the rats mature, they begin to display the deficits observed after adult decortications. In adulthood, neonatally decorticated rats are, like adult decorticate rats, inefficient eaters, grinding up large quantities of dry food during feeding, and showing impairment on tests of tongue protrusion. Interestingly neonatal operates can protrude the tongue if given special training, but the tongue movements are still inefficient (Whishaw and Kolb 1984b).

In overview, the feeding impairments of decorticate rats are not identical to those of hypothalamically damaged rats, particularly because the rats are not aphagic and do not reject food. The decorticate feeding impairments can be related to inefficient tongue and mouth use of varying degrees throughout survival and derive from damage to the anterior lateral sensorimotor and orbital frontal cortex (see Braun 1975, Kolb 1974, Kolb et al. 1977).

Notwithstanding the unique features of cortical feeding impairments, we have noted that the corticofugal fibers from the anterior lateral cortex to the brainstem take a course through the lateral hypothalamus that carries them along its lateral edge. Unilateral damage to the lateral hypothalamus on one side of the brain and cortical removal on the other produces tongue and mouth impairments and initial feeding deficits, weight loss, and striatal calcification that resembles that of decorticate animals (Whishaw and Kolb 1984a). Accordingly we have suggested that some of the impairments that comprise the lateral hypothalamic syndrome may resemble those of decortication because the damage includes corticofugal fibers (Whishaw and Kolb 1983b, 1984a).

10.4 Appearance

When compared directly with age- and sex-matched control rats, decorticate rats are identifiable. They appear about 10 percent smaller. Their fur, especially if they are adults, appears somewhat rougher. Most distinctively they do not cut their claws (figure 10.2), which become long and twisted (Whishaw et al. 1983b). Inefficient eating may contribute to reduced body weight, inefficient licking during grooming may leave fur rougher, and lack of dexterity in the use of the teeth in chewing may contribute to the rats' inability to cut their claws. A final distinctive feature is that the ears of decorticates are usually turned forward "as if the rats are paying attention" (Whishaw, unpublished observations, 1989). This may result from increased muscle tone or changes in sympathetic activation of ear muscles. The phenomenon has not been studied.

10.5 Posture

To superficial inspection decorticate rats appear to stand, rear, climb, hang from bars or cages, and sleep with normal posture. This normalcy has been observed as early as 4 to 6 hours postoperation (Vanderwolf et al. 1978).

Postural abnormalities do occur, however. When grooming, adult decorticate rats often adopt an exaggeratedly erect position, with the

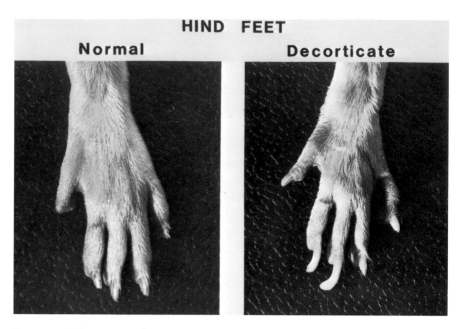

HIND FEET

Normal **Decorticate**

Figure 10.2 Photograph of a rear paw of a control and a decorticate rat. Note the short length of the claws on the control paw and the splinters on the distal edge of the claws, indicative of periodic cutting. Also note the broken claws and the length of the still unbroken claws on the paw of the decorticate rat. (Adapted from Whishaw et al. 1983.)

lumbar spine held abnormally erect or extended and the thoracic spine abnormally flexed, often coupled with an abnormal extension of the hind legs (Vanderwolf et al. 1978). This abnormality is extremely noticeable if the caudate-putamen is damaged. Abnormal posture during grooming is not noticeable in neonatal decorticates (Whishaw, unpublished observations, 1989). When walking on a flat surface or a beam, decorticates always keep their nose close to the surface they are walking on, as if less sensitive to tactile information from the distal portions of the vibrissae (Whishaw, unpublished observations, 1989). When swimming, decorticate rats tend to use the forepaws more for paddling than do normal rats, which keep the forepaws tucked up under their chin (Vanderwolf et al. 1978). This impairment is less apparent in cool water (Whishaw et al. 1981a). Ontogeny of forelimb immobility is normal in neonatal decorticate rats as is limb posture when the rats are adult. An enduring impairment occurs in all decorticates when they turn in the water: They paddle with the limb contralateral to the direction of the turn, whereas control rats make small rotary or sculling movements with the distal portions of the limb to aid their turns (Whishaw and Kolb 1984b).

When decorticate rats eat large laboratory chow food pellets (about 4 g to 6 g in size), they tend to eat the food from the floor of the cage rather than lift it with their mouth then transfer it to their forepaws (Vanderwolf et al. 1978). When they are given small food pellets they display the normal food retrieval sequence and eating posture (Whishaw et al. 1981a). When suspended by the tail or rump, decorticate rats flex their limbs so that they are frequently clasped together or clasped to the body. Normal rats extend the limbs as if to obtain an object distal to them (Whishaw et al. 1981b). Finally, decorticates can be trapped by the postures that they adopt (Whishaw et al. 1981b). If they walk into a narrow alleyway, they stop when their vibrissae touch the alley end and thus become trapped because they do not walk forward far enough to rear and turn around. They also become trapped when placed on top of cages or other objects because they back away from edges rather than lean over to climb down (figure 10.3).

Although decorticate rats show characteristic postural abnormalities, occasionally posture can be surprisingly normal. This suggests that factors other than just the lesion must be considered. The abnormal posture of eating is probably related to a difficulty in grasping large pieces of food with the mouth. Small pieces of food that are easy to grasp release more normal movements. The absence of an abnormal posture during face washing in neonatal decorticates suggests that age at operation may influence some variable such as muscle tone or spasticity. It does not, however, support a conclusion that the cortex is primarily involved in supporting posture during the behavior. With respect to swimming, the age at operation, experience, and water temperature all contribute to normal posture, and it is therefore not likely that the cortex plays a primary role in producing normal posture. This

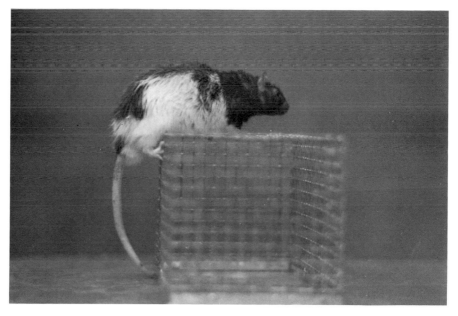

Figure 10.3 When placed on top of objects, decorticate rats back away from the edge and so become trapped and unable to climb down. (Adapted from Whishaw et al. 1981.)

conclusion seems supported by the finding that telencephalic animals can also display immobile forelimbs while swimming (Whishaw and Kolb 1984c). Thus only paddling during turning, head position during locomotion, and limb posture when suspended by the tail appear to be invariant abnormalities. Causes may include, in the first case, loss of ability to make rotary limb movement (Passingham et al. 1983), in the second case, change in tactile sensitivity (perhaps due to loss of the cortical vibrissae barrels), and in the third case, spasticity in antigravity musculature.

10.6 Activity

Hyperactivity in decorticate dogs was noted by Goltz in 1892. Hyperactivity in the rat is situation dependent, however. Vanderwolf and colleagues (1978) collected activity measures in an open field and in running wheels. In a five-minute open-field test, decorticate rats walked, reared, and turned less than did normal rats, but made more head movements while immobile. In an open field in constant light, the decorticate rats showed increased activity during the normally dark period of the animal colony room. In running wheels in a room illuminated on a 12:12-hour light-dark cycle, they were about ten times more active than were control rats in both light and dark, and again they were comparatively more active in the dark. These results were interpreted as evidence of a clear circadian rhythm in decorticates.

Using neonate and adult decorticate rats and appropriate control groups, three measures of activity were made by Kolb and Whishaw (1981). Both adult and neonate decorticates were about three times more active than their respective control groups in running wheels, but they were much less active than the rats tested by Vanderwolf and colleagues (1978). When videorecorded in a cage that had a sawdust floor, food, and water, but was under constant illumination, the incidence of grooming, drinking, rearing, walking, and postural adjustments was equal in all groups. In fact the only group difference in behavior was that the neonatal decorticate animals showed more bouts of eating. When the animals were placed in two-compartment boxes that were illuminated on one side and dark on the other, all groups spent over 90 percent of the time in the dark, and the incidence of crossing between compartments was similar, confirming a previous report by Whishaw (1974).

Four conclusions can be derived from these results: Decorticate rats (1) show a normal dark preference; (2) show evidence of a circadian rhythm, at least when tested in constant light; (3) are not hyperactive when tested in relatively normal environments; and (4) show more responsivity through locomotion to some environments (running wheels) and ambient events (decreased illumination) than do control rats. We believe that the greater activity displayed in Vanderwolf and coworkers' (1978) versus Kolb and Whishaw's (1981) study may be related to the last point. The rats in the former study were not self-subsistent on food and water and so may have been showing an exaggerated hyperactivity to their feeding schedule.

That decorticate rats have a propensity to respond with increased locomotion to some challenges is illustrated further in two studies: First, when control and decorticate rats are placed in running wheels and the lights turned on and off periodically, the decorticates become active during the dark periods (figure 10.4), whereas control rats do not (Whishaw, unpublished data, 1989). A similar dark-induced hyperactivity has been noted in an open field test (Whishaw et al. 1983). Second, Mittleman and colleagues (1990) found that decorticate rats respond to periodic feeding with exaggerated locomotion. In the experiment food-deprived rats were given a single food pellet once each minute at a food hopper at the end of a large box. In this test the decorticate rats retrieved the food pellet and then drank from a spout beside the food hopper just as did rats in the control groups. They then spent the rest of the minute running up and down the box until the next food pellet was delivered (figure 10.5). When contrasted with the behavior of rats with hippocampal or striatal lesions, the release of locomotion was distinctive.

10.7 Grooming

Rat grooming is marked by complex and distinctive organizational features that decortication has been reported to disrupt (Vanderwolf et al. 1978). The rats were habituated to an observation chamber for four days, placed in water for 60 seconds, and then observed. The decorticate rats showed all of the components and sequences of grooming observed in the normal rats. Nonetheless they made more paw-shaking and face-washing movements and fewer turns to lick the body. The duration of a sequence of grooming movements was also shorter, a few seconds versus 5 minutes for control rats. Finally, the decorticate rats walked two to three times more frequently than the control rats. The interpretation of these observations was that nonspecific ascending systems acting throughout the cerebral cortex are essential to the control of type 1 behaviors (movements such as walking and postural changes). Therefore after the loss of these afferents through cortical removal, the rats made errors in selecting appropriate type 1 movements, i.e., they walked instead of turning to groom the body.

We have reanalyzed the grooming of decorticate rats in three separate experiments. In the first (Whishaw et al. 1981a) the rats received the grooming test when wetted with water rubbed into their fur, and they were also filmed while grooming spontaneously in their home cage. The decorticate rats showed a grooming pattern when wet that was

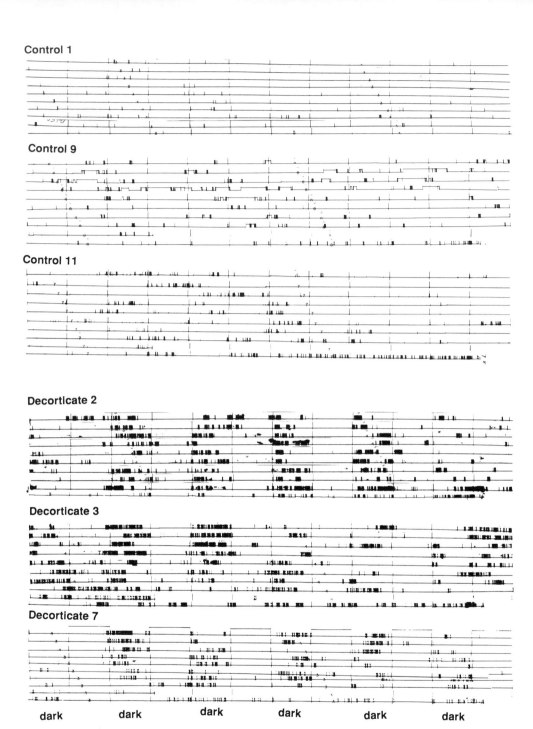

Control 1

Control 9

Control 11

Decorticate 2

Decorticate 3

Decorticate 7

dark　　　dark　　　dark　　　dark　　　dark　　　dark

Figure 10.4 Activity of control decorticate rats during light and dark portions of a 2-hour light on/off schedule. Note the increase in activity of the decorticate rats during each dark cycle. (From Whishaw, unpublished data, 1989)

Motor Systems

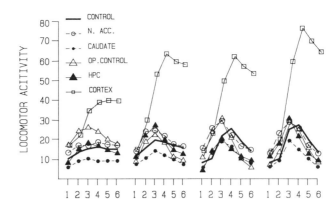

Figure 10.5 Activity of decorticate rats compared with rats having a variety of other kinds of brain lesion. Food pellets were delivered once each 60 seconds. Each figure segment is activity on six 10-second blocks of time on test sessions summarized as blocks of 5 days. Note the distinctive "release" of activity of the decorticate group. N. ACC = nucleus accumbens; OP CONTROL = control; HPC = hippocampus. (From Mittleman et al., unpublished data, 1990)

similar to that described by Vanderwolf and colleagues (1978), except that their impairments were much milder. Grooming appeared essentially normal when the dry rats spontaneously groomed in their home cages. In the second experiment we habituated wet rats to the test apparatus daily for ten days and then videotaped and scored their grooming. A summary of the sequences of movements and their probabilities are shown in figure 10.6. The preadaption procedure further reduced the abnormalities of the rats. They began the grooming sequences in the usual way, washed their face as frequently, and turned and groomed their body as frequently as did the control rats and in general devoted about as much time to grooming each part of the body as did control rats.

In the third study Berridge and Whishaw (unpublished data, 1989) examined a sequential grooming chain consisting of 10 to 25 separate actions that combine to form a structured transition between face and body grooming. This syntactic chain comprised four phases: a bout of rapid elliptical forepaw strokes performed bilaterally over the nose and mystacial vibrissae at a rate of 6 Hz to 7 Hz; a short series of 1 to 4 slower strokes of small to intermediate amplitude made unilaterally with one paw or asymmetrically with both paws at different amplitudes; a series of large-amplitude forelimb strokes, bilateral and typically asymmetrical with respect to forepaw trajectory; and tucking of the head and shifting of posture to bring the head into contact with ventral or lateral torso for a bout of body licking. On the first grooming chain of a 30-minute grooming session, decorticate rats were impaired in completions, but no more so than rats with small supplementary motor cortex

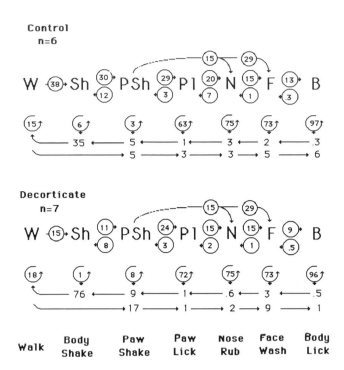

Figure 10.6 Grooming sequences in decorticate and control rats compared. Numbers indicate percentages of movement transitions from one movement to the next, as indicated by arrows. Numerical sequences at the bottom of each sequence indicate entrances into and from walking. Movements are indicated at the bottom of the figure. Note the similarity between the grooming sequencing in the two groups. The results were obtained from 30-minute recording sessions for each rat and were compiled from 8982 movements from the control rats and 9995 movements from the decorticate rats. (From Whishaw et al., unpublished data, 1989)

ablations. On the remaining chains decorticate rats' completion of this syntactic chain was not different from that of control rats. Only if the striatum was removed in addition to the cortex was order and accuracy reduced.

Two interpretations can be given to these results: First, decorticate rats are not deficient in the ability to generate and sequence grooming movements, nor are they deficient in making the postural adjustments prerequisite for successful movement transitions. The more severe impairments described by Vanderwolf and coworkers (1978) may have been due to studying the rats too soon after operation, studying rats that were not maintaining themselves normally on food and water, and studying rats that were not adequately habituated to all facets of the experimental procedure. Second, it may be the case that the cortex is in some way involved in extending the range of conditions in which optimal grooming is achieved. Thus, if placed in a novel environment, decorticate rats may display impaired grooming behaviors.

10.8   Sexual Behavior

The descriptions of the effects of cortex injury take two forms, depending on sex: For male rats (Beach 1947, p. 305), "When the extent of bilateral invasion exceeds approximately 75 percent of the total neopallial mass coital reactions are totally eliminated." In his two-factor model Beach (1940) argued that there is an arousal mechanism that is responsible for bringing the male to the threshold for copulation and an intromission and ejaculatory mechanism that regulates subsequent sexual activity. He proposed that cortex lesions abolished arousal.

We reexamined male sexual behavior after finding that a neonate decorticate rat and an adult decorticate rat had impregnated female rats with which they were housed (Kolb and Whishaw 1981). Normal female rats were paired with adult decorticate male rats, half of which had hippocampus removed in addition to neocortex (Whishaw and Kolb 1983a). One half of the male rats in each group successfully impregnated female rats, although latency to do so was about 5 days longer than it was for control rats. In a video analysis of the copulatory behavior of male decorticate rats paired with primed females, this finding was replicated (Whishaw and Kolb 1985). In addition it was observed that the decorticate rats made movements indicative of sexual interest, including treading on the female's back, passing over the female, and sniffing the female's genitals. After one successful mount the remaining copulatory patterns proceeded normally. Numbers of mounts, intromissions, ejaculations, postejaculatory songs, and the intromission and ejaculatory patterns were like those of control rats, although the decorticate rats had fewer mount bouts and showed abnormalities in the execution of some movements.

Beach's (1944) observation concerning female rats after estrogen and progesterone priming was that most of the behaviors displayed by normal rats were also displayed by the decorticate rats, but with considerable variability. Lordosis, ear wiggling, and hopping were present and even increased in frequency, whereas back kicking was reduced. The variability was illustrated by the lordosis response; females would display lordosis without the male mounting, fail to show the response when the male mounted, retain the response for more than one mount, or display the response to vaginal probes or handling. Beach interpreted these changes in behavior in terms of a reduced neural inhibition or "disinhibition," and he contrasted the female response with the absent arousal in male rats.

Using neonatally decorticated female rats, Carter and colleagues (1982) confirmed that the lesions did not eliminate female sexual behavior, but they were unable to confirm the generality of the disinhibition result. In fact lordosis in decorticate female rats given prolonged low levels of estradiol benzoate and estradiol benzoate plus progesterone was found to be reduced compared with lordosis in control rats. In addition, although the females continued to direct sniffing behavior toward the male, hopping, darting, and rejection behaviors were virtually absent. The reasons for the latter effects were not systematically investigated.

Taken together, the results of the studies on decorticate male and female rats show that the movements for sexual behavior are present, their organization resembles that of control rats, and they are functional.

10.9   Maternal Behavior

Maternal behavior was examined in two separate studies by Beach. In the first study (Beach 1937) primiparous rats deprived of cortical tissue approximately 30 days before parturition displayed poor preparatory nest building and inferior pup care when compared with control rats. In the second study (Beach 1938) comparisons were made between rats given cortical lesions at 30 days of age or adulthood. The brain-damaged animals were inferior to control rats in nest building, moving pups away from irritants, pup retrieval, cleaning pups, and pup survival. The inferiority increased with increasing lesion size. The neonatally operated rats, however, were superior to the adult operates. There were two striking findings in the experiment: First, as lesion size increased the number of pups surviving over five days decreased, and with lesions as small as 50 percent—mainly dorsolateral cortex—no pups survived. Second, there was no relation between lesion location and performance deficits on any measure. In a brief report Davis (1939) obtained similar results. Of 16 female decorticate rats, 12 became pregnant, 8 came to term, and none of these displayed cleaning, nursing, or nest building. Davis presented no histological results.

To examine decorticate maternal behavior in our rats (Whishaw, unpublished data, 1989), 8 neonatally decorticate female rats were paired with males when adult. Pup survival was monitored, nest building was rated after periodic introduction of nesting material, and pup retrieval was observed in periodic tests involving the removal of one or two pups from the nest. The ablations removed all of the cingulate and midline cortex and the dorsolateral cortex (figure 10.7). All of the rats had some cortex left ventrolaterally. Even though the removals were larger than Beach's largest removals, six of the eight rats raised litters. The decorticate rats did not always keep their litters in the corners of the plastic nesting cages as did control rats, and they did not move nesting material or construct nests as did control rats. They were slow to retrieve pups, but they usually retrieved some pups in formal tests, and the pups were occasionally found to have been moved from one portion of the nest to another.

Though none of the removals was complete, they were sufficiently large to suggest that at least some decorticate female rats will display

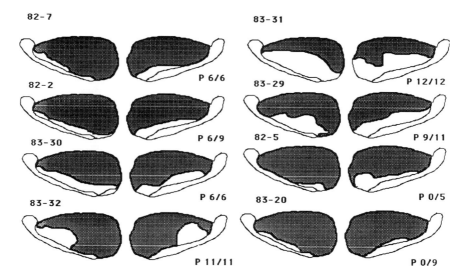

Figure 10.7 The extent of cortical removal in six female neonatally decorticate rats that raised litters of pups and two that did not. Numbers on the left indicate the rat number, whereas numbers to the right show the number of pups that were born and survived in each litter. (From Whishaw, unpublished data, 1989.)

sufficient maternal behavior or raise a litter of pups in laboratory maternity cages. Thus the limited conclusion that the neocortex is not necessary for the acts of cleaning, suckling, and otherwise caring for a litter to survival is warranted. (This supports the conclusion of Bjursten and colleagues (1976), who found that decorticate female cats could raise kittens.) It is unclear why so many of the rats were successful, as contrasted with previous studies, but the fact that the lesions were made neonatally may be a factor. Also there were many failures in the control groups in previous work, which suggests a difference in breeding populations.

Some observations on the parental behavior of male rats have also been made (Whishaw, unpublished data, 1989). Normal male rats will kill and eat rat pups when first exposed to them, but will care for them once they habituate to them (Rosenberg and Sherman 1975). We gave 28 male decorticate rats (for rat numbers and histology, see Whishaw and Kolb 1983a) three 20-minute pairings in a 30-cm^2 box with a sawdust floor. There were four 3- to 5-day-old pups in the box in the first test. Many of the male rats became agitated when they encountered the pups, orienting to them, twitching their back muscles, and hovering over them. Nine of the rats then killed one or more pups by biting them on the head or back (rats 22, 16, 14, 21, 8, 20, 54, 5, and 17 in Whishaw and Kolb 1983a). None of the rats ate a pup. These rats were then given a second test in which cold-anesthetized pups were present. None of the rats bit a pup. In the third test none of the rats bit 14-day-old pups when paired with them. After these tests we placed each male with a pregnant female and left them together after the birth of the pups. Only one of these rats killed a pup, and this occurred when the female had been removed from the cage to be weighed. In fact, although we made no systematic records, we frequently observed male rats crouching over pups in the maternal pattern described by Rosenberg and Sherman (1975). Thus male decorticate rats show many features of normal male rat parental behavior.

10.10 Other Species-Typical Behaviors

Other species-typical behaviors have been less systematically examined than those outlined above. Hoarding has been examined in a number of studies in which food has been left in an alley outside a covered home area. In none of these studies has any appreciable hoarding been observed in any decorticate rat (Whishaw 1974, Kolb and Whishaw 1981, Vanderwolf et al. 1978). The reason for the impairment is unknown. It has been observed that food-deprived decorticate rats pick up pieces of food and walk around with the food in their mouth, that they do successfully grasp pieces of food that are handed to them, and that they dodge away with the food before stopping to eat it (Whishaw, unpublished data, 1989). These behaviors are all components of hoarding (Whishaw and Tomie 1989). Thus at least some components of the hoarding response are displayed, but are not used for hoarding.

Differences between play and attack behavior in normal rats have been succinctly described. Play attacks are directed at the nape of the opponent's neck, whereas in serious fighting attacks are directed at the rump (Pellis and Pellis 1987). In a brief report Normansell and Panksepp (1984) have stated that play in juvenile decorticate rats is much the same in controls. The results of observation and video analysis of juvenile rats confirms this report (Whishaw, unpublished data, 1989). The number of pins was reduced around day 30 in decorticates as compared with control rats (figure 10.8), but some decorticate rats' behaviors were indistinguishable from the control rats'. In the experiment the most striking difference between the two groups of rats was that the decorticate rats were less likely to initiate play bouts. This aspect of play behavior is still being analyzed (Pellis and Whishaw, unpublished data, 1989).

A few observations on defensive and aggressive behavior have been made. Vanderwolf and colleagues (1978) gave paired rats foot shock in an observation box. The decorticate rats stood and boxed as did normal rats, but the incidence of the behaviors was reduced compared with controls. Using a "resident-intruder" model, Whishaw (unpublished data, 1989) observed decorticate rats as defenders or intruders. The box was 40 cm^2 with a shade umbrella in the center. A resident male was paired with a female and her pups. When decorticate rats were the resident male rats, they approached an intruder (control or decorticate) and made lateral displays as did normal rats. None of the decorticate

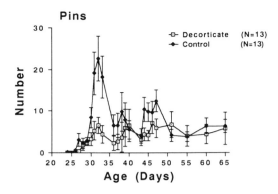

Figure 10.8 Number of pins displayed by juvenile rats at different ages during play behavior. Rats were kept in isolation and paired for 30 minutes daily in different decorticate-control combinations. Note that, with the exception of the peak activity displayed by control rats between days 30 and 35, decorticate rats were much the same as control rats. (From Whishaw, unpublished data, 1989)

rats were observed to attack intruders as did the control resident rats. When rats were first introduced into a control rat's residence, they were approached by the resident and eventually attacked. When an attack began, the intruder was immediately removed. The intruder was then reintroduced hours later. Many of the intruders, both control and decorticate, froze when reintroduced. Three decorticates displayed a dramatic collapse in which their rear end lost postural support. These preliminary observations suggest that most of the components of aggressive and defensive behavior can be expected to be found in decorticate rats (see also Whishaw and colleagues 1979).

10.11   Skilled Movements

Impairments in skilled movements are characteristic of decorticate rats. They have difficulty cutting their claws, chewing food, holding small pieces of food, protruding and using their tongue, opening puzzles, reaching, and rotating their paws to scull while swimming (see Whishaw and Kolb 1984b). It is thought that most of these impairments stem from motor cortex damage (Kolb and Whishaw 1983). Interestingly rats can show improvements in performance on some behaviors with training, as in the case of learning to drink described above. Some aspects of skilled movements survive decortication. Complete removal of the motor cortex and even complete hemidecortication spares the ballistic and grasping components of skilled reaching using the contralateral limb, while at the same time disrupting more subtle features of the movement (Whishaw and Kolb 1988). Therefore even the analysis of skilled movements requires that distinctions be made between cortical and subcortical contributions.

10.12 Learning

In contrast with the few papers on unconditioned behaviors in decorticate rats, there is a cornucopia of research on their learning abilities (table 10.1). Early studies on the cortex were conducted with the assumption that the cortex was essential for learning. Recent studies demonstrate that decorticate animals are able to learn many tasks as readily as control rats. The significance of this changed view for human rehabilitative medicine has been discussed elsewhere (Oakley 1981a, 1983a,b).

A simple classification of the results in table 10.1 suggests that decorticate rats are successful at simple associative learning (pairing a response with a single stimulus) and impaired or unable to perform conditional tasks (responding when the significance of one cue depends on another cue). Some tasks on which rats are initially impaired but eventually learn may be solved using both strategies; e.g., spatial reversals may be quickly solved using conditional information by control rats, but solved more slowly with simple associations (turn right or left) by decorticate rats. The clearest distinction between the two forms of learning comes from the swimming task.

In the swimming task (Whishaw and Kolb 1984c) rats are released from a number of points in a circular pool of water made opaque by the addition of powdered milk. In the *cue* version of the task a black platform is located in the pool so that it is clearly visible, highlighted against the white walls of the pool. The rat need only see the platform, swim to it, and climb on it and escape. In the *place* version of the task, the platform is hidden just below the surface of the water so that the only way the rat can navigate directly toward it is to determine its location relative to the ambient pool and room cues. It can also get there somewhat indirectly if it knows that the platform bears a constant relation to the wall of the pool such that it can find the platform by swimming in a circle at a given distance from the wall. All features of the two forms of the tasks are identical except for the cues used to guide performance. Decorticate rats learn the cue task, but are completely unable to perform the place task (figure 10.9). The interpretation of the experiment is that the decorticate rats can perform a simple association (swim to a visible object), but not a conditional association (swim to a place that is identified in relation to other ambient cues).

One other interpretation of the incapacities of decorticate rats in learning tasks is that they may not be able to generate or call up movements prerequisite for solving the tasks. This is best illustrated in the defensive burying paradigm (Kolb and Whishaw 1981). An electrified rod is introduced into a large box containing sawdust. When control rats investigate the prod and are shocked by it, they not only subsequently avoid further shocks but bury the rod with sawdust. The decorticate rats also successfully avoid the prod, but they do not bury it.

Table 10.1 Studies on Learning in Decorticate Rats

Task	Result	Reference
Cardiac (classical)	Success	Bloch and Lagarrigue 1968
	Success	DiCara et al. 1970
Cardiac (instrumental)	Failure	DiCara et al. 1970
One-way shock avoidance	Failure	Oakley 1979b
One-way shock avoidance (V)	Failure	Pinto-Hamuy et al. 1963
One-way shock avoidance (A)	Failure	Saavedra et al. 1963
Simple shock avoidance (V)	Mixed	Bloch and Lagarrigue 1968
One-way food approach	Success	Oakley 1979b
Habituation (A)	Success	Yeo and Oakley 1983
GO-NO GO (V)	Failure	Oakley and Russell 1979
T-maze and T-maze delay	Success	Thompson 1959
Operant FR-4-12, bar press	Failure	Oakley and Russell 1979
Operant FR-60, chain-pull	Success	Oakley 1980
Operant FR-60, bar press	Success	Oakley and Morgan 1977
Pattern discrimination (V)		Oakley 1981b
		Goldstein and Oakley 1987
acquisition	Success	
reversal	Success	
rotated obliques	Success	
Puzzles	Impaired	Kolb and Whishaw 1983
Spatial reversal		
successive reversals	Impaired	Gonzales et al. 1964
		Kolb and Whishaw 1981
		Kolb and Whishaw 1983
learning-set reversal	Impaired	Kolb and Whishaw 1981
		Kolb and Whishaw 1983
Defensive burying		
avoidance	Success	Kolb and Whishaw 1981
burying	Failure	Kolb and Whishaw 1981
Spatial navigation (swim)		
cue task	Impaired	Whishaw and Kolb 1984c
place task	Failure	Whishaw and Kolb 1984c
		Kolb et al. 1983b
Radial arm maze	Impaired	Kolb et al. 1983b

A = auditory; V = visual; Success = learned as quickly as control group;
Impaired = learned but with significant impairment; Failure = did not learn.

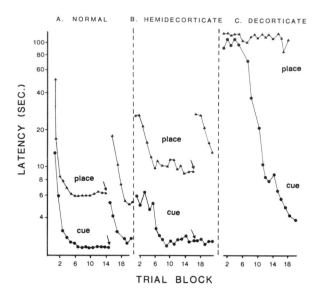

A. NORMAL   B. HEMIDECORTICATE   C. DECORTICATE

TRIAL BLOCK

Figure 10.9 Mean escape latency per trial (semilog graph) on each of four trials for rats swimming to a visible (cue) or hidden (place) platform. The rats were initially trained when normal and received first and second hemidecortications at the time indicated by the dotted lines. The arrows indicate tests on which the platform was repositioned. Note that the cue task performance survives both hemidecortication and decortication, whereas the place task performance is disrupted by hemidecortication and abolished by decortication. (Adapted from Whishaw and Kolb 1984c.)

Clearly, using one motor response they indicate that they have learned, but, apparently unable to dig, they are unable to indicate that they have learned using a different motor response. It may be the case that they fail other tasks because they are unable to generate prerequisite movements.

10.13   L'Envoi

Through improved description of deficits, some notions of cortical function have not received support. Beach's (1940) notion that the cortex is involved in arousal is negated by direct evidence that decorticate male rats engage in sexual behavior indistinguishable from that of control rats, and it is not supported in any general way by other results summarized in this review. Some textbooks include interpretations of Beach's (1940) study that indicate that the male decorticate rat, as contrasted with the female decorticate rat, is at a disadvantage because its role requires more complex behavior. The finding that males do copulate, coupled with the finding that female rats play a significant role in guiding the male's movements, negates this proposition (Whishaw and Kolb 1985).

MacLean (1982) has outlined a general theory of brain function within a comparative and evolutionary framework. The theory is vague on details, but nursing, parental care, and play are given as classes of advanced mammalian behavior (of postreptilian origin) that are distinguishable from other species-typical behaviors. The theory, supported by a study by Murphy and coworkers (1981) using hamsters, claims that midline limbic structures are essential for the expression of play behavior and integrated maternal behavior, whereas striatal and other structures are adequate for other species-typical behaviors. The general nature of this claim cannot be supported by the results of experiments with decorticate rats because they play and raise pups. Furthermore this categorization of behaviors into two classes of species-typical behavior has other difficulties: The behaviors cannot be referred to either the limbic system or striatum and brainstem, even in hamsters (Kolb and Whishaw 1985). That some species-typical behaviors consigned to the more primitive category seem impaired after decortication (hoarding and nest building), whereas others do not (grooming and sexual behavior), raises serious objections to the classification and to the theory based on such distinctions.

The Loeb-Pavlov theory that the function of the cortex is to support "learning" is difficult to reconcile with many empirical findings. Many kinds of learning survive decortication, whereas many other unconditioned behaviors, such as claw cutting, are lost. Furthermore the character of deficits in some learning tasks makes it difficult to easily parcel learning into categories that have a one-to-one relation with neural entities, as has been suggested (Oakley 1981a, table 1, p. 176).

In a theoretical directive Sperry (1952, p. 312) has argued that "motor adjustments, rather than stimulus patterns or the contents of subjective experience, figures predominantly as a proper frame of reference for understanding the organization, meaning, and significance of brain excitation." Taken seriously, this directive eliminates theories stressing classes of behavior, special attributes of the sensory environment, and theories of cognitive function and favors theories that stress movement. Among theorists that stress movement, Vanderwolf and colleagues (1978) have suggested that the cortex may be involved in the control of movement in two ways: In a more general way the cortex may regulate type 1 movements such as walking, postural adjustments, rearing, etc. (ensuring that they occur at the right time and place), and also it may play a highly specific role in the organization of some movement patterns. Unfortunately the examples illustrating these two functions— impairments of postural adjustment during grooming and immobility of the forepaws during swimming—upon reexamination are found to be displayed adequately by decorticate rats. In another vein Sherrington (Leyton and Sherrington 1917, p. 179 and Sherrington 1906, pp. 386– 387) suggested that the cortex breaks up compounds already constructed at lower centers. As noted here, however, most motor patterns are performed quite adequately by rats that have lost their cortex.

In our own analysis of decorticate rats, we have been struck by the finding that the movements they make are more subject to the stimulus condition under which the tests are conducted than are the movements of normal rats (Whishaw et al. 1981a). Consequently the reexamination of a particular behavior in changing sensory configurations is shown to be a useful way to construct a profile of an animal's motor abilities. It also shows that the capacity of decorticate rats to make movements resembling those of normal rats is greater than has been suspected.

What leaves the understanding of the cortex's function wanting is not just incomplete description. The discovery that an animal cannot perform an act after decortication is but one component of an analysis. A second involves an adequate explanation of why the deficit occurs. A third component involves getting beyond the laboratory. Rats have yet to be adequately studied in natural settings in which their brains were sculpted by evolution. For example, the pairwise relation between a male laboratory rat mating with a female in a laboratory cage may be but a caricature of the complexity of group sexual behavior in wild colonies (McClintock 1984). Accordingly acts that may appear normal in a laboratory test may be found inadequate in a more natural setting. Thus understanding of cortical function will be aided by an analysis that extends beyond simple acts performed in simple situations.

Finally, it is very likely that theories that posit one or a few functions for the cortex may be misdirected. The cortex may not simply add a new level of analysis to brain function but rather may extend the usefulness of many or all subcortical functions to allow optimal movements in an expanding range of stimulus conditions. Such an explanation of cortical function will require an extended analysis that includes all behavior.

Acknowledgment

This research was supported by grants from the Natural Sciences and Engineering Research Council of Canada.

References

Beach, F. A. (1937). The neural basis of innate behavior: I. Effects of cortical lesions upon the maternal behavior pattern in the rat. *Journal of Comparative Psychology* 24:393–438.

Beach, F. A. (1938). The neural basis of innate behavior: II. Relative effects of partial decortication in adulthood and infancy upon the maternal behavior of the primiparous rat. *The Journal of Genetic Psychology* 53:109–148.

Beach, F. A. (1940). Effects of cortical lesions upon the copulatory behavior of male rats. *Journal of Comparative Psychology* 29:193–244.

Beach, F. A. (1944). Effects of injury to the cerebral cortex upon sexually receptive behavior in the female rat. *Psychosomatic Medicine* 6:40–55.

Beach, F. A. (1947). Evolutionary changes in the physiological control of mating behavior in mammals. *Psychological Review* 54:297–315.

Bjursten, L.-M., Norrsell, K., and Norrsell, U. (1976). Behavioural repertory of cats without cerebral cortex from infancy. *Experimental Brain Research* 25:115–130.

Bloch, S., and Lagarrigue, I. (1968). Cardiac and simple avoidance learning in neodecorticate rats. *Physiology and Behavior* 3:305–308.

Braun, J. J. (1975). Neocortex and feeding behavior in the rat. *Journal of Comparative and Physiological Psychology* 89:507–522.

Bures, J., and Buresova, O. (1969). The use of Leao's spreading cortical depression in research on conditioned reflexes. *Electroencephalography and Clinical Neurophysiology* (Supplementary) 13:359–367.

Carter, C. S., Witt, D. M., Kolb, B., and Whishaw, I. Q. (1982). Neonatal decortication and adult female sexual behavior. *Physiology and Behavior* 29:763–766.

Davis, C. D. (1939). The effect of ablations of neocortex on mating, maternal behavior and the production of pseudopregnancy in the female rat and on copulatory activity in the male. *American Journal of Physiology* 127:374–380.

Descartes, R. (1664). *Traité de l'Homme*. Paris: Angot.

DiCara, L. V., Braun, J. J., and Pappas, B. A. (1970). Classical conditioning and instrumental learning of cardiac and gastrointestinal responses following removal of neocortex in rat. *Journal of Comparative and Physiological Psychology* 73:208–216.

Flourens, J. P. M. (1824). *Recherches Expérimentales sur les Propriétés et les Fonctions du Système Nerveux dans les Animaux Vertèbres*. Paris: Crevot.

Gall, J., and Spurzheim, J. (1810–1819). *Anatomie et Physiology du Système Nerveux en Général et du Cerveau en Particulier*. Paris: F. Schoell.

Goldstein, L. H., and Oakley, D. A. (1987). Visual discrimination in the absence of visual cortex. *Behavioural Brain Research* 24: 181–193.

Goltz, F. (1892). Der Hund ohne Grosshirn. Siebente Abhandlung über die Verrichtungen des Grosshirns. *Pflügers Archiv gesamte Physiologie des Menschen und der Tiere* 51:570–614.

Gonzales, R. C., Roberts, W. A., and Bitterman, M. E. (1964). Learning in adult rats with extensive cortical lesions made in infancy. *American Journal of Psychology* 77:547–562.

Grill, H. J., and Norgren, R. (1978). Neurological tests and behavioral deficits in chronic thalamic and chronic decerebrate rats. *Brain Research* 143:299–312.

Herrick, C. J. (1926). *Brains of Rats and Men*. Chicago: University of Chicago Press.

Kolb, B. (1974). Prefrontal lesions alter eating and hoarding behavior in rats. *Physiology and Behavior* 12:507–511.

Kolb, B., Sutherland, R. J., and Whishaw, I. Q. (1983a). Abnormalities in cortical and subcortical morphology after neonatal neocortical lesions in rats. *Experimental Neurology* 79:223–244.

Kolb, B., Sutherland, R. J., and Whishaw, I. Q. (1983b). A comparison of the contributions of the frontal and parietal association cortex to spatial localization in rats. *Behavioural Neuroscience* 97:13–27.

Kolb, B., and Whishaw, I. Q. (1981). Decortication of rats in infancy of adulthood produced comparable functional losses on learned and species-typical behaviors. *Journal of Comparative and Physiological Psychology* 95:468–483.

Kolb, B., and Whishaw, I. Q. (1983). Dissociation of the contributions of the prefrontal, motor, and parietal cortex to the control of movement in the rat: An experimental review. *Canadian Journal of Psychology* 37:211–232.

Kolb, B., and Whishaw, I. Q. (1985). Neonatal frontal lesions in hamsters impair species-typical behavior and reduce brain weight and neocortical thickness. *Behavioral Neuroscience* 99:691–706.

Kolb, B., Whishaw, I. Q., and Schallert, T. (1977). Behavior sequencing, sensory neglect and body weight set point following orbital frontal lesions in rats. *Physiology & Behavior* 19:93–102.

Kolb, B., Whishaw, I. Q., and van der Kooy, D. (1986). Brain development in neonatally decorticated rat. *Brain Research* 397:315–326.

Lashley, K. H. (1950). In search of the engram. *Symposia of the Society for Experimental Biology* 4:454–482.

Lassek, A. M. (1954). *The Pyramidal Tract.* Springfield, IL: Charles C. Thomas.

Lanca, A. J., Boyd, S., Kolb, B. E., and van der Kooy, D. (1986). The development of a patchy organization of the rat striatum. *Developmental Brain Research* 27:1–10.

Leyton, A. S. F., and Sherrington, C. S. (1917). Observations on the excitable cortex of the chimpanzee, orangutan, and gorilla. *Quarterly Journal of Experimental Physiology* 11:135–222.

Loeb, J. (1900). *Comparative Physiology of the Brain and Comparative Psychology.* London: J. Murray.

Lorber, J. (1968). The results of early treatment of extreme hydrocephalus. *Developmental Medicine and Child Neurology* (Supplement 16):21–29.

MacLean, P. D. (1982). On the origin and progressive evolution of the triune brain. In E. Armstrong and D. Falk (eds.), *Primate Brain Evolution: Methods and Concepts.* New York: Plenum Press, 291–316.

McClintock, M. K. (1984). Group mating in the domestic rat as a context for sexual selection: consequences for the analysis of sexual behavior and neuroendocrine responses. In J. S. Rosenberg, C. Beer, M. C. Busnel, and P. J. B. Slater (eds.), *Advances in the Study of Behavior,* Vol. 14. Orlando, FL: Academic Press, 1–50.

Mittleman, G., Whishaw, I. Q., Jones, G. H., Koch, M., and Robbins, T. W. (1990).

Cortical, hippocampal and striatal mediation of schedule-induced behaviors. *Behavioral Neuroscience* (in press).

Murphy, M. R., MacLean, P. D., and Hamilton, S. C. (1981). Species-typical behavior of hamsters deprived from birth of the neocortex. *Science* 24:459–461.

Normansell, L. A., and Panksepp, J. (1984). Play in decorticate rats. *Society for Neuroscience Abstracts* 10:612.

Oakley, D. A. (1979a). Neocortex and learning. *Trends in Neurosciences* 2:149–152.

Oakley, D. A. (1979b). Learning with food reward and shock avoidance in neodecorticate rats. *Experimental Neurology* 63:627–642.

Oakley, D. A. (1980). Improved instrumental learning in neodecorticate rats. *Physiology and Behavior* 24:357–366.

Oakley, D. A. (1981a). Brain mechanisms of mammalian memory. *British Medical Bulletin* 37:175–180.

Oakley, D. A. (1981b). Performance of decorticated rats in a two-choice visual discrimination apparatus. *Behavioural Brain Research* 3:55–69.

Oakley, D. A. (1983a). Learning capacity outside neocortex in animals and man: Implications for therapy after brain-injury. In G. C. L. Davey (ed.), *Animals Models of Human Behavior*. New York: John Wiley & Sons, 247–266.

Oakley, D. A. (1983b). The varieties of memory: A phylogenetic approach. In A. Mayes (ed.), *Memory in Animals and Humans*. Workingham: Van Nostrad Reinhold, 20–82.

Oakley, D. A., and Morgan, S. C. (1977). Fixed ratio instrumental performance in a neodecorticate rat. *IRCS Medical Science: Experimental Animals; Psychology and Psychiatry; Nervous Systems* 5:494.

Oakley, D. A., and Russell, I. S. (1979). Instrumental learning on Fixed Ratio and GO-NOGO schedules in neodecorticate rats. *Brain Research* 161:356–360.

Oakley, D. A., and Russell, I. S. (1980). Effect of prior experience on bar-pressing in rats without neocortex. *Behavioural Brain Research* 1:267–283.

Passingham, R. E., Perry, V. H., and Wilkinson, F. (1983). The long-term effects of removal of sensorimotor cortex in infant and adult rhesus monkeys. *Brain* 106:675–705.

Pavlov, I. P. (1927). *Conditioned Reflexes*. Translated by G. V. Anrep. New York: Dover Publications.

Pellis, S. M., and Pellis, V. C. (1987). Play-fighting differs from serious fighting in both target of attack and tactics of fighting in the laboratory rat *Rattus norvegicus*. *Aggressive Behavior* 13:227–242.

Pereira, S., and Russell, I. S. (1981). Learning in normal and microcephalic rats. In M. W. van Hoff and G. Mohn (eds.), *Functional Recovery from Brain Damage*. Amsterdam: Elsevier/North Holland Biomedical, 131–147.

Phillips, C. G., Zeki, S., and Barlow, H. B. (1984). Localization of function in the cerebral cortex. *Brain* 107:327–361.

Pinto-Hamuy, T., Santibanez, H. G., and Rojas, J. A. (1963). Learning and retention of a visual conditioned response in neodecorticate rats. *Journal of Comparative and Physiological Psychology* 56:19–24.

Robinson, T. E. (1983). *Behavioral Approaches to Brain Research*. New York: Oxford University Press.

Rosenberg, K. M., and Sherman, G. (1975). Influence of testosterone on pup killing in the rat is modified by prior experience. *Physiology and Behavior* 15:669–672.

Saavedra, M., Garcia, E., and Pinto-Hamuy, T. (1963). Acquisition of auditory conditioned reponses in normal and neodecorticate rats. *Journal of Comparative and Physiological Psychology* 56:31–35.

Sherrington, C. S. [1906] (1961). *The Integrative Action of the Nervous System*. New Haven, CT: Yale University Press.

Sorenson, C.A., and Ellison, G. D. (1970). Striatal organization of feeding behavior in the decorticate rat. *Experimental Neurology* 29:162–174.

Sperry, R. W. (1952). Neurology and the mind-brain problem. *American Scientist* 40:291–312.

Teitelbaum, P., and Epstein, A. N. (1962). The lateral hypothalamic syndrome: Recovery of feeding and drinking after lateral hypothalamic lesions. *Psychological Review* 69:74–90.

Thompson, R. (1959). Learning in rats with extensive neocortical damage. *Science* 129:1223–1224.

Vanderwolf, C. H., Kolb, B., and Cooley, R. K. (1978). Behavior of the rat after removal of the neocortex and hippocampal formation. *Journal of Comparative and Physiological Psychology* 92:156–175.

Whishaw, I. Q. (1974). Light avoidance in normal rats and rats with primary visual system lesions. *Physiological Psychology* 2:143–147.

Whishaw, I. Q., and Kolb, B. (1983a). Can male decorticate rats copulate? *Behavioral Neuroscience* 97:270–279.

Whishaw, I. Q., and Kolb, B. (1983b). "Stick out your tongue": tongue protrusion in neocortex and hypothalamic damaged rats. *Physiology and Behavior* 30:471–480.

Whishaw, I. Q., and Kolb, B. (1984a). We should de-emphasize the importance of the role we give to amines in the LH syndrome. *Appetite* 5:272–276.

Whishaw, I. Q., and Kolb, B. (1984b). Behavioral and anatomical studies of rats with complete or partial decortication in infancy. In S. Finger and C. R. Almli (eds.), *Early Brain Damage*. Vol. 2. New York: Academic Press, 117–138.

Whishaw, I. Q., and Kolb, B. (1984c). Decortication abolishes place but not cue learning in rats. *Behavioral Brain Research* 11:123–134.

Whishaw, I. Q., and Kolb, B. (1985). The mating movements of male decorticate rats: Evidence for subcortically generated movements by the male but regulation of approaches by the female. *Behavioural Brain Research* 17:171–191.

Whishaw, I. Q., and Kolb, B. (1988). Sparing of skilled forelimb reaching and corticospinal projections after neonatal motor cortex removal or hemidecortication in the rat: support for the Kennard doctrine. *Brain Research* 451:97–114.

Whishaw, I. Q., and Kolb, B. (1989). Tongue protrusion mediated by spared anterior ventrolateral neocortex in neonatally decorticate rats: behavioral support for the neuro-genetic hypothesis. *Behavioural Brain Research* 32:101–113.

Whishaw, I. Q., Kolb, B., and Sutherland, R. J. (1983a). The analysis of behavior in the laboratory rat. In T. E. Robinson (ed.), *Behavioral Contributions to Brain Research*. New York: Oxford University Press.

Whishaw, I. Q., Kolb, B., Sutherland, R. J., and Becker, J. B. (1983b). Cortical control of claw cutting in the rat. *Behavioral Neuroscience* 97:370–380.

Whishaw, I. Q., Nonneman, A. J., and Kolb, B. (1981a). Environmental constraints on motor abilities used in grooming, swimming, and eating by decorticate rats. *Journal of Comparative and Physiological Psychology* 95:792–804.

Whishaw, I. Q., Schallert, T., and Kolb, B. (1979). The thermal control of immobility in developing infant rats: Is the neocortex involved? *Physiology and Behavior* 23:757–762.

Whishaw, I. Q., Schallert, T., and Kolb, B. (1981b). An analysis of feeding and sensori-motor abilities of rats after decortication. *Journal of Comparative and Physiological Psychology* 95:85–103.

Whishaw, I. Q., and Tomie, J. A. (1989). Food pellet size modifies the motor behavior of foraging rats. *Psychobiology*, in press.

Yeo, A. G., and Oakley, D. A. (1983). Habituation of distraction to a tone in the absence of neocortex in rats. *Behavioural Brain Research* 8:403–409.

IV   Sensory Cortex

11 Sensory Cortex: An Introduction

Richard C. Tees

It is probably safe to say that sensitivity in no animal, with the possible exception of man, has never been investigated as thoroughly as in the rat. The story is, however, not yet complete. Large gaps still exist in our knowledge of certain aspects of sensitivity. . . . There is still much to be done before the precise cortical and subcortical contributions to various senses are disclosed. (Munn 1950)

The popularity of the rat as a species of neuroscientific study, including that which focuses on the sensory cortex, has in fact accelerated since the late 1940s. Overall since 1973 the proportion of studies performed on rodents, particularly the rat, has risen from 46 percent to 70 percent, and the proportion performed on cats has declined from 22 percent to 8 percent (Bowden 1989).

The chapters in part IV outline what is currently known about sensory/perceptual functions and the role played by specific regions of the cortex. Two of the chapters focus on the well-investigated visual system (chapter 13 by Goodale and Carey and chapter 12 by Dean), one each on the somatosensory (chapter 14 by Chapin and Lin), auditory (chapter 15 by Kelly), and gustatory cortex (chapter 16 by Braun). All of the writers examined the question of whether or not the rat is a reasonable model to study "their" specific sensory region of the cortex.

In 1958 Strumwasser reported recording from single neurons in moving rats; since then one of the major strategies used by researchers investigating the sensory cortex has been single neuron recording, and that has been the case for rodents as well as for other mammals. Nevertheless, after almost thirty-five years, the "promise" of the technique still has not been realized. In fact, as the chapters in this part demonstrate, much of the existing knowledge about the role played by the rat's cortex has been derived from lesion/behavioral studies.

Over 150 years since the introduction of phrenology a recurrent theme in neuroscience has been the contrast between the view of neural organization that stresses localization and specificity of function and the alternate view, which stresses widespread representation of functions. Much of the work that has been done in respect of recordings from single neurons seems to reflect this as a "specificity" bias. Proponents often consider an individual neuron to be a feature detector (e.g., Barlow 1972). However, it is clear that in the course of recording from single neurons in any part of the brain, most neurons do increase their firing rate in respect of many behaviors, and most neurons fire relatively rapidly sometimes in most situations. There are many possible reasons for this. The one that seems most plausible is that the brain's functions are extensively distributed (Erickson 1968). Distributed function implies that information is not encoded in the firing of single neurons and can only be "detected" when groups of related neurons are observed. The overall organization and network properties of the brain may vary in the case of different behaviors, and such variation is one aspect of what we examine in the chapters in this part.

As indicated in chapter 1, there is considerable consistency in the absolute number of neurons in a strip of constant width throughout the entire thickness of the cortex in respect of quite distinctive structural and functional areas within the brain of the rat as well as the brain of other animals, including humans (Rockel et al. 1981). The only exception to this similarity is in the case of the binocular part of area 17 of the visual cortex. In a number of primate brains there are approximately 2.5 times as many neurons as there are in the rest of its cortex and the cortex of other nonprimate species.

In any event Kaas (1987) has argued that perceptual competences are based on the coactivation of a number of (5–20) modality-specific cortical fields or modules, with the number of modules differing from species to species. Even the simplest attributes of stimuli (such as color, form, or motion) are unlikely to be based on processing within a single field, and each activated area undoubtedly makes a field-specific contribution to the overall competence. Each of the chapters in this book examines the role played by the cortical maps of specific receptor surfaces associated with processing signals in the different modalities in the rat. The five chapters in this part emphasize sensory and sensory/motor processing that is related to the signals in *one* modality. The nature of the crossmodal processing is looked at directly later in chapter 22. In Kaas's analysis and that of the authors of this part, the nature of the cortical organization of sensory and sensory/motor processing in the adult rat is treated as relatively stable and immutable. Questions related to the plasticity in these and other systems are dealt with in section VI, where, for example, the chapters by Juraska and Tees make clear that cortical organization is significantly influenced by environmental conditions.

Chapter 13 by Goodale and Carey documents the evidence that the corticofugal systems in the rodent are important in the visual control of orienting movements of the head and eyes, the visual control of target-directed locomotion, and barrier avoidance as well as the visual calibration of jumping. Goodale and Carey argue that it is important to view the visual system as a sensorimotor rather than a perceptual system. They also point out remaining gaps in our knowledge and emphasize that much of the important evidence to date is still based on lesion (behavioral) work. There have been very few studies in which electro-physiological recordings have been made while the rat is engaged in different visuomotor behaviors, and that fact in a sense has limited our description of the role played by particular parts of the rat's visual cortical system.

On the other hand Dean emphasizes in chapter 12 the evidence that suggests that different areas of the visual cortex do carry out different perceptual functions. The work Dean outlines indicates not only which perceptual cues are the focus of a particular cortical area, but begins to show what kind of computations a given area carries out in relation to these cues. The visual cortex of the rat appears to exemplify a basic form of mammalian organization in which tectocortical input is more important (relative to the geniculostriate system) than it is in primates. This organization may reflect the rodent's preoccupation with the analysis of external movement and with navigation at the expense of object recognition. Dean argues that the rat cortex may provide a good preparation for studying how "computations" involving both elementary motion perception and ambient vision can be implemented by neuronal (largely control) networks. Dean argues that the rat may offer a significant advantage for studying these problems over any species in which the visual cortex is more highly developed and thus more complex and difficult to understand.

The rat somatosensory cortex has a clarity of organization that makes it ideal for studies of the neural circuitry underlying related cortical functions. Interestingly Chapin and Lin's analysis in chapter 14 of the neuroanatomical and neurophysiological literature tends to support the proposition that typical sensory cortex functions such as feature and movement detection as well as motor/sensory gating are involved, echoing *both* Dean's and Goodale and Carey's analyses of visual cortical functions.

In his examination of the functions of the auditory cortex in chapter 15, Kelly emphasizes the number of anatomical and physiological features the rat's cortex shares with the cortex of other mammals. Kelly also provides a number of examples of differences. For instance, there seems to be little discernible effect of auditory cortical lesions in the rat on a variety of tasks, including localization. There is some reduction in performance on some localization tasks, but the ability itself to localize sound in space is not completely eliminated by such lesions. However, Kelly observes that the rat, as a relatively generalized mammal, provides an excellent basis for establishing broad principles of auditory cortical localization and placing limitations on conclusions drawn from the study of other species, particularly the cat, whose auditory system is probably highly specialized for a carnivorous existence.

Finally, in chapter 16 Braun defines and describes the gustatory cortex in the rat using a multidimensional approach. A difficulty in understanding sensory coding in the taste system, as compared to audition and vision, is the lack of clearly defined biophysical dimensions of the chemicals employed in establishing basic taste qualities. On the other hand, according to Braun, no sensory system lends itself so well to hierarchical analysis as does the gustatory system. Unlike reflexes triggered by qualitatively different auditory or visual stimuli, which are often subtle or which quickly habituate, gustatory reflexes are readily observable and persistent. Braun outlines the evidence that the cortex does not appear to be necessary for most kinds of adaptive, reactive, and regulatory processes that depend to some degree on taste information. Rather rats lacking a sensory cortex appear to lose the "association" salience or memory for tastes. The symptoms of gustatory cortex ablation of rats involves the ability to link gustatory-specific information to novel behavior patterns as well as to remember the previously learned significance of gustatory-specific cues. As does Dean, Braun emphasizes the notion that the brain can be viewed as an assembly of modules or nodes in respect of different kinds of possible sensory perceptual tasks, with some nodes more critical than others for specific tasks. Such a view salvages a localization perspective without requiring the psychologically defined categories of behavior themselves to be localized.

References

Barlow, H. B. (1972). Single units and sensation. A neuron doctrine for perceptual psychology. *Perception* 1:372–394.

Bowden, D. M. (1989). Trends in species studied by neuroscientists, 1973–1988. *Neuroscience Newsletter* 20:4–5.

Erickson, R. P. (1968). Stimulus coding in topographic and nontopographic afferent modalities: On the significance of the activity of individual sensory neurons. *Psychological Review* 75:447–465.

Kaas, J. H. (1987). The organization of neocortex in mammals: Implications for theories of brain function. *Annual Review of Psychology* 38:129–151.

Munn, N. L. (1950). *Handbook of psychological research on the rat: An introduction to animal psychology.* Boston: Houghton Mifflin.

Rockel, A. J., Hiorns, R. W., and Powell, T. P. S. (1981). The basic uniformity in structure of the neocortex. *Brain* 103:221–244.

Strumwasser, F. (1958). Long term recording from single neurons in the brains of unrestructured mammals. *Science* 127:469–470.

12 Sensory Cortex: Visual Perceptual Functions

Paul Dean

The purpose of this chapter is to review what is known about the functions of the rat's cerebral cortex in visual perception. This is an interesting problem not only for what it can tell us about neural function in a very widely used laboratory animal, but also for the light it may throw on principles of visual cortical organization common to all mammals.

The long-term goal of studying the perceptual functions of the cerebral cortex is to specify how cortical neurons cooperate to process and represent visual information. Recent developments suggest that reaching this goal requires computational theories of how such processing and representation can be carried out in principle (e.g., Marr 1982, Arbib and Hanson 1987). However, computational theories of mammalian vision are far from complete, and those that have been formulated appear not to have been used in experiments on rats. A more modest goal is therefore appropriate.

One possibility is suggested by both theoretical and empirical considerations. Simon (1969) and Marr (1982), among others, have argued that it is essential to split complex information-processing tasks into relatively independent subsystems or modules: "If a process is not designed in this way, a small change in one place has consequences in many other places. As a result the process as a whole is extremely difficult to debug or improve, whether by a human designer or in the course of natural evolution, because a small change to improve one part has to be accompanied by many simultaneous compensatory changes elsewhere" (Marr 1982, p. 102). Evidence that naturally evolved visual systems are indeed organized at least partly into modules has come from studies of cerebral cortex in primates (reviewed in, e.g., Maunsell and Newsome 1987, De Yoe and Van Essen 1988) that indicate that there are substantial differences in the extent to which different cortical areas process information about visual features such as binocular disparity, color, and direction of motion.

This chapter is therefore concerned with evidence indicating whether the perceptual functions of visual cortex are also organized in modular fashion in the rat. In particular it asks whether different areas of the visual cortex process different kinds of visual information. This kind of functional anatomy is very much a first step toward specifying the actual tasks that a particular cortical area is carrying out (e.g., De Yoe and Van Essen 1988), but nonetheless one that has to be taken. In other species much of the relevant evidence has been electrophysiological; in rats, however, there have been relatively few electrophysiological studies but many experiments investigating the effects of cortical damage on visually guided behavior. Consequently the bulk of the evidence considered here comes from behavioral experiments.

The following two sections serve as an introduction to the rest of the chapter: Section 12.1 presents a brief account of how the visual cortex is organized. Section 12.2 is concerned with problems of interpretation arising from the behavioral data and how they might be analyzed to yield inferences about perceptual functions.

12.1 Organization of the Visual Cortex in the Rat

Cytoarchitectonics
Since the pioneering work of Lashley (e.g., 1929), lesions of the rat's cortex have typically been related to cytoarchitectonic divisions. The most comprehensive recent cytoarchitectonic map—one moreover published in stereotaxic coordinates—is that of Zilles (1985) based on quantitative criteria (chapter 4 by Zilles). Three main visual areas are distinguished, and these (together with a fourth candidate area) are described briefly below at a level of detail suitable as background to studies using cortical lesions. Further discussion of the various discrepancies that exist between various cytoarchitectonic maps, and between detailed hodological or electrophysiological mapping studies, are given in Wagor et al. 1980, Montero 1981, Espinoza and Thomas 1983, Miller and Vogt 1984, Olavarria and Montero 1984, Sefton and Dreher 1985, Thomas and Espinoza 1987, and chapter 4 by Zilles.

Striate Cortex, Area Oc1
The location of area Oc1, which is also termed primary visual cortex, striate cortex, or area 17, has been established using a variety of anatomical and metabolic techniques (e.g., chapter 4 and Zilles et al. 1984) and corresponds with the results of electrophysiological mapping studies (Montero 1981, Sefton and Dreher 1985). Its lateral part, Oc1B, receives input from both eyes and contains cells responding to stimuli in the central part of the visual field (up to approximately 40° from the vertical meridian), whereas the medial segment Oc1M receives only from the contralateral eye and contains cells that respond to stimuli in the peripheral field. The major source of visual input is the dorsal lateral geniculate nucleus (LGd) of the thalamus (Figure 12.1, Zilles et al. 1984, Sefton and Dreher 1985). A factor likely to affect the organization of the rat visual cortex is that in rats, unlike primates, the LGd receives a

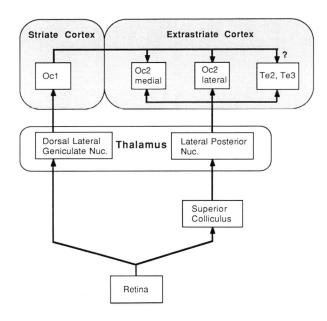

Figure 12.1 Highly schematic diagram of the rat's visual cortex to illustrate its major visual inputs. Efferent projections of extrastriate areas are not shown, nor are subcortical projections of Oc1. Further details are given in the text.

relatively small proportion of retinal input (estimated at 20–50 percent) in comparison with the superior colliculus (at least 90 percent) (Sefton and Dreher 1985). In Oc1 itself, however, the properties of cells show strong resemblances to those of striate cortex cells in the cat and monkey (Burne et al. 1984).

Extrastriate Visual Cortex: Area Oc2L

Immediately adjacent to both the lateral border and part of the rostral border of Oc1 is area Oc2L. The region of Oc2L next to the lateral border of Oc1 corresponds approximately to area 18a or the lateral peristriate cortex; the region of Oc2L situated further rostrally appears to correspond to part of what has been termed posterior parietal cortex or area 7 (e.g., Kolb and Walkey 1987). Oc1 projects to Oc2L, and an important discovery by Montero and colleagues (reviewed in Montero 1981) was that this projection is patchy, suggesting the possibility of multiple visual areas within Oc2L. Subsequent anatomical and electrophysiological studies have confirmed this suggestion, and there are now estimated to be at least four maps in the region of Oc2L immediately adjacent to Oc1 (Olavarria and Montero 1984, Thomas and Espinoza 1987). In addition this region receives afferents from the lateral posterior nucleus of the thalamus, which in turn receives a projection from the superficial retinorecipient layers of the superior colliculus (Montero 1981, Sefton and Dreher 1985). Area Oc2L thus receives visual input from both major output pathways of the retina (figure 12.1). Evidence concerning a further, direct input to Oc2L from LGd is controversial (Montero 1981, Zilles et al. 1984). The projection from the lateral posterior nucleus to Oc2L appears highly organized, in that different electrophysiologically defined maps receive from different parts of the lateral posterior nucleus (Olavarria 1979).

Extrastriate Visual Cortex: Area Oc2M

Part of area Oc2M adjoins the medial border of Oc1 and has also been termed area 18, area 18b, or the medial peristriate cortex. Further rostrally it adjoins the rostromedial boundary of Oc1 and seems to correspond better there with part of the posterior parietal cortex (area 7). Area Oc2M receives a projection from Oc1 and appears to contain at least two visual maps (Olavarria and Montero 1984, Thomas and Espinoza 1987). It also receives a projection from the lateral posterior nucleus (LP), though from a more rostral part than does Oc2L. Parts of rostral LP receive input from area Oc1, not the superior colliculus (Takahashi 1985); it is therefore possible that Oc2M receives a weaker input from the tectothalamic system than does Oc2L (see also Warton et al. 1988, in which the region of the thalamus that projects to Oc2M is called the laterodorsal nucleus).

Extrastriate Visual Cortex: Areas Te2 and Te3

There is some suggestion that the lateral posterior nucleus projects to cortical areas outside Oc2. One of these, sometimes termed area 20 (H. C. Hughes 1977, Schober 1981), appears to correspond to part of Te3 and may also receive terminals from the anterior commissure, a fiber bundle that in primates connects visual areas in the temporal lobe (Horel and Steltzner 1981). A second area to which LP projects has been described as area 36 (Coleman and Clerici 1980, Mason and Groos 1981) and appears to receive a heavier projection from the caudal, tectorecipient zone of LP than does the part of Oc2L that adjoins Oc1 (Montero 1981). Moreover, anatomical and electrophysiological techniques have identified further visual maps lateral to those in Oc2L that immediately adjoin Oc1 (Montero 1981, Olavarria and Montero 1984, Thomas and Espinoza 1987). However, whether these additional areas are located in lateral Oc2L or in, for example, Te2 is at present unclear.

Conclusions

Although there are disagreements about the precise number and locations of separate visual areas, it is clear that the rat's visual cortex is far from homogeneous, but, as in other species, contains a number of representations of visual space. The purpose of this chapter is to review evidence bearing on the issue of whether different areas of the visual cortex are performing different visual tasks. The existence of separate visual representations provides an anatomical substrate that could support such a modular organization.

12.2 Behavioral Data: Problems of Interpretation

The problems of interpreting the results of experiments using lesions to alter behavior are well known, not to say notorious. However, provided that appropriate precautions are taken, this kind of experiment can be extremely useful for beginning to specify what kind of task a given region of the brain is carrying out (for further discussion, see, e.g., Dean 1982). In the particular case of the rat's visual cortex, two precautions are especially important:

1. Care is needed in identifying which particular cortical areas have been damaged by a given lesion. This is a particular problem in rats because their visual cortex is smooth, offering none of the convenient sulcal landmarks available in cat and primate. In the absence of electrophysiological mapping it is impossible to be sure that an intended ablation of, for example, Oc1 neither spares part of Oc1 nor damages adjacent Oc2. This need not pose so great a problem for interpretation if the subsequent histological investigation of the lesion is adequate, including, for example, a cytoarchitectonic identification of spared tissue or an analysis of retrograde degeneration in the thalamus. However, these techniques are time consuming, and in any case relatively few experiments have been directly concerned with the issue of functional subdivisions in visual cortex. Thus there are a number of studies in which it is difficult to be sure whether particular cortical areas have been damaged or spared, with corresponding limitations on the inferences that can be drawn from their results.

2. Care is also needed in specifying which cues can be used to perform any given visual task. In many of the tasks used to test vision in rats, the animal is allowed (or indeed required) to move relative to the stimuli. Such movements include walking or running toward the stimuli, and scanning movements of the head (or eyes), which in some kinds of apparatus can take place as close to a stimulus as the animal chooses. These procedures, which stand in very sharp contrast to those used in human visual psychophysics, pose two major problems for the interpretation of any effects of cortical damage:

(a) What appears to be an impairment of perceptual capability—that is, whether an animal can tell two stimuli apart—may in fact be an impairment of visuomotor control or of some nonvisual process altogether (see, e.g., Christie and Russell 1985). One way to avoid this kind of false positive is to find out whether an impairment persists over alterations in the required response.

(b) Movement relative to the stimulus may create unintended visual cues, especially when the rat is allowed to come close to a stimulus and when the stimuli are about the same size as the rat, as they often are. In these circumstances there are potential optic flow, local movement, and possibly gross luminance cues available, as well as whatever stimulus features the experimenter introduces deliberately. A severe impairment in the capacity to process one of these cues may be masked by normal performance using the others. This kind of false negative may be avoided by more precise control over the animal's movements, for example, by preventing locomotion.

Taking these two constraints together, it becomes apparent that the most informative studies of rat perceptual function and cortical organization have been those of investigating "pattern" or "detail" vision, which appears in practice to mean the analysis of stationary spatial contrast in the central part of the visual field. It is these studies that have most often used restricted as opposed to very large cortical lesions and that have made some attempts to identify the stimuli controlling behavior. Accordingly these experiments are analyzed in the next section.

The results of that analysis are then used to try to interpret studies with more ambiguous results, for example, those using movement or "spatial" cues (section 12.4). In each case an attempt is made first to determine which cue other than stationary spatial contrast in the central field is likely to be guiding behavior. Then an attempt is made to assess the importance of striate and where possible different extrastriate visual areas in processing that cue. To make the text easier to follow, the impairments discussed in both sections 12.3 and 12.4 are shown schematically in table 12.1.

Section 12.5 then summarizes the results of the analyses in sections 12.3 and 12.4 and considers their significance for our understanding of whether the rat's visual cortex is organized in modular fashion. Finally, section 12.6 asks how the rat's visual cortex compares with that of other species and what that comparison can tell us about the evolution of visual cortical function.

12.3 Stationary Spatial Contrast

Performance of Normal Rats

Ever since the seminal work of Lashley over fifty years ago (e.g., Lashley 1931), one of the most popular tests of rat vision has been the two-choice "pattern" or "detail" discrimination. In this task the animal is required to discriminate between a pair of two-dimensional black-and-white patterns, usually by running or jumping toward one of them. The patterns are typically equated for mean reflectance, in the hope that they can be discriminated only by analysis of spatial contrast cues. Although square-wave gratings of differing orientation are often used, using horizontal *versus* vertical, or oblique 45° clockwise from vertical *versus* oblique 45° counterclockwise from vertical, the rat's discriminative powers are not confined to orientation. They can discriminate a wide range of figures, and indeed "one must be impressed by the similarity of the rat's discriminative behaviour to the perceptual impressions of the human observer. If a series of patterns is ranked in order of the

Table 12.1 Summary of Major Findings Discussed in Sections 12.3 and 12.4

Task	Probable Cue	Oc1	SC	"Posterior Cortex"	Decorticate	Other	
Pattern discrimination (12.3)	Stationary spatial contrast, central vision	+	0	+++	≥+++	Oc2L Oc2M Post/ Parietal Temporal	+++ ?0
Orienting (12.4)	External movement	—	++	+	?+++	Posterior cortex + Posterior parietal	?++
Locating large visual targets (12.4)	Stationary spatial contrast (central vision) + Self-produced movement	—	?+	?++	+++	—	
Navigating to invisible target (12.4)	Peripheral vision	—	+++	?++++	++++	Oc2L Posterior parietal Temporal	?0 +++ +

The four tasks are shown together with the section number of the text in which they are discussed. The *probable* cue used to solve each task is shown in the second column; as the text indicates, the uncertainty involved varies from task to task. Subsequent columns indicate the effects of lesions, measured on the following crude scale:

0   minimal or no impairment
+   clear loss
++   striking loss
+++   retraining with great difficulty
++++   total, irrecoverable loss

A dash indicates that no information is available. SC = superior colliculus. (Cortical areas as described in text.)

conspicuousness of the figures for the human eye, that order will have a high predictive value for the rate at which the rat can learn the figures. Stimuli to which the rat transfers in equivalence tests are obviously similar for man" (Lashley 1938, p. 181).

Similarities and differences between the visual capacities of rats and primates are considered further in section 12.6. Here it may be noted that although their capacity to discriminate patterns may resemble ours, their visual acuity (approximately 1 cycle/degree) is about fifty times worse (e.g., Lashley 1930, Dean 1978), and that "much of the behaviour of the rat with the jumping apparatus suggests that the figure is not a symbol indicating the correct card but is an object upon which he jumps" (Lashley 1938, p. 171).

One further feature of the rat's performance is relevant here. As mentioned in section 12.2, rats usually make head movements in discrimination learning tasks, often appearing to look directly at each stimulus in turn. This is an example of what has been rather curiously termed "vicarious trial and error" responding (for review, see, e.g., Goss and Wischner 1956), and its probable effect is to bring the image of each stimulus onto the temporal retina, which contains the area centralis and corresponds to the region of binocular overlap (e.g., Lashley 1932, Sefton and Dreher 1985). It is likely therefore that pattern discrimination learning primarily tests vision in the central part of the visual field.

Importance of Visual Cortex
It is well established that pattern discrimination learning in rats is very severely impaired by large lesions of visual cortex (for references, see, e.g., Spear and Barbas 1975, Dean 1981b). These lesions, often termed posterior cortical lesions because of their size, typically damage all of Oc1, much of Oc2L and Oc2M, and variable amounts of surrounding areas. Sparing is most likely to occur rostrally (rostral Oc2M and Oc2L, also called posterior parietal cortex) and laterally (Te2 and Te3, part of the temporal cortex). The observation that after such lesions rats usually fail completely to relearn even the simplest pattern discrimination raises the possibility of a basic perceptual deficit. This has been tested with a grating detection task in which rats were trained to stop sucking a tube when the stimulus back-projected onto a screen in front of them changed from a uniform field to a high contrast square-wave grating of the same mean luminance (Dean 1978). The problems of extraneous cues and visuomotor strategies associated with locomotion and head scanning (see section 12.2) were thus avoided. Nonetheless, after posterior cortical lesions of the kind described above, highly overtrained animals ceased to detect gratings of even low spatial frequency (0.045 cycle/degree).

Subsequent retraining was only successful in three out of four animals, took much longer than original training, and was unable to overcome what was an apparently permanent deficit in acuity (reduced to about 0.3 cycle/degree from a preoperative value of 1.0 cycle/degree). These results suggest that the integrity of the visual cortex is essential for normal detection of stationary spatial contrast (at least in the central part of the visual field where the stimuli were presented) and hence for normal form or pattern perception.

Which areas of the visual cortex are needed for this kind of vision? The following sections consider first Oc1 or striate cortex, then Oc2L or lateral peristriate cortex, and third, the remaining extrastriate areas. Finally, the implications of the evidence for the existence of multiple cortical systems in the analysis of stationary spatial contrast are summarized.

Role of the Striate Cortex, Area Oc1

As outlined in section 12.1, visual cortex receives visual input from two major sources (see figure 12.1). One is the dorsal lateral geniculate nucleus of the thalamus (LGd), which projects mainly or solely to area Oc1. The second is the superior colliculus via the lateral posterior nucleus of the thalamus to area Oc2L, and possibly also areas Oc2M, Te2, and Te3. The first question, then, concerning the role of area Oc1 is, How important is its geniculate input for the detection and hence analysis of stationary spatial contrast?

Rats with large midbrain lesions that in some cases completely destroyed the superior colliculus were only very transiently impaired on the grating detection task that produced massive impairments in animals with posterior cortical lesions (see "Performance of Normal Rats" in section 12.3). Their subsequent performance and acuity were normal (Dean 1978). Normal acuity after collicular lesions in adult rats has also been found by Cowey, Henken, and Perry (1982) and Legg and Turkish (1983). Legg and Turkish (1983) also measured spatial contrast sensitivity at a range of lower spatial frequencies and again found no collicular deficit. These results suggest that the geniculostriate input to area Oc1 carries sufficient information for normal detection of stationary spatial contrast, a conclusion consistent with numerous observations that conventional pattern discrimination tasks are unaffected by collicular damage (see references in Dean and Pope 1981).

However, these data do not indicate whether an intact geniculostriate projection is *necessary* for contrast detection, i.e., they do not indicate whether information about contrast is also conveyed by the tectocortical projection. One way of trying to answer this question is to look at the effects of lesions confined to the geniculostriate projection, for example lesions of cortical area Oc1. Such lesions have been found to have little effect on the detection of large, high-contrast, low-frequency gratings (Dean 1981a), quite unlike the very severe disruption produced by larger posterior cortical lesions that also damage surrounding extrastriate areas. Acuity is also reduced less by striate lesions (postoperative mean

0.7 cycle/degree) than by the larger lesions (0.3 cycle/degree for those animals that could be retrained). It is unlikely that these differences result from spared geniculocortical projections because lesions of the superior colliculus, which in otherwise intact animals have little effect, produce massive impairments in animals previously given lesions of Oc1 (Dean 1981a).

It therefore appears that information concerning stationary spatial contrast is conveyed to the rat's visual cortex by both the geniculostriate and tectocortical projections. This would be consistent with results obtained using pattern discriminations. In a seminal paper H. C. Hughes (1977) showed that lesions of Oc1 had much slighter effects on learning to discriminate oblique gratings than posterior cortical lesions that included both Oc1 and Oc2. Lesions of the lateral posterior nucleus, the thalamic relay of the tectocortical projection, had no effect by themselves, but worsened the Oc1 deficit. Subsequently McDaniel and Noble (1984) showed that animals with large Oc1 lesions could learn obliques; also, Goldstein and Oakley (1987) found that animals with lesions wholly or mainly within Oc1 learned a horizontal-vertical discrimination much faster than animals with larger removals.

Thus the answer to the original question concerning input is that both the geniculostriate and the tectocortical pathways carrying information about stationary spatial contrast. There is some suggestion that only the geniculostriate pathway carries information about spatial frequencies greater than 0.7 cycle/degree, because striate lesions reduced acuity to that value. Similarly McDaniel and Braucht (1984) found that animals with lesions of Oc1 were unable to discriminate upright from inverted triangles using small (4-cm) triangles, an effect that might well reflect impaired acuity. However, because of the difficulty of making precise lesions of Oc1 in the rat's smooth cortex (see section 12.1), there is always the possibility that any acuity loss arises from the invasion of extrastriate areas, thus damaging both sources of input. Perhaps the issue could be resolved by electrophysiological methods.

Role of the Lateral Peristriate Cortex, Area Oc2L
The next major question concerns which extrastriate areas handle information about stationary spatial contrast. There is strong evidence that area Oc2L, lateral peristriate cortex, is involved. In a series of studies McDaniel and coworkers have shown that lesions of Oc2L that produce little or no retrograde degeneration in the LGd severely impair or abolish the ability to discriminate oblique gratings or triangles of differing orientation (McDaniel et al. 1979, 1982, McDaniel and Braucht 1984, McDaniel and Noble 1984, McDaniel 1985, Lindsay and McDaniel 1987). Similar lesions have been found to produce more severe effects on grating detection than lesions of Oc1 (Dean 1981b): Animals with lateral peristriate lesions required longer to relearn to detect coarse

gratings, and in four out of six, their subsequently tested acuity was worse than the 0.7 cycle/degree produced by lesions of Oc1.

In contrast, damage to other areas of the extrastriate cortex have so far proved to have at worst slight effects on pattern discrimination learning (temporal lesions, damaging parts of areas Te2 and Te3, McDaniel et al. 1979 and Meyer at al. 1986; posterior parietal or medial lesions, damaging Oc2M, McDaniel and Terrell Wall 1988). It is possible that the most important part of Oc2L for analysis of stationary spatial contrast in central vision is the region immediately adjacent to the lateral border of Oc1. McDaniel and colleagues (1982) found that lesions of Oc1 that only slightly invaded adjacent Oc2L prevented relearning of an oblique-stripes discrimination. The number of errors the animals made correlated with the extent of the invasion of Oc2L. This would be consistent with the relative lack of effect of temporal lesions that invade only the lateral part of Oc2L and posterior parietal lesions that invade its rostral part (McDaniel et al. 1979, Meyer et al. 1986, McDaniel and Terrell Wall 1988).

These results suggest a critical role for area Oc2L in the processing of information about stationary spatial contrast in the central field. This in turn is consistent with area Oc2L receiving projections from both Oc1 and the lateral posterior nucleus of the thalamus, which together carry visual information relayed from both of the two major retinorecipient areas, the superior colliculus and the LGd.

Remaining Areas
Although removal of both Oc1 and Oc2L together have extremely severe effects on pattern discrimination, there are clear demonstrations that in some circumstances relearning can occur (e.g., Cowey and Weiskrantz 1971, Mize et al. 1971, Spear and Barbas 1975, Guic-Robles et al. 1982). Self-induced movement cues may sometimes be important for this relearning (Lavond et al. 1978), but it seems that they cannot always be necessary because the ability to detect gratings in the absence of such cues is eventually reacquired after posterior cortical lesions, though final performance is still very poor (see "Importance of Visual Cortex" in section 12.3).

At present it is not clear which parts of the brain mediate this residual ability. They could be entirely subcortical, though so far demonstrations of spatial vision in decorticate animals have been in circumstances where the animals either made conspicuous head movements to search for a single large target (Whishaw and Kolb 1984) or approached to within 2.5 cm of the stimuli (Goldstein and Oakley 1987), suggesting the use of cues other than stationary spatial contrast (section 12.2). Alternatively it has been suggested that areas in the temporal cortex (Te2 or Te3) that receive a projection from the lateral posterior nucleus and are often partly spared by posterior cortical lesions might be responsible for the residual contrast detection (e.g., Dean 1981b, Guic-Robles et al. 1982).

Conclusions

It appears from the evidence reviewed that the main system for detection and analysis of stationary spatial contrast comprises the pathway from retina to area Oc1 via the dorsal lateral geniculate nucleus and the projection from Oc1 to the laterally adjacent portion of Oc2L (see figure 12.1, table 12.1). The importance of the geniculostriate system for pattern or detail vision in rats was recognized by Lashley (e.g., Lashley 1931 and other references) and is consistent with the relatively large part of area Oc1 devoted to central or binocular vision (Zilles et al. 1984; for further references see, e.g., Dean Redgrave 1984b, Sefton and Dreher 1985).

In addition there appears to be a secondary system that relays spatial contrast information to Oc2L from the superior colliculus via the lateral posterior nucleus. We cannot be certain of its capacity, but there are some hints that it may not carry information about small stimuli, or spatial frequencies above 0.7 cycle/degree. It is, however, clear that for information below that spatial frequency, the secondary system can be switched in very rapidly. This conclusion is consistent with the electrophysiological data of Olavarria and Torrealba (1978) who were able to record responses to spots of light or shadows from units in Oc2L half an hour after large lesions of Oc1. It is not consistent with Lashley's belief that *only* the striate cortex is involved in pattern vision (e.g., Lashley 1931, 1939, 1942), but subsequent reanalyses of Lashley's data suggest that when the lesions are plotted more accurately (cf. section 12.2), it becomes clear that the critical region extends into the lateral peristriate area (Doty 1961, Snyder 1973).

Finally, there is a third system that can be used when both Oc1 and Oc2L are destroyed. This system does not switch in at all quickly, but rather requires (for unknown reasons) extensive training. It responds only to coarse spatial frequencies (less than 0.3 cycle/degree), and the cortical areas (if any) that comprise it are unknown.

12.4   Other Visual Features: Tasks Little Affected by Removal of Oc1 and/or Oc2L

As mentioned previously (section 12.2), it is more difficult to draw inferences concerning cortical mechanisms for analysis of features other than stationary spatial contrast. This is partly because there has been much less systematic study of such features, and partly because in the experiments that have been carried out, it is often unclear which of the multiple cues available is controlling the animal's response.

However, as a result of our understanding of the cortical systems involved in processing stationary spatial contrast, it is possible to make some progress by identifying those visual tasks in which a *different* cue is used. The assumption is that any task that can be performed without extensive training after removal of Oc1 and/or Oc2L can therefore be solved without reliance on the detection of stationary spatial contrast in the central field. The following subsections deal with some of the more common tasks that meet this criterion:

· Response to transient (suddenly appearing or moving) stimuli
· Approaching large (usually black or white) targets
· Navigating by distant spatial cues

In each case the relevant evidence is analyzed to try to answer (1) which cues are used, other than stationary spatial contrast in the visual field; (2) what is the role of the geniculostriate system in analyzing these cues; and (3) what is the role of the tectocortical systems. For reasons mentioned previously, current evidence often does not allow these questions to be answered satisfactorily. Nonetheless the importance to rats of each of the three tasks listed above (cf. section 12.6) suggests that simply defining our areas of ignorance would represent a useful step toward eventual understanding of the visual functions of the rat's cortex.

Detection of Transient Stimuli

Normal Behavior

It is easy to obtain responses to moving or suddenly appearing stimuli in laboratory rats—often too easy from the point of view of the experimenter, because an unintended movement on their part may totally disrupt the rat's performance of the task of interest. Apart from interruption of current behavior, the rat's responses to transient stimuli include orienting movements of the head, pursuit, freezing, and flight. These responses have also been observed in wild rats (e.g., Ewer 1971, Blanchard et al. 1986), and indeed it seems that transient visual stimuli are extremely important triggers of both predatory and defensive behavior in natural circumstances.

Of considerable interest for understanding how these stimuli are analyzed is the possible existence of "rules" for deciding which response is appropriate (Dean and Redgrave 1984c). For example, it appears that in some circumstances the position of the stimulus may be important, with upper-field stimuli being more likely to elicit avoidance, and lower-field stimuli, pursuit (Sahibzada et al. 1986; cf. Ingle 1982). Patterns or speed of movement may also be used: In hamsters (a rodent whose visual system seems very similar to the rat's) a "looming" stimulus elicits avoidance, whereas in *Rattus rattus* the fluttering of moths or dragonflies provokes immediate pursuit and consumption even in rats who have never seen them before (Ewer 1971). Analysis of movement is also used by gerbils (another rodent with a visual system probably similar to the rat's) to predict the future location of stimuli and so to intercept them accurately (Ingle 1982).

Role of the Striate Cortex, Area Oc1

Two main observations suggest that the geniculostriate system plays a restricted role in the processing of information about transient stimuli. First, removal of the superior colliculus severely disrupts orienting responses to such stimuli; second, posterior cortical lesions that destroy area Oc1 and surrounding cortex do not. These observations were made originally by Schneider (e.g., Schneider 1969) in hamsters, but subsequent studies have shown that rats behave very similarly (e.g., Goodale and Murison 1975, Goodale et al. 1978, Midgley and Tees 1981, Midgley et al. 1988). Hamsters with lesions of visual cortex but no collicular damage also avoid looming stimuli (Schneider et al. 1987); it is not known if this is the case for rats.

The precise nature of the deficit following lesions of the superior colliculus has been the subject of some dispute (for review, see Dean and Redgrave 1984a). However, recent studies in which the position of the animal's head was controlled and extensive training was given indicate that rats with collicular damage have difficulty detecting the onset of large bright lights in the far periphery (greater than 80° from midline) and small dim lights more centrally (Overton et al. 1985, Overton and Dean 1988). These observations are consistent with much other evidence in rodents (Goodale and Milner 1982, Ingle 1982, Dean and Redgrave 1984a, Mlinar and Goodale 1984) that the superior colliculus receives more information about the peripheral field than does the geniculostriate projection and that this difference becomes more marked the further peripherally you go.

Does the geniculostriate system play any role in the analysis of transients? It seems a plausible candidate for the system that mediates detection of transients in the absence of the superior colliculus, and in gerbils it has been shown that lesions of the striate cortex after previous destruction of the superior colliculus abolish detection of transients anywhere in the visual field (Mlinar and Goodale 1984, cf. Ingle 1982). However, its importance in the intact animal is unclear because experiments investigating response to transient stimuli after lesions of Oc1 have either reported no effect (Overton et al. 1985) or have damaged surrounding areas (see next subsection).

The Role of Extrastriate Cortex

The above evidence indicates that pathways besides the geniculostriate projection carry information about transient stimuli and indeed carry information about small stimuli and stimuli in the far periphery that is not conveyed by the geniculostriate projection. Given the effects of lesions of the superior colliculus, either alone or in combination with striate lesions, it seems likely that these extrastriate pathways originate in the superior colliculus. The question is whether they are entirely subcortical or whether the important projection is from superior colliculus to extrastriate cortex via the lateral posterior nucleus. The following evidence is relevant:

1. Although posterior cortical lesions do not affect responding to all transient stimuli, there is some suggestion that they may have more subtle effects. Rats' sensitivity to small dim light flashes may be reduced by rather small lesions that spare most of Oc2L (Overton and Dean 1988). In gerbils somewhat larger lesions affect accuracy of response to moving stimuli, as if the direction and velocity of movement were ignored (Ingle 1982).

2. Standard lesions of posterior cortex often spare parts of both temporal cortex (Te2, Te3) and posterior parietal cortex (rostral Oc2L and Oc2M) that probably receive projections from the lateral posterior nucleus. Midgley and Tees (1981) report that responsiveness to patterns of light flashes is reduced if the lesions are extended rostrally to include posterior parietal cortex. Overton (1986) similarly found that two animals with lesions of Oc1 that additionally destroyed all of rostral Oc2L and Oc2M had difficulty detecting light onset both peripherally and more centrally. These observations may be related to the finding of Scheff and Wright (1977) that flash-evoked potentials could still be recorded in the parietal region after large posterior cortical removals.

3. Remarks about the behavior of decorticate rats suggest that some form of response to transients can be mediated entirely by subcortical pathways (e.g., Vanderwolf et al. 1978, Whishaw and Kolb 1984). However, no systematic studies appear to have been undertaken.

These data suggest that (1) parts of the tectocortical pathway probably are important for processing information about suddenly appearing or moving stimuli, and (2), more speculatively, rostral Oc2L and Oc2M (the posterior parietal cortex) might be a critical region of the extrastriate cortex dealing with information about transient stimuli from both striate cortex and the superior colliculus. However, the lack of appropriate psychophysical studies prevents any precise understanding of the role of different cortical areas in the analysis of movement.

Approach to Large Targets

Normal Behavior

The ability of rats to navigate accurately toward visible targets that differ in luminance from their background has been investigated in runways (e.g., with black versus white discriminations), jumping stands, and swimming pools. Usually the direction of the target is the variable of interest, but the jumping stand has been exploited to study the perception of distance as well. One curious feature of the rat's performance in these tasks is that, despite a visual acuity of about 1 cycle/degree, prolonged training may be required for targets smaller than about 6° to 8° across (references in Dean 1981c). This may relate to the rat's use of such targets in natural surroundings as escape routes: If the target is in fact a hole, it must be big enough for the rat to get through.

As mentioned in section 12.2, there may be up to four separate cues available to the animal in this kind of task: (1) stationary spatial contrast, (2) movement of the image across the retina resulting from head or eye movements, (3) movement of the image across the retina resulting from approaching the stimuli, and (4) whole-field luminance. This last cue appears not to be much used by normal rats, but can be used by animals with extensive cortical damage; in fact whole field luminance appears to be processed mainly subcortically (e.g., Bauer and Cooper 1964, Cooper et al. 1972, Miller and Cooper 1974, Meyer and Meyer 1977; see also Bloch-Rojas et al. 1964, Horel 1968, Kolb and Whishaw 1981, Goetsch and Isaac 1983, Gray and LeVere 1980). Accordingly, from the viewpoint of understanding cortical function, it is versions of the target-approach task in which whole-field luminance cannot be used that are of interest. These are usually versions in which the animal must make its choice at some distance from the stimuli.

Behavior of Animals with Posterior Cortical Lesions
A number of studies indicate that even when required to choose a large target at some distance from them, rats with large lesions of Oc1 and Oc2L are still much less impaired than on pattern discrimination learning. In the jumping stand, rats with large lesions to Oc1 and Oc2L that failed all tests for pattern discrimination could still learn a black-white discrimination and show signs of depth discrimination when jumping to a single target (Lashley 1931). Accurate jumping to a light source after posterior cortical lesions has also been reported by Ferrier and Cooper (1976). In a conventional discrimination box, Birch and colleagues (1978) required rats to choose while at least 10 cm away from the stimuli. Subsequent tests suggested strongly that this procedure prevented the use of whole-field luminance cues. Nonetheless animals with posterior neocortical lesions learned a black-white discrimination as rapidly as did normal animals.

It is unlikely that the animals were using stationary spatial contrast to perform these tasks. Animals with similar lesions require very extensive retraining to detect 0.045 cycle/degree grating subtending about 90° (see "Performance of Normal Rats" in section 12.3), and attempts to speed relearning by substituting a 0.026-cycle/degree grating (each bar subtending 20°) or a single dark bar subtending 38° were not successful (Dean 1978). The sizes of the stimuli producing rapid learning in the black-white discriminations were in the range of 20° to 50°.

A more plausible cue is movement of the image across the retina produced by either moving toward the stimulus, where this is possible, or by head scanning. As mentioned previously, rats often do make head movements, as if looking at the stimuli, when solving visual discriminations in conventional testing situations (e.g., Goss and Wischner 1956, Steele Russell et al. 1979). One likely effect of these head movements is to move the retinal image of a stimulus into the central visual field. The use of self-produced movement cues to separate figure from ground is a primitive competence, observed, for example, in flies (Horridge 1987). The arguments that rats with posterior cortical lesions can use self-produced movement cues to approach large targets accurately are

1. The task that produced very severe deficits of large targets after posterior cortical damage was the one in which scanning head movements did not occur (because the animals were sucking a tube when the stimuli were presented).

2. Ability to detect externally produced movement has been demonstrated to survive posterior cortical ablation (see introduction to section 12.4).

3. Use of self-produced movement cues by animals with lesions of posterior cortex have been invoked to explain the otherwise curious fact that in some circumstances they can relearn to discriminate horizontal from vertical gratings, but not between oblique gratings (Lavond et al. 1978).

4. Braun and colleagues (1970) trained rats to approach one stimulus door through which a deep compartment lined with checkered paper was visible and to avoid another door showing a two-dimensional drawing of the same scene. The former but not the latter stimulus would afford motion parallax cues. Rats with posterior cortical lesions learned the discrimination, though they showed no signs of learning a horizontal-vertical discrimination.

In summary there is reasonable evidence that rats with large posterior cortical lesions are soon able to detect external movement after operation, but require extensive retraining to use stationary cues in central vision. This suggests that their ability to relearn rapidly black-white discriminations, for example, depends on the use of self-produced movement cues in the central field.

Role of the Striate Cortex, Area Oc1
Unravelling the contributions of different parts of the visual system to the processing of self-produced motion cues is particularly difficult because of the inevitable presence of stationary cues. An impairment might be concealed by judicious switching from one cue to another. This is probably one reason why studies of the effects of lesions of the superior colliculus on the approach to large targets have in the past produced a wide variety of results (e.g., Lashley 1937, Schneider 1969, Goodale and Murison 1975, Dean and Key 1981, Dean and Pope 1981),

though in these cases there were additional sources of variance: In some studies the lesions invaded surrounding structures and/or impaired the production of head movements.

More recently Ellard and associates (1984, 1986) have studied the ability of gerbils to jump to targets of differing distance. This ability was impaired after collicular damage, even though head movements increased in frequency. In conjunction with the evidence that collicular damage in a number of rodents has little effect on the processing of stationary spatial contrast in the central field ("Importance of Visual Cortex," section 12.3), this result raises the possibility that the geniculostriate system in rodents may not carry sufficient information for the normal analysis of self-produced movement cues. This would be consistent with data concerning the detection of externally produced transients ("Detection of Transient Stimuli," section 12.4) and speculations that the superior colliculus plays an important role in "ambient" vision (e.g., Trevarthen 1968; see section 12.6). However, alternative explanations of a collicular deficit in depth perception, such as an effect via disturbed vergence movements of the eyes (Lawler and Cowey 1986), need to be explored.

Whether area Ocl carries any information necessary for analysis of self-induced motion is unclear. Studies of the effects of lesions confined to Ocl on the use of these cues have not yet been carried out.

Role of Extrastriate Areas
Although it has been argued that rats with posterior neocortical lesions can use self-produced motion cues, it does not follow that they are completely unimpaired. Ellard and colleagues (1986) have reported that in gerbils lesions of striate cortex with some invasion of surrounding peristriate areas affect judgment of distance in a way difficult to explain solely by the inability to use stationary cues. If so, then there are grounds for suspecting that the tectocortical projection may play a part in the analysis of self-produced motion cues.

To what extent remnants of this projection also mediate the residual abilities still found after lesions of Ocl and Oc2L remains to be determined. It is possible that some of these can be mediated subcortically. Whishaw and Kolb (1984) report that, although very impaired, decorticate rats eventually learn to swim accurately toward a black platform visible in a tank of white liquid. When placed in the tank, they "made head movements characteristic of search behavior and then swam directly to the platform" (p. 133).

Navigation by Distant Visual Cues

Normal Behavior
Early observers of the rat's visually guided behavior were impressed by their reliance on distant visual cues, even when much closer cues were

available (e.g., Hebb 1938, Lashley 1938). Hebb required rats to find food behind one of four barriers placed on a table. The correct barrier was large and white, with the smaller incorrect barriers and the surface of the table painted black. After the task had been learned, the table was rotated so that a black barrier occupied the previous position of the white one. The rats continued to visit the same place, apparently uninfluenced by a local cue that seemed extremely conspicuous to the experimenter.

The general issue of place-learning in rats has once more become a focus of experimental interest, primarily because of the possible involvement of the hippocampus in the construction of spatial maps (for references, see, e.g., Foreman and Stevens 1987). Two main types of apparatus have been used: the radial maze, in which food is concealed at the end of each arm (e.g., Olton and Samuelson 1976), and the water maze, in which a platform is concealed beneath the surface of an opaque liquid (Morris 1981). The targets in these tasks are invisible, and it has been demonstrated unequivocally that rats can use distant visual cues to remember their locations (e.g., Suzuki et al. 1980, Morris 1984).

It is not clear, however, how these distant cues are processed. They might be fixated sequentially or processed in peripheral vision as either stationary or self-produced movement cues. Lines and Milner (1985) have provided some evidence that peripheral vision (presumably in the upper field) may be important in the water maze, in that rats appear to acquire information about the distant visual cues when they are swimming rather than when they are making exploratory head movements after reaching the platform.

Role of the Striate Cortex, Area Oc1
A number of studies have indicated that lesions of the superior colliculus impair learning in both the radial maze and the water maze (Dean and Key 1981, Foreman and Stevens 1982, Milner and Lines 1983, Lines and Milner 1985). Lines and Milner (1985) found that even after extensive training rats with such lesions showed no improvement in the accuracy of their initial heading in the water maze and suggested that the improvement in speed that they show in finding the target "must be attributable to nonspecific factors such as more systematic search strategies, rather than any real spatial awareness" (p. 714). They also found that allowing normal rats 1 or 60 seconds on the platform did not significantly affect performance, suggesting that the disruption of orienting movements caused by collicular lesions to such movements was irrelevant to the deficit. As mentioned above, it seems rather that normal animals process information about distant cues while they are swimming.

These results suggest that the geniculostriate system does not carry information adequate for learning to use distant visual cues. If these cues are indeed processed via peripheral vision, this would be consistent with the demonstration that collicular lesions severely impair detection of light onset in the periphery ("Detection of Transient Stimuli," section 12.4). Lines and Milner (1985) argue that a "peripheral scotoma seems a most unlikely explanation" (of their results), because their animals with lesions of the superior colliculus showed evidence of light detection in their lateral visual fields. However, perimetric studies indicate that the deficit produced by collicular destruction is very severe in the far periphery (at 120° even large bright stimuli are not detected) and less so more centrally (at 40° only small dim stimuli are not detected) ("Detection of Transient Stimuli," section 12.4). Thus the collicular deficit is better described as a peripheral amblyopia, which might well allow the detection of sudden flashing lights but not of the cues needed for the water maze (which in Lines and Milner's study comprised such items as curtains, two doors, a window, and a metal cupboard).

The effects of lesions confined to area Oc1 appear not to have been tested on radial or water mazes; the "striate" ablations of McDaniel and Brown (1984) extensively damaged Oc2M. It is therefore not known whether the geniculostriate system carries any information essential for their performance. However, both behavioral and electrophysiological evidence suggests that in rodents striate cortex plays a lesser role in peripheral vision than the superior colliculus ("Approach to Large Targets," section 12.4; Dean and Redgrave 1984b).

Role of Extrastriate Areas
The above evidence suggests that the superior colliculus plays an important part in processing distant visual cues, but does not indicate whether cortical (via the lateral posterior nucleus) or subcortical projections from the colliculus are involved. Two pieces of evidence suggest that it is the cortical projections that matter. First, subcortical systems alone seem to be incapable of mediating performance on the water bath: Whishaw and Kolb (1984) found no evidence of learning whatever in decorticate rats, and indeed they suggest that the use of distant spatial cues in general is a major component of cortical function. Second, posterior cortical lesions that include targets of the tectocortical system impair learning on the radial maze (Goodale and Dale 1981, Foreman and Stevens 1982) and indeed produce similar impairments when combined with eye removal, suggesting that visual pathways surviving the cortical lesions are not useful in this task.

Further experiments provide clues to which parts of this pathway are important:

1. Lesions of Oc2L similar to those that severely impair pattern discrimination do not affect retention of the radial maze task (McDaniel and Brown 1984).

2. Radial maze performance is affected by lesions of Oc1 that also invade Oc2M (McDaniel and Brown 1984). Similarly, posterior parietal

lesions that damage rostral Oc2L and Oc2M impair learning of both the radial maze and the water maze (Kolb and Walkey 1987). In the water maze, rats with posterior parietal lesions fail to achieve normal performance even after extensive practice, making persistent errors in heading angle (compare the effects of collicular lesions—see previous subsection). They are also unable to learn to find the platform when its position, varying from trial to trial, is advertised by a large black rectangle hung on the wall of the tank behind it—a different kind of distant cue, but one still likely to appear in the upper visual field of a swimming rat. A role for Oc2M in the processing of information from peripheral vision is consistent with electrophysiological evidence that visual maps in this area emphasize the peripheral field (Montero 1981, Espinoza and Thomas 1983). There is also evidence that Oc2M might serve to integrate spatial cues from different modalities (Pinto-Hamuy et al. 1987, cf. Goodale and Dale 1981).

3. Two of the areas usually spared by large posterior cortical lesions are Te2 and Tc3 in the temporal cortex, both of which probably receive projections from the lateral posterior nucleus. Recently Meyer and co-workers (1986) have found that lesions of these areas retard learning in a variant of the black-white task in which the stimuli were placed above the part of the apparatus to which the rats directed their response (stimulus-response discontiguity). Lesions of the superior colliculus can produce similar impairments (Milner et al. 1979). It seems unlikely that the temporal lesions affected processing of stationary cues in central vision because they had no effect on a pattern discrimination, whereas lesions of Oc1 and Oc2L prevented pattern learning but had no effect on the black-white discontiguous task (Meyer et al. 1986). Thus temporal cortex may also be involved in processing information from peripheral vision. However, the effects of temporal lesions on performance in the radial or water mazes seem to have been investigated.

In summary, current evidence suggests that the projection from the superior colliculus to extrastriate visual cortex via the lateral posterior nucleus is important for tasks involving nagivation using distant cues, whereas the role of the geniculostriate system is unclear. Of the extrastriate areas so far investigated, posterior parietal cortex (rostral Oc2L and Oc2M) and possibly temporal cortex (Te2 and Te3) are implicated in processing distant cues.

12.5 Modularity of the Rat Visual Cortex

The point of reviewing the evidence in sections 12.3 and 12.4 was to see whether different parts of the rat visual cortex carried out different perceptual functions, i.e., whether the visual cortex was organized into relatively independent subsystems or modules. The evidence concerning each of the areas described in section 12.1 can be summarized as follows (cf. table 12.1):

1. *Striate Cortex, Area Oc1* This area appears to be part of the main system for the analysis of stationary spatial contrast in the central field. It is not part of the main system for the detection of transient stimuli: As a back-up system it performs very poorly in the far periphery and is insensitive to small dim flashes more centrally. Whether it is nonetheless capable of sophisticated analysis of motion (either externally or self-produced) in the central field is unclear. The emphasis of striate cortex on central vision is consistent both with electrophysiological studies (for references, see, e.g., Dean and Redgrave 1984b) and with the high proportion of it devoted to the binocular field (Zilles et al. 1984).

2. *Extrastriate Visual Cortex, Area Oc2L* The behavioral data raise the possibility that lateral Oc2L, which adjoins the lateral border of Oc1, is functionally distinct from rostral Oc2L, which adjoins the rostral border of Oc1.

Lateral Oc2L appears to be part of both the main (geniculostriate) and the secondary (tectocortical) systems for analysis of stationary spatial contrast in central vision. It seems to be less critical for the detection of movement or the use of peripheral cues for navigation, though whether it plays *any* role in movement or peripheral vision is not known. Lateral Oc2L contains several visual maps; in those adjacent to the border with Oc1 the receptive fields are fairly small and central vision emphasized (Montero 1981, Espinoza and Thomas 1983).

Rostral Oc2L is usually removed together with rostral Oc2M in a "posterior parietal" lesion.

3. *Extrastriate Visual Cortex, Area Oc2M* There is weak evidence to suggest that rostral Oc2M and rostral Oc2L may be involved in the detection of transient stimuli throughout the visual field and stronger evidence for their involvement in the analysis of peripheral cues for navigation. They appear not to be required for analysis of stationary spatial contrast in central vision. Maps in Oc2M tend to emphasize the peripheral field (Montero 1981, Espinoza and Thomas 1983).

4. *Temporal Cortex, Areas Te2 and Te3* There is some suggestion that temporal cortex may be involved in peripheral—not central—vision. Maps in this region have very large receptive fields (Montero 1981, Espinoza and Thomas 1983), but their precise location with respect to the border between Oc2L and the temporal cortex is not clear.

The limitations of the evidence available have been sufficiently criticized in previous sections. Nonetheless, as far as it goes, this evidence does favor the view that different areas of the visual cortex are carrying out different perceptual functions. Indeed there are hints of very marked changes in emphasis between cortical areas. We may now be in a position where understanding of visual cortical function in rats would advance very rapidly with further electrophysiological and behavioral experimentation (provided the latter concentrated on precise control of both stimulus presentation and location of lesion).

This work would indicate not only which perceptual cues a particular cortical area concentrates on, but also would start to show what is done with those cues—that is, what computations a given area carries out (DeYoe and Van Essen 1988; cf. section 12.1). Understanding of this kind is obviously important for understanding neural function in rats, but it may also be crucial for any attempt to interest those who work in vision in other species. As mentioned in section 12.1, rats are not studied for their own sake alone, but also for what they can tell us about general biological principles—in this case common principles of visual cortical organization in mammals. The final section considers what those principles are likely to be.

12.6   Comparative Issues: Functions of Rat Vision

The evidence reviewed in sections 12.3 and 12.4 suggests that there may be substantial differences in cortical organization between rats and primates. In particular the effects of damage to the geniculostriate system are relatively mild in the rat; in primates, by contrast, the effects are very severe—so much so in fact that for many years destruction of striate cortex was thought to result in almost total blindness (see, e.g., Humphrey and Weiskrantz 1971, Keating and Dineen 1982).

This difference may not be surprising given what is known of the anatomy of the visual pathways in the two animals: In macaque monkeys about 90 percent of retinal ganglion cells project into the geniculostriate system with 10 percent projecting to the superior colliculus (Perry and Cowey 1984, Perry et al. 1984), whereas in rats 90 percent of retinal ganglion cells project to the superior colliculus and perhaps 20 percent to 50 percent to the dorsal lateral geniculate nucleus (Sefton and Dreher 1985). Thus in primates visual cortex is dominated by geniculostriate input (e.g., Snyder 1973, Diamond 1976), but in rats the influence of the tectocortical projection (via the thalamus) is more important. Comparative studies indicate that this latter organization is also characteristic of hedgehogs, squirrels, and tree shrews, and that it may correspond to a relatively early stage in the evolution of visual cortex (Diamond and Hall 1969, Diamond 1973, 1976). Thus the original source of visual information to the neocortex may well have been the tectocortical projection; the geniculostriate system appeared later and achieved preeminence only in certain evolutionary lines.

This kind of argument suggests that understanding the rat's visual cortex could be important because it will offer insights into a form of basic visual processing that still predominates in many mammalian species and in any case forms the simple foundations on which the complex superstructure of the geniculostriate systems must be erected (cf. Brooks 1985). Is it possible at present to give any indication about what this basic processing might be?

It is clear from both laboratory-based and ethological studies that a major use of vision by rats is to detect predators and prey, based primarily on sudden movement in the visual field. It is probably for effective detection of predators that rats have laterally placed eyes giving a total field of view of about 320° (A. Hughes 1977). Movement detection is obviously of fundamental biological importance, and not surprisingly many nonmammalian vertebrates also use vision for this purpose. In their case the optic tectum seems to be the critical neural structure (e.g., Ewert 1984), just as in rats the homologous superior colliculus is involved ("Detection of Transient Stimuli," section 12.4). Thus one basic process for the tectocortical system might be the analysis of externally produced movement (cf. Frost et al. 1988). This would be consistent with evidence that in primates cortical area MT receives visual input from the superior colliculus via the pulvinar (e.g., Diamond 1976, Rodman et al. 1985), and that area MT is specialized for the analysis of movement (e.g., Maunsell and Newsome 1987).

Other major uses of vision by rats are not so clear, either from laboratory-based or ethological studies. Indeed it often seems to be implicitly assumed that vision in rats is essentially similar to (though clearly not as good as) our own. However, as mentioned in sections 12.3 and 12.4, various observers have been impressed by the apparent oddities of rat vision, such as its being more concerned with a spatial location than the properties of the object located there, and its use of those properties as indicants of safe passage (can it be jumped on or run through?) rather than of the objects' intrinsic qualities. Lashley (1938) suggested that "it seems possible that in the lower mammals there is . . . a qualitative difference in the visual perception of the environment or a qualitatively different organization of visual activity. In this organization the distinctive feature would be the dominance of the perception of spatial relations rather than of the visual properties of objects" (p. 347).

These remarks indicate that the second major use of vision in rats is a broad range of activities that may be loosely classified as navigation, or getting from one place to another (see also Finlay and Sengelaub 1981, Ingle 1981, Goodale 1983). If so, the tectocortical projection may be concerned not only with the analysis of externally produced motion, but also with visual processing relevant for navigation. This suggestion is clearly related to Trevarthen's (1968) argument that in primates the visual midbrain mediates "ambient" vision. Ambient vision has relatively "low angular resolution for stationary features, low sensitivity to relative position, orientation, luminance or hue, but high sensitivity to change in any of these attributes" (p. 328), whether externally or self-produced. It operates over the entire visual field, and its function is to provide sufficient information about the three-dimensional space surrounding the body to govern locomotion or postural adjustments. It characterizes the vision of "primitive active vertebrates" (p. 328), a view shared by Horridge (1987), who argues that in evolutionary terms ambient vision is primitive to object recognition. Additional evidence for a collicular role in ambient vision is provided by Humphrey's (1974) very striking demonstration that almost complete removal of striate cortex can virtually destroy a monkey's capacity to recognize objects, but still allows the exercise of some basic navigational skills (for further discussion of the mechanisms underlying primate ambient vision, see, e.g., Ungerleider and Mishkin 1982, Bruce et al. 1986, DeYoe and Van Essen 1988).

Perhaps, therefore, studying the rat's visual cortex can provide important insights into the visual computations necessary for navigation. This is by no means a trivially simple procedure. On the contrary, navigation involves a number of competencies, such as (1) those that answer the question "where to go" including use of (a) distant visual cues and spatial maps to reach invisible targets, and (b) size and shape to assess visible targets; (2) those that answer the question "how to get there," such as use of stationary, motion parallax, and optic flow cues to (a) plan a trajectory, (b) avoid obstacles, and (c) follow winding routes such as those provided by branches, etc. Indeed it may be because navigation is complex that the organization of the rat's visual cortex is complex: For example, the different component processes may be reflected in the existence of different visual mappings on the cortical surface.

In summary, then, visual cortex in the rat appears to exemplify a basic form of mammalian organization in which the tectocortical input is more important relative to the geniculostriate system than it is in primates. This organization may reflect a preoccupation with the analysis of external movement and with navigation at the expense of object recognition. It is therefore possible that the rat's visual cortex will prove to be a good preparation for studying how the computations involved in both elementary motion perception and in ambient vision can be implemented by neuronal networks. Indeed at our present stage of knowledge rats may offer a significant advantage for studying these problems over species in which the visual cortex is more highly developed and thus more complex and difficult to understand.

Acknowledgments

It is a pleasure to thank Dr. Peter Redgrave for his critical reading of the manuscript and expert assistance in the preparation of the diagrams.

References

Arbib, M. A., and Hanson, A. R. (eds.) (1987). *Vision, Brain and Cooperative Computation.* Cambridge, Mass.: MIT Press.

Bauer, J. H., and Cooper, R. M. (1964). Effects of posterior cortical lesions on performance of a brightness discrimination task. *Journal of Comparative Physiological Psychology* 58:84–92.

Birch, M. P., Ferrier, R. J., and Cooper, R. M. (1978). Reversal set formation in the visually decorticate rat. *Journal of Comparative Physiological Psychology* 92:1050–1061.

Blanchard, R. J., Flannelly, K. K., and Blanchard, D. C. (1986). Defensive behaviors of laboratory and wild *Rattus norvegicus*. *Journal of Comparative Psychology* 100:101–107.

Bloch-Rojas, S., Toro, A., and Pinto-Hamuy, T. (1964). Cardiac versus somatomotor conditioned responses in neodecorticate rats. *Journal of Comparative Physiological Psychology* 58:233–236.

Braun, J. J., Lundy, E. G., and McCarthy, F. V. (1970). Depth discrimination in rats following removal of visual neocortex. *Brain Research* 20:283–291.

Brooks, R. A. (1985). A robust layered control system for a mobile robot. M.I.T. Artificial Intelligence Laboratory, A.I. Memo 864.

Bruce, C. J., Desimone, R., and Gross, C. G. (1986). Both striate cortex and superior colliculus contribute to visual properties of neurons in superior temporal polysensory area of macaque monkey. *Journal of Neurophysiology* 55:1057–1075.

Burne, R. A., Parnevelas, J. G., and Lin, C.-S. (1984). Response properties of neurons in the visual cortex of the rat. *Experimental Brain Research* 53:374–383.

Christie, D., and Steele Russell, I. (1985). Visuomotor strategies in pattern discrimination learning in rats. *Behavioural Brain Research* 16:9–18.

Coleman, J., and Clerici, W. J. (1980). Extrastriate projections from thalamus to posterior occipital-temporal cortex in rat. *Brain Research* 194:205–209.

Cooper, R. M., Blochert, K. P., Gillespie, L. A., and Miller, L. G. (1972). Translucent occluders and lesions of posterior neocortex in the rat. *Physiology and Behaviour* 8:693–697.

Cowey, A., Henken, D. B., and Perry, V. H. (1982). Effects on visual acuity of neonatal or adult tectal ablation in rats. *Experimental Brain Research* 48:149–152.

Cowey, A., and Weiskrantz, L. (1971). Contour discrimination in rats after frontal and striate cortical ablations. *Brain Research* 30:241–252.

Dean, P. (1978). Visual acuity in hooded rats: effects of superior collicular or posterior neocortical lesions. *Brain Research* 156:17–31.

Dean, P. (1981a). Grating detection and visual acuity after lesions of striate cortex in hooded rats. *Experimental Brain Research* 43:145–153.

Dean, P. (1981b). Visual pathways and acuity in hooded rats. *Behavioural Brain Research* 3:239–271.

Dean, P. (1981c). Are rats short-sighted? Effects of stimulus distance and size on visual detection. *Quarterly Journal of Experimental Psychology* 33B:69–76.

Dean, P. (1982). Visual behavior in monkeys with inferotemporal lesions. In D. J. Ingle,

M. A. Goodale, and R. J. W. Mansfield (eds.), *Analysis of Visual Behavior*. Cambridge, Mass.: MIT Press, 67–109.

Dean, P., and Key, C. (1981). Spatial deficits on radial maze after large tectal lesions in rats: possible role of impaired scanning. *Behvioural and Neural Biology* 32:170–190.

Dean, P., and Pope, S. G. (1981). Visual discrimination learning in rats with lesions of superior colliculus: door-push and approach errors in modified jumping stand. *Quarterly Journal of Experimental Psychology* 33B:141–157.

Dean, P., and Redgrave, P. (1984a). The superior colliculus and visual neglect in rat and hamster. I. Behavioural evidence. *Brain Research Review* 8:129–141.

Dean, P., and Redgrave, P. (1984b). The superior colliculus and visual neglect in rat and hamster. II. Possible mechanisms. *Brain Research Review* 8:143–153.

Dean, P., and Redgrave, P. (1984c). The superior colliculus and visual neglect in rat and hamster. III. Functional implications. *Brain Research Review* 8:155–163.

DeYoe, E. A., and Van Essen, D. C. (1988). Concurrent processing streams in monkey visual cortex. *Trends in Neuroscience* 11:215–226.

Diamond, I. T. (1973). The evolution of the tectal-pulvinar system in mammals: structural and behavioural studies of the visual system. *Symposium of the Zoological Society of London* 33:205–233.

Diamond, I. T. (1976). Organization of the visual cortex: comparative anatomical and behavioral studies. *Federal Proceedings* 35:60–67.

Diamond, I. T., and Hall, W. C. (1969). Evolution of neocortex. *Science* 164:251–262.

Doty, R. W. (1961). Functional significance of the topographical aspects of the retino-cortical projection. In R. Jung and H. Kornhuber (eds.), *The Visual System: Neurophysiology and Psychophysics*. Berlin: Springer Verlag, 228–245.

Ellard, C. G., Goodale, M. A., and Timney, B. (1984). Distance estimation in the Mongolian gerbil: the role of dynamic depth cues. *Behavioural Brain Research* 14:29–39.

Ellard, C. G., Goodale, M. A., Scorfield, D. M., and Lawrence, C. (1986). Visual cortical lesions abolish the use of motion parallax in the Mongolian gerbil. *Experimental Brain Research* 64:599–602.

Espinoza, S. G., and Thomas, H. C. (1983). Retinotopic organization of striate and extrastriate visual cortex in the hooded rat. *Brain Research* 272:137–144.

Ewer, R. F. (1971). The biology and behavior of a free-living population of black rats (*Rattus rattus*). *Animal Behaviour Monograph* 4:127–174.

Ewert, J.-P. (1984). Tectal mechanisms that underlie prey-catching and avoidance behaviors in toads. In H. Vanegas (ed.), *Comparative Neurology of the Optic Tectum*. New York: Plenum Press, 274–416.

Ferrier, R. J., and Cooper, R. M. (1976). Striate cortex ablation and spatial vision. *Brain Research* 106:71–85.

Finlay, B. L., and Sengelaub, D. R. (1981). Toward a neuroethology of mammalian vision: ecology and anatomy of rodent visuomotor behavior. *Behavioural Brain Research* 3:133–149.

Foreman, N., and Stevens, R. (1982). Visual lesions and radial maze performance in rats. *Behavioural and Neural Biology* 36:126–136.

Foreman, N., and Stevens, R. (1987). Relationships between the superior colliculus and the hippocampus: Neural and behavioral considerations. *Behavioural Brain Science* 10:101–152.

Frost, B. J., Cavanagh, P., and Morgan, B. (1988). Deep tectal cells in pigeons respond to kinematograms. *Journal of Comparative Physiology A* 162:639–647.

Goetsch, V. L., and Isaac, W. (1983). The effect of occipital ablation on visual sensitivity in young and old rats. *Physiological Psychology* 11:173–177.

Goldstein, L. H., and Oakley, D. A. (1987). Visual discrimination in the absence of visual cortex. *Behavioural Brain Research* 24:181–193.

Goodale, M. A. (1983). Vision as a sensorimotor system. In T. E. Robinson (ed.), *Behavioral Approaches to Brain Research*. New York: Oxford University Press, 41–61.

Goodale, M. A., and Dale, R. H. I. (1981). Radial-maze performance in the rat following lesions of posterior neocortex. *Behavioural Brain Research* 3:273–288.

Goodale, M. A., Foreman, N. P., and Milner, A. D. (1978). Visual orientation in the rat: A dissociation of deficits following cortical and collicular lesions. *Experimental Brain Research* 31:445–457.

Goodale, M. A., and Milner, A. D. (1982). Fractionating orientation behavior in rodents. In D. J. Ingle, M. A. Goodale, and R. J. W. Mansfield (eds.), *Analysis of Visual Behavior*. Cambridge, Mass.: MIT Press, 267–299.

Goodale, M. A., and Murison, R. C. C. (1975). The effects of lesions of the superior colliculus on locomotor orientation and the orienting reflex in the rat. *Brain Research* 88:243–261.

Goss, A. E., and Wischner, G. J. (1956). Vicarious trial and error and related behavior. *Psychological Bulletin* 53:35–54.

Gray, T., and LeVere, T. E. (1980). Infant posterior neocortical lesions do not induce visual responses in spared anterior neocortex. *Physiological Psychology* 8:487–492.

Guic-Robles, E., Venable, N., Acevedo, I., Aramburu, B., and Pinto-Hamuy, T. (1982). Recovery of visual pattern discrimination by rats without visual cortex when trained by fading procedure. *Physiological Psychology* 10:175–185.

Hebb, D. O. (1938). Studies of the organization of behavior. I. Behavior of the rat in a field orientation. *Journal of Comparative Psychology* 25:333–351.

Horel, J. A. (1968). Effects of subcortical lesions on brightness discrimination acquired by rats without visual cortex. *Journal of Comparative Physiological Psychology* 65:103–109.

Horel, J. A., and Stelzner, D. J. (1981). Neocortical projections of the rat anterior commissure. *Brain Research* 220:1–12.

Horridge, G. A. (1987). The evolution of visual processing and the construction of seeing systems. *Proceedings of the Royal Society of London B* 230:279–292.

Hughes, A. (1977). A schematic eye for the rat. *Vision Research* 19:569–588.

Hughes, H. C. (1977). Anatomical and neurobehavioral investigations concerning the thalamo-cortical organization of the rat's visual system. *Journal of Comparative Neurology* 175:311–336.

Humphrey, N. K. (1974). Vision in a monkey without striate cortex: a case study. *Perception* 3:241–255.

Humphrey, N. K., and Weiskrantz, L. (1971). Vision in monkeys after removal of the striate cortex. *Nature* 215:595–597.

Ingle, D. J. (1981). New methods for analysis of vision in the gerbil. *Behavioural Brain Research* 3:151–173.

Ingle, D. J. (1982). Organization of visuomotor behaviors in vertebrates. In D. J. Ingle, M. A. Goodale, and R. J. W. Mansfield (eds.), *Analysis of Visual Behavior*. Cambridge, Mass.: MIT Press, 67–109.

Keating, E. G., and Dineen, J. (1982). Visuomotor transforms of the primate tectum. In D. J. Ingle, M. A. Goodale, and R. J. W. Mansfield (eds.) *Analysis of Visual Behavior.* Cambridge, Mass.: MIT Press, 335–365.

Kolb, B., and Walkey, J. (1987). Behavioural and anatomical studies of the posterior parietal cortex in the rat. *Behavioural Brain Research* 23:127–145.

Kolb, B., and Whishaw, I. Q. (1981). Decortication of rats in infancy or adulthood produced comparable functional losses on learned and species-typical behaviors. *Journal of Comparative Physiological Psychology* 95:468–483.

Lashley, K. S. (1929). *Brain Mechanisms and Intelligence.* Chicago: University of Chicago Press.

Lashley, K. S. (1930). The mechanism of vision: III. The comparative visual acuity of pigmented and albino rats. *Journal of Genetic Psychology* 37:481–484.

Lashley, K. S. (1931). The mechanism of vision: IV. The cerebral areas necessary for pattern vision in the rat. *Journal of Comparative Neurology* 53:419–478.

Lashley, K. S. (1932). The mechanism of vision: V. The structure and image-forming power of the rat's eye. *Journal of Comparative Psychology* 13:173–200.

Lashley, K. S. (1937). The mechanism of vision: XIV. Visual perception of distance after injuries to the cerebral cortex, colliculi, or optic thalamus. *Journal of Genetic Psychology* 51:189–207.

Lashley, K. S. (1938). The mechanism of vision: XV. Preliminary studies of the rat's capacity for detail vision. *Journal of General Psychology* 18:123–193.

Lashley, K. S. (1939). The mechansim of vision: XVI. The functioning of small remnants of the visual cortex. *Journal of Comparative Neurology* 70:45–67.

Lashley, K. S. (1942). The mechanism of vision: XVII. Autonomy of the visual cortex. *Journal of Genetic Psychology* 60:197–221.

Lavond, D., Hata, M. G., Gray, T. S., Geckler, C. I., Meyer, P. M., and Meyer, D. R. (1978). Visual form perception is a function of the visual cortex. *Physiological Psychology* 6:471–477.

Lawler, K. A., and Cowey, A. (1986). The effects of pretectal and superior collicular lesions on binocular vision. *Experimental Brain Research* 63:402–408.

Legg, C. R., and Turkish, S. (1983). Flicker sensitivity changes after subcortical visual system lesions in the rat. *Behavioural Brain Research* 10:311–324.

Lindsay, J. F., Jr., and McDaniel, W. F. (1987). Neural tissue transplants in rats with lateral peristriate lesions: II. Behavior. *Medical Science Research* 15:655–656.

Lines, C. R., and Milner, A. D. (1985). A deficit in ambient visual guidance following superior colliculus lesions in rats. *Behavioural Neuroscience* 99:707–716.

Marr, D. C. (1982). *Vision*. San Francisco: Freeman.

Mason, R., and Groos, G. A. (1981). Cortico-recipient and tecto-recipient visual zones in the rat's lateral posterior (pulvinar) nucleus: an anatomical study. *Neuroscience Letters* 25:107–112.

Maunsell, J. H. R., and Newsome, W. T. (1987). Visual processing in monkey extrastriate cortex. *Annual Review of Neuroscience* 10:363–401.

McDaniel, W. F. (1985). Functions of the posterior neocortex of the rat. *IRCS Journal of Medical Science* 13:286–289.

McDaniel, W. F., and Braucht, G. S. (1984). Pattern discrimination acquisition and performance following regionally limited posterior neocortical ablations. *IRCS Journal of Medical Science* 12:1086–1087.

McDaniel, W. F., and Brown, R. G. (1984). Radial maze performance following restricted posterior neocortical lesions. *IRCS Journal of Medical Science* 12:807–808.

McDaniel, W. F., Coleman, J., and Lindsay, J. F., Jr. (1982). A comparison of lateral peristriate and striate neocortical ablations in the rat. *Behavioural Brain Research* 6:249–272.

McDaniel, W. F., and Noble, L. M. (1984). Visual pattern discrimination following bilateral striate or lateral peristriate neocortical injuries. *IRCS Journal of Medical Science* 12:1084–1085.

McDaniel, W. F., and Terrell Wall, T. (1988). Visuospatial functions in the rat following injuries to striate, peristriate, and parietal neocortical areas. *Psychobiology* 16:251–260.

McDaniel, W. F., Wildman, L. D., and Spears, R. H. (1979). Posterior association cortex and visual pattern discrimination in the rat. *Physiological Psychology* 7:241–244.

Meyer, D. R., and Meyer, P. M. (1977). Dynamics and bases of recoveries of functions after injuries to the cerebral cortex. *Physiological Psychology* 5:133–165.

Meyer, P. M., Meyer, D. R., and Cloud, M. D. (1986). Temporal neocortical injuries in rats impair attending but not complex visual processing. *Behavioural Neuroscience* 100:845–851.

Midgley, G. C., and Tees, R. C. (1981). Orienting behavior by rats with visual cortical and subcortical lesions. *Experimental Brain Research* 41:316–328.

Midgley, G. C., Wilkie, D. M., and Tees, R. C. (1988). Effects of superior colliculus lesions on rats' orienting and detection of neglected visual cues. *Behavioural Neuroscience* 102:93–100.

Miller, L. G., and Cooper, R. M. (1974). Translucent occluders and the role of visual cortex in pattern vision. *Brain Research* 79:45–59.

Miller, M. W., and Vogt, B. A. (1984). Direct connections of rat visual cortex with sensory, motor, and association cortices. *Journal of Comparative Neurology* 226:184–202.

Milner, A. D., Goodale, M. A., and Morton, M. C. (1979). Visual sampling after lesions of the superior colliculus in rats. *Journal of Comparative Physiological Psychology* 93:1015–1023.

Milner, A. D., and Lines, C. R. (1983). Stimulus sampling and the use of distal visual cues in rats with lesions of the superior colliculus. *Behavioural Brain Research* 8:387–401.

Mize, R. R., Wetzel, A. B., and Thompson, V. E. (1971). Contour discrimination in the rat following removal of posterior neocortex. *Physiological Behaviour* 6:241–246.

Mlinar, E. J., and Goodale, M. A. (1984). Cortical and tectal control of visual orientation in the gerbil: evidence for parallel channels. *Experimental Brain Research* 55:33–48.

Montero, V. M. (1981). Comparative studies on the visual cortex. In C. N. Woolsey (ed.), *Cortical Sensory Organisation: Vol. 2 Multiple Visual Areas.* Clifton, N.J.: Humana Press, 33–81.

Morris, R. G. M. (1981). Spatial localization does not require the presence of local cues. *Learning and Motivation* 12:239–260.

Morris, R. G. M. (1984). Developments of a water-maze procedure for studying spatial learning in the rat. *Journal of Neuroscience Methods* 11:47–60.

Olavarria, J. (1979). A horseradish peroxidase study of the projections from the lateroposterior nucleus to three lateral peristriate areas in the rat. *Brain Research* 173:137–141.

Olavarria, J., and Montero, V. M. (1984). Relation of callosal and striate-extrastriate cortical connections in the rat: Morphological definition of extrastriate visual areas. *Experimental Brain Research* 54:240–252.

Olavarria, J., and Torrealba, F. (1978). The effect of acute lesions of the striate cortex on the retinotopic organization of the lateral peristriate cortex in the rat. *Brain Research* 151:386–391.

Olton, D. S., and Samuelson, R. J. (1976). Remembrance of places passed: spatial memory in rats. *Journal of Experimental Psychology: Animal Behaviour Proceedings* 2:97–116.

Overton, P. (1986). *The visuo-motor functions of the superior colliculus, and its crossed descending efferent projection, in the rat.* Unpublished doctoral dissertation, University of Sheffield, England.

Overton, P., and Dean, P. (1988). Detection of visual stimuli after lesions of the superior colliculus in the rat: deficit not confined to the far periphery. *Behvioural Brain Research* 31:1–15.

Overton, P., Dean, P., and Redgrave, P. (1985). Detection of visual stimuli in far periphery by rats: possible role of superior colliculus. *Experimental Brain Research* 59:559–569.

Perry, V. H., and Cowey, A. (1984). Retinal ganglion cells that project to the superior colliculus and pretectum in the macaque monkey. *Neuroscience* 12:1125–1137.

Perry, V. H., Oehler, R., and Cowey, A. (1984). Retinal ganglion cells that project to the dorsal lateral geniculate nucleus in the macaque monkey. *Neuroscience* 12:1101–1123.

Pinto-Hamuy, T., Olavarria, J., Guic-Robles, E., Morgues, M., Nassal, O., and Petit, D. (1987). Rats with lesions in anteromedial extrastriate cortex fail to learn a visuosomatic conditional response. *Behavioural Brain Research* 25:221–231.

Rodman, H. R., Gross, C. G., and Albright, T. A. (1985). The effect of striate cortex and superior colliculus lesions on visual responses in MT. *Society of Neuroscience Abstracts* 11:1246.

Sahibzada, N., Dean, P., and Redgrave, P. (1986). Movements resembling orientation or avoidance elicited by electrical stimulation of the superior colliculus in rats. *Journal of Neuroscience* 6:723–733.

Scheff, S. W., and Wright, D. C. (1977). Behavioral and electrophysiological evidence for cortical reorganization of function in rats with serial lesions of the visual cortex. *Physiological Psychology* 5:103–107.

Schneider, G. E. (1969). Two visual systems. *Science* 163:895–902.

Schneider, G. E., Carman, L. S., and Ayres, S. (1987). Superior colliculus function in visually elicited "fear" and in scanning movements in Syrian hamsters. *Society of Neuroscience Abstracts* 13:871.

Schober, W. (1981). Efferente und afferente Verbindungen des Nucleus lateralis posterior thalami ("Pulvinar") der Albinoratte. *Zeitschrift für mikroskopische-anatomische Forschung Leipzig* 95:827–844.

Sefton, A. J., and Dreher, B. (1985). Visual System. In G. Paxinos (ed.), *The Rat Nervous System, Vol. 1 Forebrain and Midbrain.* Sydney: Academic Press, 169–221.

Simon, H. A. (1969). *The Sciences of the Artificial.* Cambridge, Mass.: MIT Press.

Snyder, M. (1973). The evolution of mammalian visual mechanisms. In R. Jung (ed.), *Handbook of Sensory Physiology, Vol. 7, Part 3B, Central Processing of Visual Information,* Berlin: Springer Verlag, 693–712.

Spear, P. D., and Barbas, H. (1975). Recovery of pattern discrimination ability in rats receiving serial or one-stage visual cortex lesions. *Brain Research* 94:337–346.

Steele Russell, I., Bookman, J. F., and Mohn, G. (1979). Interocular transfer of visual learning in the rat. In I. Steele Russell, M. W. Van Hof, and G. Berlucchi (eds.), *Structure and Function of Cerebral Commissures*. Macmillan: London, 164–181.

Suzuki, S., Augerinos, G., and Black, A. H. (1980). Stimulus control of spatial behavior on the eight-arm maze in rats. *Learning and Motivation* 11:1–18.

Takahashi, T. (1985). The organization of the lateral thalamus of the hooded rat. *Journal of Comparative Neurology* 231:281–309.

Thomas, H. C., and Espinoza, S. G. (1987). Relationships between interhemispheric cortical connections and visual areas in hooded rats. *Brain Research* 417:214–224.

Trevarthen, C. B. (1968). Two mechanisms of vision in primates. *Psychologische Forschung* 31:299–337.

Ungerleider, L. G., and Mishkin, M. (1982). Two cortical visual systems. In D. J. Ingle, M. A. Goodale, and R. J. W. Mansfield (eds.), *Analysis of Visual Behavior*. Cambridge, Mass.: MIT Press, 549–586.

Vanderwolf, C. H., Kolb, B., and Cooley, R. K. (1978). Behavior of the rat after removal of the neocortex and hippocampal formation. *Journal of Comparative Physiological Psychology* 92:156–175.

Wagor, E., Mangini, N. J., and Pearlman, A. L. (1980). Retinopathic organization of striate and extrastriate visual cortex in the mouse. *Journal of Comparative Neurology* 193:187–202.

Warton, S. S., Dyson, S. E., and Harvey, A. R. (1988). Visual thalamocortical projections in normal and enucleated rats: HRP and fluorescent dye studies. *Experimental Neurology* 100:23–39.

Whishaw, I. Q., and Kolb, B. (1984). Decortication abolishes place but not cue learning in rats. *Behavioural Brain Research* 11:123–134.

Zilles, K. (1985). *The Cortex of the Rat. A Stereotaxic Atlas*. Berlin: Springer Verlag.

Zilles, K., Wree, A., Schleicher, A., and Divac, I. (1984). The monocular and binocular subfields of the rat's primary visual cortex: A quantitative morphological approach. *Journal of Comparative Neurology* 226:391–402.

13 The Role of Cerebral Cortex in Visuomotor Control

Melvyn A. Goodale and David P. Carey

Although scientists have been studying the visual functions of the rat's cerebral cortex for more than fifty years, very little of this work has been concerned with the role of the cortex in visuomotor behavior. The few studies that have looked at the visual control of movement in this animal have concentrated not on the cortex but on the superior colliculus. This is not too surprising because in other species, such as monkey and cat, the superior colliculus has long been implicated in the initiation and control of eye and head movements. Moreover, in the rat, nearly all the retinal ganglion cells project to this midbrain structure, and less than 40 percent of them have collateral projections to the dorsal lateral geniculate nucleus (Dreher et al. 1985, Linden and Perry 1983, Martin 1986). However, the main reason that cortical contributions to visuomotor behavior have rarely been studied in the rat (or in any other animal for that matter) is related to philosophy rather than anatomy or physiology. For the past 50 or more years, visual research in experimental psychology and physiology has been driven by the belief (usually implicit) that vision (particularly cortically mediated vision) provides the organism with some sort of perceptual representation of the external world. Even the recent emphasis on independent and parallel processing within the visual system has paid scant attention to the motor outputs of the different processing "modules" and has concentrated instead on investigating the ways in which the algorithms within these different modules or channels are brought to bear on the retinal image (see Dean, chapter 12, Livingstone and Hubel 1988, Tees, chapter 22, Ungerleider and Mishkin 1982). In other words the visual system (particularly the pathway to the cerebral cortex) has been regarded as a piece of perceptual machinery in which the different processing modules contribute to a complex, but essentially monolithic, representation of the external world on which the organism can act.

With such a perspective it is understandable why most research on the visual functions of the cerebral cortex has been concerned not with visuomotor behavior but with sensory processing, perception, and memory. The motor act, insofar as it has been considered at all by researchers studying visual cortex, has been seen as part of the province of motor physiology or the psychology of motor skills rather than visual science. In fact, with the notable exception of eye movements (which have been studied a great deal in cat, monkey, and human), the visual system of mammals has been studied almost entirely with respect to the organization of its sensory inputs, with little attention being paid the organization of the motor acts that such sensory inputs eventually direct.

Although studies of visual discrimination learning have provided a great deal of information about the perceptual boundaries of rodent vision and its neural substrate (see Dean, chapter 12), much of the research in this tradition has lost sight of the evolutionary context in which all types of visual systems have developed. As one of us has argued elsewhere (Goodale 1983a, 1988), vision evolved not to provide the organism with a unified percept of the world in which it lives but to control the movements that the animal makes in that world. Natural selection operates at the level of overt behavior. It is interested not in how well an animal "sees" the world in which predators and prey can be found but only in how well the animal avoids the predators and catches the prey. Indeed an argument can be made that it was not a visual system that evolved but a *visuomotor* system. If this is the case, the functional architecture of such a system can be fully understood only by studying its motor outputs as well as its sensory inputs.

The purpose of our chapter then is to review the rather limited amount of work that has been carried out on the visuomotor functions of the cerebral cortex in the rat and other rodents, comparing the results where possible to those obtained with monkey and cat. The general thesis of the chapter is that cerebral cortex participates in the control of visuomotor behavior in part by modulating the functions of phylogenetically older retinofugal pathways, such as those to the superior colliculus.

Several categories of visuomotor behavior are considered in this chapter, including orientation movements, escape, target-directed locomotion, barrier avoidance, and jumping. The emphasis is on detailed descriptions of the movements, most of which are derived from film or videotapes of the animals' behavior rather than on more abstract notions such as spatial navigation and cognitive maps. In other words many of the experiments we present attempt to deal with the visual control of these movements in much the same way that other investigators have dealt with the visual control of eye movements—by recording the movements directly and relating them to the spatial and temporal characteristics of the visual stimulus eliciting and/or controlling those movements. For eye movements such an approach has lead to real progress in working out the way in which particular visuomotor system transforms sensory input into motor output. The study of the neural substrates of visually guided head movements, limb movements, and whole-body movements in the rat and other rodents hold a similar promise for the understanding of other kinds of sensorimotor transformations.

13.1 The Role of the Cortex in Orienting Behavior

The Two Visual Systems Hypothesis

The superior colliculus (or optic tectum, as it is usually called in non-mammalian vertebrates) has long been implicated in what Hess et al. (1946) termed the *visual grasp reflex,* the rapid shift in gaze that brings a stimulus originally located in the visual periphery into central vision where it can be scrutinized in more detail. The most explicit statement of this idea was made by Schneider (1969) who argued, largely on the basis of his own experiments with the Syrian hamster, for a functionally dichotomous visual system—a retinotectal system that enables the animal to "localize" a stimulus in visual space and a geniculostriate system that allows the animal to "identify" that object. Even though the two visual systems hypothesis was put forward nearly twenty years ago, it remains the most influential account of how the visual system is organized. Unfortunately the functions attributed to the two anatomical subdivisions reflect old prejudices about the role of the cortex and subcortical structures in visual processing (for a discussion of this issue, see Goodale 1983a). Cortically based vision is treated as a purely perceptual system and the problem of how sensory inputs are used to control the different patterns of motor output produced by the animal is not dealt with directly. The superior colliculus is relegated to the more primitive and reflexive task of "orienting" the animal toward the stimulus to be perceived. Even the term "orientation behavior," which sounds as though it might refer to a specific set of visually guided movements, refers instead to "localizing" a stimulus by means of any one of a multitude of very different motor outputs, only some of which are now known to depend on collicular circuitry. In fact, as we demonstrate below, even those behaviors that involve collicular pathways are often modulated by the cortex.

The Visual Grasp Reflex Reconsidered

Before discussing the role of the cortex in orientation behavior, it is worth pointing out that the two-step process implied by Schneider's hypothesis—first localizing (or orienting toward) a visual stimulus and then identifying it—presupposes that central vision is more acute than peripheral vision. Although this is certainly true of the monkey and cat, it is not necessarily the case in the rat and other rodents. The variation in ganglion cell density across the rat's retina is relatively small, ranging from a low of about 1000 cells/mm^2 to a high of only 6000 cells/mm^2 (Dreher et al. 1984). This ratio of 6 : 1 stands in striking contrast to the figures for the cat—a center/periphery ratio of approximately 80 : 1 with a ganglion cell density in the area centralis of about

8600 cells/mm^2 (Rowe and Stone 1976)—and the figures for the monkey—a ratio of more than 300 : 1 with a foveal density of 80,000 to 100,000 ganglion cells/mm^2 (van Buren 1963, Rolls and Cowey 1970).[1] In addition the size of the dendritic trees of ganglion cells in the rat, which reflect the size of the receptive field centers of these cells, does not vary with ganglion cell density across the retina (Dreher et al 1985). This observation is congruent with electrophysiological studies; despite the fact that a larger proportion of Oc1 is devoted to the projection of the central versus the peripheral visual field (Montero 1981, Zilles et al. 1984), there is no apparent increase in the receptive field size of single units with increasing retinal eccentricity (Shaw et al. 1975, Wiesenfeld and Kornel 1975). In the cat and monkey, of course, there are dramatic increases in receptive field size as one moves from central portions of the visual map in the striate cortex to the periphery (Gatass et al. 1985, Hubel and Wiesel 1974, Tusa et al. 1978). It is also worth noting that recent work on ganglion cell density in the Syrian hamster—the animal that Schneider (1969) used in his original experiments—has revealed a distribution that is even more uniform than that of the rat, with a maximal center/periphery ratio of only 2 : 1 (Sengelaub et al. 1983).

Thus, in the rat and hamster, it is unlikely that the act of bringing a stimulus into a position in front of the animal's head serves the purpose of identifying that stimulus visually. Instead it is more likely in these species that the animal is positioning the stimulus so that it can locomote toward it or grasp it with its mouth and forelimbs. The stimulus would also now be in a convenient position for olfactory, gustatory, and tactile exploration. In the case of more distal stimuli, the animal may be positioning the stimulus in the binocular portion of the visual field (which extends some 50° to 80° in front of the animal) so that the distance of the stimulus can be estimated on the basis of retinal disparity cues or convergence. In short the term *visual grasp reflex* may be something of a misnomer when applied to the rat and other animals with relatively undifferentiated retinae.

Cortical and Collicular Control of Orienting: Parallel Channels to the Hindbrain?

Whatever might be going on when an animal turns its head (or eyes) toward a food object or some other visual stimulus, it is one of the classes of orientation behavior that Schneider and others have argued depends on retinotectal projections. Lesions of the superior colliculus that extend into the deeper layers of this structure result in a reduction in the number of head turns made to visual stimuli in rats (Goodale et al. 1978, Goodale et al. 1975, Goodale and Murison 1975, Marshall 1978, Midgley and Tees 1981), Mongolian gerbils (Goodale and Milner 1982, Mlinar and Goodale 1984), and Syrian hamsters (Mort et al. 1980, Schneider 1967, 1969). The story is more complicated than this, however. If only the superficial layers of the superior colliculus are destroyed, thereby eliminating the direct retinal input, much of an animal's ability to orient toward food objects is retained (Casagrande and Diamond 1974, Ingle 1982). These results suggest that remaining inputs to the deep layers of the colliculus, originating either from the visual cortex or from other subcortical visual areas, are sufficient to mediate well-organized orientation movements. Whatever the substrate might be for the residual orientation behavior in these animals, the role of the highly organized retinotectal projection becomes less clear (see Edwards 1980, Harting et al. 1973, and Albano and Wurtz 1982 for a discussion of this problem).

The picture is further complicated by the fact that close examination of the deficits in animals with large lesions of the superior colliculus that include both the superficial and the deeper layers reveals considerable sparing of orientation ability in the central portions of the visual field. Thus rats and gerbils with large collicular lesions are able to turn their heads toward small lights or food objects presented within a portion of the anterior visual field extending some 45° to the right and left of the midline axis (Goodale et al. 1978, Goodale and Milner 1982, Mlinar and Goodale 1984). Similar observations have been made in the cat (Sprague and Meikle 1965), tree shrew (Casagrande and Diamond 1974), and monkey (Albano and Wurtz 1982). These observations suggest that pathways quite separate from the tectofugal systems are capable of mediating the head and eye movements that constitute an orienting response, at least to stimuli that occur within the central portion of the visual field.

There is some evidence to suggest that projections from visual cortical areas are involved in this extratectal control. In the monkey, for example, Schiller and colleagues (1980) have demonstrated that although complete lesions of the superior colliculus result in a moderate reduction in the accuracy, frequency, and velocity of saccadic eye movements, an additional lesion of the frontal eye fields (area 8) results in a dramatic and relatively permanent loss of visually triggered saccades. In an earlier study Mohler and Wurtz (1977) showed that saccadic eye movements to visual targets by the monkey could be abolished by combined lesions of the striate cortex and the superior colliculus, whereas lesions of either structure alone had much smaller effects on the generation of saccades. A similar pattern of results can be seen with respect to the generation of oriented head turns in at least one rodent species, the Mongolian gerbil. Ingle (1982) and Mlinar and Goodale (1984) have observed that the residual ability to make head turns toward visual stimuli after complete lesions of the superior colliculus was abolished when an additional lesion was made in the striate cortex of these animals. These results and those obtained in the monkey suggest that structures receiving input from the geniculostriate pathway, such as area 17 itself as well as the frontal eye fields, are capable of mediating the orientation behavior (either head movements or saccadic eye movements) that survives collicular ablation, and that these pathways may play an important role in the organization of orientation behavior in the intact animal.

In a number of different mammals, including rodents, both the superior colliculus and the neocortex send projections to common targets in the pons and medulla (see, for example, Burne et al. 1981, Redgrave et al. 1987, Wiesendanger and Wiesendanger 1982a,b). One group of nuclei in the rat receiving dual input from the colliculus and the cortex are those making up the pontine reticular formation, particularly the nucleus reticularis pontis oralis and caudalis (Redgrave et al. 1987), which form part of a region commonly referred to in monkey as the paramedian pontine reticular formation, or PPRF (see Buttner-Ennever and Henn 1976). These converging inputs to the pons are illustrated schematically in figure 13.1. In the cat and monkey the PPRF has long been implicated in the production of visually triggered head and eye movements. Units have been isolated in the PPRF of the cat that fire in conjunction with spontaneous head movements (e.g., Siegel and McGinty 1977) and axons originating in the PPRF of this species appear to synapse on the alpha motor neurons that innervate the neck musculature (Anderson et al. 1971, Peterson et al. 1975). Anatomical studies have also demonstrated projections from the PPRF to the abducens nuclei and/or closely adjacent regions in both the cat (Graybiel 1977) and the monkey (Buttner-Ennever and Henn 1976). Moreover a large number of studies in the monkey have shown a precise relationship between the discharge of different types of cells in the PPRF (the so-called burst cells, pause cells, and tonic cells) and the generation of saccadic eye movements (e.g., Hepp and Henn 1979, Van Gisbergen et al. 1981) and head movements (Lestienne et al. 1981) that constitute a

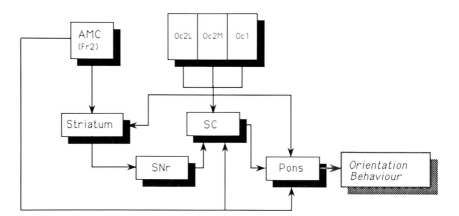

Figure 13.1 Schematic representation of corticofugal pathways that may be involved in the mediation of orientation behavior. The arrows represent single-synapse pathways, although nothing is implied about bifurcating or collateral axons. AMC = anteromedial cortex, part of Fr2 in Zilles's (1985) nomenclature; SC = Superior colliculus; SNr = substantia nigra, pars reticulata. Oc1, Oc2L, and Oc2M refer to different visual areas in the posterior neocortex (see Dean, chapter 12, and Zilles, chapter 4, for details).

shift in gaze.[2] Thus the PPRF may represent a common neural site through which both retinotectal and retinogeniculocortical systems can operate in the control of visually triggered orientation movements of the head and/or eyes. There are also converging inputs from visual cortical areas and the superior colliculus on the dorsolateral pontine nuclei and the nucleus reticularis tegmenti pontis in the rat, both of which provide a possible route for cortical and collicular input to the cerebellar circuits involved in orientation movements of the head and eyes (Burne et al. 1981).

If two such channels to brainstem nuclei exist—one cortical, the other collicular—it is no longer a puzzle why lesions of the superior colliculus result in only a partial disruption of orienting movements. Nor is it surprising that subsequent lesions of the striate cortex wipe out the residual orienting ability of the collicular animals (e.g., Mlinar and Goodale 1984). One problem remains, however. Unlike the work on rat and gerbil (or tree shrew, cat, and monkey, for that matter), none of the work on Syrian hamsters, including Schneider's original study, has given any indication of spared orienting behavior following collicular lesions (Mort et al. 1980, Schneider 1967, 1969). One major difference between the hamster work and the work on rats and gerbils lies in the technique used to make the collicular lesions. Rather than removing the tectal laminae by direct aspiration or destroying them with electrolytic or radiofrequency lesions, investigators working with hamsters have used a vibrating knife to undercut the superior colliculus, thereby transecting the pathways originating from the deep collicular layers. The possibility exists therefore that they may have interrupted corticofugal pathways traveling through the tegmentum on their way to the pontine nuclei.

The cortical projection system to the pontine nuclei may be particularly concerned with orientation movements of the head and eyes to stimuli in the central portions of the visual field since movements in this part of the field are most often spared after large lesions of the superior colliculus. This may represent the emergence of a cortically based visuomotor system for the control of orienting movements within the operating space directly in front of the animal. Whatever the function of this system might be, it appears to have been integrated with a phylogenetically older tectofugal system that mediates orienting movements to salient stimuli throughout the entire visual field.

The Effects of Cortical Lesions on Orientation Behavior
Although the notion of two parallel visuomotor channels to pontine nuclei can account for the fact that lesions of the superior colliculus result in only partial deficits in orientation behavior, it also implies that deficits in orienting should follow lesions restricted to visual cortical areas. Such deficits, however, might be expected for other reasons as well. Like other mammals, rodents have a number of projections from

the cortex to the superior colliculus itself (see figure 13.1). One of the most prominent of these is the occipitotectal projection that originates in Oc1 and the surrounding cortex and terminates in a retinotopic fashion on the superficial and intermediate layers of the superior colliculus in both rat (Lund 1964, 1966, Olavarria and van Sluyters 1982) and hamster (Rhoades and Chalupa 1978). Corticotectal projections have also been described in the rat from a number of other regions of the visual cortex including parts of the anteromedial cortex, corresponding to a portion of Zilles's (1985) area Fr2, that are thought to be homologous with the frontal eye field or area 8 in the monkey (Beckstead 1979, Kolb 1984, Leonard 1969, Tehovnik et al. in press, Wyss and Sripanidkulchai 1984). A possible role for these corticotectal inputs in the control of orientation behavior is discussed later in this section.

In addition to the direct projections from the cortex to the superior colliculus, there is evidence of a cortico-striato-nigro-tectal projection system on both rat (Faull et al. 1986, Williams and Faull 1985) and hamster (Rhoades et al. 1982). As figure 13.1 indicates, some of these projections arise in Oc1 and surrounding cortical areas and are relayed via the striatum and substantia nigra pars reticulata to the deeper layers of the superior colliculus. Other projections to this system originate in the anteromedial cortex and terminate directly on the dendrites of striatonigral neurons (Somogyi et al. 1981). The role of the cortico-striato-nigro-tectal circuit in visually guided behavior is not well understood. Electrophysiological studies in both monkey (Hikosaka and Wurtz 1985a,b) and rat (Chevalier, Deniau, Thierry, and Feger 1981, Chevalier, Thierry, Shibazaki, and Feher 1981, Chevalier et al. 1985, DiChiara et al. 1979) have shown that the nigral input to the colliculus is largely tonic and inhibitory. Although the striatal input to the nigrotectal cells is also largely inhibitory (Crossman et al. 1973, Dray et al. 1976, Feltz 1971, Precht and Yoshida 1971), it is likely that in this case the inhibition is more phasic because the spontaneous activity of striatal units is typically very low (Dray 1980). Because it has been shown that activation of the striatum can disinhibit tectal cells (Chevalier et al. 1985), the possibility exists that the anteromedial cortex and other visual cortical areas may exert some control over orientation behavior via this double-inhibitory route to the superior colliculus. Although there is little behavioral work on the system as a whole in either the monkey or the rat, Wurtz and Hikosaka (1986) have argued, on the basis of the known anatomy and behavioral electrophysiology in the monkey, that the cortico-striato-nigro-tectal system (particularly the circuit involving area 8) may play a role in the initiation of saccades to remembered targets or in the production of saccadic eye movements in the absence of direct sensory guidance.[3]

Although the effects of lesions in the visual areas of the cortex on orientation behavior (while the superior colliculus is still intact) cannot be attributed with certainty to interruptions of the corticotectal, corticopontine, or cortico-striato-nigro-tectal pathways (or to interruptions in any one of a myriad of other output pathways), the presence of deficits in visually triggered head movements following cortical lesions would suggest that the mechanisms controlling visual orientation behavior in the rodent are not entirely mediated by retinotectal circuitry.[4]

In a recent study on gerbils by Mlinar and Goodale (1984), subtle deficits in orientation behavior were observed following large lesions of the posterior neocortex that included area Oc1 and extended well into Oc2M and Oc2L.[5] The gerbils in this study were trained to enter the center of a circular arena via a tunnel located beneath the arena (figure 13.2). As soon as they emerged from the tunnel exit, a small light (subtending either 1° or 5° of visual angle) was illuminated. The light marked the location of a hidden sunflower seed that could be recovered by the gerbil. The head turns and locomotor behavior of the gerbil were

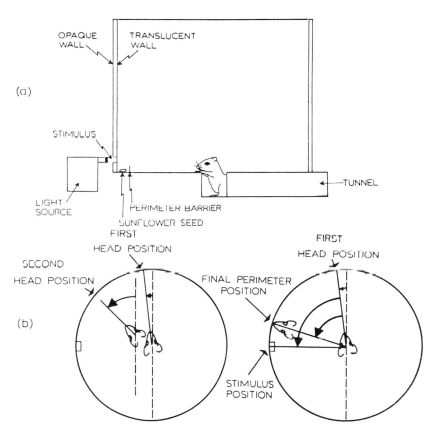

Figure 13.2 Schematic diagram (not to scale) of apparatus used in experiment by Mlinar and Goodale (1984) to test orientation movements in the Mongolian gerbil. (A) Cross section of the perimeter. (B) Overhead view illustrating the calculation of the angles that represent initial head turn amplitude, final perimeter position, and stimulus position. The dashed lines represent the reference axes used for each calculation. The amplitude of the initial head turn was defined as the difference between the first and second head positions. The final perimeter position and the stimulus position were also calculated with reference to the first head position.

videotaped and analyzed by means of a computer-assisted digitizing system. Sham-operated animals typically produced a sequence of head turns before running quickly and accurately toward the light that marked the position of the sunflower seed. On many trials they appeared to be scanning the arena because their initial head turn was made into the visual half-field away from the target, and yet they rarely ran into that half-field but instead turned back in the correct direction. Moreover, even though their initial head turn toward the target nearly always undershot its position, they made one or more additional head turns to bring the target into a position directly ahead of them. In contrast the animals with lesions of the posterior neocortex rarely produced more than a single head turn. As a result they would frequently undershoot the position of the target (particularly if it was located more peripherally) or would even run into the visual half-field opposite the target if their head turn had been made into that half-field. *Thus although animals with posterior neocortex lesions were capable of making head turns in this situation, they seemed unable to make any further adjustments in their orientation to the target.* As figure 13.3 illustrates, the tendency for the head turn to determine the ultimate trajectory followed by the animals in the group was reflected in a tight correlation between head-turn amplitude and final perimeter position. One must speculate that these animals were "victims" of their basic collicular circuitry and, in the absence of cortical modulation, could no longer modify their orientation behavior. As we indicated above, however, it is difficult to determine whether the deficit in these animals was due to an interruption in the corticotectal projections to the superior colliculus, the cortico-striato-

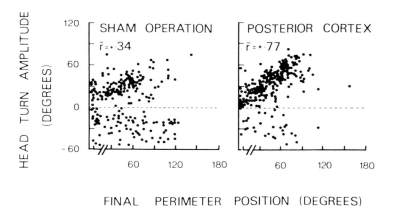

FINAL PERIMETER POSITION (DEGREES)

Figure 13.3 Scatterplots illustrating the relationship between the amplitude of the initial head turn and the final perimeter position for gerbils with sham operations and lesions of the posterior neocortex (areas 17, 18a, and 18b) in the experiment by Mlinar and Goodale (1984). Each point represents a single trial. Head turns and locomotor responses made into the same visual half-field are plotted above the dashed line; head turns and locomotor responses that were made into opposite visual half-fields are plotted below the line. Mean correlations between head turn amplitude and final perimeter position are also indicated.

nigro-tectal projections to the superior colliculus, or the corticopontine projections to the premotor nuclei that receive converging inputs from the superior colliculus.

There are other sorts of deficits following lesions of the posterior neocortex that are more easily attributed to disruptions of the cortico-tectal rather than the cortico-striato-nigro-tectal or corticopontine pathways. Ingle (1977a, 1981), for example, observed that bilateral lesions of the primary visual cortex in the gerbil abolished the animal's ability to make "anticipatory overshoots" when turning its head toward moving visual targets. Instead of making larger head turns for stimuli moving into the temporal visual field as normal gerbils do (Ingle et al. 1979), gerbils with visual cortical lesions simply turned toward the initial position of the target. In other words, they behaved like frogs and toads (Ingle 1982), "precortical" vertebrates that do not show anticipatory orienting but instead rely on the speed of their response and their wide and sticky tongue to catch their prey. The absence of anticipatory overshoots in the gerbils with cortical lesions suggests that information about the direction (and perhaps the velocity) of target movement is no longer available to the collicular circuitry mediating the orienting movements. One possible source of this motion information in the intact animal is the corticotectal projection originating from Oc1. There have been a number of demonstrations in the cat (Wickelgren and Sterling 1969) and the rabbit (Graham et al. 1982) that the directional selectivity of motion-sensitive units in the superior colliculus is abolished or substantially reduced following ipsilateral ablation of the striate cortex. Moreover elegant experiments in the cat by Palmer and Rosenquist (1974) have demonstrated that the directional selectivity is conferred on the collicular units by cells in layer 5 of the striate cortex that project directly to the colliculus via the corticotectal pathway. In the hamster too there is evidence that the directional selectivity of collicular units is lost following removal of the striate cortex (Rhoades and Chalupa 1978). Although a number of studies have found directionally selective units in the superior colliculus of the rat (Fukada and Iwama 1978, Siminoff et al. 1966), they appear to be less numerous and less sharply tuned than those in the hamster. In contrast to the work on cats and hamsters, Humphrey (1968) found no effect of cortical ablation on the receptive-field characteristics of collicular units in the rat. It should be pointed out, however, that unlike Fukada and Iwama (1978) and Siminoff and colleagues (1966), Humphrey (1968) found no evidence for directionally selective units in the rat colliculus, which makes it unlikely that he would have found changes after cortical ablation. Although it is true that the amplitude of the light-evoked potential in the superior colliculus has been shown to be reduced after ablation of the ipsilateral posterior neocortex in the rat (Goodale 1973), this says nothing about the contribution of this cortical area to directional tuning of collicular cells. It may be that the receptive-field properties of some of the directionally selective cells in the rat's colliculus, like those in the ground squirrel (Michael 1972), do not depend entirely on cortical input; Hughes (1980), for example, has found evidence for a small number of directionally selective units in the optic nerve of the rat, a finding that suggests that some of the directional tuning of the collicular units may be provided by direct retinal input. Although there have been no electrophysiological studies of the effects of cortical ablation on the receptive-field characteristics of collicular cells in the gerbil, recent work by Ellard (personal communication, 1989) has shown that some of the collicular units in this species, like those in the rat and hamster, are also motion sensitive.

Deficits in orientation behavior have also been reported in the rat following lesions of the anteromedial cortex (part of Fr2), which, as mentioned above, contains a region thought to be homologous with the frontal eye field of primates (Kolb 1984). In many ways the deficits are similar to those reported in monkeys (and humans) with lesions in this area (for an example of deficits in monkeys, see Schiller et al. 1980; for an example of deficits in humans, see Guitton et at. 1985). Thus rats with unilateral lesions of the anteromedial cortex show a contralateral neglect and, like monkeys and humans with similar lesions, often fail to orient to visual, auditory, and tactile stimuli presented on the side contralateral to the lesion (Cowey and Bozek 1974, Crowne 1983, Crowne and Pathria 1982). Moreover, like monkeys and humans, there is often complete recovery from this orienting deficit several weeks later. Rats with bilateral lesions, again like monkeys with similar lesions, show less dramatic deficits than animals with unilateral lesions; they show no impairment in orientation movements of the head in a hole-board test or during a visual distraction test (Foreman 1983a,b). Recent work by Sinnamon and Charman (1988) indicates that the anteromedial cortex in the rat may play an inhibitory role in the control of head movements by suppressing responses to salient stimuli. In their experiments rats with unilateral and bilateral lesions had difficulty in withholding orienting head movements to unrewarded positions in a learned orientation task even though they had no difficulty in making orienting movements to rewarded sites. This dissociation is reminiscent of that experienced by patients with frontal eye field lesions who could make saccades toward visual targets in either hemifield, but had trouble learning to make saccades *away* from the targets (Guitton et al. 1985).

In addition to the lesion studies, there have also been a number of stimulation and recording experiments that point to a role for portions of the anteromedial cortex of rats in orientation behavior. Contraversive eye movements have been reported following electrical stimulation of the medial precentral region of the anteromedial cortex (Donoghue and Wise 1982; Hall and Lindholm 1974), the region that projects to the superior colliculus (Beckstead 1979, Leonard 1969). Head movements have also been observed following stimulation of this region, and the sites from which such movements can be elicited appear to be topographically organized (Sinnamon and Galer 1984). In an electrophysiological study of the anteromedial cortex (Kanki et al. 1983), the activity of some of the neurons was found to be correlated with head movements, in particular directions. Like the lesion studies then, these experiments have revealed an organization in a region of the rat's anteromedial cortex similar to that found in the frontal eye fields of the monkey. At present, however, it is difficult to conclude very much about how this cortical area is contributing to the control of orientation behavior in the rat. The fact that some of the lesion work (Sinnamon and Charman 1988) points to an inhibitory role for this area, permitting the animal to override the tendency to orient to salient stimuli, suggests that the mechanisms involved represent a fairly high-order modulation of the orientation networks.

Multiple Channels in the Control of Orientation Behavior?
The work of orientation behavior outlined in the previous section shows that the behavior of orienting the head and/or eyes to a discrete visual target depends on a complicated interaction between several visuomotor pathways (see figure 13.1). Although the tectofugal system can mediate head turns and eye movements to stimuli occurring anywhere throughout the entire visual field, output from the geniculostriate pathway and its cortical targets appears to play an important role in the control of orienting movements to stimuli in the central portion of the visual field. The cortical control of these orienting movements may involve direct projections to premotor nuclei in the pontine reticular formation that parallel those from the superior colliculus. In addition to this parallel input to the pons, information from the geniculostriate system may modulate collicular output via direct corticotectal projections, particularly in the case of moving visual stimuli. Finally, cortical modulation of collicular processing may also depend on cortico-striato-nigro-tectal projections. It is clear that the superior colliculus is neither necessary nor sufficient for the production of all orienting movements and that several different cortical projection systems may contribute to this class of behaviors.

13.2 The Role of the Cortex in Visually Elicited Escape

Although there is surprisingly little work on visually guided escape in any mammalian species (but see Blanchard et al. 1986, Merker 1980, Schneider et al. 1987), work in the frog has shown that descending tectofugal projections paly a fundamental role in this important behavior (Ingle 1982). Recent work in our laboratory (Ellard and Goodale 1988) has shown that gerbils with bilateral lesions of the superior colliculus or its descending ipsilateral projections to tegmentum and pons no longer attempt to escape from rapidly looming visual stimuli. Although we have not tested gerbils with lesions of Oc1 in this situation, similar lesions in the hamster do not appear to affect visually driven escape (Schneider et al. 1987). There is, however, a modification of the typical pattern of escape in the gerbil that might depend on cortical pathways. If a safe haven (a small tube) is provided in the test arena, the gerbil after 5 minutes' exposure to the situation will often head for the tube when the looming visual stimulus is presented, no matter what direction the gerbil is facing in the arena, even if it must run toward rather than away from the threatening stimulus (Ellard 1988, Ellard and Goodale 1988). It is possible that this behavior, which involves remembering the location of the safe haven even when it is not in view, may involve cortical modulation of the basic visually elicited escape mechanism in which the colliculus is the major player.

13.3 The Role of the Cortex in Visually Guided Locomotion

Locomotion toward Targets

Although visually guided locomotion toward a target was originally subsumed under the term *orientation behavior* in Schneider's (1969) original discussion of collicular function, a number of later studies have shown that rats (Dyer et al. 1976, Goodale et al. 1978, Goodale and Murison 1975) and gerbils (Goodale and Milner 1982, Mlinar and Goodale 1984) with complete lesions of the superior colliculus are capable of locomoting accurately toward discrete visual targets, provided they have already brought the target into the central portion of their visual field. Even hamsters with undercut colliculi can locomote efficiently toward visual targets (Mort et al. 1980). Similar observations have been made following large collicular lesions in tree shrew (Casagrande and Diamond 1974) and cats (Tunkl and Berkley 1974). In short any deficit in locomotion that has been observed in animals with collicular lesions appears to have been due to a failure to turn toward a stimulus that was initially presented in the peripheral visual field. Once the stimulus is located in the anterior field, the animal has no trouble locomoting accurately toward it.

In contrast to the performance of animals with collicular lesions, animals with visual cortical lesions (Oc1 with some involvement of Oc2M and Oc2L) can show large deficits on this task. Goodale and Murison (1975), for example, found that rats with such lesions failed to approach a low-contrast target door under visual control, even when it was located well within the anterior portion of the visual field. Although posterior neodecorticate gerbils show no evidence for a deficit in visually guided locomotion to high-contrast targets (Goodale and Milner 1982), gerbils with the same kind of lesions behaved like the posterior neodecorticate rats described above when faced with the task of running to a target hole in an arena covered with a vertical black and white grating; i.e., they ran forward from the arena entrance until they encountered the wall opposite, where they appeared to search for the opening using their vibrissae (Goodale 1983b). These results suggest that cortical mechanisms (probably dependent on geniculate input) play an important role in disembedding targets from the visual array during locomotion, particularly when the acuity demands are high. The routes by which these cortical mechanisms access the motor programs controlling target-directed locomotion are not known. It is clear, however, that although cortical circuitry is involved, the retinotectal system is not an essential participant in the mediation of this behavior. What remains a puzzle is how the animal locomotes accurately to high-contrast targets in the absence of visual cortex (Goodale and Milner 1982). Are other cortical regions involved, or is the superior colliculus by itself capable of mediating visually guided locomotion when the acuity demands are not too high? Dean (chapter 12) argues that because animals with large lesions of the posterior neocortex are still sensitive to self-produced visual motion, this information may be used to separate a target from its background, particularly if it is a large, high-contrast target.

Locomotion around Barriers
In the real world rodents often have to avoid barriers, such as a clump of vegetation, as they run toward a food item or conspecific they have spotted. Although there have been few laboratory investigations of barrier avoidance in mammals, the work that has been carried out indicates that both cortex and pretectal mechanisms may be involved. Whereas gerbils with collicular lesions could successfully negotiate a barrier (a piece of transparent plastic covered with vertical black bars and subtending some 80° of visual angle) placed between them and a high-contrast visual target, animals with lesions of the posterior neocortex (including Oc1 and parts of the surrounding cortex) often collided with the barrier or failed to go around it as efficiently as could normal animals (Goodale 1983b). Not only would the posterior decorticate animals run into the barrier when the target was located behind it, they would also run toward it on about one-half of the trials in which the target was not obscured by the barrier but was instead in plain view on other side of it. The reasons for the deficit in these animals are unclear. The terminal fields of a number of different thalamic nuclei were aspirated and the observed deficits could have arisen from the disruption of any one of a number of different visuomotor pathways, including the reciprocal projections from the cortex to the pretectum, a structure that has been shown to play a role in barrier avoidance in both the gerbil (Goodale 1983b) and the frog (Ingle 1977b).

Finally, it is interesting to speculate about the role of the striatum in the avoidance of barriers. As was discussed previously, Wurtz and Hikosaka (1986) have argued that in the monkey, the cortico-striato-nigro-tectal circuit may play a role in organizing saccades to remembered targets. What about remembered barriers? Hoff and Ingle (1988) have recently shown that frogs escaping from a visual threat will avoid jumping into an area where an obstacle was recently seen, even when that obstacle has been removed by the experimenter. They went on to show that lesions of the striatum abolished this tendency to avoid remembered obstacles, but had no effect on the frogs' ability to avoid obstacles in plain view (Ingle and Hoff 1988). Instead of appealing to a striato-nigro-tectal circuit (or its homolog in the frog), Ingle and Hoff (1988) suggest that striatal projections to the ventromedial tegmentum are responsible for this behavior via direct tegmental projections to the medulla and cord. Similar experiments could be easily carried out in rodents and might shed light on the role of the striatum (and its cortical inflow) in mediating different kinds of visually guided behavior in these animals.

The Visual Calibration of Jumping

Both rats (Russel 1932) and gerbils (Ellard et al. 1984) can jump accurately from one surface to another over a wide range of distances. Ellard and colleagues (1984) have shown that the gerbil uses a number of static and dynamic depth cues to calibrate the amplitude of the required jump in this situation, and the final estimate of the distance to be jumped is a weighted average of these different cues. One of the most important distance cues in this situation is the retinal motion that is generated by the series of vertical translation movements of the head (or head bobs) that the gerbil produces just before it jumps. Work by Ellard and associates (1986) has shown that even though gerbils with lesions of Oc1 (with minimal involvement of areas Oc2L and Oc2M) continued to produce head bobs when they were placed on the jumping apparatus, their jumps were far less accurate than those of sham-operated animals (figure 13.4). The variance in their landing position was much higher than that of the sham-operated animals, and they missed the landing platform completely on nearly half the trials. Because Oc1 in rat (Parnavelas et al. 1981, Shaw et al. 1975, Wiesenfeld and Kornel 1975), mouse (Drager 1975, Mangini and Pearlman 1980), and hamster (Tiao and Blakemore 1976) contains a high proportion of motion-sensitive cells, it is likely that the same is true of the gerbil and that the lesions abolished the ability of these animals to make use of motion cues in the calibration of jump amplitude. It is equally likely, however, that the use of other cues such as retinal disparity and loom was also disrupted by the cortical lesions.

The fact that the jump produced by animals with striate lesions showed some relation to the size of the gap between the two platforms, however badly those jumps may have been calibrated, suggests that the animals were still capable of using some kind of distance cue. One possibility was retinal image size, a very salient cue in this situation because the size of the landing platform remained constant from trial to trial. Normal gerbils make ready use of this learned distance cue in

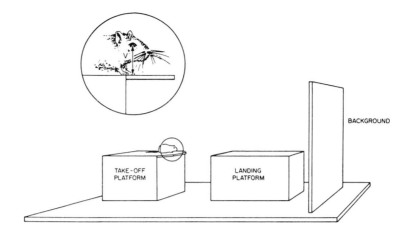

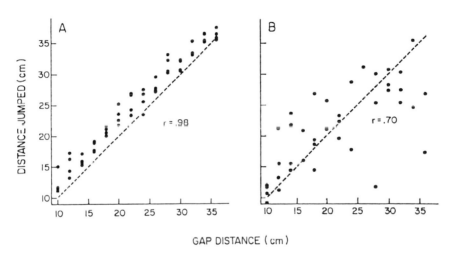

Figure 13.4 The diagram shows the jumping situation employed by Ellard and associates (1984, 1986) and Carey and colleagues (1987). The inset indicates that vertical (V) translation movements of the head were measured with respect to the eye. The graphs show distance jumped as a function of gap distance in the experiment by Ellard and colleagues (1986). Each point represents the performance of an animal on a single trial. The x,y axis represents the leading edge of the landing platform. Overall correlations for each group are also shown. (A) Sham operate group. (B) Visual cortex group (Oc1 with some invasion of 18a and 18b).

calibrating their jumps (Goodale et al. 1989). This was demonstrated by the use of "probe" trials, where landing platforms smaller or larger than the standard training platform were inserted randomly among regular training trials. With small probe platforms (which, on the basis of their smaller retinal image, would appear further away than they actually were) normal gerbils overjumped the edge of the platform; with large probe platforms (which would appear closer) they underjumped and often fell short of the platform's edge. We have recently shown that although the landing positions of gerbils with complete lesions of Oc1, extending in this case well into Oc2M and Oc2L, were more variable than those of sham-operated animals (as they had been in the earlier study), they were just as sensitive as normal animals to the retinal image size manipulation, overjumping with small probe platforms and underjumping with larger ones (Carey et al. 1987). The effect of this manipulation for both sham-operated animals and animals with lesions of Oc1 is shown in figure 13.5.

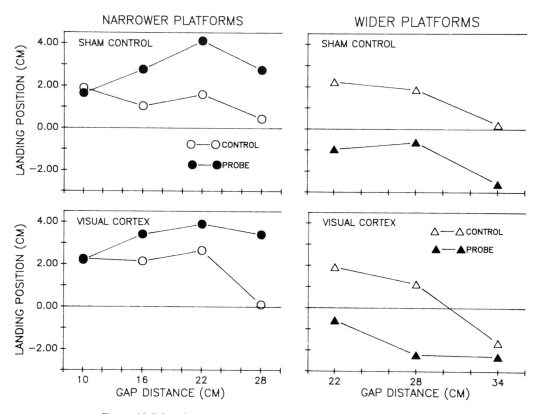

Figure 13.5 Landing position as a function of gap distance for probe and control trials in the experiment by Carey and colleagues (1987). Positive scores indicate an overjump; negative scores an underjump. Except for the fact that the landing platform on probe trials was smaller or larger than the standard platform used on control trials, there were no other differences between the trials. The task was essentially similar to that depicted in figure 13.4.

The fact that these animals could use the differences in retinal image size to calibrate the amplitude of their jumps might seem surprising given the fact that rats (Lashley 1939) and monkeys (Kluver 1941) with striate lesions could not discriminate between two stimuli differing in size when they were equated for luminous flux (the total amount of light falling on the retina).[6] In the Carey and colleagues (1987) study, however, the gerbils could not have been using luminous flux cues because the testing environment were brightly lit and the amount of incident light at the end of the take-off platform did not vary systematically with platform distance. To have been sensitive to changes in the distance of the platform (as indicated by changes in the visual angle subtended by that platform), the visuomotor system calibrating the jump amplitude in these animals must have been capable of disembedding the platform from the rest of the visual array. Furthermore this system, which must be extrageniculate, would have needed to use the size of this disembedded image to compute the distance of the required jump. What is interesting is that same kind of information apparently could not be used by rats with similar lesions to choose the bigger (or smaller) of two stimuli in a traditional discrimination paradigm (Lashley 1939). The difference between these two situations is largely one of response requirements: In one case the animal uses retinal image size as a variable in an algorithm that, once calibrated, solves for distance on the basis of an invariant law of physics; in the other the animal is asked very arbitrarily to approach one stimulus and not the other. In the former case the invariant nature of the distance/image-size relationship is one that a lot of vertebrates (and other organisms as well) are likely to use for programming ballistic movements and could be quite "hard-wired," phylogenetically ancient (Collett and Harkness 1982), and relatively independent of cortical modulation. In the latter case the attachment of "value" to a particular stimulus is arguably much more "cognitive" and may therefore depend on quite plastic cortical mechanisms.

13.4 Is There a Role for the Cortex in Visually Guided Reaching?

In the monkey there is ample evidence that visual areas in the cerebral cortex have an important role to play in visually guided reaching and grasping (for comprehensive reviews see Humphrey 1979 and Hyvarinen 1985). Whereas Krieg's area 7 in the rat (corresponding to the most rostal parts of Oc2L and Oc2M) is thought to be analogous to the posterior parietal region of primates (Kolb and Walkey 1987) and receives visual inputs from the primary visual cortex (Montero et al. 1973) and the lateral posterior nucleus (Hughes 1977), there have been no studies of the effects of lesions in this area on visually guided reaching with the forelimbs in this species. Since the early work of Peterson and colleagues on paw preference in the rat (Peterson 1934, Peterson and

Fracarol 1938), a good number of studies have examined the role of the cortex and the basal ganglia in skilled forelimb reaching in this animal (Castro, chapter 24). But despite the fact that a number of the lesions used in these studies included the rostral parts of areas Oc2L and Oc2M, the effects of these lesions on the *visual control* of forelimb reaching was not examined. As it turns out, there may have been no effect anyway because recent work by Whishaw and Tomie (1989) has revealed that in the normal rat it is olfaction rather than vision that provides the distal-stimulus control of reaching in this animal. In the study occluding the eyes had no effect on the rats' ability to reach for food pellets, whereas removing the olfactory bulbs resulted in near-random reaches at all possible locations. But although area 7 might not play a role in the visual control of skilled reaching movements in the rat, this region may still contribute to other visuomotor behaviors such as eye and head movements as well as whole-body movements. Unfortunately there have been no studies of these particular patterns of behavior following lesions restricted to area 7 that are comparable to the detailed work on the effects of lesions in the anteromedial cortex, Oc1, or the superior colliculus. Finally, it should be emphasized that other rodents, such as gerbils and squirrels, that are diurnal or crepuscular may be more dependent on visual information to guide reaching and grasping movements with the forepaws. For a review of how ecological constraints might affect the evolution of rodent visual systems, see Finlay and Sengelaub (1981).

The only clear demonstrations of what might be considered visual deficits following lesions of the parietal area in the rat are disruptions in performance on place and landmark navigation tasks (e.g., Kolb and Walkey 1987) and complex mazes (e.g., Kolb et al. 1983). Unfortunately in none of this work was any attention paid to visuomotor control per se. Instead the focus was on the effects of such lesions on spatial navigation or motor learning. Thus on the basis of work carried out to date, it is difficult to conclude anything about the role of the parietal cortex in the visuomotor behavior of rats (or any other rodent).

13.5 Conclusions

Throughout this chapter we have tried to emphasize the importance of treating the visual system as a sensorimotor rather than a perceptual system. Without denying that there are many "visuocognitive" functions that are independent of any particular motor act, we would maintain that a complete understanding of vision and the visual pathways demands close attention to the motor outputs of the system as well as to the sensory inputs. The two visual systems hypothesis was an important first step in this direction, but it was not sufficiently precise about the motor behavior mediated by different visual pathways. As we tried to show, it is not enough to talk about localizing or identifying a visual stimulus; one has to come to grips with how the pattern of electromagnetic radiation dancing on the retina is transformed into different patterns of motor behavior.

Visual cortex has traditionally been considered part of the perceptual machinery of the visual system, and as we have seen, the two-visual-systems story did little to change that view. For this reason there have been relatively few studies of the visuomotor functions of different cortical areas. This has been particularly true of the rat, perhaps because it has been regarded as a much less "visual" animal than the cat or monkey. Nevertheless, as we tried to document, there is ample evidence that corticofugal systems in the rodent (such as the corticopontine, corticotectal, and cortico-striato-nigro-tectal pathways) play an important role in the visual control of the orienting movements of the head and eyes, the visual control of target-directed locomotion and the avoidance of barriers, and the visual calibration of jumping. Much of this control is exercised through modulation of other retinofugal systems such as the superior colliculus and its outputs, as is the case for cat and monkey as well. There are many other behaviors, however, such as visually elicited escape, for which a possible cortical contribution has not been investigated in any detail. Moreover, even for those visuomotor behaviors in which the cortex has been shown to be involved, most evidence has come from lesions (and rather large lesions at that). There have been very few studies in which electrophysiological recordings have been made of units in the visual cortex (and other retinofugal targets) while the rat is engaged in different visuomotor behaviors. Indeed it is paradoxical that work on the neural substrates of visuomotor behavior is so-called lower vertebrates, such as the frog and toad, as well as work on higher mammals, such as the monkey, should be so much more sophisticated than that carried out on the rat, an animal whose phylogeny at least would place it somewhere in between these two points on the vertebrate line. Given the resurgence of interest in the anatomical organization of the cortex in the rat and its ontogenetic development, one can only hope that the study of cortical contributions to visuomotor control take advantage not only of the new information about how the visual cortex is organized but of the new technologies that are emerging for the measurement of motor behavior.

Notes

Much of the research described in this chapter was supported by Grant #A6313 from the Natural Sciences and Engineering Research Council of Canada to M. A. Goodale.

1. It should be pointed out that the resolution acuity of the eye cannot be predicted from ganglion cell density alone. One must also know the focal length of the eye. Since the rat eye is so much smaller than the cat eye. for example, it would have to have a much higher ganglion cell density to achieve the same resolution acuity. Since it does not, the rat has far poorer acuity than the cat.

2. Although there have been a number of studies demonstrating the existence of spinal projections from the n. reticularis pontis oralis and caudalis in the rat (e.g., Satoh 1979), there appears to be no work in rodents on projections from this region to the abducens or any other cranial nerve nuclei that might be involved in the production of eye movements. There are also no recording studies that have looked at the activity of cells in these region with respect to eye movements in these animals. Rats are certainly capable of making quite large eye movements; spontaneous saccades of up to 15° have been observed (Fuller 1985). In addition, electrical stimulation of the superior colliculus in rats (with immobilized heads) evokes conjugate eye movements of similar magnitude and has revealed a topographic organization similar to that observed in other mammals (McHaffie and Stein 1980). Similar electrical stimulation studies of the striate cortex and other visual cortical areas have not been attempted in the rat.

3. Behavioral work on striatal and nigral circuitry in the rat has paid little attention to the cortico-striato-nigro-tectal projections and has been focused much more on the well-known dopaminergic projections from substantia nigra pars compacta to striatum. It has been repeatedly demonstrated in both the rat (and the cat), for example, that a unilateral lesion of the striatum or its dopaminergic input (by local intracerebral infusion of 6-OHDA into pars compacta of the substantia nigra or electrolytic lesions of the same structure) results in a persistent failure of the animal to orient to stimuli (tactile, somesthetic, olfactory, and visual) presented on the contralesional side (Dunnett and Iversen 1982; Feeney and Wier 1979; Ljunberg and Ungerstedt 1976; Marshall et al. 1980). It is entirely possible of course that this deficit in orientation, which has sometimes been characterized as "sensory inattention" or "neglect," is due to the fact that the superior colliculus ipsilateral to the striatal lesion may be continually inhibited by nigrotectal inputs that are no longer subject to inhibition from striatonigral inputs. In short, the lesion may have removed the first part of the double-inhibitory circuit that has been shown to modulate tectal activity (Chevalier et al. 1985). Indirect evidence for this conclusion comes from recent experiments on rats with this kind of lesion that have been given systemic injections of apomorphine, a dopaminergic-receptor blocker, and then a unilateral lesion of the ipsilateral superior colliculus (DiChiara et al. 1982). Apomorphine typically produces forced contraversive circling in animals with unilateral nigrostriatal lesions, and it is usually thought that this is due to supersensitivity of the dopaminergic-receptors in the denervated striatum (Ungerstedt 1971). In the experiments by DiChiara and associates (1982), however, an additional lesion of the ipsilateral superior colliculus was found to reduce or even reverse the contraversive circling normally elicited by peripheral administration of apomorphine. This result suggests that the striatal neurons sensitive to dopamine-agonists are intimately connected with the striato-nigro-tectal system and that the circling behavior is due to a massive disinhibition of the superior colliculus ipsilateral to the nigrostriatal lesion.

4. A possibility that we have not discussed in that damage to cortical circuits that receive input from the superior colliculus (via the lateral posterior thalamic nucleus) could result in deficits in orientation behavior. The projection fields of this part of the lateral posterior nucleus (Perry 1980) are certainly contiguous with those cortical regions that contribute to the three corticofugal projections we have just described. Although a lesion study by Hughes (1977) suggested that the lateral posterior nucleus may support visual discrimination learning in rats in the absence of Oc1 (via its projections to the remaining cortex), there have been no studies of orientation behavior following lesions of this structure. In the monkey, however, there have been a number of studies of orientation behavior following lesions of the pulvinar, a structure thought to be homologous with the rodent lateral posterior nucleus. In none of these experiments was there any evidence of deficits in visual orientation behavior (Bender and Baizer 1986; Ungerleider and Christensen 1977, 1979). Even the prolonged fixation times that were observed by Ungerleider and Chris-

tensen (1979) during the scanning of a complex visual scene were probably due to the fact that the corticotectal tract was damaged when heat was used to lesion the pulvinar because monkeys with kainic acid lesions in the same region show no changes in their saccadic eye movements (Bender and Baizer 1986). At the same time, electrophysiological studies have revealed cells in the monkey pulvinar that correlate with saccadic eye movements and shifts in visual attention (e.g., Petersen, et al. 1987). Thus while the tectal route to the cortex via the lateral posterior nucleus/pulvinar undoubtedly plays some role in visually guided behavior, its contribution is not well understood, particularly in rodents.

5. For the sake of consistency we have used the nomenclature introduced by Zilles (1985) to refer to the striate cortex and to the medial and lateral extrastriate regions in the rat. Such divisions of the visual cortex in the gerbil must be regarded as tentative until comparable anatomical and physiological studies are carried out in this species.

6. Some researchers (Dean 1981; McDaniel et al. 1982) have argued that destriate rats are capable of much more than Lashley's original experiments might indicate. They have pointed out that the lesions in Lashley's experiments extended far beyond the boundaries of the striate cortex, and that when lesions are restricted to Oc1 the impairments are far less impressive. In fact it appears to be the degree of damage to the lateral extrastriate cortex (Oc2L and possibly other areas as well) that leads to the kind of deficit observed by Lashley (1939). Dean (chapter 12) has concluded that lesions of Oc1 that do not invade surrounding cortical areas "have little effect on the detection of large, high contrast, low frequency gratings." This kind of explanation, however, cannot account for the findings of Carey and associates (1987). All the gerbils in this study had very large lesions that extended well beyond the boundaries of Oc1 and invaded the lateral extrastriate cortex, much like the extensive lesions made by Lashley.

References

Albano, J. E., and Wurtz, R. H. (1982). Deficits in eye position following ablation of monkey superior colliculus, pretectum, and posterior-medial thalamus. *Journal of Neurophysiology* 48:318–337.

Anderson, M. E., Yoshida, M., and Wilson, V. J. (1971). Influence of superior colliculus on cat neck motoneurons. *Journal of Neurophysiology* 34:898–919.

Beckstead, R. M. (1979). An autoradiographic examination of corticocortical and subcortical projections of the mediodorsal projection (prefrontal) cortex in the rat. *Journal of Comparative Neurology* 184:43–62.

Bender, D. B., and Baizer, J. S. (1986). Effects of kainic acid lesions of the pulvinar on saccadic eye movements in monkeys. *Society of Neuroscience Abstracts* 12(2):1039.

Blanchard, R. J., Flannelly, K. J., and Blanchard, D. C. (1986). Defensive behaviors of laboratory and wild *Rattus norvegicus*. *Journal of Comparative Psychology* 100:101–107.

Burne, R. A., Azizi, S. A., Mihailoff, G. A., and Woodward, D. J. (1981). The tectopontine projection in the rat with comments on visual pathways to the basilar pons. *Journal of Comparative Neurology* 202:287–307.

Buttner-Ennever, J. A., and Henn, V. (1976). An autoradiographic study of the pathways from the pontine reticular formation involved in horizontal eye movements. *Brain Research* 108:155–164.

Carey, D. P., Booth, L. A., and Goodale, M. A. (1987). Can gerbils with lesions of primary visual cortex use retinal image size to estimate distance in a jumping task? *Society for Neuroscience Abstracts* 13(1):629.

Casagrande, V. A., and Diamond, I. T. (1974). Ablation study of the superior colliculus in the tree shrew (*Tupaia glis*). *Journal of Comparative Neurology* 156:207–238.

Chevalier, G., Deniau, J. M., Thierry, A. M., and Ferger, J. (1981). The nigro-tectal pathway. An electrophysiological re-investigation in the rat. *Brain Research* 213:253–263.

Chevalier, G., Thierry, A. M., Shibazaki, T., and Feher, J. (1981). Evidence for a GABA-ergic inhibitory nigrotectal pathway in the rat. *Neuroscience Letters* 21:67–70.

Chevalier, G., Vacher, S., Deniau, J. M., and Desban, M. (1985). Disinhibition as a basic process in the expression of striatal functions. I. The striato-nigral influence on tecto-spinal/tectodiencephalic neurons. *Brain Research* 334:215–226.

Collett, T. S., and Harkness, L. I. K. (1982). Depth vision in animals. In D. J. Ingle, M. A. Goodale, and R. W. J. Mansfield (eds.), *Analysis of visual behavior*. Cambridge, Mass.: M.I.T. Press, 111–176.

Cowey, A., and Bozek, T. (1974). Contralateral 'neglect' after unilateral dorsomedial prefrontal lesions in rats. *Brain Research* 72:53–63.

Crossman, A. R., Walker, R. J., and Woodruff, G. N. (1973). Picrotoxin antagonism of gamma-aminobutyric acid inhibitory responses and synaptic inhibition in the rat substantia nigra. *British Journal of Pharmacology* 49:696–698.

Crowne, D. P. (1983). The frontal eye field and attention. *Psychological Bulletin* 93(2):232–260.

Crowne, D. P., and Pathria, M. H. (1982). Some effects of unilateral frontal lesions in the rat. *Behavioural Brain Research* 6:25–39.

Dean, P. (1981). Grating detection and visual acuity after lesions of striate cortex in hooded rats. *Experimental Brain Research* 43:145–153.

DiChiara, G., Porceddu, M. L., Morelli, M., Mulas, M. L., and Gessa, G. L. (1979). Evidence for a gabaergic projection from the substantia nigra to the ventromedial thalamus and to the superior colliculus in the rat. *Brain Research* 176:273–284.

DiChiara, G., Morelli, M., Imperato, A., and Porceddu, M. L. (1982). A re-evaluation of the role of superior colliculus in turning behaviour. *Brain Research* 237:61–77.

Donoghue, J. P., and Wise, S. P. (1982). The motor cortex of the rat: Cytoarchitecture and microstimulation mapping. *Journal of Comparative Neurology* 212:76–88.

Drager, U. C. (1975). Receptive fields of single cells and topography in mouse visual cortex. *Journal of Comparative Neurology* 160:269–290.

Dray, A. (1980). The physiology and pharmacology of mammalian basal ganglia. *Progress in Neurobiology* 14:221–335.

Dray, A., Gonye, T. J., and Oakley, N. R. (1976). Caudate stimulation and substantia nigra activity in the rat. *Journal of Physiology (London)* 259:825–849.

Dreher, B., Potts, R. A., Ni, S. Y. K., and Bennett, M. R. (1984). The development of heterogeneities in distribution and soma sizes of rat retinal ganglion cells. In J. Stone, B. Dreher, and D. H. Rapaport (eds.), *Development of visual pathways in mammals*. New York: Alan R. Liss, 39–58.

Dreher, B., Sefton, A. J., Ni, S. Y. K., and Nisbett, G. (1985). The morphology, number, and distribution of the class I cells in the retina of the albino and hooded rat. *Brain, Behavior, and Evolution* 26:10–48.

Dunnett, S. B., and Iversen, S. D.(1982). Sensorimotor impairments following localized kanic acid and 6-hydroxydopamine lesions of the neostriatum. *Brain Research* 248:121–27.

Dyer, R. S., Marino, M. F., Johnson, C., and Kruggel, T. (1976). Superior colliculus lesions do not impair orientation to pattern. *Brain Research* 112:176–179.

Edwards, S. B. (1980). The deep cell layers of the superior colliculus: Their reticular characteristics and structural organization. In J. A. Hobson and M. A. B. Brazier (eds.), *The reticular formation revisted: Specifying functions for a non-specific system*. New York: Raven Press, 193–209.

Ellard, C. G. (1988). Visually elicited avoidance in the Mongolian gerbil. *Society for Neuroscience Abstracts* 14(2):832.

Ellard, C. G., and Goodale, M. A. (1988). A functional analysis of the collicular output pathways: A dissociation of deficits following lesions of the dorsal tegmental decussation and the ipsilateral collicular efferent bundle in the Mongolian gerbil. *Experimental Brain Research* 71:307–319.

Ellard, C. G., Goodale, M. A., MacLaren Scorfield, D., and Lawrence, C. (1986). Visual cortical lesions abolish the use of motion parallax in the Mongolian gerbil. *Experimental Brain Research* 64:599–602.

Ellard, C. G., Goodale, M. A., and Timney, B. (1984). Distance estimation in the Mongolian gerbil: The role of dynamic depth cues. *Behavioural Brain Research* 14:29–39.

Faull, R. L. M., Nauta, W. J. H., and Domesick, V. B. (1986). The visual cortico-striato-nigral pathway in the rat. *Neuroscience* 19:1119–1132.

Feeney, D. M., and Wier, C. S. (1979). Sensory neglect after lesions of substantia nigra or lateral hypothalamus: Differential severity and recovery of function. *Brain Research* 178:329–348.

Feltz, P. (1971). Gamma aminobutyric acid and a caudato-nigral inhibition. *Canadian Journal of Physiological Pharmacology* 49:1113–1115.

Finlay, B. L., and Sengelaub, D. R. (1981). Toward a neuroethology of mammalian vision: Ecology and anatomy of rodent visuomotor behavior. *Behavioural Brain Research* 3:133–149.

Foreman, N. (1983a). Distractibility following simultaneous bilateral lesions of the superior colliculus or medial frontal cortex in the rat. *Behavioural Brain Research* 8:177–194.

Foreman, N. (1983b). Head-dipping in rats with superior colliculus, medial frontal cortical and hippocampal lesions. *Physiology and Behavior* 30:711–717.

Fukada, Y., and Iwama, K. (1978). Visual receptive-field properties of single cells in the rat superior colliculus. *Japanese Journal of Physiology* 28:385–400.

Fuller, J. H. (1985). Eye and head movements in the pigmented rat. *Vision Research* 25:1121–1128.

Gattass, R., Sousa, A. P. B., and Covey, E. (1985). Cortical areas of the Macaque: Possible substrates for pattern recognition mechanisms. In C. Chagas, R. Gattass, and C. Gross (eds.), *Pattern recognition mechanisms*. Berlin: Springer Verlag, 1–19.

Goodale, M. A. (1973). Cortico-tectal and intertectal modulation of visual responses in the rat's superior colliculus. *Experimental Brain Research* 17:75–86.

Goodale, M. A. (1983a). Vision as a sensorimotor system. In T. Robinson (ed.), *Behavioral approaches to brain research*. New York: Oxford University Press, 41–61.

Goodale, M. A. (1983b). Neural mechanisms of visual orientation in rodents: Targets versus places. In A. Hein and M. Jeannerod (eds.), *Spatially oriented behavior* New York: Springer Verlag, 35–61.

Goodale, M. A. (1988). Modularity in visuomotor control: From input to output. In Z. Pylyshyn (ed.), *Computational processes in human vision: An interdisciplinary perspective*. Norwood, New Jersey: Ablex, 262–285.

Goodale, M. A., Ellard, C. G., and Booth, L. (1989). The role of image size and retinal motion in the computation of absolute distance by the Mongolian gerbil (*Meriones unguiculatus*). *Vision Research,* in press.

Goodale, M. A., Foreman, N. P., and Milner, A. D. (1978). Visual orientation in the rat: A dissociation of deficits following cortical and collicular lesions. *Experimental Brain Research* 31:445–447.

Goodale, M. A., and Milner, A. D. (1982). Fractionating orientation behavior in the rodent. In D. J. Ingle, M. A. Goodale, and R. J. Mansfield (eds.), *Analysis of visual behavior*. Cambridge, Mass.: MIT Press, 267–299.

Goodale, M. A., Milner, A. D., and Rose, J. E. V. (1975). Susceptibility to startle during ongoing behavior following collicular lesions in the rat. *Neuroscience Letters* 1:333–337.

Goodale, M. A., and Murison, R. C. C. (1975). The effects of lesions of the superior colliculus on locomotor orientation and the orienting reflex in the rat. *Brain Research* 88:243–255.

Graham, J., Berman, N., and Murphy, E. H. (1982). Effects of visual cortical lesions on receptive-field properties of single units in superior colliculus of the rabbit. *Journal of Neurophysiology* 47:272–286.

Graybiel, A. (1977). Direct and indirect preoculomotor pathways of the brainstem: An autoradiographic study of the pontine reticular formation in the cat. *Journal of Comparative Neurology* 175:37–78.

Guitton, D., Buchtel, H. A., and Douglas, R. M. (1985). Frontal lobe lesions in man cause difficulties in suppressing reflexive glances and in generating goal-directed saccades. *Experimental Brain Research* 58:455–472.

Hall, R. D., and Lindholm, E. P. (1974). Organization of motor and somatosensory neocortex in the albino rat. *Brain Research* 66:23–38.

Harting, J. K., Hall, W. C., Diamond, I. T., and Martin, G. F. (1973). Anterograde degeneration study of the superior colliculus in *Tupaia glis*: Evidence for a subdivision between superficial and deep layers. *Journal of Comparative Neurology* 148:361–386.

Hepp, K., and Henn, V. (1979). Neuronal activity preceding rapid eye movements in the brainstem of the alert monkey. In R. Granit and G. Pompeiano (eds.), *Progress in brain research, Vol. 50. Amsterdam: Elsevier, 645–652.*

Hess, S., Burgi, S., and Bucher, J. (1946). Motor function of tectal and tegmental area. *Monatsschrift fur Psychiatrie und Neurologie* 112:1–52.

Hikosaka, O., and Wurtz, R. H. (1985a). Modification of saccadic eye movements by GABA-related substances. I. Effect of muscimol and bicuculline in the monkey superior colliculus. *Journal of Neurophysiology* 53:266–291.

Hikosaka, O., and Wurtz, R. H. (1985b). Modification of saccadic eye movements by GABA-related substances. II. Effects of muscimol in the monkey substantia nigra pars reticulata. *Journal of Neurophysiology* 53:292–308.

Hoff, K. vS., and Ingle, D. J. (1988). Frogs have short-term memory of obstacles. *Society for Neuroscience Abstracts* 14(1):692.

Hubel, D. H., and Wiesel, T. N. (1974). Uniformity of monkey striate cortex: A parallel relationship between field size, scatter and magnification factor. *Journal of Comparative Neurology* 158:295–306.

Hughes, A. (1980). Directional units in the rat optic nerve. *Brain Research* 202:196–200.

Hughes, H. C. (1977). Anatomical and neurobehavioral investigations concerning the thalamo-cortical organization of the rat's visual system. *Journal of Comparative Neurology* 175(3):311–335.

Humphrey, D. R. (1979). On the cortical control of visually directed reaching: Contributions of nonprecentral motor areas. In R. E. Talbott and D. R. Humphrey (eds.), *Posture and movement* New York: Raven Press, 51–112.

Humphrey, N. K. (1968). Responses to visual stimuli of units in the superior colliculus of rats and monkeys. *Experimental Neurology* 20:312–340.

Hyvarinen, J. (1985). Posterior parietal lobe of the primate brain. *Physiological Reviews* 62(3):1060–1123.

Ingle, D. J. (1977a). Role of visual cortex in anticipatory orientation toward moving targets by the gerbil. *Society for Neuroscience Abstracts* 3:68.

Ingle, D. J. (1977b). Detection of stationary objects by frogs (*Rana pipiens*) after ablation of optic tectum. *Journal of Comparative and Physiological Psychology* 91:1359–1364.

Ingle, D. J. (1981). New methods for analysis of vision in the gerbil. *Behavioural Brain Research* 3:151–173.

Ingle, D. J. (1982). Organization of visuomotor behaviors in vertebrates. In D. J. Ingle, M. A. Goodale, and R. W. J. Mansfield (eds.), *Analysis of visual behavior*. Cambridge, Mass.: M.I.T. Press, 67–109.

Ingle, D. J., Cheal, M., and Dizio, P. (1979). Cine analysis of visual orientation and pursuit by Mongolian gerbil. *Journal of Comparative and Physiological Psychology* 93:919–928.

Ingle, D., and Hoff, K. vS. (1988). Neural mechanisms of short-term memory in frogs. *Society for Neuroscience Abstracts* 14(1):692.

Kanki, J. P., Martin, T. L., and Sinnamon, H. M. (1983). Activity of neurons in the anteromedial cortex during rewarding brain stimulation, saccharin consumption and orienting behavior. *Behavioural Brain Research* 8:69–84.

Kluver, H. (1941). Visual functions after removal of the occipital lobes. *Journal of Psychology* 11:23–45.

Kolb, B. (1984). Functions of the frontal cortex of the rat: a comparative review. *Brain Research Reviews* 8:65–98.

Kolb, B., Sutherland, R. J., and Whishaw, I. Q. (1983). A comparison of the contributions of the frontal and parietal association cortex to spatial localization in rats. *Behavioral Neuroscience* 97(1):13–27.

Kolb, B., and Walkey, J. (1987). Behavioral and anatomical studies of the posterior parietal cortex in the rat. *Behavioural Brain Research* 23:127–145.

Lashley, K. S. (1939). The mechanism of vision. XVI. The functioning of small remnants of the visual cortex. *Journal of Comparative Neurology* 70:45–67.

Leonard, C. M. (1969). The prefrontal cortex of the rat. I. Cortical projections of the mediodorsal nucleus. II. Efferent connections. *Brain Research* 12:321–343.

Lestienne, F., Whittington, D. A., and Bizzi, E. (1981). Single cell recording from the pontine reticular formation in monkeys: Behavior of preoculomotor neurons during eye-head coordination. In A. F. Fuchs and W. Becker (eds.), *Progress in oculomotor research*. Amsterdam: Elsevier, 325–334.

Linden, R., and Perry, V. H. (1983). Massive retinotectal projection in rats. *Brain Research* 272:145–149.

Livingstone, M., and Hubel, D. H. (1988). Segregation of form, color, movement, and depth: Anatomy, physiology, and perception. *Science* 240:740–749.

Ljunberg, T., and Ungerstedt, U. (1976). Sensory inattention produced by 6-hydroxydo-pamine-induced degeneration of ascending dopamine neurons in the brain. *Experimental Neurology* 53:585–600.

Lund, R. D. (1964). Terminal distribution in the superior colliculus of fibers originating in the visual cortex. *Nature* 264:1283–1285.

Lund, R. D. (1966). The occipitotectal pathway of the rat. *Journal of Anatomy (London)* 100:51–62.

Mangini, N., and Pearlman, A. L. (1980). Laminar distribution of receptive field properties in the primary visual cortex of the mouse, *Mus musculus. Journal of Comparative Neurology* 193:203–222.

Marshall, J. F. (1978). Comparison of the sensorimotor dysfunctions produced by damage to lateral hypothalamus or superior colliculus in the rat. *Experimental Neurology* 58:203–217.

Marshall, J. R., Berrios, N., and Sawyer, S. (1980). Neostriatal dopamine and sensory inattention. *Journal of Comparative and Physiological Psychology* 94:833–846.

Martin, P. R. (1968). The projection of different retinal ganglion cell classes to the dorsal lateral geniculate nucleus in the hooded rat. *Experimental Brain Research* 62:77–88.

McDaniel, W. F., Coleman, J., and Lindsay, J. F., Jr. (1982). A comparison of lateral peristriate and striate neocortical ablations in the rat. *Behavioral Brain Research* 6:249–272.

McHaffie, J. G., and Stein, B. E. (1980). Control of eye movements in rat superior colliculus. *Society for Neuroscience Abstracts* 6:476.

Merker, B. (1980). *The sentinel hypothesis: A role for the mammalian superior colliculus.* Unpublished doctoral thesis. Cambridge, Mass.: M.I.T. Press.

Michael, C. R. (1972). Functional organization of cells in the superior colliculus of the ground squirrel *Journal of Neurophysiology* 35:833–846.

Midgley, G. C., and Tees, R. C. (1981). Orienting behavior by rats with visual cortical and subcortical lesions. *Experimental Brain Research* 41:316–328.

Mlinar, E. J., and Goodale, M. A. (1984). Cortical and tectal control of visual orientation in the gerbil: Evidence for parallel channels. *Experimental Brain Research* 55:33–48.

Mohler, C. W., and Wurtz, R. H. (1977). Role of striate cortex and superior colliculus in visual guidance of saccadic eye movements in monkeys. *Journal of Neurophysiology* 40:74–94.

Montero, V. M. (1981). Comparative studies on the visual cortex. In N. Woolsey (ed.), *Cortical sensory organization*, Vol. 2. Clifton, N.J.: Humana Press, 33–81.

Montero, V. M., Bravo, H., and Fernandez, V. (1973). Striate-peristriate cortico-cortical connections in the albino and gray rat. *Brain Research* 53:202–207.

Mort, E., Cairns, S., Hersch, H., and Finlay, B. (1980). The role of the superior colliculus in visually-guided locomotion and visual orientation in the hamster. *Physiological Psychology* 8:20–28.

Olavarria, J., and van Sluyters, R. C. (1982). The projection from striate and extrastriate cortical areas to the superior colliculus in the rat. *Brain Research* 242:332–336.

Palmer, L. A., and Rosenquist, A. C. (1974). Visual receptive fields of single striate cortical units projecting to the superior colliculus in the cat. *Brain Research* 67:27–42.

Parnavelas, J. G., Burne, R. A., and Lin, C.-S. (1981). Receptive field properties of neurons in the visual cortex of the rat. *Neuroscience Letters* 27:291–296.

Perry, V. H. (1980). A tectocortical visual pathway in the rat. *Neuroscience* 5:915–927.

Peterson, G. M. (1934). Mechanisms of handedness in the rat. *Comparative Psychology Monographs* 9(46):1–67.

Peterson, G. M., and Fracarol, C. (1938). The relative influence of the locus and mass of destruction upon the control of handedness by the cerebral cortex. *Journal of Comparative Neurology* 68:173–190.

Peterson, B. W., Maunz, R. A., Pitts, N. G., and Mackel, R. C. (1975). Patterns of projection and branching of the reticulospinal neurons. *Experimental Brain Research* 23:333–351.

Peterson, S. E., Robinson, D. L., and Morris, J. D. (1987). Contributions of the pulvinar to visual spatial attention. *Neuropsychologia* 25:97–105.

Precht, W., and Yoshida, M. (1971). Blockage of caudate-evoked inhibition of neurons in the substantia nigra by picrotoxin. *Brain Research* 32:229–233.

Redgrave, P., Mitchell, I. J., and Dean, P. (1987). Descending projections from the superior colliculus in rat: a study using orthograde transport of wheatgerm-agglutinin conjugated horseradish peroxidase. *Experimental Brain Research* 68:147–167.

Rhoades, R. W., and Chalupa, L. M. (1978). Functional and anatomical consequences of neonatal visual cortical damage in superior colliculus of the Golden hamster. *Journal of Neurophysiology* 4(6):1466–1494.

Rhoades, R. W., Kuo, D. C., Polcer, J. D., Fish, S. E., and Voneida, T. J. (1982). Indirect visual cortical input to the deep layers of the hamster's superior colliculus via the basal ganglia. *Journal of Comparative Neurology* 208:39–254.

Rolls, E. T., and Cowey, A. (1970). Topography of the retina and striate cortex and its relationship visual acuity in Rhesus monkeys and Squirrel monkeys. *Experimental Brain Research* 10:298–310.

Rowe, M. H., and Stone, J. (1976). Properties of ganglion cells in the visual streak of the cat's retina. *Journal of Comparative Neurology* 167:99–126.

Russell, J. T. (1932). Depth discrimination in the rat. *Journal of Genetic Psychology* 40:136–159.

Satoh, K. (1979). The origin of reticulospinal fibers in the rat: An HRP study. *Journal für Hirnforschung* 20:313–332.

Schiller, P. H., True, S. D., and Conway, J. L. (1980). Deficits in eye movements following frontal eye-field and superior colliculus ablations. *Journal of Neurophysiology* 44:1175–1189.

Schneider, G. E. (1967). Contrasting visuomotor functions of tectum and cortex in the Golden hamster. *Psychologische Forschung* 31:52–62.

Schneider, G. E. (1969). Two visual systems: Brain mechanisms for localization and discrimination are dissociated by tectal and cortical lesions. *Science* 163:895–902.

Schneider, G. E., Carman, L. S., and Ayres, S. (1987). Superior colliculus function in visually elicited "fear" and in scanning movements in Syrian hamsters. *Society for Neuroscience Abstracts* 13:871.

Sengelaub, D. R., Windrem, M. S., and Finlay, B. L. (1983). Increased cell number in the adult hamster retinal ganglion cell layer after early removal of one eye. *Experimental Brain Research* 52:269–276.

Shaw, C., Yinon, U., and Auerbach, E. (1975). Receptive fields and response properties of neurons in the rat visual cortex. *Vision Research* 15:203–208.

Siegel, J. M., and McGinty, D. J. (1977). Pontine reticular formation neurons: Relationship of discharge to motor activity. *Science* 196:678–680.

Siminoff, R., Schwassman, H. O., and Kruger, L. (1966). An electrophysiological study of the visual projection to the superior colliculus of the rat. *Journal of Comparative Neurology* 127:435–444.

Sinnamon, H. M., and Charman, C. S. (1988). Unilateral and bilateral lesions of the anteromedial cortex increase perseverative head movements of the rat. *Behavioural Brain Research* 27:145–160.

Sinnamon, H. M., and Galer, B. S. (1984). Head movements elicited by electrical stimulation of the anteromedial cortex of the rat. *Physiology and Behavior* 33:185–190.

Somogyi, P., Bolam, J. P., and Smith, A. D. (1981). Monosynaptic cortical input and local axon collaterals of identified striatonigral neurons. A light and electron microscopic study using the Golgi-peroxidase transport-degeneration procedure. *Journal of Comparative Neurology* 195:567–584

Sprague, J. M., and Meikle, T. H., Jr. (1965). The role of the superior colliculus in visually-guided behavior. *Experimental Neurology* 11:115–146.

Tehovnik, E. J., Spence, S. J., and Saint-Cyr, J. A. (in press). Efferent projections of the anteromedial cortex of the rat as described by phaseolus vulgaris leucoagglutinin immunohistochemistry. *Behavioural Brain Research*.

Tiao, Y.-C., and Blakemore, C. (1976). Functional organization in the visual cortex of the Golden hamster. *Journal of Comparative Neurology* 168:459–482.

Tusa, R. J., Palmer, L. A., and Rosenquist, A. C. (1978). The retinotopic organization of area 17 (striate cortex) in the cat. *Journal of Comparative Neurology* 177:213–236.

Tunkl, J. E., and Berkley, M. A. (1974). Form discrimination and localization performance in cats with superior colliculus ablations. *Society for Neuroscience Abstracts*, p. 454.

Ungerleider, L. G., and Christensen, C. A. (1977). Pulvinar lesions in monkeys produce abnormal eye movements during visual discrimination training. *Brain Research* 136:189–196.

Ungerleider, L. G., and Christensen, C. A. (1979). Pulvinar lesions in monkeys produce abnormal scanning of a complex visual array. *Neuropsychologia* 17:493–501.

Ungerleider, L. G., and Mishkin, M. (1982). Two cortical visual systems. In D. J. Ingle, M. A. Goodale, and R. W. J. Mansfield (eds.), *Analysis of visual behavior*. Cambridge, Mass. M.I.T. Press, 549–586.

Ungerstedt, U. (1971). Postsynaptic supersensitivity after 6-hydroxydopamine induced degeneration of the nigro-striatal dopamine system. *Acta Physiologica Scandinavica*, Suppl. 367:69–93.

van Buren, J. M. (1963). *The retinal ganglion cell layer*. Springfield, Ill.: Thomas.

Van Gisbergen, J. A. M., Robinson, D. A., and Gielen, S. (1981). A quantitative analysis of generation of saccadic eye movements by burst neurons. *Journal of Neurophysiology* 45:417–442.

Whishaw, I., and Tomie, J. (1989). Olfaction directs skilled forelimb reaching in the rat. *Behavioural Brain Research* 32(2):11–22.

Wickelgren, B. G., and Sterling, P. (1969). Influence of visual cortex on receptive fields in the superior colliculus of the cat. *Journal of Neurophysiology* 32:16–23.

Wiesendanger, R., and Wiesendanger, M. (1982a). The corticopontine system in the rat. I. Mapping of corticopontine neurons. *Journal of Comparative Neurology* 208:215–226.

Wiesendanger, R., and Wiesendanger, M. (1982b). The corticopontine system in the rat. II. The projection pattern. *Journal of Comparative Neurology* 208:227–238.

Wiesenfeld, Z., and Kornel, E. E. (1975). Receptive fields of single cells in the visual cortex of the hooded rat. *Brain Research* 94:401–412.

Williams, M. N., and Faull, R. L. M. (1985). The striatonigral projection and nigrotectal neurons in the rat. A correlated light and electron microscopic study demonstrating a monosynaptic striatal input to identified nigrotectal neurons using a contingent degeneration and horseradish peroxidase procedure. *Neuroscience* 14:991–1010.

Wurtz, R. H., and Hikosaka, O. (1986). Role of the basal ganglia in the initiation of saccadic eye movements. In H.-J. Freund, U. Buttner, B. Cohen, and J. Noth (eds.), *Progress in brain research*, Vol. 64. Amsterdam: Elsevier, 175–190.

Wyss, J. M., and Sripanidkulchai, K. (1984). The topography of the mesencephalic and pontine projections from the cingulate cortex of the rat. *Brain Research* 293:1–15.

Zilles, K. (1985). *The cortex of the rat: A stereotaxic atlas*. New York: Springer Verlag.

Zilles, K., Wree, A., Schleicher, A., and Divac, I. (1984). The monocular and binocular subfields of the rat's primary visual cortex: A quantitative morphological approach. *Journal of Comparative Neurology* 226:391–402.

14 The Somatic Sensory Cortex of the Rat

John K. Chapin and Chia-Sheng Lin

The mechanism by which circuitry in the cerebral neocortex processes sensory information has been an important issue in neuroscience for many years. The traditional approach to studying the function of different cortical areas has been to define functional divisions in the cortex based on a number of criteria, including cytoarchitecture, electrophysiological maps, neuroanatomical connectivity, receptive field properties, and behavior. If one wishes to study the neural circuit mechanisms underlying higher information processing functions, it is very beneficial to utilize a cortical area that is very clearly organized and in which it is possible to accurately reference the same regions using a variety of different neuroanatomical and neurophysiological techniques. As this chapter describes, the rat somatosensory cortex is a structure whose clarity of organization lends itself very easily to such a multipronged approach. As such it may prove ideal for studies of neural circuit mechanisms of cortical function.

Though this chapter can provide only limited background information on the structure and function of the rodent somatosensory cortex, it will serve as a basis for the understanding of the functional organization of this cortical region. In the course of this review, we pay special attention to several global issues. First, possible homologies with other species, particularly primates, are explored. Although the rodent cortex clearly has developed considerable fine specialization in its own right, it appears that certain structural and functional homologies can be established. Second, hypotheses are developed to explain the mechanism by which the circuit organization in this region may support the physiological responses that have been observed at the single-neuron level. These in turn may elucidate the mechanisms of sensory processing in this region.

14.1 Cytoarchitectural Divisions

Definition of Somatosensory Cortex
The rodent S-I cortex has been the subject of numerous cytoarchitectural studies, beginning with those of Droogleever Fortuyn (1914) and Rose

(1912) in rat and Lorente de Nó (1922) in mouse. Although the region could not at the time be definitively identified as the somatosensory cortex, it was known to be a sensory cortical area because of its "koniocortical" cytoarchitecture, characterized by a granule cell-rich cortical layer IV. With the advent of evoked potential mapping techniques, it became possible to define cortices according to their sensory submodality as well as their representation of the body. In his pioneering studies, Woolsey (1947, 1952, 1958) used these techniques to map the topographic organization of the somatosensory cortices of rats as well as of cats, rabbits, monkeys, and other mammals. The rough body representations found in the S-I cortices of all these species were oriented similarly, with the animal's head lying ventrolaterally on the convexity of the cerebral hemisphere and facing rostrally, and the hind extremities located dorsomedially, near the sagittal fissure. In the rat, the body map ("ratunculus") thus defined (figure 14.1) faces forward, its paws, nose and perioral regions being rostral, with the back and caudal head regions occupying the caudal S-I cortex. One striking feature is the degree to which the rat S-I cortex is dominated by its massive representation of the whiskers on the face, in particular each mystacial vibrissa occupying a clearly distinct subzone within the rat S-I cortex. More detailed mapping studies are described in section 14.2.

In comparison with the S-I cortex, very little is known about the S-II cortex in rodents. Krieg (1947) defined area 40 (S-II in the Brodmann map) as a small area just caudal and lateral to the caudolateral edge of S-I.

Cytoarchitectonic Description of the S-I Cortex

The system for cytoarchitectural subdivision of the neocortex devised by Brodmann (1909) has become the standard not only for the human cortex but also for apes, monkeys, and other mammalian species. Although attempts to specify homologies between cortical subregions become increasingly difficult with phylogenetic distance, several workers have recognized the importance of defining bases for comparing the cortices of rodents with those of primates. The first detailed effort to delineate the cytoarchitectonic regions of the rat cortex in terms of the Brodmann scheme was that of Krieg (1946a,b, 1947). In keeping with Brodmann, he divided the rat S-I cortex into areas 3, 1, and 2, arrayed in that order from the rostromedial edge to the caudolateral edge of the S-I cortex. It appears, however, that this homology cannot be supported, partly because it tends to break up the single representation of the body into two zones. Krieg's areas 2 and 2a, for example, contain the entire head representation, whereas area 3 contains the body and limb representations. Because both Krieg's areas 2 and 3 exhibit highly granular cytoarchitecture, they could together be homologous with area 3b in primates.

Caviness's (1975) more recent attempt to apply Brodmann-type hom-

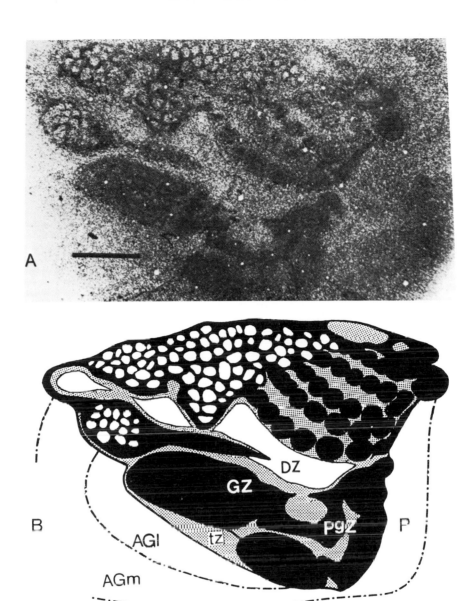

Figure 14.1 Topography of cytoarchitectonic zones in the rat S-I cortex. (A) A thionin-stained 75-μm section cut tangentially through layer IV of a flattened cortex. The granular zones (GZs) appear as dark patches surrounded by lighter, dysgranular cortex. Left = rostral; up = lateral; bar = 1 mm. (B) Schematic drawing of the cytoarchitectural zones visible in figure 14.1A. Granular zones (GZs) shown as black areas, some containing center sparse barrels. Perigranular zones (PGZs) defined as stippled area surrounding GZs, except in transitional zones (TZs) just rostral to S-I. Dysgranular zones (DZs) lie in center of S-I. Medial and lateral frontal agranular areas (mAG and lAG) lie rostral to S-I.

ologies in the rodent (in this case, mouse) cortex appears to have been more successful. He defined all of the S-I cortex as area 3, except the dysgranular zone (our definition given below), which is contained within area 1. He also defined a rostrolateral "visceral" area (Caviness and Frost 1980), calling it area 3i. An updated map of this type has been constructed by Zilles and associates (1980); Zilles and Wree (1985); and Zilles, Wree, and Dausch (chapter 5) using computer cytoarchitectonic analysis. In Zilles's scheme the S-I cortex is divided into three areas: (1) *Par1* contains most of the head representation and part of the forelimb representation in some coronal sections; (2) *HL* appears to contain the representations of the hindpaw, hindlimb, and back and part of the forelimb in some coronal sections; and (3) *FL* contains most of the forepaw and part of the forelimb representation. The central dysgranular zone that we have studied appears to be contained mainly within the HL and FL areas.

Identification of direct homologies with the primate cortex may be very difficult. The cytoarchitectonically defined areas 3, 1, and 2 in the primate appear as mediolateral strips. Each of these areas is relatively homogeneous, and each tends to contain separate and complete body maps (see Kaas 1982 for review). In contrast the rodent S-I cortex features a fine structure that is cytoarchitecturally heterogeneous on the scale of fractions of millimeters. As Woolsey and Van der Loos (1970) pointed out, layer IV in the rodent S-I cortex exhibits distinct aggregations of granule cells, whose shape engendered the name "barrels." These barrels lie within a less granular cortical matrix called barrel septa. The fact that this fine, discontinuous microstructure is contained within a single body representation in the rodent S-I cortex indicates an organizational plan fundamentally different from that in primates.

As an alternative nomenclature for cytoarchitectonically dividing the rat S-I cortex we have proposed the terms *granular, perigranular,* and *dysgranular* zones. These zones can be seen in figure 14.1A, which shows a photograph of a Nissl-stained histological section cut through layer IV in a plane tangential to the surface of the rat S-I cortex. The granular zones (GZs) are visible as dark granular aggregates, surrounded by lighter-colored, less granular cortex. Figure 14.1B shows a drawing of the same section with the GZs colored black. The GZs appear to float in a matrix of less granular cortex consisting of relatively large dysgranular zones (DZs) and transitionally dysgranular regions just surrounding the GZs, which we call perigranular zones (PGZs). There is also a "transitional zone" (TZ) forming the border between the S-I cortex and rostrally adjacent "lateral agranular" (primary motor) cortex. The following are cytoarchitectural descriptions of these zones:

Granular Zones
In general the GZs are characterized by a markedly granular layer IV. This "koniocortical" cytoarchitecture identifies it, of course, as primary

sensory cortex and thus might be thought of as a discontinuous homolog of the primate area 3b. The GZs in rat are also characterized by a clear division of layer V into a cell-sparse and fiber-rich layer Va and a richly pyramidal layer Vb. In the lateral and caudal parts of the S-I, these consist mainly of medium-size pyramids. However, along the rostromedial edge of the S-I (which overlaps somewhat with the electrically excitable motor cortex), layer Vb contains mainly large pyramidal cells that are actually more numerous than in the rostrally adjacent area 4 (Krieg 1946b).

Modern study of the granular regions of the rodent S-I cortex was precipitated by Woolsey and Van der Loos (1970), who observed barrels in Nissl-stained sections cut tangentially through layers III and IV in the granular regions of the S-I cortex of the mouse. These barrels were especially prominent in the caudomedial S-I, which contains the mystacial vibrissae representation. Each of these large barrels corresponds to a single vibrissa on the mystacial pad. Each contains about 2000 cells (Pasternak and Woolsey 1975) consisting of mainly nonpyramidal and a few pyramidal cells.

Although these structures had been observed previously (Lorente de Nó 1922), this rediscovery provoked a great deal of interest, resulting in part from the suggestion that the barrels represented the first cytoarchitecturally visible example of a *cortical column*. As originally defined by Mountcastle (1957), such columns were vertically oriented cortical regions that formed the exclusive representation of a single discrete region of the cutaneous periphery. Accordingly it was established that each large barrel in the posteromedial subregion corresponded to a single whisker on the mystacial vibrissae pad on the face. The notion that the barrels represented sensory thalamocortical receiving zones was reinforced by Killackey (1973) and Lee and Woolsey (1975a,b), who showed that the barrels correlated with high thalamocortical innervation density. This unique organization has been elegantly demonstrated with the succinic dehydrogenase stain (Dawson and Killackey 1987) and also with cytochrome oxidase (Wong-Riley and Welt 1980; also see figure 14.2).

Barrellike structures were subsequently described in a number of other mammals (Woolsey et al. 1975b), including the rat (Welker 1971, 1976). Welker and Woolsey (1974) pointed out that the rat cortex contains true barrels in the rostrolateral S-I (which represent perioral and nasal regions), but not in the posteromedial barrel subfield (PMBSF), which contains large barrels in the mouse, each representing a single vibrissa. In the rat this region contains center-filled aggregates of granule cells rather than true center-sparse barrels. The remainder of the rat S-I cortex is also dominated by granular aggregates rather than barrels.

Despite these differences it appears that barrellike structures do not represent mutually exclusive cytoarchitectural types, but may be more simply related to the thickness of layer IV. It appears that thin but

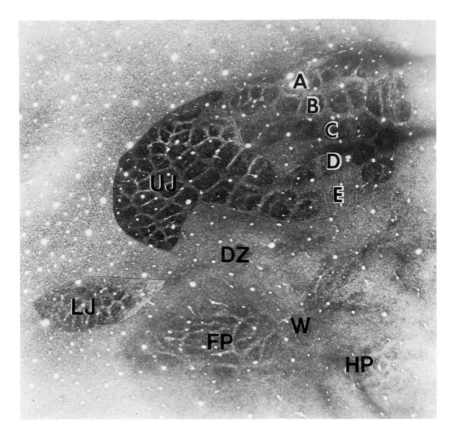

Figure 14.2 Photomicrograph of a tangential section through layer IV of a rat's flattened S-I cortex reacted with cytochrome oxidase. A–E = rows of mystacial vibrissae; UJ = upper jaw; LJ = lower jaw; DZ = dysgranular zone; FP = forepaw; W = wrist; HP = hindpaw.

densely packed granular layers tend to exhibit barrels, while thicker granular layers tend to exhibit granular aggregate-type morphology. Closer examination reveals that the barrels and granular aggregates are fundamentally similar structures: the center-sparse barrels in superficial layer IV tend to overlie "bases" of aggregated granular cells in deep layer IV. For this reason tangential sections cut just deep to the barrels in the perioral and nose regions of the rat S-I reveal aggregates of granule cells. Conversely tangential sections cut through layer IV just superficial to the granular aggregates in the vibrissae or paw areas reveal faint center-sparse barrels. We have therefore consolidated the cortical regions exhibiting both barrel and granular aggregate-type cytoarchitecture under the single classification of GZ.

Perigranular Zones and Dysgranular Zones
In tangential sections such as in figure 14.1A, the GZs appear as islands floating in a sea of less granular cortex, which we have further subdivided as follows: PGZs consist of 100-μm– to 300-μm–wide strips of

transitionally granular cortex just surrounding the GZs. The DZs are 1-mm– to 2-mm–wide strips of dysgranular cortex lying centrally within the S-I cortex (interposed between the body and head representations) and also laterally (between the S-I and S-II cortices). This division between the PGZs and DZs is based not only on this cytoarchitectural criterion but also was suggested by results of neuroanatomical and neurophysiological experiments, which are discussed in sections 14.2 and 14.3.

The central DZ, referred to as area 1 by Krieg, appears markedly less stratified than the surrounding GZs, an effect produced chiefly by its paucity of layer IV granule cells. Thus the supragranular layers present a pale, uniform appearance, and the plexiform layer Va is much less conspicuous. Overall the cytoarchitecture of the DZ is quite similar to the "posterior parietal" cortex (Krieg's area 7), which lies just caudal to the S-I cortex in the rat.

The PGZs consist of narrow strips of lightly granular cortex interposed between the GZs and the DZs. We have distinguished between the PGZs and the distinctly different *transitional zone* (TZ), which occupies the transitionally dysgranular border between the granular S-I and frontal agranular fields. Unlike the PGZs within the S-I, this TZ contains a prominently pyramidal layer Vb similar to that of the rostrally adjacent lateral agranular zone (Krieg's area 4).

The rodent S-I cortex has figured importantly in studies concerned with the role of the periphery in determination of the pattern of brain development. This work was initiated by Van der Loos and Woolsey (1973), who showed that the destruction of vibrissa follicles in the newborn mouse markedly changed the cytoarchitectural pattern ultimately observed in the cortex of the adult mouse. Specifically destruction of a row of vibrissae follicles at birth prevented normal development of a corresponding row of GZs (barrels) in the S-I cortex, which was replaced by a single narrow band of cells. In a subsequent series of studies, Killackey and his colleagues demonstrated that this disruption of cortical cytoarchitecture is attributable to similar disruptions of the vibrissae representations, first in the trigeminal nuclei and then in the ventrobasal thalamus (see Killackey 1980). Overall these findings emphasize the developmental plasticity of the cortical cytoarchitectonic pattern and demonstrate the importance of the periphery in determining this pattern.

14.2 Electrophysiological Mapping of the Somatosensory Cortex

The most definitive mappings of sensory cortical regions, including the S-I and S-II cortices, have been provided by electrophysiological techniques. This approach originated with the evoked potential maps of Woolsey (1947b, 1952, 1958), who definitively located the S-I cortex in a number of species, including monkey, cat, rabbit, and rat. The "Mammunculi" of all of these species, including rodents, consist of an S-I cortical map of the cutaneous periphery with the hindquarters located dorsomedially near the sagittal fissure, and with the head located ventrolaterally over the convexity of the parietal cortex. The distal paws and mouth are rostral and the trunk caudal. A cortical "taste" area has been defined in the rostrolateral corner of the S-I cortex (Benjamin and Akert 1959; see chapter 16 by Braun). A second representation of the body is contained in the S-II cortex, lying along the posterolateral edge of the S-I cortex.

Unit Cluster Mapping of the S-I Cortex

More recently several workers have utilized unit cluster recording to map the S-I cortex in anesthetized animals, including rats. Hall and Lindholm (1974) and Welker (1971, 1976) defined a ratunculus that had a similar overall orientation, but greater detail. Furthermore Welker (1976) definitively correlated the cortical regions exhibiting cutaneous, hair, or vibrissae receptive fields with the barrels (in this case referring to all granular regions of the S-I). These granular regions were made more visible in tangential sections through layer IV of flattened cortex. In contrast, in these anesthetized animals no sensory responses of any kind could be recorded in the DZ. For this reason Sur and colleagues (1978), in a mapping study of the S-I cortex of the squirrel (whose S-I cortex is somewhat similar to that of the rat), referred to the DZ as the "unresponsive zone" (UZ).

A number of other studies have used unit cluster recording to map the S-I cortex of anesthetized rats (Angel and Lemmon 1975, Waite and Taylor 1978, Sanderson et al. 1981). The resultant papers have all reinforced the general notion of a single unique representation for each body part. However, the question of whether complete multiple representations exist corresponding to different somatosensory submodalities remains unresolved. Some evidence for the separation of cutaneous submodalities has been provided by Pidoux and Verley (1981), who reported that the mystacial vibrissae and the common fur surrounding them project to different subregions in the S-I cortex. This finding has been more recently echoed by Sharp and colleagues (1988), who used 2-deoxyglucose (2-DG) uptake to map the cortical and subcortical regions responding to either vibrissae or common fur stimulation. Although the vibrissae stimulation produced 2-DG uptake in S-I cortical barrels and in the S-II cortex, stimulation of the common fur dorsally adjacent to the vibrissae labeled the intervening area between the S-I and S-II.

We (Chapin and Lin 1984) have used single-unit recording techniques to map the representation of cutaneous and also muscle-joint somatosensory modalities in the S-I cortex of awake and freely moving rats as well as anesthetized rats. Quantitative measurements of the properties of cutaneous receptive fields in S-I showed that adjacent neurons exhibited differences in response threshold, adaptability, frequency response, and overall RF size and shape. Nevertheless the size and location of the "centers" of the receptive fields were quite constant and were similar to those seen in multiple-unit recordings. The same was true of receptive fields of single neurons recorded in awake animals and through different anesthetic states.

Figure 14.3 illustrates our map of the cutaneous periphery in the rat S-I. Receptive fields in layer IV of the GZs tended to be discrete and of cutaneous modalities. As such a single, finely detailed, continuous map of the cutaneous periphery was definable within the GZs themselves. Receptive fields in the PGZs were larger and more diffuse, but because they covered roughly the same skin areas as the receptive fields in the most closely adjacent GZs, they fit into the same body map. Neurons in the DZs were unresponsive to any sensory stimuli in the anesthetized animal.

In chronically implanted, awake, freely moving animals the cutaneous receptive fields were larger and more volatile than in anesthetized animals, but the accuracy of the map was clearly preserved by the fact that the locations of the RF centers were unchanged. Neurons in the PGZs and DZs in the awake animals exhibited a multimodal convergence of cutaneous and joint movement receptive fields within single vertical penetrations, or even on single neurons. Directionally specific

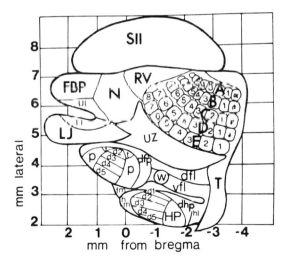

Figure 14.3 Composite map of the cutaneous representation in the S-I cortex of the anesthetized rat, determined by microelectrode mapping. Abbreviations, from caudal to rostral body regions: T = trunk; hl = hindlimb; HP = hindpaw; dhp = dorsal hindpaw; d1–5 = digits 1–5 of hindpaw; hm = hindlimb muscle; vfl = ventral forelimb; dfl = dorsal forelimb; w = wrist whiskers; dfp = dorsal forepaw; p = palm; d2–5 = digits 2–5 of forepaw; t = thumb (pollux); UZ = zone unresponsive in anesthetized recordings; A–E, 1–8 = rows (from dorsal to ventral) and numbers (from caudal to rostral) of mystacial vibrissae; RV = rostral small vibrissae; N = nose; FBP = frontobuccal pads; UL = upper lip; LL = lower lip; LJ = lower jaw.

and bilateral cutaneous receptive fields were also observed in the DZs. It was concluded that DZs are more associational or integrative areas within the S-I, but they could not be shown to comprise a distinct and separate body representation. The rat S-I cortex therefore appears to contain, within a single overall body map, both granular and dysgranular cytoarchitectonic zones. Not only are different sensory modalities subserved within this map, but also different levels of physiological complexity and anesthesia sensitivity.

Overlap of S-I with Electrically Excitable M-I Cortex

The representation of body movements in the motor cortex in the rat, as originally shown by Woolsey (1952, 1958), is oriented in a mirror image to the sensory map in the S-I cortex. Thus the head and back areas of the two maps are farthest from each other, whereas the paw areas adjoin and actually overlap. This overlap, originally described by Hall and Lindholm (1974), has been for the most part confirmed by many authors (Sapienza et al. 1981, Donoghue and Wise 1982, and Sanderson et al. 1983). The M-I/S-I overlap area occupies an approximately 1.0-mm–wide strip running obliquely along the rostromedial edge of the S-I. The overlap covers most of the S-I hindpaw representation and about half of the forepaw representation. In an investigation of the M-I/S-I–forepaw overlap region, we (Chapin and Woodward 1986), noticed that the overlap is coextensive with the representation of the glabrous skin on the palmar surface of the forepaw. We also observed that the predominant motor effect of microstimulating in this overlap region is to produce shoulder flexion and wrist extension, both of which are elemental movements that typically occur just before forepaw contact on the ground during locomotion. Finally, neurons recorded in this area were found to discharge just before footfall. Thus the M-I/S-I–forepaw overlap region contains neural circuits that receive sensory input from the forepaw upon foot contact and also appear to be involved in the control of the forelimb movements that produce the foot contact. The neurophysiological implications of this sensorimotor juxtaposition are discussed further in section 14.4.

Body Map in the S-II Cortex

A map of S-II has been defined electrophysiologically by Welker and Sinha (1972). In a more recent reexamination, Carvell and Simons (1986, 1987) report that the body representation in the S-II is a mirror image of that in S-I. Thus the face representations of S-I and S-II adjoin each other (though there is an intervening DZ along the S-I/S-II border). One interesting problem encountered when mapping the S-II cortex is that its location is quite caudal and lateral, rendering it difficult to differentiate from the primary auditory cortex (A-I). This difficulty may not be simply due to cytoarchitectural vagueness. Carvell and Simons (1986, 1987) suggest an overlap of somatosensory and auditory function in this region. In this the trunk and limb representations are coextensive with cortical regions responding to auditory stimuli, but the face representation is not.

14.3 Axonal Connections of the Rodent Somatosensory Cortex

The following sections briefly review our current knowledge about the morphology of somatosensory cortical neurons and their thalamocortical and cortico-cortical axonal connections. A major issue is the striking difference in the pattern of these connections in the GZs as compared with the PGZs and DZs. Concomitantly we attempt to construct a model of the information flow within this system. One particularly important general hypothesis to be developed is that sensory information is processed in both serial and parallel models in the rat S-I cortex. The parallel model is supported by the observation that granular and dysgranular subzones receive information from different afferent systems. Alternatively the serial model is supported by the recognition that sensory information in the S-I cortex appears to flow through a series of relatively clearly defined "processing levels." Ultimately the information from the different ascending pathways and cortico-cortical systems appears to be integrated, supporting the idea that the rat S-I cortex may subserve higher-order sensory processing functions.

Morphology of Neurons in S-I Cortex

Dendrites
The morphological characteristics of neurons in the mouse barrel has been described in detail using Golgi impregnations. Woolsey and colleagues (1975a) and Simons and Woolsey (1984) have described two nonpyramidal types of neurons, types I and II, which appear to correspond respectively to the stellate and short-axon neurons of Lorente de Nó (1922) and to the spiny and aspiny stellates of White (1978). (It is presumed that some of these may also have been pyramidal neurons.) About 85 percent of these layer IV neurons had dendritic fields restricted to a single barrel. Most of the remaining 15 percent of neurons whose dendrites extended into multiple barrels had somata in the septa between barrels. The axons of both cell types also tended to be restricted within a single barrel (Harris and Woolsey 1983).

Synapses
White (1976) has described the ultrastructure of these neurons and their synaptic contacts. Approximately 90 percent of all synapses within the barrel were asymmetric, of which only about 20 percent were derived from the thalamus (Keller et al. 1985). All thalamocortical synapses were asymmetric. The sides of the barrels contained densely packed cell bodies, high concentrations of myelinated axons, and large-diameter

dendrites, many of which were apical dendrites of layer V pyramidal neurons. The barrel hollows contained a much greater concentration of synaptic contacts, though only a few of these were derived in part from thalamocortical axon terminations. For instance, Benshalom and White (1986) reported that only 17 percent of asymmetric synapses on the dendrites of spiny stellate neurons come from the thalamus (Benshalom and White 1986). These thalamocortical synapses are regularly distributed at about 5-μm intervals on spines along the dendrites of spiny stellate cells (White and Rock 1979).

More recently White and his colleagues have combined such EM observation of degenerating thalamocortical synapses with the use of retrograde transport of horseradish peroxidase as a means of identifying the postsynaptic pyramidal neurons in terms of their projection zones. The proportion of thalamically derived synapses was found to differ among different classes of pyramidal cells whose apical or basilar dendrites could be observed in layer IV. For example, thalamocortical synapses accounted for 7 percent to 20 percent of all synapses on corticothalamic neurons, but only 0.3 percent to 0.9 percent of synapses on corticostriatal cells and 1.5 percent to 6.8 percent of synapses on cortico-cortical cells (White and Hersch 1982).

Overall these findings emphasize the relative importance of cortico-cortical connections within the S-I cortex. In particular the relatively weak thalamic input on layer V corticofugal pyramidal neurons is consistent with the notion that these neurons represent a higher processing level in the cortex.

Thalamocortical Inputs

Inputs from the Ventral Posterior Thalamus

To a large extent the functional differentiation of sensory cortical areas has been defined by their input from specific thalamic nuclei. Thus the S-I cortex of higher mammals is thought of as receiving inputs primarily from the ventral posterior (VP) thalamus (often called "ventrobasal" (VB) in nonprimates). This input from the VP thalamus to the S-I cortex in the rat has been known since Gurdjian's (1927) work. In the mouse, Lorente de Nó (1922) attached the name *glomeruli* to the plexes of thalamocortical axon terminations within barrels. Retrograde tracer studies have demonstrated a highly topographic organization of neuronal clusters in the VP thalamus projecting to discrete cortical regions (Saporta and Kruger 1974). When viewed in three dimensions these clusters are not spherical, but appear as *curvilinear arrays* (Saporta and Kruger 1976, 1977). These may correspond to the *barreloids* that have been observed in the face region of the rat VP thalamus (Van der Loos 1976) and that have a one-to-one relation with cortical barrels (Belford and Killackey 1978).

Axonal projections to the S-I cortex from the VP thalamus are sharply segregated according to cytoarchitectonic subzone. Thalamocortical axons ascend to the cortex in segregated bundles and terminate mainly within single GZs, especially within the layer IV granular aggregates (Killackey 1973, Lu and Lin 1986). Less dense terminations are found in layers I, II, and III. Observations of single thalamocortical axons stained either with Golgi impregnation (Lorente de Nó 1922) or with horseradish peroxidase (Jansen and Killackey, 1987, Bernardo and Woolsey 1987) indicate that most such axons terminate richly within a single barrel and to a lesser extent in other layers within the same "column."

Inputs from the Posterior Thalamus

The PO thalamic projections to the S-I cortex terminate mainly in the DZs and PGZs (Killackey and Ebner 1973, Herkenham 1980). The PO also contributes sparse terminals in layers I and V in the GZs. By using the anterograde transport of horseradish peroxidase (HRP) and Phaseolus vulgaris leucoagglutinin (PHA-L), we (Lu and Lin 1986, 1989) have confirmed these projections and have also found that the PO projects widely to several cortical areas, including the DZs and PGZs in the S-I, S-II, posterior parietal cortex, and the primary and secondary motor cortices. Retrograde studies (Lin and Chapin 1981) have confirmed that the major source of thalmocortical afferents to the DZs and PGZs is the PO.

The dorsolateral region of the rostral PO is cytoarchitectonically indistinguishable from the rostrally adjacent VL. Because the DZs, and also the agranular motor cortex, largely contain neurons exhibiting deep (proprioceptive) receptive fields, it is conceivable that this rostral subregion of the PO may be a thalamic relay for deep receptor information. In fact the homologous thalamic region (VPS) in cats (Dykes et al. 1986) and monkeys (Jones and Friedman 1982) exhibits deep and proprioceptive receptive fields and projects to area 3a.

Inputs from Other Thalamic Nuclei

Two other thalamic regions also project to the S-I cortex. Herkenham (1980) described *nonspecific* inputs originating in the ventrolateral (VL) and ventromedial (VM) thalamic nuclei, which mainly terminate diffusely in layer I throughout the S-I cortex. This is to be contrasted with a *specific* projection from the VL described by Donoghue and colleagues (1979). This specific VL input appears to differ from the nonspecific in that it has dense terminations in layers III and V throughout the M-I cortex and (most important for our purposes) also the S-I/M-I overlap zone. This partial overlap in the rat of inputs from the VL and VP thalamic nuclei may represent a midpoint in the evolutionary trend toward separation of these inputs, which is almost complete in primates. It is instructive to note that in the opossum the VL and VP thalamocortical projections are overlapped throughout the parietal cortex (Killackey and Ebner 1973). Additional nonspecific inputs arise from the intralaminar thalamic nuclei that project sparsely and diffusely to layers V and VI of the S-I cortex (Herkenham 1978a,b).

Corticofugal Outputs

Outputs to Motor Control Structures

A large descending corticofugal fiber system emanates from the deep layers of the rat S-I cortex and projects to a variety of sensory and motor regions throughout the brain and spinal cord. Because many of these outputs are generally coextensive with similar outputs from the rostrally adjacent M-I cortex, many of the reports on this subject have not adequately differentiated between M-I and S-I sources for descending projections. The following discussion therefore is mainly limited to those studies in which descending projections of the S-I cortex were definitively identified.

The corticospinal tract (CST) in the rat has been extensively studied using light microscopic techniques (Brown 1971), EM techniques (Barnard and Woolsey 1956), and electrophysiology (Shapovalov 1975). Below the pyramidal decussation the CST in rat takes an anomalous course through the ventralmost quadrant of the dorsal columns (Douglas and Barr 1950, Goodman et al. 1966). There is also a ventrally placed, uncrossed CST (Vahlsing and Feringa 1981). The CST in the rat appears to originate from two separate cortical regions, one rostrally placed in the second motor area, i.e., Neafsey's SMA (Neafsey and Sievert 1982), and one more caudally, in the M-I fore- and hindlimb areas including the S-I/M-I overlap zone (Hicks and D'Amato 1977). This is consistent with the neurophysiological findings of Elger and associates (1977), who also demonstrated the existence of direct corticomotoneuronal connections in the rat.

Considerable work has also characterized the descending corticofugal projections from the S-I and M-I cortices to brainstem and telencephalic regions (Wise et al. 1979). All of these projection systems have been shown to emanate from neurons in layer V (except for corticothalamic fibers that derive from layer VI). In general those projections that descend the farthest (e.g., the CST) originate in the deepest part of layer V. Though it is not our intention to review this literature in detail, the following studies on the various corticofugal fiber systems descending from the frontal and parietal cortices can be consulted:

Corticorubral connections in the rat were demonstrated by Brown (1974). Gwyn and Flumerfelt (1974) differentiated between cortical and cerebellar afferents to the red nucleus. *Corticoreticular* and *corticobulbar* projections in the rat have been described by Valverde (1962) and Zimmerman (1964), but no detailed study of the precise termination pattern has yet appeared. *Corticotectal* projections were shown by Wise and Jones (1977). These terminate predominantly in the deep layers of the superior colliculus. *Corticopontine* projections in the rat have been extensively studied by Mihailoff and coworkers (1978) and Wiesendanger and Wiesendanger (1982a,b). *Corticostriatal* systems were originally described in the rat by Webster (1961) and later were confirmed by Donoghue and Kitai (1979) and Knowles and colleagues (1980).

Corticofugal projections to somatosensory relay nuclei (Zimmerman 1964) are of particular interest because they may subserve modulation of sensory inflow, a topic discussed in detail in section 14.4. Direct S-I cortical terminations within the dorsal column nuclei have been observed by Kosinski (personal communications 1986). These corticofugal systems from S-I and M-I could subserve the modulation of sensory inflow through the dorsal column nuclei (Dawson 1958, Guzman-Flores et al. 1962, Shin and Chapin 1989).

Outputs to the Somatosensory Thalamus
Corticothalamic projections from the S-I cortex terminate in a topographically reciprocal pattern in the VPL thalamus (Catsman-Berrevoets and Kuypers 1981). For the most part these are derived from layer VI neurons, though some appear to be collaterals of corticofugal axons of layer V neurons (Wise and Jones 1977). S-I corticothalamic projections also terminate in the PO, intralaminar, and reticular thalamic nuclei (Jones and Leavitt 1974).

McAllister and associates (1977) and McAllister and Wells (1981) have shown at the EM level that lemniscal afferents terminate on VPL proximal dendrites and contain round vesicles. Cortical afferents on the other hand terminate on distal dendrites and also contain round vesicles. And third class of afferents (probably from the nucleus reticularis thalami (nRT)) terminate on both proximal and distal dendrites and contain flat vesicles. Akers and Killackey (1979) point out that barreloids, which appear transiently in early development, receive trigeminothalamic afferents, whereas the surrounding cell-sparse matrix receives corticothalamic afferents.

Cortico-cortical Connections
The pattern of connections within a cortical region defines its modes of processing. Cortico-cortical connections within the rat S-I vary markedly according to cytoarchitectonic subregion. In particular the DZs and (to a lesser extent) the PGZs tend to strongly and reciprocally interconnect with ipsilateral and contralateral cortical regions. In contrast the GZs are for the most part immune from any but short-distance cortico-cortical connections.

Contralateral Connections
Several workers have studied the callosal connections of S-I in rodents (Wise and Jones 1976, 1978, Akers and Killackey 1978). They have shown (through use of degeneration or through tracer transport studies)

that callosal connections terminate mainly in the DZs and PGZs, but are extremely sparse in the GZs. The callosal projections terminate in layers II, III, deep layer I, and sparsely in layers V and VI. They originate mainly from pyramidal neurons in layers II through VI in DZs and PGZs in the contralateral side.

Ipsilateral Connections

The frontal agranular cortex (containing the M-I and M-II cortices) maintains a strong and topographically organized system of interconnections with the S-I. As with the contralateral connections, Akers and Killackey (1978) showed, using degeneration techniques, that these ipsilateral connections favor the DZs and PGZs over the GZs. More recently we have examined the topography of such connections through use of several retro- and orthograde transported tracers (Chapin and Woodward 1982, Chapin et al. 1987). Overall the interconnections between the S-I and M-I cortices were shown to follow a roughly mirror-image pattern, the division line forming along the rostromedial edge of the S-I cortex. Strong projections from the M-I cortex were observed in deep layers of the GZs, representing the palmar and plantar surfaces of the fore- and hindpaws. Both retrograde and orthograde tracer injections in the M-I cortex just rostral to the M-I/S-I border resulted in columnar patterns of labeling in the PGZs just caudolateral to the forepaw and hindpaw GZs.

The more rostral M-II (or *supplementary motor area*, Neafsey and Sievert 1982) maintained a separate though more diffusely topographic interconnection pattern with the S-I cortex. Finally, we have also observed connections between the S-I and S-II cortices (Lin and Chapin 1981). Again these connections primarily involve the PGZs and DZs.

Connections Within the S-I

Cortico-cortical connections within the S-I can be subdivided into intracolumnar and extracolumnar connections. The pattern of intracolumnar connections in the S-I is not well understood. However, it is clear that within a given column there is a general downward flow of sensory information from thalamocortical termination zones in the superficial layers to the deep layers. This was suggested by Ryugo and Killackey (1975), who reported that lesions in superficial S-I layers cause degeneration in subjacent layer V. Furthermore we (Chapin et al. 1987) observed that axons coursing from HRP-filled cortico-cortically projecting pyramidal neurons in layers II through IV tend to descend and collateralize in layer V before traveling to terminate in other cortical areas.

Extracolumnar intracortical connections vary markedly according to cytoarchitectonic subregion. In particular a much stronger system of interconnections was found within the DZs and PGZs than in the GZs (Chapin et al. 1987). For example, discrete tracer injections in the PGZs produced "walls" of labeling that sharply demarcated the edges of adjacent GZs. Although the GZs themselves were only sparsely labeled, basilar dendrites of pyramidal neurons in adjacent PGZs extended about 0.5 mm into the GZs. Because these dendrites are in a good position to receive inputs from the VP thalamus, they represent one path through which this thalamic sensory information might be transmitted to the PGZs. (According to White and Hersch 1982, direct VP inputs on pyramidal neuron dendrites terminals are less common than indirect inputs relayed through intrinsic stellate cells.) Further transmission to the DZs might be subserved by a topographically organized system of reciprocal interconnections that was found between the PGZs and DZs.

In coronal sections labeling produced by relatively distant injections of either retro- or orthograde tracers generally appeared in a columnar distribution and was localized in PGZs and DZs. Within these zones orthograde labeling consisted of vertically oriented axons emitting collateral sprays of terminals in all layers. Retrograde neuronal labeling was greatest in superficial layers. These identified cortico-cortical projection neurons consisted exclusively of pyramidal cells, except for a few horizontal cells in layer I. Proximal to the injection site, labeling tended to spread out from these columns into supra- and infragranular layers in adjacent GZs.

Summary and Conclusion
Figure 14.4 schematically illustrates the major conclusions drawn from these hodological studies. The fact that thalamocortical inputs from the VP (terminating in GZs) are segregated from inputs from the PO (terminating in the PGZs and DZs) suggests a parallel processing of the modalities represented by these two afferent systems. However, the conception of GZs and DZs as independent areas operating in parallel

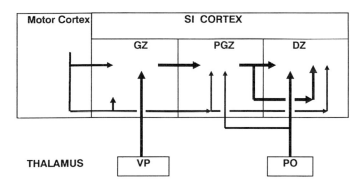

Figure 14.4 Simplified schematic drawing summarizing the major thalamocortical and cortico-cortical connections of the three different cytoarchitectonic subdivisions in the S-I cortex. Sizes of the arrows indicate approximate strength of connections, and arrow placement indicates layers of axonal flow. VP = ventroposterior thalamic nucleus; PO = posterior thalamic nucleus; GZ = granular zones; PGZ = perigranular zones; DZ = dysgranular zones.

seems to be contradicted by the marked differences in the cortico-cortical connectivity of these areas. Whereas the GZs mainly receive inputs only from closely adjacent GZs (or from M-I, along the S-I/M-I border), the DZs receive inputs from many zones including the GZs (via PGZs) in the S-I, the M-I, and M-II cortices, the S-II cortex, and the contralateral S-I. Thus the DZs should be considered as much higher-order processing zones than the GZs.

The pattern of inputs to the DZs and PGZs suggests that these regions could function to integrate deep/proprioceptive sensory information (derived via the PO thalamus) with "motor" information derived from the M-I and M-II cortices. The cutaneous information derived from the GZs/PGZs may also be suited to movement, especially if the processing in the GZs/PGZs extracts features of stimulus movement on the skin, hair, or whiskers. These hypotheses about function derived from neuroanatomical findings are expanded upon in the next section, which reviews the neurophysiology of the rat somatosensory cortex.

14.4 Neurophysiological Studies

Recent years have seen a marked increase in the number and scope of electrophysiological investigations using the rodent S-I cortex. In addition to electrophysiological mapping (section 14.2), much work has been devoted to single-unit studies, especially involving receptive field analysis and iontophoresis. Furthermore the rodent S-I cortex has now been studied extensively in the in vitro slice preparation. ˙

Our major aim in reviewing the neurophysiological literature is to correlate functional characteristics of this system with possible neuroanatomical substrates. Major issues that are developed include correlation of (1) electrophysiological and morphological characteristics of neurons, (2) receptive fields and neuroanatomical circuitry within specific subregions and layers of the S-I cortex, and (3) neurotransmitter systems and effects of drugs on this circuitry.

Cell Electrophysiology of S-I Cortex Neurons

The electrophysiological properties of intracellulary recorded S-I cortical neurons have been studied by Connors and colleagues (1982) in the rat and by McCormick and colleagues (1985) in the guinea pig. In the latter Lucifer yellow was used, allowing neurons to be identified as to cell type. Three distinct classes of neurons were found:

1. *Regular spiking cells* are spiny pyramidal neurons located in layers II through VI. They exhibit relatively long-duration action potentials (about 0.8 ms at one-half amplitude). These neurons also show prominent afterhyperpolarizations following spike trains, evoked either by intracellularly applied current or by stimulation of afferent pathways.

2. *Bursting cells* are spiny pyramidal cells, recorded mainly in layer IV and upper layer V. These typically emit all-or-none bursts of three to five spikes, which appear to depend on a relatively hyperpolarized state because they are lost when the neuron is depolarized to near spiking threshold.

3. *Fast-spiking cells* are aspiny or sparsely spiny stellate cells with bitufted or radial dendritic arrangements and are found in layers II through VI. They are characterized by short-duration action potentials (0.32 ms) and display little or no frequency adaptation. They are powerfully activated by synaptic excitation and exhibit little or no inhibition.

Single-Unit Studies

Somatic Sensory Responses in the Rat S-I

As was indicated in section 14.3, the best-known source of afferents to the S-I cortex is the dorsal column-lemnisco-thalamic system. This sensory information originates mainly in low-threshold cutaneous afferents and ascends rapidly, relaying through as few as two synapses (dorsal column or trigeminal nuclei, and VP thalamus) before reaching the cortical level. As Mountcastle (1957) pointed out, the short-latency, highly reliable sensory responses that form the basis of most recordings in the S-I cortex appear to reflect inputs ascending through this system (in rat, Angel and Berridge 1974). Nevertheless other types of responses can be recorded in the S-I cortex that may be derived from other afferent systems, such as the spinothalamic or spinocervical systems.

Evidence for spinothalamic-type input to neurons in the S-I has been provided by Lamour and associates (1983a,b), who reported the existence of specifically nociceptive responses in the deep layers of the rat S-I cortex. We (Chapin et al. 1981) have found additional support for such extralemniscal inputs in experiments in which single units in the rat S-I cortex were recorded in both awake and anesthetized animals. In awake rats electrical and natural punctate stimulation of the periphery (forepaw) evoked a series of separable response components in S-I cortical neurons. These response components were categorized as (1) *E1a*, a sharp excitatory peak at 7 ms to 15 ms latency poststimulus, (2) *E1b*, a broader excitatory peak, variably seen in the 15 ms to 50 ms poststimulus latency epoch, (3) *I1*, an inhibitory response of variable magnitude lasting for 20 ms to 200 ms after the initial excitatory responses and (4) *E2*, an excitatory peak typically beginning about 200 ms poststimulus and lasting for 50 ms to 100 ms. Of these the E1a peak was observed in most neurons in awake animals, whereas the E1b, I1, and E2 peaks were less commonly seen. In rats anesthetized with halothane (and most other anesthetics), the E1b and E2 peaks were almost never observed. In fact, when these peaks were observed in awake animals, it was possible to reversibly abolish them by transiently administering halothane anesthesia. Typically the E1b peak was replaced by an I1 inhibitory period commencing just after the E1a peak.

A subsequent experiment shed light on the possible pathways subserving these responses. Figure 14.5 shows the results of an experiment involving the recording of a neuron in the forepaw area of the S-I cortex of a rat lightly anesthetized with pentobarbital (from Chapin and Woodward 1986). This neuron responded to stimulation of the forepaw and also to low-current stimulation through an electrode stereotaxically implanted in the contralateral cuneate nucleus. When this region of the cuneate nucleus was subsequently lesioned by passing DC current through the same electrode, the E1a response peak in the cortical neuron was abolished. Interestingly a slightly higher current of paw stimulation was then able to produce an excitatory peak at roughly the same latency as the E1b peak normally seen only in awake animals. This result suggests that the E1a peak is derived from sensory information transmitted through the dorsal column nuclei, but that the E1b peak may be at least partially extralemniscal. It is well known that transmission through extralemniscal systems (e.g., spinothalamic tracts) may be blocked at the spinal level during anesthesia. However, these inputs may be further blocked at the cortical level by the I1 inhibition that normally follows the E1a peak. This suggests that the presence or

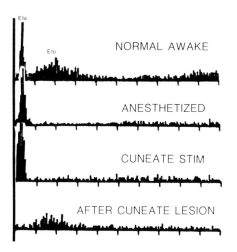

Figure 14.5 Short latency responses of S-I cortical neurons are dependent on the dorsal column nuclei. (A) Poststimulus histogram showing typical S-I cortical neuronal response to forepaw stimulation in the awake condition. Two excitatory responses are visible, including a narrow short latency peak (E1a) and a broader longer latency peak (E1b). (B) Histogram showing response of an S-I cortex neuron to similar stimulation in a pentobarbital anesthetized rat, in which E1b peak is selectively lost. (C) Response of the same neuron to microstimulation of the cuneate nucleus. (D) Response of the same neuron to forepaw stimulation after placement of a small electrolytic lesion in the cuneate nucleus. A small response in the E1b latency range is uncovered by this lesion. bins = 1ms; X-axis ticks = 25 ms; Y-axis automatically scaled to constant instantaneous firing rate per bin.

absence of this peak in various behavioral conditions may depend on a competition between this excitatory input and post-E1a peak inhibition.

Frequency Responses of S-I Neurons

Frequency response has traditionally been used as a criterion for classification of peripheral receptors and also as a means for investigating the central processing of inputs from these receptors. Frequency responses of S-I cortical neurons have been investigated in anesthetized rats by Angel (1967) and in awake (curarized-treated) rats by Simons (1978). Simons observed a generally narrower range of frequency response among regular spiking neurons than among fast-spiking neurons (mainly in layer IV), which could follow frequencies up to at least 40 Hz. The lower-frequency response of the regular spiking neurons is probably caused by the afterhyperpolarizations characteristic of these neurons (McCormick et al. 1985), but may also be related to the actions of inhibitory interneurons. In any case this phenomenon appears to explain the observation that slowly adapting cutaneous responses are relatively rare in the rat S-I cortex, whereas they are common in the dorsal column nuclei and the VP thalamus. It should also be noted that anesthesia strongly decreases the frequency response of neurons in the S-I cortex (Chapin et al. 1981).

Receptive Field Properties

Receptive field (RF) analysis is one of the most useful methods for determining how input information is processed as it ascends through successive levels of a sensory system. In general the results of RF analyses in the rat S-I cortex have paralleled those carried out in other species such as cats (Mountcastle 1957) and monkeys (Mountcastle and Powell 1959).

Cutaneous RFs of single neurons in the rat S-I cortex were originally studied by McComas and Wilson (1967) and Angel (1967). In general these authors reported very small, discrete RFs, corresponding to either single whiskers or small regions of hairy skin on the limbs and trunk, or glabrous skin on the ventral surfaces of the paws. Other investigators (e.g., Waite and Taylor 1978) have reported larger RFs, including even bilateral RFs (Armstrong-James and George 1985). It now appears that several factors influence the size of RFs recorded in the rodent S-I cortex. These include anesthetic state, vertical and horizontal location in cortex, the physical parameters of the sensory stimulus, and the method for analysis of the RF.

What Determines RF Size?

Most evidence suggests that RF sizes may be determined by a balance of excitatory and inhibitory influences around the RF peripheries. Thus increasing stimulus intensity might enlarge the RFs, whereas *lateral* or *surround* inhibition might sharpen the RF boundaries. It is important, however, to distinguish postexcitatory inhibition, which tends to be strongest in the RF center, from lateral inhibition, which is strongest at the edge of the RF. We have observed in the rat S-I cortex that the "infield" postexcitatory inhibition is much stronger than lateral inhibition (unpublished data, 1989). Nevertheless it is possible to demonstrate lateral inhibition in the rat (and other species) S-I cortex by preceding a sensory stimulus to the center of a RF with a stimulus on the periphery of the RF. This sort of lateral inhibition has been shown by Armstrong-James (1975), who observed it in adult rats, but not in infant rats.

The notion that anesthetic state may influence RF size in the rodent S-I cortex has been suggested by several authors, beginning with Armstrong-James (1975), who mentioned that the single-whisker RFs found in urethane-anesthetized rats may have been made more discrete by the anesthetic. In experiments in which the same neurons were recorded under both awake and halothane-anesthetized conditions, we found that RFs that were small and stable under anesthesia became larger and more nonspecific after the animals became conscious (Chapin et al. 1981, Chapin and Lin 1984). The anesthetic had stronger effects on the more volatile peripheries of the RFs than the more reliable centers. Thus the locations of the RF centers were relatively immutable, and, as such, the essential body map in the S-I cortex became clearer. Other changes induced by the anesthetic included decreased frequency response, increased postexcitatory inhibition, and the loss of longer latency responses that are normally observed in awake conditions.

Laminar Organization of RFs

Serial processing of somatosensory information in the rodent S-I cortex is reflected in the fact that RFs vary markedly in size as a function of cortical layer (Simons 1978, Simons and Woolsey 1979). Using quantitative techniques we (Chapin 1986) have shown that RFs in layer V can be several times larger than those immediately superjacent in layer IV. In the vibrissae area, for example, single-whisker receptive fields were found in layer IV just above RFs in layer V that covered the whole mystacial whisker pad. RFs in layers II, III, and VI were also found to be larger than in layer IV, but still not nearly as large as in layer V. Layer V RFs were also more complex in that they sometimes contained multiple peaks. Nevertheless the major RF centers were maintained throughout the column.

The increased size and complexity of RFs in layer V suggests that a major portion of their responses may be derived from cortico-cortical, rather than thalamocortical, inputs. This notion is supported neuroanatomically by the fact that few thalamocortical synapses appear on layer V pyramidal neurons (Benshalom and White 1986) and also by the observation that layer V receives especially dense cortico-cortical terminations from adjacent cortical regions. We have also provided neurophysiological support for this hypothesis in a study (Guise and

Chapin 1986) in which the sizes of layer V neuronal receptive fields in the S-I vibrissae area were diminished by lesions made in adjacent cortical regions. These experiments also made use of stimulating microelectrodes placed about 3 mm distant in the barrelfield region. Stimulation at low current (10–20μA) through these microelectrodes typically produced robust responses in neurons with large RFs recorded in layer V. When the same electrode was subsequently used to electrolytically lesion the barrel previously stimulated, the layer V neurons selectively lost the ability to respond to stimulation of the whisker corresponding to the lesioned barrel.

This result emphasizes the strength and importance of cortico-cortical fiber systems within the rat S-I cortex. The relative unimportance of direct thalamocortical inputs to the discharge of these layer V neurons was illustrated by the fact that they typically responded only slightly more to stimulation of their central whisker (i.e., the whisker represented by that barrel) than to other, even quite distant whiskers. These findings are consistent with the suggestion based on neuroanatomical findings (section 14.3) that the flow of information from layer IV to layer III to layer V in the GZs involves a large amount of convergence and constitutes the most important circuit for integrative processing in the lemniscal system.

RFs across Cytoarchitectonic Subzones of the S-I

RFs in the PGZs are similar to those in the GZs in that they can be found in anesthetized animals and respond to mainly cutaneous submodalities. They tend to be larger, however, than those in the GZs. We have observed this in the PGZs surrounding the paw areas (Chapin and Lin 1984) and also in the PGZs (or *septa*) surrounding the barrels in the vibrissae area in the rat S-I cortex (Uhr et al. 1982, Uhr and Chapin 1983). This physiological finding parallels the neuroanatomical observations (section 14.3) that (1) cortico-cortical terminations are much stronger in the PGzs than in the GZs, and (2) basilar dendrites of large layer III pyramidal neurons in the PGZs spread into the layer IV granular aggregates of multiple adjacent GZs. As such these neurons are in a position to receive thalamocortical inputs (directly or indirectly through interneurons) from several adjacent GZs.

In comparison with the GZs and PGZs, the DZs contain RFs that are larger, more complex, and more likely to respond to proprioceptive inputs. Neurons in the DZs of anesthetized animals are typically unresponsive to any applied stimuli. In awake animals the majority of neurons in the DZs respond to (1) muscle stretch, (2) manipulation of limbs around joints and/or cutaneous stimulation. The proprioceptive sensory properties appear to be derived from the dorsolateral subregion of the PO thalamus, which provides the major thalamic input to this region. The cutaneous sensory properties are probably derived from the PGZs, whose cortico-cortical connections terminate in columnar zones within topographically related subregions in the DZs. Because the PGZs themselves receive a convergence of cutaneous inputs from the GZs, the DZs may be thought of as a site for "tertiary" convergence of cutaneous information (Chapin and Lin 1984). This notion is further supported by the fact that the DZs also receive profuse callosal connections.

The level of associational convergence indicated by this connection pattern appears to be reflected in the higher complexity of receptive fields recorded in the DZs. As an example, we (Guise and Chapin 1985) have recorded neurons in the DZ whisker area that possessed bilateral RFs that responded preferentially when the head passed through an aperture of a certain shape. Such RFS were not typically found in the GZs or PGZs. Similarly neurons with multimodal RFs were common in the limb areas of the DZs, but not in the GZ limb areas. These multimodal neurons responded to the movement of limbs around certain joints and also to cutaneous touch of the skin of the same limb.

In conclusion, the size and complexity of RFs recorded across different layers and cytoarchitectonic subzones appear to be predicted by their neuroanatomical connections. Thus from a knowledge of the information content of the inputs that converge on a region, it may be possible to discern the computational problem that is "solved" by that region. To further approach this question, however, it is necessary to define the actual behavioral conditions under which the input information is *used* by the neurons in that region.

Reorganization of S-I Cortical Maps after Peripheral Nerve Damage

Much recent attention has been devoted to cortical reorganization phenomena that have been observed following transection of peripheral nerves or amputations of digits (see reviews by Merzenich et al. 1983 and Wall and Kaas 1985). The general finding of these studies has been that the S-I cortical areas representing the damaged nerve or digit becomes electrophysiologically silent immediately after the injury. However, over weeks or months of recovery these silent areas become occupied by new or expanded representations of adjacent body regions, as verified by receptive field mapping in anesthetized animals (monkeys, Merzenich et al. 1983; rats, Wall and Egger 1971 and Wall and Kaas 1985). These phenomena have been generally interpreted as indicating either a sprouting of thalamocortical or cortico-cortical connections or a gradual unmasking of normally silent functional connections. However, more recent studies in which receptive fields were examined in awake or lightly anesthetized animals have demonstrated that such neurons begin to respond to stimulation of adjacent peripheral regions immediately after peripheral injury (Rasmusson and Turnbull 1983). It is conceivable therefore that a portion of the expansion of adjacent parts of the body map into the lesioned silent area in observed in anesthetized animals may be attributed to an unmasking of cortio-cortical inputs from adjacent cortico-cortical regions.

Behavioral Modulation of Sensory Transmission

We have investigated the issue of behavioral control of sensory transmission in a series of studies in which single neurons were recorded in the S-I cortical forepaw area of awake, freely moving rats. State-dependent changes in afferent transmission to these neurons was tested by stimulating through electrodes chronically implanted under the skin of the forepaw.

Arousal versus Movement-Dependent Sensory Gating

We have shown (Chapin and Woodward 1981) that arousal in the absence of movement is associated with a slight increase in sensory responsiveness of S-I cortical neurons, coupled with a decrease in spontaneous behavior. In contrast motor behavior is associated with a powerful suppression of the sensory input to the same neurons. Furthermore this movement-related suppression of sensory responsiveness is not generalized, but is expressed selectively on certain classes of neurons during certain particular phases of forelimb movement (Chapin and Woodward 1982a,b, Chapin 1987). For example, though most neurons recorded in the S-I forepaw area possess RFs covering the palmar surface of the forepaw, only about half of these respond when the forepaw touches the ground during running (type I neurons). Many of those that do not respond to footfall (type II neurons) do respond when the palm is touched with a probe while the forelimb is moving through the air in the swing phase of stepping. The differences between these neuronal types could relate to the fact that footfall is an *expected* event, whereas paw contact with objects during the swing phase might be considered as *unexpected*. When electrical stimulation of the forepaw is used to further investigate the timing of this modulation, it is found that sensory transmission to these cortical neurons is selectively modulated over the forelimb step cycle. Although the sensory responses of most neurons are strongly suppressed when averaged over the whole step cycle, most cells also exhibit short, phasic periods of facilitation (or "disinhibition") of afferent input. The type I neurons (which only respond at footfall) do so because their sensory input is phasically facilitated just before the footfall event, but is suppressed during all other phases. Conversely, sensory inputs to type II neurons (which do not respond to footfall) are either tonically suppressed throughout the whole step cycle or are facilitated during the early swing phase.

At what level in the somatosensory pathway to the S-I cortex does this gating occur? More recent studies involving recordings in the VPL thalamus and cuneate nuclei have suggested that the strong suppression of E1a (lemniscal) responses mainly occurs at the cortical level, whereas the E1b responses are subject to strong suppression at thalamic or prethalamic levels (Shin and Chapin 1986; 1987).

Possible Circuits Underlying Movement-Related Gating

The above results indicate that the cortical circuitry may be subject to influences temporally correlated with relatively specific limb movements. The neuroanatomical literature (section 14.3) suggests two possible sources for such "motor" biasing: (1) cortico-cortical inputs from the motor cortex, and/or (2) thalamocortical inputs from the VL or PO carrying motor or proprioceptive sensory information.

Physiological correlates of such inputs were sought in a study (Chapin and Woodward 1986) in which S-I and M-I cortical neurons in awake, moving rats were tested for *motor correlates,* as well as proprioceptive and cutaneous RFs. As expected, most neurons in the M-I cortex discharged during, just before, and in correlation with sudden limb movements. Surprisingly a large number of neurons in the S-I cortex exhibited similar *movement correlates,* sometimes in the absence of any sensory RF that could explain this neuronal activity during movement. Furthermore these bursts of firing occurred during the same step cycle phases as the sensory gating observed among neurons in the same area.

These findings are consistent with the hypothesis that the modulation may be produced by excitatory actions of motor cortical projections onto inhibitory neurons in S-I during certain step cycle phases. Alternatively the movement-correlated activity may have resulted from afferent activity, which for some reason could not be evoked passively. These might in turn inhibit (in a phase-dependent manner) sensory responses of other S-I cells. Whatever the cause, these results indicated a complex integration of facilitory and inhibitory influences shaping the spontaneous activity and sensory responses of S-I cells. The much greater variety of neuronal properties seen during active movement, as compared with passive testing of sensory responses during rest, has reinforced the view of this region as a site for sensorimotor integration.

Physiology of Neurotransmitters in the S-I Cortex

A growing number of investigators have begun to use the rodent S-I cortex as a useful model for studies designed to elucidate the role of various neurotransmitters in cortical function. Here we briefly summarize the results of in vitro and in vivo studies on neurotransmitters and neuromodulators in this region.

Neurotransmitter Basis of Conventional Inhibition

The ionic and neurotransmitter basis of inhibitory responses in in vitro slices of the rodent somatosensory cortex have been investigated by Connors and colleagues (1988). Pyramidal neurons in layers II and III were recorded intracellularly during electrical stimulation of the deep cortical layers. This typically produced three separable responses: an initial, brief excitatory postsynaptic potential (EPSP), followed by a fast IPSP (f-IPSP), which itself was followed by a longer-lasting inhibition (l-IPSP). Iontophoretic studies suggested that both the fast and long IPSPs were traceable to the actions of the neurotransmitter γ-amino-butyric acid (GABA). Because the f-IPSP was blocked by bicuculline, it was assumed to be mediated through GABA$_A$ receptors, which act by increasing membrane chloride conductance. In the rat S-I cortical slice, this had slightly *depolarizing* effects on pyramidal neurons while promoting a powerful depression of neuronal excitability in which both spontaneous and evoked neuronal discharge were inhibited.

The l-IPSP was different in that it was bicuculline insensitive, but mimicked by baclofen, suggesting that it was mediated by GABA$_B$ receptors, which increase potassium conductance. These effects were more subtle in that they selectively decreased the steady-state firing rate, while slightly enhancing the transient responses to strong stimulation.

The resolution of three different types of IPSPs suggests a fairly complex role for the inhibitory neurotransmitter GABA in the rat S-I cortex. Nevertheless clear effects of GABA or its agonists have been shown in in vivo studies. For example, Dykes and associates (1984) have shown that receptive fields in cat S-I cortex are sharpened by local iontophoresis of GABA agonists.

Neurotransmitter Basis of Conventional Excitation
Glutamate and aspartate are the most extensively studied excitatory neurotransmitters in the cortex. Recently these effects have been found to be mediated by at least three distinct receptor subtypes, all of which exist in the rat S-I cortex (Cotman and Iversen 1987). These include *kainate* and *quisqualate*, which produce rapid, sodium-dependent depolarizing responses and appear to mediate the conventional fast EPSP (MacDermott and Dale 1987). A third receptor is that for N-methyl-D-aspartate (NMDA), which plays a role in generating slow EPSPs (MacDermott and Dale 1987) and synaptic potentiation (Collingridge and Bliss 1987). Jones and Baughman (1988) have investigated the neurotransmitter basis of EPSPs in layer V pyramidal neurons recorded intracellularly in the rat visual cortex slice. EPSPs evoked from gray and white matter stimulation were all strongly reduced by broad spectrum antagonists of glutamate-aspartate receptors. Specific NMDA antagonists were used to demonstrate that excitation through the layer II, III to layer V pathway is mediated directly through NMDA and also non-NMDA (kainate and/or quisqualate) receptors.

Effects of Neuromodulators on RFs
Various other pharmacological agents have been shown to be capable of modifying RFs in the rodent S-I cortex. This reflects the fact that RF organization is determined to a large extent by interactions between

excitatory and inhibitory effects. Lamour and coworkers (1988) have shown that direct iontophoresis of glutamate on S-I cortical neurons in the rat can enhance the strength of somatosensory responses in the cortex and can also uncover new RFs. In addition the GABA antagonist bicuculline was shown to enlarge RFs by as much as nine times. Lamour and associates (1983, 1988) also showed that acetylcholine (ACh) tends to enhance somatic sensory responsiveness of such S-I cortical neurons, but that this enhancement is much slower than that of glutamate. The monoamine norepinephrine has also been shown to sharpen RFs in the rat S-I (Waterhouse and Woodward 1980), apparently by increasing the efficacy of both GABA and glutamate neurotransmitters. These results overall suggest that somatosensory RFs are dynamic and are subject to changes in behavioral state.

14.5 Functional Studies

What is the function of the rodent somatosensory cortex? This question has been addressed in a substantial literature dealing with the behavioral effects of lesions in various subregions of the S-I and S-II cortices. Though interpretation of results of many of the early studies suffered because inadequate identification of the lesion sites, the rat S-I cortex has more recently been recognized as a useful structure for lesion experiments. As Finger and colleagues (1978) pointed out, lesion sites in the S-I can be verified by taking advantage of the histological configuration of GZs (especially barrels) and also through electrophysiological mapping.

In general agreement with similar studies carried out in other species, clear functional differences have been found between the S-I and S-II cortices. Whereas lesions in both regions impair performance in tactile sensory tasks, the discrimination of *passively* delivered tactile stimuli appears to selectively involve the S-II cortex (Norsell 1978). In contrast the S-I cortex appears to be more selective for performance in tasks that require movement such as palpation, haptic exploration, "active touch," tactile placing, hopping, etc. (Brooks and Peck 1939, Finger and Frommer 1968, Hicks and D'Amato 1970, 1975, Gruenthal et al. 1980).

This "motor" component of the functionality of the S-I cortex might be expected given the fact that it slightly overlaps with the M-I cortex in the rat. This overlap is a source of confusion, however, when interpreting the results of lesions. Do lesions in the S-I/M-I area corss through two adjacent zones whose functions are purely sensory and motor? Or, alternatively, does this region support an integrated sensorimotor function? Wall (1970) has argued for the latter notion by pointing out that lesions limited to the dorsal columns do not produce lasting deficits in passive tactile recognition, but mainly result in sensorimotor deficits, such as in active touch, or use of tactile cues to trigger movement.

Answers to some of these problems have been provided in a study in rat carried out by Hutson and Masterson (1986). They investigated the effects of S-I cortical (barrelfield) lesions on different tasks involving sensory detection using a single vibrissa. Tasks involving passive detection of an oscillating airstream were found to be unaffected by small barrelfield lesions and also larger cortical lesions involving the S-I cortex and adjacent regions. In contrast even small lesions in the appropriate barrelfield subregion abolished the ability of blinded animals to jump a gap in an elevated runway after actively palpating the far side with its vibrissa. The possibility that coincident damage to motor cortical areas could have caused these effects was easily discounted because of the fact that the S-I and M-I cortical representations of the vibrissae are relatively distant from each other. More likely the S-I cortical damage prevented the motor regions from receiving sensory information necessary to coordinate appropriate motor responses. As these authors have pointed out, future experimentation into the functional importance of sensory processing in the S-I cortex should involve behavioral tasks in which different sensory requirements are cross-attached to different motor requirements.

14.6 Conclusion

The neuroanatomical and neurophysiological literature reviewed here tends to generally support the sensorimotor hypothesis of S-I cortex function. Structurally the S-I cortex appears well suited for integration of cutaneous and proprioceptive somatosensory submodalities with information from the motor cortex. Whereas the afferent systems ascending to the S-I cortex are modality and space specific, and their termination pattern in layer IV granular aggregate zones is finely topographic, subsequent cortical processing tends to mix this information. This "higher" level of processing is accomplished through the massive convergence of cortico-cortical terminations on neurons in infragranular and (to a lesser extent) supragranular cortical layers. Further convergence occurs in subsequent projections to the PGZs and DZs, where processed cutaneous information from the GZs mixes with information from proprioceptive afferent systems and with projections from motor cortex. Thus cutaneous and proprioceptive sensory information is integrated with input containing "motor" information from the motor cortex. This integration is reflected generally in greater complexity and size of receptive fields and specifically in sensorimotor properties of neurons recorded during motor behavior. The computations to be expected from this selection of inputs would include such typical sensory cortex functions as feature extraction and movement detection. However, the convergence of motor and proprioceptive inputs could support a motor-sensory gating function. These are in fact the sorts of properties that have been observed in the neurons of this region (see section 14.4).

As a global hypothesis, therefore, we suggest that the rat S-I cortex may function as a multistage processor that "recognizes" sensorimotor situations. Corticofugal outputs from this processor inform the motor systems and other brain regions of salient features detected from the sensorimotor environment. These may be finally used to coordinate subsequent movement or may enter into consciousness.

Acknowledgment

This work was supported by UPHS grants NS-26722, AA-06965, AA-00089, and NS-06233.

References

Akers, R. M., and Killackey, H. P. (1978). Organization of corticocortical connections in the parietal cortex of the rat. *Journal of Comparative Neurology* 181:513–538.

Akers, R. M., and Killackey, H. P. (1979). Segregation of cortical and trigeminal afferents to the ventrobasal complex of the neonatal rat. *Brain Research* 161:527–532.

Angel, A. (1967). Cortical responses to paired stimuli applied peripherally and at sites along the somatosensory pathway. *Journal of Physiology (London)* 191:427–448.

Angel, A., and Berridge, D. A. (1974). Pathway for the primary evoked somatosensory cortical response in the rat. *Journal of Physiology (London)* 240:35–36P.

Angel, A., and Clarke, K. A. (1973a). Fine somatotopic representation of the forelimb area of the ventrobasal thalamus of the albino rat. *Journal of Physiology (London)* 233:43–44P.

Angel, A., and Clarke, K. A. (1973b). An analysis of the representation of the forelimb in the ventro-basal thalamic complex of the albino rat. *Journal of Physiology (London)* 249:399–424.

Angel, A., and Lemon, R. N. (1975). Sensorimotor cortical representation in the rat and the role of the cortex in the production of sensory and myoclonic jerks. *Journal of Physiology (London)* 248:465–488.

Armstrong-James, M. (1975). The functional status and columnar organization of single cells responding to cutaneous stimulation in neonatal rat somatosensory cortex SI. *Journal of Physiology (London)* 246:501–538.

Armstrong-James, M., and George, M. (1985). Bilateral synchronous firing and receptive fields of single units in Sm1 neocortex of the althesin-anesthetized rat. *Journal of Physiology (London)* 360:27P.

Armstrong-James, M., and Fox, K. (1987). Spatiotemporal convergence and divergence in the rat S1 "barrel" cortex. *Journal of Comparative Neurology* 263:265–281.

Barnard, J. W., and Woolsey, C. M. (1956). A study of localization in the corticospinal tracts of monkey and rat. *Journal of Comparative Neurology* 105:25–50.

Belford, G. R., and Killackey, H. P. (1978). Vibrissae representation in subcortical trige-minal centers of the neonatal rat. *Journal of Comparative Neurology* 183:305–322.

Benjamin, R. M., and Akert, K. (1959). Cortical and thalamic areas involved in taste discrimination in the albino rat. *Journal of Comparative Neurology* 11:231–259.

Benshalom, G., and White, E. L. (1986). Quantification of thalamocortical synapses with spiny stellate neurons in layer IV of mouse somatosensory cortex. *Journal of Comparative Neurology* 253:303–314.

Bernardo, K. L., and Woolsey, T. A. (1987). Axonal trajectories between mouse somato-sensory thalamus and cortex. *Journal of Comparative Neurology 258:542–564.*

Brodmann, K. (1909). Vergleichende Lockalisationslehre der Großhirnrinde in ihren Prin-zipien dargestellt auf Grund des Zellenbaus. Leipzig: J. A. Barth.

Brooks, C. M., and Peck, M. E. (1939). Effect of various cortical lesions on development of placing and hopping reactions in rats. *Journal of Neurophysiology* 3:66–73.

Brown, L. T., Jr. (1971). Projections and terminations of corticospinal tract in rodents. *Exp. Brain Res.* 13:432–450.

Brown, L. T., Jr. (1974). Corticorubral projections in the rat. *J. Comp. Neurol.* 154:149–168.

Carvell, G. E., and Simons, D. J. (1986). Somatotopic organization of the second soma-tosensory area (SII) in the cerebral cortex of the mouse. *Somatosensory Reserach* 3:213–237.

Carvell, G. E., and Simons, D. J. (1987). Thalamic and corticocortical connections of the second somatic sensory area of the mouse. *Journal of Comparative Neurology* 265:409–427.

Catsman-Berrevoets, C. E., and Kuypers, H. G. J. M. (1981). A search for corticospinal collaterals to thalamus and mesencephalon by means of multiple retrograde fluorescent tracers in cat and rat. *Brain Research* 218:15–33.

Caviness, V. S., Jr. (1975). Architectonic map of neocortex of the normal mouse. *Journal of Comparative Neurology* 164:247–264.

Caviness, V. S., and Frost, D. O. (1980). Tangential organization of thalamic projections to the neocortex in the mouse. *Journal of Comparative Neurology* 194:335–367.

Chapin, J. K., and Woodward, D. J. (1981). Modulation of sensory responsiveness of single somatosensory cortical cells during movement and arousal behaviors. *Experimental Neurology* 72:164–178.

Chapin, J. K., and Woodward, D. J. (1982a). Somatic sensory transmission to the cortex during movement: I. Gating of single cell responses to touch. *Experimental Neurology* 78:654–669.

Chapin, J. K., and Woodward, D. J. (1982b). Somatic sensory transmission to the cortex during movement: II. Phasic modulation over the locomotor step cycle. *Experimental Neurology* 78:670–684.

Chapin, J. K., and Woodward, D. J. (1982c). Cortico-cortical connections between physiologically and histologically defined zones in the rat SI and MI cortices. *Society for Neuroscience Abstracts* 8:434.

Chapin, J. K., Waterhouse, B. D., and Woodward, D. J. (1981). Differences in cutaneous sensory response properties of single somatosensory cortical neurons in awake and halothane anesthetized rats. *Brain Research Bulletin* 6:63–70.

Chapin, J. K., and Lin, C.-S. (1984). Mapping the body representation in the SI cortex of anesthetized and awake rats. *Journal of Comparative Neurology* 229:199–213.

Chapin, J. K. (1986). Laminar differences in sizes, shapes, and response profiles of cutaneous receptive fields in the rat SI cortex. *Experimental Brian Research* 262:549–559.

Chapin, J. K., and Woodward, D. J. (1986). Distribution of somatic sensory and active-movement neuronal discharge properties in the MI-SI cortical border area in the rat. *Experimental Neurology* 91:502–523.

Chapin, J. K. (1987). Modulation of cutaneous sensory transmission during movement: possible mechanism and biological significance. In S. P. Wise and E. V. Evarts (eds.), *Neural and Behavioral Approaches to Higher Brain Function*. New York: John Wiley & Sons.

Chapin, J. K., Guise, J. L., and Sadeq, M. (1987). Cortico-cortical connections within the primary somatosensory (SI) cortex of rat. *Journal of Comparative Neurology* 263:326–346.

Collingridge, G. L., and Bliss, T. V. P. (1987). NMDA receptors—their role in long-term potentiation. *Trends in Neuroscience* 10:288–293.

Connors, B. W., Gutnick, M. J., and Prince, D. A. (1982). Electrophysiological properties of neocortical neurons *in vitro*. *Journal of Neurophysiology* 48:1302–1320.

Connors, B. W., Malenka, R. C., and Silva, L. R. (1988). Two inhibitory postsynaptic potentials, and $GABA_A$ and $GABA_B$ receptor-mediated responses in neocortex of rat and cat. *Journal of Physiology (London)* 406:443–468.

Cotman, C. W., and Iversen, L. L. (1987). Excitatory amino acids in the brain—focus on NMDA receptors. *Trends in Neuroscience* 10:263–280.

Dawson, G. D. (1958). The central control of sensory inflow. *Proceedings of the Royal Society of Medicine* 51:531–535.

Dawson, D. R., and Killackey, H. P. (1987). The organization and mutability of the forepaws and hindpaw representations in the somatosensory cortex of the neonatal rat. *Journal of Comparative Neurology* 256:246–256.

Donoghue, J. P., Kerman, K. L., and Ebner, F. F. (1979). Evidence for two organizational plans within the somatic sensory-motor cortex of the rat. *Journal of Comparative Neurology* 183:647–664.

Donoghue, J. P., and Kitai, S. T. (1981). A collateral pathway to the neostriatum from corticofugal neurons of the rat sensory-motor cortex: an intracellular HRP study. *Journal of Comparative Neurology* 201:1–13.

Donoghue, J. P., and Wise, S. P. (1982). The motor cortex of the rat: Cytoarchitecture and microstimulation mapping. *J. Comp. Neurol.* 212:76–88.

Douglas, A., and Barr, M. L. (1950). The course of the pyramidal tract in rodents. *Revue Canadian Biology* 9:118–122.

Droogleever Fortuyn, A. B. (1914). Cortical cell-lamination of the hemispheres of some rodents. *Archs of Neurological Psychiatry* (Mott's) 6:221–354.

Dykes, R. W., Landry, P., Metherate, R., and Hicks, T. P. (1984). Functional role of GABA in cat primary somatosensory cortex: Shaping receptive fields of cortical neurons. *Journal of Neurophysiology* 52:1066–1093.

Dykes, R. W., Herron, P., and Lin, C. S. (1986). Ventroposterior thalamic regions projecting to cytoarchitectonic areas 3a and 3b in the cat. *Journal of Neurophysiology* 56:1521–1541.

Elger, C. E., Speckmann, E. J., Caspers, H., Janzen, R. W. C. (1977). Cortico-spinal connections in the rat. I. Monosynaptic and polysynaptic responses of cervical motoneurons to epicortical stimulation. *Experimental Brain Research* 28:385–404.

Finger, S., and Frommer, G. P. (1968). Effects of somatosensory thalamic and cortical lesions on roughness discriminations in the albino rat. *Physiology and Behavior* 3:83–89.

Finger, S., Simons, D., and Posner, R. (1978). Anatomical, physiological, and behavioral effects of neonatal sensorimotor cortex ablation in the rat. *Experimental Neurology* 60:347–373.

Goodman, D. C., Jarrard, L. E., and Nelson, J. F. (1966). Corticospinal pathways and their sites of termination in the albino rat. *Anatomical Record* 154:462.

Gruenthal, M., Finger, S., Berenbeim, J., Pollock, D., and Hart, T. (1980). A delayed lesion effect following sensorimotor cortex ablation in adult rats. *Experimental Neurology* 69:4–21.

Guise, J. L. U., and Chapin, J. K. (1985). Receptive fields of vibrissae-driven units in the awake rat SI cortex: effects of active movement and anesthetics. *Society for Neuroscience Abstracts* 15:752.

Guise, J. L. U., and Chapin, J. K. (1986). Influence of local cortico cortical circuits on layer V receptive fields in the rat SI barrelfield. *Society for Neuroscience Abstracts* 16:1433.

Gurdjian, E. S. (1927). The diencephalon of the albino rat. Studies on the brain of the rat. No. 2. *Journal of Comparative Neurology* 43:1–114.

Guzman-Flores, C., Buendia, N., Anderson, C., and Lindsley, D. B. (1962). Cortical and reticular influences upon evoked responses in dorsal column nuclei. *Experimental Neurology* 5:37–46.

Gwyn, D. G., and Flumerfelt, B. A. (1974). A comparison of the distribution of cortical and cerebellar afferents in the red nucleus of the rat. *Brain Research* 69:130–135.

Hall, R. D., and Lindholm, E. P. (1974). Organization of motor and somatosensory neocortex in the albino rat. *Brain Research* 66:23–38.

Harris, R. M., and Woolsey, T. A. (1983). Computer assisted analyses of barrel neuron axons and their putative synaptic contacts. *Journal of Comparative Neurology* 220:63–79.

Herkenham, M. (1978a). Intralaminar and parafascicular efferents to the striatum and cortex in the rat; an autoradiographic study. *Anatomical Record* 190:420.

Herkenham, M. (1978b). The connections of the nucleus reuniens thalami: Evidence for a direct thalamo-hippocampal pathway in the rat. *Journal of Comparative Neurology* 177:589–610.

Herkenham, M. (1980). Laminar organization of thalamic projections to the rat neocortex. *Science* 207:532–535.

Hicks, S. P., and D'Amato, C. J. (1970). Motor-sensory and visual behavior after hemispherectomy in newborn and mature rats. *Experimental Neurology* 29:416–438.

Hicks, S. P., and D'Amato, C. J. (1975). Motor-sensory cortex-corticospinal system and developing locomotion and placing in rats. *American Journal of Anatomy* 143:1–42.

Hicks, S. P., and D'Amato, C. J. (1977). Locating corticospinal neurons by retrograde axonal transport of horseradish peroxidase. *Experimental Neurology* 56:410–420.

Hutson, K. A., and Masterson, R. B. (1986). The sensory contribution of a single vibrissa's cortical barrel. *Journal of Neurophysiology* 56:1196–1223.

Jansen, K. F., and Killackey, H. P. (1987). Terminal arbors of axons projecting to the somatosensory cortex of the adult rat: I. The normal morphology of specific thalamocortical afferents. *Journal of Neuroscience* 7:3529–3543.

Jones, K. A., and Baughman, R. W. (1988). NMDA- and non-NMDA-receptor components of excitatory synaptic potentials recorded from cells in layer V of rat visual cortex. *Journal of Neuroscience* 8(9):3522–3534.

Jones, E. G., and Friedman, D. P. (1982). Projection pattern of functional components of thalamic ventrobasal complex upon monkey somatosensory cortex. *Journal of Neurophysiology* 48:521–544.

Jones, E. G., and Leavitt, R. Y. (1974). Retrograde axonal transport and the demonstration of non-specific projections to the cerebral cortex and striation from the thalamic intralaminar nuclei in the rat, cat, and monkey. *J. Comp. Neurol.* 154:349–378.

Kaas, J. H. (1982). The segregation of function in the nervous system: Why do sensory systems have so many subdivisions? In W. P. Neff (ed.), *Contributions to Sensory Physiology*. New York: Academic Press, 201–280.

Keller, A., White, E. L., and Cipolloni, P. B. (1985). The identification of thalamocortical axon terminals in barrels of mouse SmI cortex using immunohistochemistry of anterogradely transported lectin (Phaseolus vulgaris-leucoagglutinin). *Brain Research* 343:159–165.

Killackey, H. P. (1973). Anatomical evidence for cortical subdivisions based on vertically discrete thalamic projections from the ventral posterior nucleus to cortical barrels in the rat. *Brain Research* 51:326–331.

Killackey, H. P. (1980). Pattern formation in the trigeminal system of the rat. *Trends in Neuroscience* pp. 303–305.

Killackey, H., and Ebner, F. (1973). Convergent projection of three separate thalamic nuclei on to a single cortical area. *Science* 179:283–285.

Killackey, H. P., and Leshin, S. (1975). The organization of specific thalamocortical projections to the posteromedial barrel subfield of the rat somatic sensory cortex. *Brain Research* 86:469–472.

Knowles, S. E., Lin, C.-S., Chapin, J. K., and Woodward, D. J. (1980). Cells of origin and axonal branching patterns of the corticostriate pathway in rat. *Society for Neuroscience Abstracts* 6:324.

Krieg, W. J. S. (1946a). Connections of the cerebral cortex. I. The albino rat. A. Topography of the cortical areas. *Journal of Comparative Neurology* 84:221–275.

Krieg, W. J. S. (1946b). Connections of the cerebral cortex. I. The albino rat. B. Structure of the cortical areas. *Journal of Comparative Neurology* 84:277–323.

Krieg, W. J. S. (1947). Connections of the cerebral cortex. I. The albino rat. C. Extrinsic connections. *Journal of Comparative Neurology* 86:267–394.

Lamour, Y., Willer, J. C., and Guilbaud, G. (1983a). Rat somatosensory (SmI) cortex: I. Characteristics of neuronal responses to noxious stimulation and comparison with responses to non-noxious stimulation. *Experimental Brain Research* 49:35–45.

Lamour, Y., Guilbaud, G., and Willer, J. C. (1983b). Rat somatosensory (SmI) cortex: II. Laminar and columnar organization of noxious and non-noxious inputs. *Experimental Brain Research* 49:46–54.

Lamour, Y., Dutar, P., Jobert, A., and Dykes, R. W. (1988). An iontopheretic study of somatosensory neurons in rat granular cortex serving the limbs: a laminar analysis of glutamate and acetylcholine effects on receptive-field properties. *Journal of Neurophysiology* 60:725–750.

Lee, K. J., and Woolsey, T. A. (1975a). The relationship of peripheral innervation density (vibrissae) to cortical neuron number (barrels) in the mouse. *Anatomical Record* 99:349–353.

Lee, K. J., and Woolsey, T. A. (1975b). A proportional relationship between innervation density and cortical neuron number in the somatosensory system of the mouse. *Brain Research* 99:349–353.

Lin, C. S., and Chapin, J. K. (1981). Some connections of SI and SII in the rat. *Society for Neuroscience Abstracts* 7:254.

Lorente de Nó, R. (1922). La corteza del raton, Trab. Lab. *Invest. Biol.* (Madrid) 20:41–78.

Lu, S. M., and Lin, C.-S. (1986). Cortical projection patterns of the medial division of the nucleus posterior thalamus in the rat. *Society for Neuroscience Abstracts* 12:1434.

Lu, S. M., and Lin., C.-S. (1989). Afferent patterns from the posterior nucleus to the barrels. (In preparation).

Lund, R. D., and Webster, K. E. (1967a). Thalamic afferents from the dorsal column nuclei. An experimental anatomical study in the rat. *Journal of Comparative Neurology* 130:301–312.

MacDermott, A. B., and Dale, N. (1987). Receptors, ion channels and synaptic potentials underlying the integrative actions of excitatory amino acids. *Trends in Neuroscience* 10:280–284.

McAllister, J. P., Fekete, D. M., Wells, J., and Ryugo, D. K. (1977). The relationship of cytoarchitecture and dendritic morphology to afferent input within the thalamic ventral tier nuclei of the rat. *Society for Neuroscience Abstracts* 3:487.

McAllister, J. P., and Wells, J. (1981). The structural organization of the ventral postero-lateral nucleus in the rat. *Journal of Comparative Neurology* 197:271–301.

McComas, A. J., and Wilson, P. (1967). Some properties of pyramidal tract cells in the rat somatosensory cortex. *Journal of Physiology* 188:35P.

McCormick, D. A., Connors, B. W., Lighthall, J. W., and Prince, D. A. (1985). Comparative electrophysiology of pyramidal and sparsely spiny stellate neurons of the neocortex. *Journal of Neurophysiology* 54:782–806.

Merzenich M. M., Kaas, J. H., Wall, J. T., Nelson, R. J., Sur, M., and Felleman, D. J. (1983). Topographic reorganization of somatosensory cortical areas 3b and 1 in adult monkeys following restricted deafferentation. *Neuroscience* 8:33–55.

Mihailoff, G. A., Burne, R. A., and Woodward, D. J. (1978). Projections of the sensorimotor cortex to the basilar pontine nuclei in the rat: An autoradiographic study. *Brain Research* 145:347–354.

Mountcastle, V. B. (1957). Modality and topographic properties of single neurons of cat's somatic sensory cortex. *Journal of Neurophysiology* 20:408–418.

Mountcastle, V. B., and Powell, T. P. S. (1959). Neural mechanisms subserving cutaneous sensibility, with special reference to the role of afferent inhibition in sensory perception and discrimination. *Bulletin Johns Hopkins Hospital* 105:201–232.

Neafsey, E. J., and Sievert, S. (1982). A second forelimb area exists in the rat frontal cortex. *Brain Research* 232:151–156.

Norsell, U. (1978). Sensory defects caused by lesions of the first (SI) and second (SII) somatosensory areas of the dog. *Experimental Brain Research* 32:181–195.

Pasternak, J. F., and Woolsey, T. A. (1975). The number, size, and spatial distribution of neurons in lamina IV of mouse SmI neocortex. *Journal of Comparative Neurology* 160:291–306.

Pidoux, B., and Verley, R. (1981). Projections onto the cortical somatic barrel field from ipsilateral/vibrissae in adult rodents. *Electroencephalography and Clinical Neurophysiology* 46:715–726.

Rasmusson, D. D., and Turnbull, B. G. (1983). Immediate effects of digit amputation on SI cortex in the racoon: unmasking of inhibitory fields. *Brain Research* 288:368–370.

Rose, M. (1912). Histologische Lokalisation der Grosshirnrinde bei kleinen Säugetieren (Rodentia, Insectivora, Chiroptera). *J. Psychol. Neurol., Lpz.* 19:389–479.

Ryugo, R., and Killackey, H. P. (1975). Corticocortical connections of the barrel field of rat somatosensory cortex. *Society for Neuroscience Abstracts* 1:126.

Sanderson, K. J., Welker, W. I., and Shambes, G. M. (1981). Sensory and motor maps in rat somatic sensorimotor cortex. *Abstract, Australian Neuroscience Meeting* p. S77.

Sanderson, K. J., Welker, W., Shambes, G. M. (1983). Reevaluation of motor cortex and of sensorimotor overlap in cerebral cortex of albino rats. *Brain Research* 292:251–260.

Sapienza, S., Talbi, B., Jacquemin, J., and Albe-Fessard, D. (1981). Relationship between input and output of cells in motor and somatosensory cortices of the chronic awake rat. A study using glass micropipettes. *Experimental Brain Research* 43:47–56.

Saporta, S., and Kruger, L. (1974). The pattern of ventrobasal neuron projections to rat somatosensory cortex studied by retrograde axonal transport of horseradish peroxidase. *Society for Neuroscience Abstracts* 1:407.

Saporta, S., and Kruger, L. (1976). Quantitative study of thalamocortical projections of the ventrobasal complex in the rat. *Anatomical Record* 184:522.

Saporta, S., and Kruger, L. (1977). The organization of thalamocortical relay neurons in the rat ventrobasal complex studied by the retrograde transport of horseradish peroxidase. *Journal of Comparative Neurology* 174:187–208.

Shapovalov, A. I. (1975). Neuronal organization and synaptic mechanisms of supraspinal motor control in vertebrates. *Review of Physiology, Biochemistry and Pharmacology* 72:1–54.

Sharp, F. R., Gonzalez, M. F., Morgan, C. W., Morton, M. T., and Sharp, J. W. (1988). Common fur and mystacial vibrissae parallel sensory pathways: 14 C 2-deoxyglucose and WGA-HRP studies in the rat. *Journal of Comparative Neurology* 270:446–469.

Shin, H.-C., and Chapin, J. K. (1986). Inhibition of somatosensory transmission during movement is less at the thalamic than the cortical level. *Society for Neuroscience Abstracts* 12:564.

Shin, H.-C., and J. K. Chapin (1987). Movement correlated modulation of sensory transmission to single units in the VPL thalamus. *Society for Neuroscience Abstracts* 13:875.

Shin, H.-C., and Chapin, J. K. (1989). Mapping effects of motor cortex stimulation on single neurons in the dorsal column nuclei of rat: direct responses and afferent modulation. *Brain Research Bulletin* 22:245–252.

Simons, D. J. (1978). Response properties of vibrissa units in rat SI somatosensory neocortex. *Journal of Neurophysiology* 41:798–808.

Simons, D. J., and Woolsey, T. A. (1979). Functional organization in mouse barrel cortex. *Brain Research* 165:327–332.

Simons, D. J., and Woolsey, T. A. (1984). Morphology of Golgi- Cox-impregnated barrel neurons in rat SmI cortex. *Journal of Comparative Neurology* 230:119–132.

Sur, M., Nelson, R. J., and Kaas, J. H. (1978). The representation of the body surface in somatosensory area I of the grey squirrel. *Journal of Comparative Neurology* 179:425–450.

Uhr, J. L., Chapin, J. K., and Woodward, D. J. (1982). Variation in receptive field size across layer IV in rat barrelfield cortex. *Society for Neuroscience Abstracts* 8:465.

Uhr, J. L., and Chapin, J. K. (1983). Contribution of thalamo- cortical and cortico-cortical connections to receptive field properties in rat SI cortex. *Society for Neuroscience Abstracts* 9:652.

Vahlsing, H. L., and Feringa, E. R. (1981). A ventral uncrossed corticospinal tract in the rat. *Experimental Neurology* 70:282–287.

Valverde, F. (1962). Reticular formation of the albino rat's brain stem. Cytoarchitecture and corticofugal connections. *Journal of Comparative Neurology* 119:25–54.

Van der Loos, H. (1976). Barreloids in mouse somatosensory thalamus. *Neuroscience Letters* 2:1–6.

Van der Loos, H., and Woolsey, T. A. (1983). Somatosensory cortex: structural alterations following early injury to sense organs. *Science* 179:395–398.

Waite, G. D., and Taylor, P. K. (1978). Removal of whiskers in young rats causes functional changes in cerebral cortex. *Nature* 274:600–602.

Wall, P. D. (1970). The sensory and motor role of impulses traveling in the dorsal columns towards cerebral cortex. *Brain* 93:505–524.

Wall, J. T., and Egger, M. D. (1971). Formation of new connexions in adult rat brain after partial deafferentation. *Nature* 232:542–545.

Wall, J. T., and Kaas, J. H. (1985). Cortical reorganization and sensory recovery following nerve damage and regeneration. In C. Cotman (ed.), *Synaptic Plasticity.* New York: Guilford, 231–260.

Waterhouse, B. D., and Woodward, D. J. (1980). Interaction of norepinephrine with cerebrocortical activity evoked by stimulation of somatosensory afferent pathways in the rat. *Experimental Neurology* 67:11–34.

Webster, K. E. (1961). Cortico-striate interrelationships in the albino rat. *Journal of Anatomy (London)* 95:532–544.

Welker, C. (1971). Microelectrode delineation of fine grain somatotopic organization of SmI cerebral neocortex in albino rat. *Brain Research* 26:259–275.

Welker, C. (1976). Receptive fields of barrels in the somatosensory neocortex of the rat. *Journal of Comparative Neurology* 166:173–190.

Welker, C., and Sinha, M. M. (1972). Somatotopic organization of SmII cerebral neocortex in albino rat. *Brain Res.* 37:132–136.

Welker, C., and Woolsey, T. A. (1974). Structure of layer IV in the somatosensory neocortex of the rat: description and comparison with the mouse. *Journal of Comparative Neurology* 158:437–454.

Welker, W., Sanderson, K. J., and Shambes, G. M. (1983). Patterns of afferent projections to transitional zones in the somatic sensorimotor cerebral cortex of albino rats. *Brain Research* 292:261–267.

White, E. L. (1976). Ultrastructure and synaptic contacts in barrels of mouse SI cortex. *Brain Research* 105:229–251.

White, E. L. (1978). Identified neurons in mouse SMI cortex which are post-synaptic to thalamocortical axon terminals: A combined Golgi–electron microscopic and degeneration study. *J. Comp. Neurol.* 181:627–662.

White, E. L., and Rock, M. P. (1979). Distribution of thalamic input to different dendrites of a spiny stellate cell in mouse sensorimotor cortex. *Neuroscience Letters* 15:115–119.

White, E. L., and Hersch, S. M. (1982). A quantitative study of the thalamocortical and other synapses involving the apical dendrites of corticothalamic projection cells in mouse SmI cortex. *Journal of Neurocytology* 11:137 157.

Wiesendanger, R., and Wiesendanger, M. (1982a). The corticopontine system in the rat. I. Mapping of corticopontine neurons. *Journal of Comparative Neurology* 208:214–226.

Wiesendanger, R., and Wiesendanger, M. (1982b). The corticopontine system in the rat. II. The projection pattern. *Journal of Comparative Neurology* 208:227–238.

Wise, S. P., and Jones, E. G. (1976). The organization and postnatal development of the commissural projection of the rat somatic sensory cortex. *Journal of Comparative Neurology* 168:313–343.

Wise, S. P., and Jones, E. G. (1977). Cells of origin and terminal distribution of descending projections of the rat somatic sensory cortex. *Journal of Comparative Neurology* 175:129–158.

Wise, S. P., and Jones, E. G. (1978). Developmental studies of thalamocortical and commissural connections in the rat somatic sensory cortex. *Journal of Comparative Neurology* 178:187–208.

Wise, S. P., Murray, E. A., and Coulter, J. D. (1979). Somatotopic organization of corticospinal and corticotrigeminal neurons in the rat. *Neuroscience* 4:65–78.

Wong-Riley, M. T. T., and Welt, C. (1980). Histochemical changes in cytochrome oxidase of cortical barrels following vibrissal removal in neonatal and adult mice. *Proceedings of the National Academy of Sciences* USA 77:2333–2337.

Woolsey, C. N. (1947). Patterns of sensory representation in the cerebral cortex. *Federation Proceedings* 6:437–441.

Woolsey, C. N. (1952). Patterns of localization in sensory and motor areas of the cerebral cortex. In *Milbank Memorial Fund: The biology of mental health and disease*. New York: P. B. Hoeber, ch. 14.

Woolsey, C. N. (1958). Organization of somatic sensory and motor areas of the cerebral cortex. In H. F. Harlow and C. N. Woolsey, (eds.) *Biological and Biochemical Bases of Behavior*. Madison: University of Wisconsin Press, 63–82.

Woolsey, T. A., and Van der Loos, H. (1970). The structural organization of layer IV in the somatosensory region (SI) of mouse cerebral cortex. The description of a cortical field composed of discrete cytoarchitectonic units. *Brain Research* 17:205–242.

Woolsey, T. A., Dierker, M. L., and Wann, D. F. (1975a). Mouse SmI cortex: qualitative and quantitative classification of Golgi- impregnated barrel neurons. *Proceedings of the National Academy of Sciences* 72:2165–2169.

Woolsey, T. A., Welker, C., and Schwartz, R. H. (1975b). Comparative anatomical studies of the SmI face cortex with special reference to the barrels. *Journal of Comparative Neurology* 164:79–94.

Zilles, K., and Wree, A. (1985). Cortex: Areal and laminar structure. In G. Paxinos (ed.), *The Rat Nervous System: Vol. 1, Forebrain and Midbrain*. New York: Academic Press.

Zilles, K., Zilles, B., and Schleicher, A. (1980). A quantitative approach to cytoarchitectonics. VI. The areal pattern of the cortex of the albino rat. *Anatomy and Embryology (Berlin)* 159:335–360.

Zimmerman, R. A., Chambers, W. W., and Liu, C. N. (1964). An experimental study of the anatomical organization of the corticobulbar system in the albino rat. *J. Comp. Neurol.* 123:301–323.

15 Rat Auditory Cortex

Jack B. Kelly

The laboratory rat, *Rattus norvegicus*, is well suited for neuroanatomical, electrophysiological, and behavioral investigations of the central auditory system. Structures within the auditory pathway are well developed and easily accessible for the introduction of chemicals, placement of electrodes, or surgical intervention. The rat's behavioral audiogram reveals pure-tone sensitivity typical of small mammals and shows no indication of sensory abnormalities or degenerative disorders. The lower limit of hearing for the albino rat is 0.25 kHz, and the upper limit is 80 kHz, with maximum sensitivity between 8 kHz and 38 kHz. Both absolute thresholds and minimum audible angles for sound localization are similar to those found in pigmented wild rats (Heffner and Heffner 1985a,b, Kelly and Masterton 1977). The rat is easily trained in a variety of behavioral tasks and is therefore convenient for psychophysical tests of sensory capacity or general assessment of auditory ability. It is useful for developmental studies because its central nervous system is relatively immature at birth and early experimental treatment is possible (Kelly 1986). The rat has also been used to advantage in studies of the effects of aging on the central auditory system (Vaughan 1976, 1977, Vaughan and Peters 1974).

Despite the advantages of using the rat, there are still relatively few studies of its auditory cortex (see Webster 1985 for an earlier review). Only recently has the basic organization of the primary auditory cortex become apparent, and many questions concerning both the structure and function of the auditory cortex remain unanswered. This chapter reviews what is known about the auditory cortex in the rat, including neuroanatomical, neurophysiological, and behavioral data, and draws comparisons where appropriate with data from other species.

15.1 Organization of the Auditory Cortex

The auditory cortex of the rat is made up of several distinct cytoarchitectonic zones situated in the posterolateral neocortex (Krieg 1946, Zilles 1985, Zilles and Wree 1985, and Zilles, chapter 4). The main auditory area, designated area 41 by Krieg and Te1 by Zilles, is characterized by a large number of stellate cells in cortical layer IV and an increased density of myelinated fibers entering the middle cortex layers (koniocortex). This area is surrounded by several less granular, less heavily myelinated regions, the precise number and limits of which are still undetermined. These secondary areas include 20, 36, and 39 of Krieg and Te2 and Te3 of Zilles (figure 15.1A,B).

The rat's auditory cortex receives projections from the medial geniculate body and related intralaminar nuclei in the posterior thalamus (Lashley 1941, Waller 1934). On the basis of the pattern of thalamocortical projections, the auditory cortex can be subdivided into a central core that is more or less coextensive with Te1 (area 41) and a surrounding belt region that includes secondary cortical areas as indicated in figure 15.1C (LeDoux et al. 1985, Patterson 1977, Ryugo 1976). The core auditory cortex receives fibers from the ventral division of the medial geniculate, which in turn receives afferents from the central nucleus of the inferior colliculus (LeDoux et al. 1985, LeDoux et al. 1984, Patterson 1977, Ryugo 1976, Vaughan 1983, Vaughan and Foundas 1982). There is general agreement that this thalamic projection is topographic, but the issue of precisely which areas of the ventral medial geniculate project to which areas of core auditory cortex is unresolved (Patterson 1977, Ryugo 1976). The ventrocaudal part of the belt auditory cortex receives fibers from the dorsal division of the medial geniculate. This projection is probably also topographic, but the detailed connections are unknown (Patterson 1977, Ryugo 1976).

Both core and belt regions receive projections from the medial division of the medial geniculate and the neighboring posterior intralaminar nucleus. Although the fibers from the medial division to the auditory cortex overlap topographically with those from the ventral and dorsal subdivisions, they have a different pattern of terminal distribution within the cortical laminae. Fibers from the ventral and dorsal subdivisions terminate primarily in layer IV and the lower part of layer III, whereas axons from the medial subdivision terminate mainly in layers I and VI (Patterson 1977, Ryugo 1976, Ryugo and Killackey 1974). The total cortical area receiving projections from the medial division extends beyond the combined target zones of the ventral and dorsal subdivisions (Guldin and Markowitsch 1983, LeDoux et al. 1984, Patterson 1977, Ryugo 1976) and may include part of the second somatosensory cortex (LeDoux et al. 1984). It should be pointed out, however, that the medial division of the medial geniculate has input from the spinal cord as well as the auditory midbrain (LeDoux et al. 1987b), so that it is unclear without corroborating physiological evidence to what extent this projection is auditory, somatosensory, or a combination of both modalities. Unlike the other main subdivisions of the medial geniculate, the medial division has substantial projections to subcortical structures including the corpus striatum and lateral amygdala (Patterson 1977, Ryugo 1976, Ryugo and Killackey 1974, LeDoux et al. 1984, 1985). A similar but more

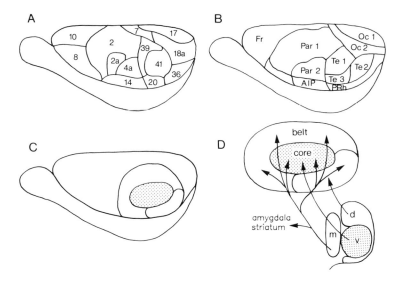

Figure 15.1 (A) Cytoarchitectonic subdivisions of the neocortex according to Krieg (1946). The central auditory area, area 41, is surrounded by a number of additional areas, 20, 36, and 39, with presumed auditory function. (B) Cytoarchitectonic areas according to Zilles (1985). The central auditory area, designated Te1, is surrounded by several additional areas, Te2, Te3, and PRh. (C) Auditory core and belt areas as defined by thalamocortical connections (derived from Patterson 1977 and Ryugo 1976). The location of the core area is indicated by shading. The auditory belt is indicated by a solid line showing the extent of the thalamocortical projection from the medial division of the medial geniculate and the location of the ventrocaudal belt region that receives a projection from the dorsal division of the medial geniculate. (D) A schematic summary of the main thalamocortical projections from the medial geniculate to the auditory cortex. The ventral division of the medial geniculate projects to the core auditory cortex, the dorsal division projects to the ventrocaudal belt region, and the medial division projects diffusely to both core and belt. In addition the medial division projects to the lateral amygdala and the corpus striatum. AIP = agranular insular cortex, posterior part; d = dorsal division of the medial geniculate; Fr = frontal cortex; m = medial division of the medial geniculate, Oc = occipital cortex; Par = parietal cortex; PRh = perirhinal cortex; Te = temporal cortex; v = ventral division of the medial geniculate.

extensive projection from the auditory thalamus to subcortical telencephalic structures (lateral amygdala and putamen) has been described in the primitive Virginia opossum, suggesting the possibility of a progressive evolution of auditory cortical projections in mammalian phylogeny (Kudo et al. 1986). A schematic view of the rat's auditory cortex as defined by cytoarchitecture and thalamocortical connections is shown in figure 15.1C,D.

The descending connections of the auditory cortex include projections to medial geniculate, inferior colliculus, and other subcortical structures. The medial geniculate projections arise from deep cortical layers (layer VI, Land et al. 1984 and LeDoux et al. 1985) and generally reciprocate the afferent thalamocortical projections, i.e., cortical areas that receive terminals from a particular location in the thalamus typically send projections back to the same thalamic site. Detailed analysis of the thalamocortical connections with combined anterograde and retrograde transport techniques, however, reveals zones of nonreciprocity in the medial geniculate body. Thus retrograde labeling of cell bodies is not precisely coextensive with areas of terminal labeling (Winer and Larue 1987). Projections to the inferior colliculus originate from large and middle-sized pyramidal cells in layer V and terminate in the dorsal cortex and external nucleus of the inferior colliculus (Beyerl 1978, Coleman and Clerici 1987, Coleman et al. 1984, Druga and Syka 1984, Faye-Lund 1985, Land et al. 1984, Syka and Popelar 1984). The perirhinal and suprarhinal cortical areas located between the core auditory cortex and the rhinal fissure give rise to projections to the lateral amygdala and parts of the corpus striatum (LeDoux et al. 1987a).

Azizi and colleagues (1985) have described a corticopontine cerebellar pathway in the rat that provides auditory input to the paraflocculus of the cerebellum. The cells of origin of this pathway are located in the belt cortex dorsal and ventral to the core auditory area (area 41 or Te1). A small injection of tritiated leucine into the dorsal belt region results in labeling of terminals in the lateral zone of the middle pons, an area that is known to project to the paraflocculus, whereas an injection directly into the auditory core itself does not result in labeling in the pontine gray. Electrical stimulation of either the dorsal or ventral belt regions results in neural responses in the paraflocculus that resemble those produced by acoustical stimulation.

The commissural connections of the auditory cortex arise from pyramidal and possibly nonpyramidal cells located in cortical layers II through VI. In layer V these cells can be distinguished from those projecting to the inferior colliculus on the basis of their morphology and laminar distribution. The commissural cells are smaller and more heterogeneous in form and tend to have a greater representation in the superficial parts of layer V than do the pyramidal cells projecting to the inferior colliculus (Games and Winer 1988). The terminals of callosal fibers to area 41 or Te1 are distributed in a trilaminar fashion to layers

I through III, the superficial part of layer V and layer VI. Projections to belt areas appear more bilaminar because of the thinning of layer IV in these regions and the consequent merging of the terminal fields in layers I through III and V (Vaughan 1983). Most of the callosal terminals form asymmetric synapses with apical dendritic spines or basal dendrites of pyramidal cells (Cipolloni and Peters 1983).

The terminals of thalamic fibers projecting to the auditory cortex are unevenly distributed across the cortical surface. A lesion of the ventral medial geniculate results in a patchy distribution of degenerating fibers with areas of relatively dense degeneration alternating with areas of sparse degeneration in cortical layers III and IV (Vaughan 1983, Vaughan and Foundas 1982). Lateral reconstructions from serial sections through the auditory cortex reveal several rostrocaudally oriented bands (200 μm to 1400 μm wide) of dense terminal degeneration interposed by bands (100 μm to 700 μm) of sparse terminal degeneration. Callosal fibers are also unevenly distributed across the cortical surface. Following transection of the corpus callosum, areas of dense terminal degeneration alternate with areas of relatively sparse degeneration within the auditory cortex, forming bands that run in a dorsoventral direction, i.e., at right angles to the rostrocaudally oriented bands of thalamocortical terminals (Cipolloni and Peters 1979, Vaughan 1983). Vaughan (1983) emphasizes that the difference between areas of dense and sparse terminal degeneration in the rat auditory cortex is not great and that all areas receive some projection from both callosal and thalamic sources. Combined lesions of corpus callosum and medial geniculate result in a relatively homogeneous pattern of degeneration within the auditory cortex.

In summary, the rat's auditory cortex can be subdivided into a core of koniocortex (Te1 or area 41) surrounded by a belt of cytoarchitectonically distinct secondary areas. The core and belt areas can be distinguished on the basis of their thalamocortical projections, but the precise topography of the projections is not known. The auditory cortex has descending projections to the medial geniculate, inferior colliculus, and other subcortical structures as well as callosal connections to the auditory cortex in the opposite hemisphere.

15.2 Electrophysiological Studies

The auditory cortex can be defined electrophysiologically by the distribution and pattern of neural responses (either slow waves or action potentials) elicited by acoustic stimulation. In the anesthetized animal an acoustically responsive area can be identified in posterolateral neocortex that is roughly coextensive with auditory cortex as defined by cytoarchitecture and neural connections (Azizi et al. 1985, LeMesserier 1948, Sally and Kelly 1988a, Scheel 1984, Syka et al. 1981, Woolsey 1952). The auditory cortex can be subdivided according to physiological criteria into a primary area (A-I) and other adjoining areas that have so far not been explored in detail (Sally and Kelly 1988a, Kelly and Sally 1988). Although A-I corresponds generally to the core auditory cortex (area 41 or Te1), as defined by neuroanatomy, a precise correlation between physiological and neuroanatomical subfields has not yet been established.

Single neurons in A-I are characterized by short-latency (8–14 ms), transient bursts of action potentials narrowly tuned to sound frequency. Each cell or group of cells can be associated with a characteristic frequency (CF, the frequency at which a neural response has its lowest excitatory sound pressure level). By mapping the CFs of a large number of neurons at different positions across the cortical surface it is possible to determine the frequency organization of the auditory cortex in individual animals. In the rat's A-I the representation of sound frequency is tonotopic with high frequencies located rostrally and low frequencies caudally (Sally and Kelly 1988a). The CFs cover most of the rat's hearing range, and the lowest thresholds for single neurons match closely the area of best sensitivity in the rat's behavioral audiogram. The distribution of characteristic frequencies for neurons within A-I of a single rat is shown in figure 15.2.

Neurons at different dorsoventral positions within A-I have similar CFs. Thus for each rostrocaudal location there is a dorsoventrally oriented contour that represents a single sound frequency, i.e., an isofrequency contour. In the rat the isofrequency contours usually extend about 1 mm across the cortical surface. Although some minor variations are noted in individual cases, the general location and orientation of the frequency maps and isofrequency contours are similar across animals.

The tonotopicity of the rat's primary auditory cortex is similar to that found in other mammals, but there are differences among species in the specific orientation of the frequency axis. For example, among rodents high frequencies are represented dorsally in the rabbit (McMullen and Glaser 1982) and caudally in the squirrel (Luethke et al. 1988, Merzenich et al. 1976) and guinea pig (Hellweg et al. 1977, Redies and Creutzfeldt 1987) rather than rostrally as in the rat. Among carnivores high-frequency responses are found within the rostral part of A-I in the cat (Brugge and Reale 1985, Imig and Morel 1983, Merzenich et al. 1975, Reale and Imig 1980) and dog (Tunturi 1950, 1960) but in the dorsal part of A-I in the ferret (Kelly et al. 1986, Phillips et al. 1988). Rotation of the tonotopic axis of A-I is also found in the marsupial possum (Gates and Aitkin 1982), tree shrew (Oliver et al. 1976), bushbaby (Brugge 1982), marmoset (Aitkin et al. 1986, Aitkin et al. 1988), owl monkey (Imig et al. 1977), macaque monkey (Merzenich and Brugge 1973), little brown bat (Suga 1965), and mustached bat (Suga and Jen 1976). Thus, even for species within the same taxonomic order, the map of sound frequency in A-I might be rotated as much as 180° relative to the major

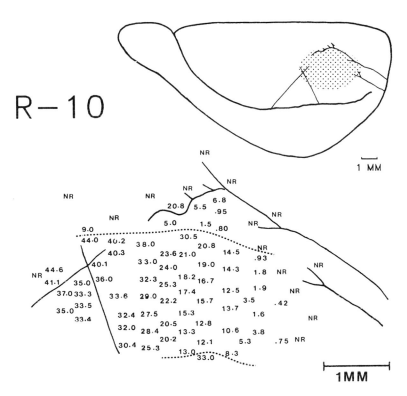

Figure 15.2 Distribution of characteristic frequencies (CF) of neurons within the auditory cortex of a single rat, R-10. The shading on the lateral surface of the neocortex in the upper half of the figure indicates the area of cortical tissue explored during this experiment. In the lower half of the figure the CFs of neurons at each cortical location are expressed in kHz. The solid lines represent blood vessels that served as landmarks during the mapping experiment, and the dotted lines indicate the boundaries between primary and secondary auditory cortex. High frequencies are represented rostrally and low frequencies caudally with isofrequency lines extending dorsoventrally. NR indicates no response. The scales in the upper and lower halves of the figure are equivalent to 1 mm. (From Sally and Kelly 1988a)

cortical landmarks. Nevertheless in the rat, as in every other species examined to date, the primary auditory cortex is tonotopically organized with an extended frequency representation down isofrequency contours.

The representation of high frequencies occupies a larger proportion of the cortical surface than does the representation of low frequencies, at least when sound frequency is expressed on a logarithmic scale. Approximately 80 percent of the rat's primary auditory cortex is devoted to the upper three octaves of the audiogram (above 8 kHz), with the remaining 20 percent devoted to the lower four octaves. The disproportionate representation of high frequencies can also be seen in the relation between CF and cortical position shown in figure 15.3. Each cell's CF is plotted as a function of the distance of the cell from the caudal boundary of A-I in four animals (rats 10, 13, 20, and 32 from Kelly and Sally 1988 and Sally and Kelly 1988a). The curvilinear form of the data is very similar to that reported for A-I in the guinea pig (Hellweg et al. 1977) and gray squirrel (Merzenich et al. 1976). The emphasis on high-frequency representation is also seen in cat (Merzenich et al. 1975), monkey (Merzenich and Brugge 1973), and ferret (Kelly et al. 1986). Thus the pattern of frequency representation within the rat's A-I probably reflects a general feature of mammalian auditory cortex, rather than an exaggeration of cortical representation associated with specialization of hearing at particular frequencies as in the case of the mustached bat (Suga 1984).

The tuning curves of cells in the rat's primary auditory cortex (i.e.,

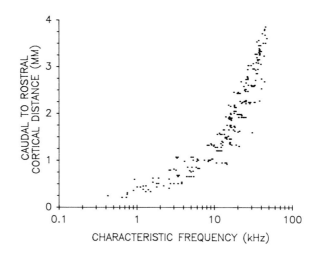

Figure 15.3 Characteristic frequency (CF) of cortical neurons as a function of the distance of the recording site from the caudal boundary of A-I. Cortical distance was measured in millimeters from a line drawn parallel to the isofrequency contours on maps from four individual cases (R-10, R-13, R-20, R-32). Because the results of the measurements were similar for the four cases, they were combined to produce a single figure. (Data from Kelly and Sally 1988 and Sally and Kelly 1988a)

curves defined by a cell's threshold for excitation across a range of sound frequencies) are similar to those found in A-I of other mammals. They are typically V-shaped with progressively narrower frequency response at lower sound pressure levels (figure 15.4A). In general, high-frequency neurons are more narrowly tuned than are low-frequency neurons. This relation can be seen by plotting Q10 (a measure of the narrowness of tuning) for a large number of neurons with different CFs, where Q10 is defined as the characteristic frequency divided by the bandwidth of the cell's response 10 dB above threshold. The distribution of Q10 for single neurons in A-I of the rat is shown in figure 15.4B. The maximum Q10 increases monotonically with sound frequency in a manner similar to that found in the primary auditory cortex, A-I, of the cat (Sally and Kelly 1988a, Phillips and Irvine 1981).

Most neurons in the rat's auditory cortex have monotonic rate-intensity functions, i.e., as sound pressure is increased above threshold the probability of firing increases up to some asymptotic level. The dynamic ranges of neurons with monotonic rate-intensity functions are typically between 5 dB and 35 dB, but in some cases are as great as 60 dB. Other cells exhibit nonmonotonic rate-intensity functions, i.e., the probability of firing increases up to a maximum and then decreases with additional sound pressure increments. The pattern of these rate-intensity functions is diverse: Some cells are completely inhibited whereas others show a reduction in firing that plateaus with further increase in sound pressure. Nonmonotonic cells are often "tuned" to specific sound pressures, but

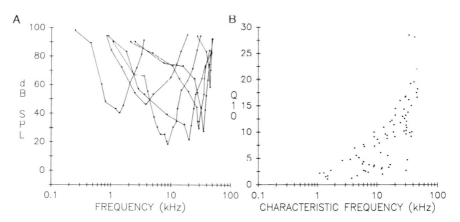

Figure 15.4 (A) Tuning curves for neurons in A-I of the rat. Each point represents the excitatory threshold in dB SPL at various sound frequencies. The solid lines describe the limits of sensitivity for each cell. The curves are V-shaped and narrowly tuned to sound frequency. The lowest threshold for each cell defines its characteristic frequency (CF). (B) Narrowness of tuning as determined by Q10 values for single neurons in the rat's A-I. The Q10 is defined as a cell's CF divided by the bandwidth of its tuning curve 10 dB above threshold. A large Q10 represents relatively narrow tuning to sound frequency. The maximum Q10 at any given sound frequency increases monotonically over the range from 1 kHz to 40 kHz. (Adapted from Sally and Kelly 1988a.)

Kelly: Auditory Cortex

the narrowness of tuning is variable from cell to cell. The dynamic range of nonmonotonic responses is usually 30 dB to 40 dB, but can be as great as 80 dB (Phillips and Kelly 1989).

Over 95 percent of the cells in the rat's primary auditory cortex are sensitive to binaural input (Kelly and Sally 1988). The majority of cells exhibit either binaural summation or suppression. Approximately 35 percent of the cells show binaural summation, i.e., a sound presented to either the contralateral or ipsilateral ear alone produces excitation, and stimulation of both ears together results in an increased probability of response (EE/F cells according to the classification scheme of Aitkin et al. 1975). Forty-two percent of the cells show binaural suppression, i.e., the probability of firing is increased by contralateral stimulation, is uninfluenced by ipsilateral stimulation alone, but is greatly reduced by binaural stimulation (EO/I cells). Approximately 18 percent of the cells exhibit a mixture of summation and suppression: They are excited by binaural stimulation when the ipsilateral sound pressure level is low, but are inhibited as the sound pressure in the ipsilateral ear is increased in a fashion similar to that described by Reale and Kettner (1986) for the cat.

Cells with different binaural response properties are not uniformly distributed across the cortical surface. There is a tendency for cells with similar binaural response characteristics to be grouped together (figure 15.5), although there is considerable variability among individual animals in the spatial distribution of binaural response types. In many cases cortical areas exhibiting binaural summation and suppression appear to cut across isofrequency contours to form rostrocaudally oriented bands. A similar grouping of binaural response types is found in the cat (Imig and Adrian 1977, Imig and Brugge 1978, Imig and Reale 1981, Reale and Kettner 1986, Middlebrooks et al. 1980, Middlebrooks and Zook 1983) and ferret (Judge and Kelly 1988) and may be a general feature of the organization of the primary auditory cortex.

In the cat combined mapping and tract tracing studies have shown that areas of A-I with predominantly EE/F cells receive callosal projections from the auditory cortex in the opposite hemisphere, whereas areas with EO/I cells receive projections primarily from the anterior and posterior fields of the auditory cortex in the same hemisphere (Imig and Brugge 1978, Imig and Reale 1981). Comparable studies have not been done in the rat, but the uneven distribution of binaural response types and the patchy distribution of callosal fibers to A-I suggest the possibility of a similar relationship. It should be pointed out, however, that the correspondence of binaural classes and callosal projections in the rat is far from obvious. According to Cipolloni and Peters (1979, 1983) the callosal fibers are distributed in dorsoventrally oriented bands, whereas the binaural areas described by Kelly and Sally (1988) tend to have a rostrocaudal orientation.

All three major binaural response types—summation, suppression,

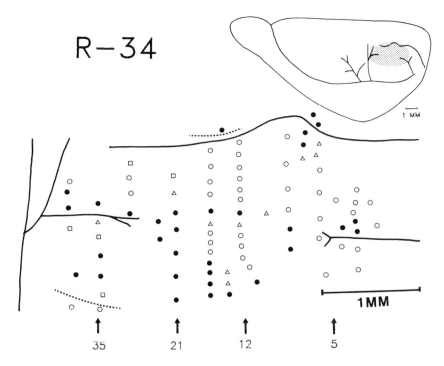

Figure 15.5 The distribution of binaural response types within A-I of a single rat (R-34). The area mapped is indicated by shading on the lateral surface of the rat's neocortex in the upper right of the figure. The lower half of the figure shows the binaural response types at specific locations within that area. Solid circles represent summation responses (EE/F), open circles represent suppression responses (EO/I), triangles represent mixed responses, and squares represent other responses. Solid lines indicate blood vessels, and dotted lines indicate the boundaries between primary and secondary auditory cortex. The approximate position and CFs of selected isofrequency contours are shown by arrows at the bottom of the figure. CF is expressed in kHz. The scales in the upper and lower parts of this figure represent 1 mm. (Adapted from Kelly and Sally 1988.)

and mixed—are represented at each sound frequency within the rat's hearing range. However, the proportional distribution of binaural summation and suppression responses is frequency dependent. There is a tendency toward a larger percentage of binaural suppression responses at high frequencies and summation responses at low frequencies as shown in figure 15.6. A similar distribution is seen among cells in the central nucleus of the rat's inferior colliculus (Kelly et al. 1989). Thus it seems likely that this distribution of responses is the product of binaural interaction patterns established in the rat's lower brainstem (Inbody and Feng 1981, Irvine 1986, Sally and Kelly 1988b). The distribution is consistent with the suggestion of Brugge and Geisler (1978) that there is differential representation of binaural interaction types by frequency within the medial and lateral subdivisions of superior olivary complex.

Microelectrode mapping studies have shown that acoustically responsive regions do exist outside the boundaries of physiologically defined

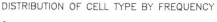

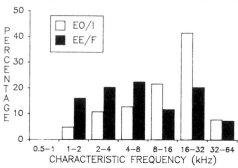

Figure 15.6 The distribution of binaural interaction class by characteristic frequency. Cells in the summation category (EE/F) are shown as shaded bars, and those in the suppression category (EO/I) are indicated by unshaded bars. These data are expressed as the percentage of cells within each category found at different sound frequencies. There is a tendency toward a higher proportion of EE/F responses at low frequencies and EO/I responses at high frequencies. (Data from Kelley and Sally 1988.)

A-I (Horikawa et al. 1988, Kelly and Sally 1988, Sally and Kelly 1988a). Both dorsal and ventral to A-I there are cells whose CFs are inconsistent with the prevailing isofrequency trends within A-I. Also, caudal to A-I there are cells with high-frequency CFs, suggesting the possibility of a second auditory field. Most other mammals, including other small rodents (squirrels, rabbits, and guinea pigs), have multiple auditory fields that are tonotopically organized. In some cases the frequency representation is a mirror-image reversal of the map in A-I (Hellweg et al. 1977, Leuthke et al. 1988, McMullen and Glaser 1982). Leuthke and associates (1988) have demonstrated at least three fields outside A-I in the auditory cortex of the squirrel. Multiple tonotopic fields are probably also present in the rat auditory cortex (Horikawa et al. 1988).

In summary, recent electrophysiological investigations have established a framework for understanding the basic organization of the auditory cortex in the rat. However, much remains to be discovered. The response properties of acoustically driven cells outside A-I are largely unexplored. The possible correspondence between auditory cortical subdivisions as defined by neurophysiological and neuroanatomical criteria, and the interconnections among different auditory areas must still be examined. Additional studies with combined electrophysiological and neuroanatomical techniques are needed to provide a more nearly complete understanding of the organization of the auditory cortex in the rat.

15.3 Behavioral Studies of Cortical Function

Behavioral studies of the auditory cortex in the rat have dealt mostly with sound localization. The rationale for this approach has come from the fact that ablation of the auditory cortex in other mammalian species results in severe sound localization deficits. In the cat bilateral ablation of the auditory cortex results in a complete inability to localize brief sounds in tasks requiring an approach response (Neff 1968, Neff et al. 1975, Neff et al. 1956, Strominger 1969). Dogs, monkeys, and ferrets also suffer impairments in sound localization following bilateral ablation of the auditory cortex (Heffner 1978, Heffner and Masterton 1975, Kavanagh and Kelly 1987, 1988, Wegener 1964). Furthermore unilateral lesions of the auditory cortex in cats, ferrets, and squirrel monkeys result in impaired sound localization in the field contralateral to the side of the lesion (Jenkins and Masterton 1982, Jenkins and Merzenich 1984, Kavanagh and Kelly 1983, 1987, Thompson and Cortez (1983). Jenkins and Merzenich (1984) and Kavanagh and Kelly (1987) have shown that these contralateral deficits can be produced by lesions restricted to the primary auditory cortex (A-I) alone.

In contrast, studies with the albino rat reveal little impairment in sound localization following bilateral ablation of the auditory cortex. In tests with two sound sources positioned symmetrically on the right and left of midline, rats are still capable of accurate localization following complete bilateral destruction of the auditory cortex (Kelly 1980, Kelly and Glazier 1978, Kelly and Judge 1985, Kelly and Kavanagh 1986). As shown in figure 15.7, only minor deficits in performance are found with short duration (65-ms) pure-tone pulses of various frequencies from 2 kHz to 32 kHz (Kavanagh and Kelly 1986). Similar results are obtained with single clicks and brief noise bursts (Kelly 1980). Bilateral destruction of the medial geniculate body, which disrupts the thalamic projections to the auditory cortex, also fails to produce an incapacity for sound localization. Severe deficits are found only if the lesions extend caudally and medially to include the brachium of the inferior colliculus and the neighboring lateral tegmentum (Kelly and Judge 1985).

Tests of lateral field sound localization reveal no substantial deficits following either bilateral or unilateral ablation of the auditory cortex (Judge and Kelly 1983), but do show that normal rats have considerable difficulty localizing sounds within a field (Kavanagh and Kelly 1986). In a seven-choice apparatus with loudspeakers positioned at equal intervals between +90° and −90° azimuth, normal rats localize a single click at performance levels of only about 40 percent correct response (14.3 percent would be expected by chance alone). In this situation bilateral auditory cortical lesions fail to produce deficits beyond those already expected from studies of two-choice (left versus right) sound localization. Furthermore unilateral destruction of the auditory cortex does not result in exclusively contralateral impairments as might be expected from studies with other mammals.

The difficulty that normal rats experience with seven-choice localization is probably due to the fact that rats have very poor acuity in the lateral fields (Kavanagh and Kelly 1986). The minimum audible angle

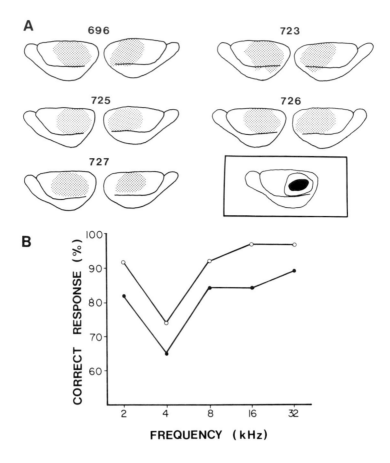

Figure 15.7 (A) The extent of damage to the auditory cortex in rats tested in behavioral studies of sound localization. Lesions are shown as a shaded area in the lateral reconstruction of left and right hemispheres of five rats from Kelly and Kavanagh 1986. For comparison the location of core and belt auditory cortex as defined by Ryugo (1976) is indicated on the same standardized lateral view of the rat brain in the lower right-hand panel. (B) Performance of normal and brain-damaged rats in a two-choice (left versus right) test of sound localization. The stimuli were 65-ms tone pulses at frequencies between 2 kHz and 32 kHz. The sound pressure level at each frequency was 40 dB above absolute threshold. The performance level expected by chance in this situation is 50 percent correct response. Open circles indicate the average performance of normal animals at each of the five frequencies; filled circles represent the average performance of animals with bilateral ablation of the auditory cortex. (From Kelly and Kavanagh 1986.)

for a single click around 0° azimuth is about 12.5°, but is in excess of 60° for left and right lateral fields. Indeed rats show no clear indication of being able to distinguish separate positions of a single click within the same lateral field. This result precludes any further investigation of the effects of cortical lesions on lateral field localization. The *normal* rat appears to be deficient in precisely the aspect of sound localization that depends most on the primary auditory cortex in cat and ferret.

There have been relatively few studies of the effects of cortical lesions on sound localization in lissencephalic mammals other than the rat. Nevertheless the data suggest that the rat might not be the only species that is capable of sound localization after the destruction of the auditory cortex. Complete bilateral decortication of the Virginia opossum has little effect on the ability to detect a change in the spatial location of a noise burst or to identify its position in space (Ravizza and Masterton 1972). The minimum audible angle for discriminating left from right is elevated relative to normal, but performance at angles above 30° speaker separation is unaffected. The minimum audible angle for detecting a shift in elevation is unaffected by decortication. These data do not rule out the possibility that severe impairments would emerge in other tests, for example, ones requiring an approach response, but neither do they contradict the idea that sound localization is still possible following ablation of the auditory cortex.

Ravizza and Diamond (1974) have examined the effects of auditory cortical lesions in two other primitive mammals, the hedgehog (*Paraechinus hypomelas*) and the bushbaby (*Galago senegalensis*), both of which have a lissencephalic neocortex. In a six-choice apparatus with loudspeakers positioned at equal intervals between +60° and −60° azimuth, *normal* hedgehogs have difficulty maintaining high performance levels when the duration of the acoustic stimulus (a noise burst) is less than about 500 ms. Performance levels are around 60 percent correct at durations as brief as 25 ms, a result that suggests that hedgehogs, like rats, have difficulty with lateral field localization. Bilateral ablation of the auditory cortex results in impaired performance at very brief durations, but it is not clear whether the impairments are due to midline or lateral field deficits or to more general behavior problems.

Bushbabies are capable of maintaining a high level of performance in a six-choice apparatus even with very brief stimulus durations. After bilateral ablation of the auditory cortex there is a reduction in performance at durations less than about 500 ms, but even with noise bursts as brief as 25 ms performance levels are around 50 percent correct, well above chance in this test situation. It is impossible to determine from these data whether the reduction in performance is due to midline or lateral field deficits, but the results suggest that bushbabies, like rats, retain some ability to localize sounds after bilateral destruction of the auditory cortex.

Complete bilateral destruction of the auditory cortex in the rat produces no obvious abnormality in conditioned autonomic responses or conditioned emotional responses to auditory stimuli (LeDoux et al. 1984, Romanski et al. 1988). There are no discernible effects of auditory cortical lesions on conditioning of arterial blood pressure, heart rate, freezing, or drink suppression. On the other hand bilateral lesions of the medial geniculate body reduce the magnitude of conditioned emotional and autonomic responses to sound (LeDoux et al. 1984, LeDoux et al. 1986). This result is attributed to the substantial subcortical projections from the auditory thalamus to the lateral amygdala and corpus striatum in the rat (LeDoux et al. 1987a, LeDoux et al. 1985). Birt and coworkers (1978) found that rats with large bilateral lesions of the auditory cortex do have difficulty learning a differential response (head movement) to 1-kHz versus 4-kHz tone bursts. Smaller lesions that produce degeneration restricted largely to the ventral division of the medial geniculate have no obvious effect on the development of this conditioned response.

The relative lack of permanent behavioral deficits after lesions of the auditory cortex in the rat raises the question of the functional significance of the cortex for hearing. It is unlikely that the rat's auditory cortex is without some essential contribution. A more challenging interpretation is that studies so far have failed to use appropriate tests for detecting a deficit. Experiments with cats and monkeys have revealed impairments following auditory cortical lesions in several aspects of hearing other than simple conditioning or the ability to localize sounds in space. For example, cats and monkeys with bilateral lesions of the auditory cortex have long-lasting impairments in the ability to discriminate between temporal patterns of sound frequency, e.g., high-low-high versus low-high-low tone sequences (Colavita et al. 1974, Diamond and Neff 1957, Jerison and Neff 1953, Kelly 1973, Kelly and Whitfield 1971, Neff et al. 1975, Strominger et al. 1980, Wegener 1976) and tone duration (Scharlock et al. 1965). Also, ablation of the auditory cortex in monkeys produces deficits in discrimination of speech sounds, [i] versus [u], and species-specific monkey vocalizations—the "coo" calls produced by Japanese macaques (Dewson et al. 1969, Heffner and Heffner 1984, 1986, 1989a,b). Tees (1967) and Patchett (1977) have shown that rats are capable of temporal pattern discriminations and that the ability is disrupted by restricted auditory stimulation during early development (see Tees, chapter 22). There are no studies, however, of the effects of auditory cortical lesions on these tasks in the rat. Thus it is possible that the functional significance of the auditory cortex in the rat lies in the ability to process temporally or spectrally complex acoustic signals. Additional behavioral studies of the effects of cortical lesions are necessary before the role of the auditory cortex can be determined.

In summary, behavioral studies indicate that the rat's auditory cortex is not essential for the localization of sounds in space. Nor is the auditory cortex essential for conditioned emotional responses to sounds. The possible role of the rat's auditory cortex in other aspects of audition, such as the perception of complex sounds or the discrimination of tonal patterns, has not been systematically investigated. There is currently little basis for speculation about the possible functional specialization of physiologically and/or neuroanatomically defined subdivisions of the auditory cortex in the rat.

15.4 Conclusions

1. Anatomically the rat's auditory cortex can be subdivided into a central core and a surrounding belt region, both of which receive direct projections from the medial geniculate body. The core area receives a topographic projection from the ventral division of the medial geniculate, and the ventrocaudal belt region receives a parallel projection from the dorsal division of the medial geniculate. The medial division of the medial geniculate sends fibers to both core and belt auditory cortex.

2. Cell bodies in the deep layers of the auditory cortex send fibers back to the medial geniculate body. The terminal fields of these efferent fibers largely overlap the thalamic areas that gave rise to the cortical projections, but there are also prominent zones of nonreciprocity in the medial geniculate. Large pyramidal cells in layer V of the auditory cortex project directly to the inferior colliculus and terminate in both the dorsal cortex and external nucleus. Other descending projections include fibers to the lateral amygdala, corpus striatum, and the lateral pontine region. Callosal fibers originate from a morphologically heterogeneous cell population in cortical layers II through V and project to layers I through III, V, and VI of the auditory cortex in the opposite hemisphere.

3. Physiologically the auditory cortex can be subdivided into a tonotopically organized A-I and an additional surrounding zone, which has not yet been examined in detail. Within the rat's A-I, responses are typically short-latency and narrowly tuned to sound frequency. Characteristic frequencies range from 0.42 kHz to 47.1 kHz with a disproportionately large area of the cortical surface devoted to the upper octaves. High frequencies are represented rostrally and low frequencies caudally with isofrequency contours extending dorsoventrally.

4. Cells in the auditory cortex exhibit various binaural response patterns including summation (EE/F), suppression (EO/I), and mixed summation and suppression. Each of these binaural response types is represented across the entire range of sound frequencies (CFs) with a tendency toward a higher proportion of EO/I cells at high frequencies and EE/F cells at low frequencies. Cells with the same binaural response characteristic are grouped together to form discrete areas of binaural representation within A-I. There is some indication that these areas are continuous across isofrequency contours forming rostrocaudally ori-

ented binaural bands, but the pattern of banding is quite variable from case to case.

5. Complete bilateral destruction of the auditory cortex in the rat results in only minor impairments in the ability to localize sounds in space. Minimum audible angles for sound localization are elevated slightly, but localization at larger angles is still possible. Also there is no discernible effect of auditory cortical lesions on conditioned emotional or autonomic responses to sounds. Thus the auditory cortex is not essential for either of these aspects of hearing. Behavioral evidence regarding the role of the auditory cortex in the perception of temporal patterns or complex acoustic signals is lacking for the rat, although deficits have been reported for other species. Further behavioral studies are needed to determine the essential functional contribution of the rat's auditory cortex to the perception of sound.

References

Aitkin, L. M., Kudo, M., and Irvine, D. R. F. (1988). Connections of the primary auditory cortex in the common marmoset, *Calithrix jacchus jacchus*. *Journal of Comparative Neurology* 268:235–248.

Aitkin, L. M., Merzenich, M. M., Irvine, D. R. F., Clarey, J. C., and Nelson, J. E. (1986). Frequency representation in the auditory cortex of the common marmoset (*Callithrix jacchus jacchus*). *Journal of Comparative Neurology* 252:175–185.

Aitkin, L. M., Webster, W. R., Veale, J. L., and Crosby, D. C. (1975). Inferior colliculus. I. Comparison of response properties of neurons in central, pericentral and external nuclei of the cat. *Journal of Neurophysiology* 38:1196–1207.

Azizi, S. A., Burne, R. A., and Woodward, D. J. (1985). The auditory corticopontocerebellar projection in the rat: inputs to the paraflocculus and midvermis. An anatomical and physiological study. *Experimental Brain Research* 59:36–49.

Beyerl, B. D. (1978). Afferent projections to the central nucleus of the inferior colliculus in the rat. *Brain Research* 145:209–223.

Birt, D., Nienhuis, R., and Olds, J. (1978). Effects of bilateral auditory cortex ablation on behavior and unit activity in rat inferior colliculus during differential conditioning. *Journal of Neurophysiology* 41:705–715.

Brugge, J. F. (1982). Auditory cortical areas in primates. In C. N. Woolsey (ed.), *Cortical Sensory Organization, Vol. 3, Multiple Auditory Areas*. Clifton, N.J.: Humana Press, 59–70.

Brugge, J. F., and Geisler, C. D. (1978). Auditory mechanisms of the lower brain stem. *Annual Review of Neuroscience* 1:363–394.

Brugge, J. F., and Reale, R. A. (1985). Auditory cortex. In A. Peters and E. G. Jones (eds.), *Cerebral Cortex, Vol 4, Association and Auditory Cortices*. New York: Plenum Press, 229–266.

Cipolloni, P. B., and Peters, A. (1979). The bilaminar and banded distribution of the callosal terminals in the posterior neocortex of the rat. *Brain Research* 176:33–47.

Cipolloni, P. B., and Peters, A. (1983). The termination of callosal fibres in the auditory cortex of the rat. A combined Golgi-electron microscope and degeneration study. *Journal of Neurocytology* 12:713–726.

Colavita, F. B., Szeligo, F. V., and Zimmer, S. D. (1974). Temporal pattern discrimination in cats with insular-temporal lesions. *Brain Research* 79:153–156.

Coleman, J. R., and Clerici, W. J. (1987). Sources of projections of the inferior colliculus in the rat. *Journal of Comparative Neurology* 262:215–226.

Coleman, J., Rainer, R., and Clerici, W. J. (1984). Projection pattern of the rat auditory cortex. *Society for Neuroscience Abstracts* 10:247.

Dewson, J. H. III, Pribram, K. H., and Lynch, J. C. (1969). Effects of ablations of temporal cortex upon speech sound discrimination in the monkey. *Experimental Neurology* 24:579–591.

Diamond, I. T., and Neff, W. D. (1957). Ablation of temporal cortex and discrimination of auditory patterns. *Journal of Neurophysiology* 20:300–315.

Druga, R., and Syka, J. (1984). Ascending and descending projections of the inferior colliculus in the rat. *Physiologica Bohemoslovia* 33:31–42.

Faye-Lund, H. (1985). The neocortical projection to the inferior colliculus in the albino rat. *Anatomy and Embryology* 173:53–70.

Games, K. D., and Winer, J. A. (1988). Layer V in rat auditory cortex: projection to the inferior colliculus and contralateral cortex. *Hearing Research* 34:1–26.

Gates, G. R., and Aitkin, L. M. (1982). Auditory cortex in the marsupial possum (*Trichosurus vulpecula*). *Hearing Research* 7:1–11.

Guldin, W. O., and Markowitsch, H. J. (1983). Cortical and thalamic afferent connections of the insular and adjacent cortex of the rat. *Journal of Comparative Neurology* 215:135–153.

Heffner, H. E. (1978). Effects of auditory cortex ablation on the discrimination of brief sounds. *Journal of Neurophysiology* 41:963–976.

Heffner, H. E., and Heffner, R. S. (1984). Temporal lobe lesions and perception of species-specific vocalizations by macaques. *Science* 226:75–76.

Heffner, H. E., and Heffner, R. S. (1985a). Hearing in two cricetid rodents: wood rat (*Neotoma floridana*) and grasshopper mouse (*Onychomys leucogaster*). *Journal of Comparative Psychology* 99:275–288.

Heffner, H. E., and Heffner, R. S. (1985b). Sound localization in wild Norway rats (*Rattus norvegicus*). *Hearing Research* 19:151–155.

Heffner, H. E., and Heffner, R. S. (1986). Effect of unilateral and bilateral auditory cortex lesions on the discrimination of vocalizations by Japanese macaques. *Journal of Neurophysiology* 56:683–701.

Heffner, H. E., and Heffner, R. S. (1989a). Cortical deafness cannot account for the inability of Japanese macaques to discriminate species-specific vocalizations. *Brain and Language* 36:275–285.

Heffner, H. E., and Heffner, R. S. (1989b). Effect of restricted lesions on absolute thresholds and aphasia-like deficits in Japanese macaques. *Behavioral Neuroscience* 103:158–169.

Heffner, H. E., and Masterton, R. B. (1975). Contribution of auditory cortex to sound localization in the monkey (*Macaca mulatta*). *Journal of Neurophysiology* 38:1340–1358.

Hellweg, F. C., Koch, R., and Vollrath, M. (1977). Representation of the cochlea in the neocortex of guinea pigs. *Experimental Brain Research* 29:467–474.

Horikawa, J., Ito, S., Hosokawa, Y., Homma, T., and Murata, K. (1988). Tonotopic representation in the rat auditory cortex. *Proceedings of the Japan Academy* 64 (Series B):260–263.

Imig, T. J., and Adrian, H. O. (1977). Binaural columns in the primary auditory field (AI) of the cat auditory cortex. *Brain Research* 138:241–257.

Imig, T. J., and Brugge, J. F. (1978). Sources and terminations of callosal axons related to binaural and frequency maps in primary auditory cortex of the cat. *Journal of Comparative Neurology* 182:637–660.

Imig, T. J., and Morel, A. (1983). Organization of the thalamocortical auditory system in the cat. *Annual Review of Neuroscience* 6:95–120.

Imig, T. J., and Reale, R. A. (1981). Ipsilateral corticocortial projections related to physiological maps of the cat's cortex. *Journal of Comparative Neurology* 203:1–14.

Imig, T. J., Ruggero, M. A., Kitzes, L. M., Javel, E., and Brugge, J. F. (1977). Organization of auditory cortex in the owl monkey (*Aotes trivirgatus*). *Journal of Comparative Neurology* 171:111–128.

Inbody, S. B., and Feng, A. S. (1981). Binaural response characteristics of single neurons in the medial superior olivary nucleus of the albino rat. *Brain Research* 210:361–366.

Irvine, D. R. F. (1986). *The Auditory Brainstem: A Review of the Structure and Function of Auditory Brainstem Processing Mechanisms* (Progress in Sensory Physiology, Vol. 7). Berlin: Springer Verlag.

Jenkins, W. M., and Masterton, R. B. (1982). Sound localization: effects of unilateral lesions in central auditory pathways. *Journal of Neurophysiology* 47:987–1016.

Jenkins, W. M., and Merzenich, M. M. (1984). Role of cat primary auditory cortex for sound localization behavior. *Journal of Neurophysiology* 52:819–847.

Jerison, H. J., and Neff, W. D. (1953). Effect of cortical ablation in the monkey on discrimination of auditory patterns. *Federation Proceedings* 12:237.

Judge, P. W., and Kelly, J. B. (1983). The effects of auditory cortical lesions on seven-choice sound localization by the rat. *Society for Neuroscience Abstracts* 9:956.

Judge, P. W., and Kelly, J. B. (1988). Topographic organization of binaural neurons in the primary auditory cortex of the ferret. *Society for Neuroscience Abstracts* 14:651.

Kavanagh, G. L., and Kelly, J. B. (1983). The effects of auditory cortical lesions on seven-choice sound localization by ferrets. *Society for Neuroscience Abstracts* 9:956.

Kavanagh, G. L., and Kelly, J. B. (1986). Midline and lateral field sound localization in the albino rat (*Rattus norvegicus*). *Behavioral Neuroscience* 100:200–205.

Kavanagh, G. L., and Kelly, J. B. (1987). Contribution of auditory cortex to sound localization by the ferret (*Mustela putorius*). *Journal of Neurophysiology* 57:1746–1766.

Kavanagh, G. L., and Kelly, J. B. (1988). Hearing in the ferret (*Mustela putorius*): Effects of primary auditory cortical lesions on thresholds for pure tone detection. *Journal of Neurophysiology* 60:879–888.

Kelly, J. B. (1973). The effects of insular and temporal lesions in cats on two types of auditory pattern discrimination. *Brain Research* 62:71–87.

Kelly, J. B. (1980). Effects of auditory cortical lesions on sound localization by the rat. *Journal of Neurophysiology* 44:1161–1174.

Kelly, J. B. (1986). The development of sound localization and auditory processing in mammals. In R. N. Aslin (ed.), *Advances in Neural and Behavioral Development*. Norwood, N.J.: Ablex Press, 205–234.

Kelly, J. B., and Glazier, S. J. (1978). Auditory cortex lesions and discrimination of spatial location by the rat. *Brain Research* 145:315–321.

Kelly, J. B., Glenn, S. L., and Beaver, C. (1989). Frequency and binaural response characteristics of single neurons in the rat's inferior colliculus. *Association for Research in Otolaryngology Abstracts* 12:36.

Kelly, J. B., and Judge, P. W. (1985). The effects of medial geniculate lesions on sound localization by the rat. *Journal of Neurophysiology* 53:361–372.

Kelly, J. B., Judge, P. W., and Phillips, D. P. (1986). Representation of the cochlea in primary auditory cortex of the ferret (*Mustela putorius*). *Hearing Research* 24:111–116.

Kelly, J. B., and Kavanagh, G. L. (1986). The effects of auditory cortical lesions on pure tone sound localization by the albino rat. *Behavioral Neuroscience* 100:569 575.

Kelly, J. B., and Masterton, R. B. (1977). Auditory sensitivity of the albino rat. *Journal of Comparative and Physiological Psychology* 91:930–936.

Kelly, J. B., and Sally, S. L. (1988). Organization of auditory cortex in the albino rat: binaural interactions. *Journal of Neurophysiology* 59:1756–1769.

Kelly, J. B., and Whitfield, I. C. (1971). Effects of auditory cortical lesions on discriminations of rising and falling frequency modulated tones. *Journal of Neurophysiology* 34:802–816.

Krieg, W. J. S. (1946). Connections of the cerebal cortex. I. The albino rat. A. The topography of the cortical areas. *Journal of Comparative Neurology* 84:221–275.

Kudo, M., Glendenning, K. K., Frost, S. B., and Masterton, R. B. (1986). Origin of mammalian thalamocortical projections. I. Telencephalic projections of the medial geniculate body in the opossum (*Didelphis virginiana*). *Journal of Comparative Neurology* 245:176–197.

Land, P. W., Rose, A. R., Harvey, A. R., and Liverman, S. A. (1984). Neonatal auditory cortex lesions result in aberrant crossed corticotectal and corticothalamic projections in rats. *Developmental Brain Research* 12:126–130.

Lashley, K. S. (1941). Thalamocortical connections of the rat's brain. *Journal of Comparative Neurology* 75:67–121.

LeDoux, J. E., Farb, C., Ruggiero, D. A., and Reis, D. J. (1987a). Thalamic and cortical auditory pathways converge in the rat amygdala. *Neuroscience Abstracts* 13:1467.

LeDoux, J. E., Iwata, J., Pearl, D., and Reis, D. J. (1986). Disruption of auditory but not visual learning by destruction of intrinsic neurons in the rat medial geniculate body. *Brain Research* 371:395–399.

LeDoux, J. E., Ruggiero, D. A., Forest, R., Stornetta, R., and Reis, D. J. (1987b). Topographic organization of convergent projections to the thalamus from the inferior colliculus and the spinal cord in the rat. *Journal of Comparative Neurology* 264:123–146.

LeDoux, J. E., Ruggiero, D. A., and Reis, D. J. (1985). Projections to the subcortical forebrain from anatomically defined regions of the medial geniculate body in the rat. *Journal of Comparative Neurology* 242:182–213.

LeDoux, J. E., Sakaguchi, A., and Reis, D. J. (1984). Subcortical efferent projections of the medial geniculate nucleus mediate emotional responses conditioned to acoustic startle. *Journal of Neuroscience* 4:683–698.

LeMesserier, D. H. (1948). Auditory and visual areas of the cerebral cortex of the rat. *Federation Proceedings* 7:70.

Leuthke, L. E., Krubitzer, L. A., and Kaas, J. H. (1988). Cortical connections of electrophysiologically and architectonically defined subdivisions of auditory cortex in squirrels. *Journal of Comparative Neurology* 268:181–203.

McMullen, N. T., and Glaser, E. M. (1982). Tonotopic organization of rabbit auditory cortex. *Experimental Neurology* 75:208–220.

Merzenich, M. M., and Brugge, J. F. (1973). Representation of the cochlear partition on the superior temporal plane of the macaque monkey. *Brain Research* 50:275–296.

Merzenich, M. M., Kaas, J. H., and Roth, G. L. (1976). Auditory cortex in the grey squirrel: tonotopic organization and architectonic fields. *Journal of Comparative Neurology* 166:387–402.

Merzenich, M. M., Knight, P. L., and Roth, G. L. (1975). Representation of the cochlea within the primary auditory cortex in the cat. *Journal of Neurophysiology* 38:231–249.

Middlebrooks, J. C., Dykes, R. W., and Merzenich, M. M. (1980). Binaural response specific bands in primary auditory cortex (AI) of the cat: Topographic organization orthogonal to isofrequency contours. *Brain Research* 181:31–48.

Middlebrooks, J. C., and Zook, J. M. (1983). Intrinsic organization of the cat's medial geniculate body identified by projections to binaural response-specific bands in the primary auditory cortex. *Journal of Neuroscience* 3:203–224.

Neff, W. D. (1968). Behavioral studies of auditory discrimination: localization of sound in space. In A. V. S. de Reuck and J. Knight (eds.), *Hearing Mechanisms in Vertebrates*. London: Churchill Press, 207–231.

Neff, W. D., Diamond, I. T., and Casseday, J. J. (1975). Behavioral studies of auditory discrimination: central nervous system. In W. D. Keidel and W. D. Neff (eds.), *Handbook of Sensory Physiology* (Volume 5, Pt. 2). Berlin: Springer Verlag, 307–400.

Neff, W. D., Fisher, J. D., Diamond, I. T., and Yela, M. (1956). Role of auditory cortex in discrimination requiring localization of sound in space. *Journal of Neurophysiology* 19:500–512.

Oliver, D. L., Merzenich, M. M., Roth, W. C., Hall, W. C., and Kaas, J. H. (1976). Tonotopic organization and connections of primary auditory cortex in the tree shrew. *Anatomical Record* 184:491.

Patchett, R. F. (1977). Auditory pattern discrimination in albino rats as a function of auditory restriction at different ages. *Developmental Psychology* 13:168–169.

Patterson, H. A. (1977). An anterograde degeneration and retrograde axonal transport study of the cortical projections of the rat medial geniculate body. Doctoral dissertation, Boston University.

Phillips, D. P., and Irvine, D. R. F. (1981). Responses of single neurons in physiologically defined primary auditory cortex (AI) of the cat: frequency tuning and responses to intensity. *Journal of Neurophysiology* 45:48–58.

Phillips, D. P., Judge, P. W., and Kelly, J. B. (1988). Primary auditory cortex in the ferret (*Mustela putorius*): neural response properties and topographic organization. *Brain Research* 443:281–294.

Phillips, D. P., and Kelly, J. B. (1989). Coding of tone-pulse amplitude by single neurons in auditory cortex of albino rats (*Rattus norvegicus*). *Hearing Research* 37:269–279.

Ravizza, R., and Diamond, I. T. (1974). Role of auditory cortex in sound localization: a comparative ablation study of hedgehog and bushbaby. *Federation Proceedings* 33:1917–1919.

Ravizza, R. J., and Masterton, B. (1972). Contribution of neocortex to sound localization in opossum (*Didelphis virginiana*). *Journal of Neurophysiology* 35:344–356.

Reale, R. A., and Imig, T. J. (1980). Tonotopic maps of auditory cortex in the cat. *Journal of Comparative Neurology* 192:265–292.

Reale, R. A., and Kettner, R. E. (1986). Topography of binaural organization in primary auditory cortex of the cat: Effects of changing interaural intensity. *Journal of Neurophysiology* 56:663—682.

Redies, H., and Creutzfeldt, O. D. (1987). The auditory thalamocortical system in the guinea pig. *Neuroscience Supplement* 22:2153P.

Romaneski, L. M., Xagoraris, A. E., Reis, D. J., and LeDoux, J. E. (1988). Destruction of perirhinal and neocortical projection targets of the acoustic thalamus does not disrupt fear conditioning. *Society for Neuroscience Abstracts* 14:1227.

Ryugo, D. K. (1976). An attempt towards an integration of structure and function in the auditory system. Doctoral dissertation, University of California, Irvine.

Ryugo, D. K., and Killackey, H. P. (1974). Differential telencephalic projections of the medial and ventral divisions of the medial geniculate body of the rat. *Brain Research* 82:173–177.

Sally, S. L., and Kelly, J. B. (1988a). Organization of the auditory cortex in the albino rat: sound frequency. *Journal of Neurophysiology* 59:1627–1638.

Sally, S. L., and Kelly, J. B. (1988b). The effects of superior olivary complex lesions on binaural interaction in the auditory cortex of the albino rat. *Society for Neuroscience Abstracts* 14:1096.

Scharlock, D. P., Neff, W. D., and Strominger, N. L. (1965). Discrimination of tone duration after bilateral ablation of cortical auditory areas. *Journal of Neurophysiology* 28:673–681.

Scheel, M. (1984). Isofrequency laminae in the medial geniculate body of the rat as shown by injections of WGA-HRP into auditory cortex. *Neuroscience Letters* [*Supplement*] 18:S245.

Strominger, N. L. (1969). Localization of sound in space after unilateral and bilateral ablation of auditory cortex. *Experimental Neurology* 25:521–533.

Strominger, N. L., Oesterreich, R. E., and Neff, W. D. (1980). Sequential auditory and visual discriminations after temporal lobe ablation in monkeys. *Physiology and Behavior* 24:1149–1156.

Suga, N. (1965). Functional properties of auditory neurones in the cortex of echolocating bats. *Journal of Physiology (London)* 181:671–700.

Suga, N. (1984). The extent to which biosonar information is represented in the bat auditory cortex. In G. M. Edelman, W. E. Gall, and W. M. Cowan (eds.), *Dynamic Aspects of Cortical Function*. New York: John Wiley, 315–374.

Suga, N, and Jen, P. H.-S. (1976). Disproportionate tonotopic representation for processing species-specific CF-FM sonar signals in the mustached bat auditory cortex. *Science* 194:542–544.

Syka, J., Druga, R., Popelar, J., and Kalinova, B. (1981). Functional organization of the inferior colliculus. In Josef Syka and Lindsay Aitkin (eds.), *Neuronal Mechanisms of Hearing*. New York: Plenum Press, 137–154.

Syka, J, and Popelar, J. (1984). Inferior colliculus in the rat: neuronal responses to stimulation of the auditory cortex. *Neuroscience Letters* 51:235–240.

Tees, R. C. (1967). Effects of early auditory restriction in the rat on adult pattern discrimination. *Journal of Comparative and Physiological Psychology* 63:389–393.

Thompson, G. C., and Cortez, A. M. (1983). The inability of squirrel monkeys to localize sound after unilateral ablation of auditory cortex. *Behavioral Brain Research* 8:211–216.

Tunturi, A. R. (1950). Physiological determination of the arrangement of afferent connections to the middle ectosylvian auditory area of the dog. *American Journal of Physiology* 162:489–502.

Tunturi, A. R. (1960). Anatomy and physiology of the auditory cortex. In G. L. Rasmussen and W. F. Windle (eds.), *Neural Mechanisms of the Auditory and Vestibular Systems*. Springfield, Ill.: Charles C. Thomas, 181–200.

Vaughan, D. W. (1976). Membranous bodies in the cerebral cortex of aging rats: an electron microscopic study. *Journal of Neuropathology and Experimental Neurology* 35:152–166.

Vaughan, D. W. (1977). Age-related deterioration of pyramidal cell basal dendrites in rat auditory cortex. *Journal of Comparative Neurology* 171:501–515.

Vaughan, D. W. (1983). Thalamic and callosal connections of the rat auditory cortex. *Brain Research* 260:181–189.

Vaughan, D. W., and Foundas, S. (1982). Synaptic proliferation in the auditory cortex of the young adult rat following callosal lesions. *Journal of Neurocytology* 11:29–51.

Vaughan, D. W., and Peters, A. (1974). Neuroglial cells in the cerebral cortex of rats from young adulthood to old age: an electron microscopic study. *Journal of Neurocytology* 3:405–429.

Waller, W. H. (1934). Topographic relations of cortical lesions to thalamic nuclei in the albino rat. *Journal of Comparative Neurology* 60:237–270.

Webster, W. R. (1985). The auditory system. In G. Paxinos (ed.), *The Rat Nervous System. Vol. 2. Hindbrain and Spinal Cord*. New York: Academic Press, 153–184.

Wegener, J. G. (1964). Auditory discrimination behavior of brain damaged monkeys. *Journal of Auditory Research* 4:227–254.

Wegener, J. G. (1976). Auditory and visual discrimination following lesions of the anterior supratemporal plane in monkeys. *Neuropsychologia* 14:161–173.

Winer, J. A., and Larue, D. T. (1987). Patterns of reciprocity in auditory thalamocortical and corticothalamic connections: study with horseradish peroxidase and autoradiographic methods in the rat medial geniculate body. *Journal of Comparative Neurology* 257:282–315.

Woolsey, C. N. (1952). Patterns of localization in sensory and motor areas of the cerebral cortex. In C. N. Woolsey (ed.), *The Biology of Mental Health and Disease*. London: Cassell and Company.

Zilles, K. (1985). *The Cortex of the Rat. A Stereotaxic Atlas*. Berlin: Springer Verlag.

Zilles, K., and Wree, A. (1985). Cortex: areal and laminar structure. In G. Paxinos (ed.), *The Rat Nervous System. Vol. I. Forebrain and Midbrain*. New York: Academic Press, 375–392.

16   Gustatory Cortex: Definition and Function

J. Jay Braun

16.1   Defining the Gustatory Cortex

In 1982 we published a comprehensive review and analysis of anatomical, physiological, and behavioral research concerning the rat's gustatory cortex (Braun et al. 1982b). This chapter is in part an update of the
previous paper. The rat's gustatory cortex (GC) is defined here by
characterizing its boundaries, internal organization, anatomical context,
afferent and efferent connections, and the consequences of GC ablation.
The second half of the chapter addresses functional considerations regarding gustatory cortical involvement in taste-guided behavior.

Boundaries

The most important recent finding with regard to defining the boundaries of the GC is its unequivocal localization within the agranular
insular cortex (Kosar et al. 1986a). If one is inclined to define *neocortex*
as the dorsal pallium, above the rhinal sulcus, then this area would
continue to be properly designated as "gustatory *neocortex*" as labeled
in so many previous publications (e.g., Braun et al. 1982b). On the other
hand, if one insists on six distinct layers, then the lack of layer 4, which
defines the "agranular" area, clearly indicates that the more general
term, *cortex,* is most appropriate. I use the latter term here in deference
to the taxonomic preference exhibited in this book.

The seminal work of Benjamin and Pfaffmann (1955) portrayed the
"taste nerve area" as distinctly dorsal to the rhinal sulcus within the
ventral somatosensory representation for the face. However, Benjamin
and Akert (1959) later acknowledged that according to *behavioral* measures of reactivity to quinine hydrochloride, the most critical area extended ventrally to the upper margin of the rhinal sulcus.

Fundamental disagreements concerning the exact location and extent
of the cortical taste area persisted up to the time of our previous review,
where they are described in more detail (Braun et al. 1982b). At that
time it was becoming evident from behavioral studies that insular cortex
adjacent to the rhinal sulcus was especially involved in the learning and
retention of behaviors guided by gustatory cues, whereas a more dorsal

area within the somatosensory representation of the face was not (e.g., Braun et al. 1981, Lasiter and Glanzman 1982). As Benjamin and Akert (1959) had suggested, a thin strip of cortex spanned by the middle cerebral artery, immediately dorsal to the rhinal sulcus, seemed especially important for taste-guided behavior. Further supporting the importance of this cortical area for taste processes, it was noted that *taste-specific* unit responses—unconfounded by tactile or temperature responses—appear to be restricted to the insular area (Yamamoto et al. 1984b).

Kosar et al. (1986a,b) recently provided confirmation and closure regarding the anatomical location of the GC. Procedurally they recorded multiunit activity and used with small electrolytic lesions to mark the exact locations of areas defining the effective modes (taste, tactile, temperature) of tongue stimulation. The cortical taste area was found to be clearly located within the agranular insular cortex, distinctly ventral to the primary somatosensory cortex, in Krieg's (1946) area 14. In addition it was found to be distinct from areas identified as responsive to oral tactile or temperature stimuli, being immediately ventral to the latter, which were located in granular cortex.

Emmers's (1966) original observations concerning separate cortical projections for tactile and gustatory tongue information were thus elegantly supported by Kosar and colleagues (1986a,b) and extended to include an interdigitated area receiving tongue temperature information. The authors flatly state that in sixteen preparations, "gustatory responses were *never* recorded within granular cortex, but could only be elicited within the dorsal agranular insular cortex" (Kosar et al. 1986a, p. 336). Although noting some variation between rats in the exact position of the dorsal agranular boundary, they point out that, "in *every* case this boundary coincided with the shift in functional properties from tongue temperature to gustatory sensibility" (Kosar et al. 1986a, p. 337).

While these recent studies more precisely define the dorsal margin of the GC, definitions of other dimensions remain somewhat vague. Kosar and associates (1986a) point out and discuss, for example, the problems associated with specifying the A-P boundaries, especially the posterior margin. In addition they indicate the GC to be limited to Krieg's (1946) area 14, and they do not discuss area 13, a thin strip of neocortex immediately adjacent to and overlapping somewhat the rhinal sulcus (Zilles's area AIV?). In a separate autoradiography study of axonal projections from the gustatory thalamus, the most intense labeling clearly encompassed the dorsal lip of the rhinal sulcus at caudal levels, while appearing to be focused above the rhinal sulcus rostrally (Kosar et al. 1986b, fig. 2, p. 346). Thus involvement of Krieg's area 13 in the caudal representation of GC is suggested. In addition the orientation of the long axis of the GC as indicated by these data seems to conform better in some respects to that delineated by Yamamoto and associates

(1985a, fig. 5, p. 1362) than it does to their own electrophysiological data (Kosar et al. 1986a, fig. 7, p. 338).

However, despite minor problems regarding the defining boundaries of GC, there is substantial agreement concerning a distinct focus of a population of gustatory-specific cortical neurons (figure 16.1).

Chemotopic Organization

The work summarized above makes it clear that the mode of sensation called "taste" has, by electrophysiological criteria, a collective, localized, and apparently unconfounded representation in the insular cortex. The next question we ask concerns how taste representation is organized within the rat's GC.

Yamamoto and colleagues (1985b) classified areas of an arbitrary grid superimposed on the GC according to the predominant taste response characteristic of samples of units in each area. Although different taste stimuli might converge to varying degrees on single taste-specific neurons, individual neurons typically could be classified as most responsive to a specific quality, and they observed a certain degree of what Halpern (1967) has called *chemotopic* organization. That is, maximum sensitivity to sucrose, salt, acid, and quinine was found to be differentially distrib-

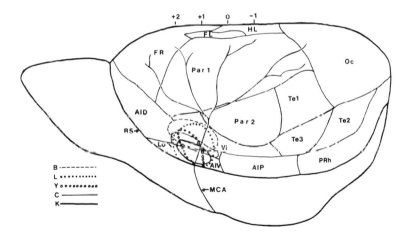

Figure 16.1 Composite (and approximate) superimposition of several descriptions of the location of the gustatory neocortex on a slightly modified camera drawing of a lateral view of the rat cortex as portrayed by Zilles (chapter 4). B is the original definition of the area as portrayed by Benjamin and Pfaffmann (1955); L represents the lesion boundaries as defined in a recent study (Lasiter et al. 1985c); Y is the "ventral" taste area electrophysiologically explored by Yamamoto and colleagues (1984b—see especially figure 2); C is from Cechetto and Saper (1987, figure 6); K represents the findings of Kosar and associates (1986a). Some authors use bregma as a zero reference point (e.g., "C"), as indicated by the millimeter marks atop the figure, and others use the intersection of the rhinal sulcus (RS) and the middle cerebral artery (MCA) as a reference point for the gustatory cortical area (e.g., Y and K). AID, V and P = anterior insular dorsal, ventral and posterior, respectively; FR = frontal; Par = parietal; Te = temporal; Oc = occipital; PRh = perirhinal; FL and HL = front and hind leg areas, respectively; Lo = lateral orbital.

uted within the GC. Sucrose and quinine had fairly segregated representations at opposite ends of the cortical taste area, with salt and acid having relatively wider representation throughout the GC area.

Chemotopic organization accounts for the observation that lesions of the GC that effectively eliminated learned aversions to quinine and sucrose stimuli were insufficient to eliminate an equivalent learned aversion to an acid stimulus (Kiefer et al. 1984). The sparing of this aversion was based on either slight sparing of acid-relevant cortex, or on distinctive odor cues associated with the acid stimulus. Because relatively subtle olfactory stimuli associated with taste cues appear to become salient *following* GC ablation (Braun 1983), it is unlikely that such cues were the basis for postoperative sparing of the acid aversion habit in Kiefer and colleagues' (1984) study. Therefore these results and those of Yamamoto (1985a) indicate that qualitative gustatory representation within GC is segregated spatially to some degree.

Anatomical Context

With regard to potential functional considerations, the modern map of the anterolateral cortex is especially interesting. The classical maps of the rat cortex by Woolsey (1958), Hall and Lindholm (1974), and Welker (1971) had left this area undesignated. Woolsey's diagrams of somatosensory neocortex representing the heads of monkeys, cats, and rats portrayed the tongue protruding backward into the representation of the mouth. This picture suggested possible visceral representation of the alimentary track adjacent to the back of the somatosensory tongue area, a suggestion supported by Cechetto and Saper's (1987) elegant study of viscerotopic cortical organization in the rat. In the contiguous juxtaposition of visceral, olfactory, somatosensory face and tongue, and gustatory cortical areas, one can now begin to see anatomical foundations for functional integration of systems that clearly are interrelated psychologically.

To summarize, the GC overlies the anterior claustrum and is bounded ventrally by piriform (olfactory) cortex beneath the rhinal sulcus, anteriorly by what may be an olfactory area *dorsal* to the rhinal sulcus (Eichenbaum et al. 1980, Leonard 1972), and dorsocaudally by an extensive viscerotopic area (Cechetto and Saper 1987). In figure 16.1 the lateral orbital area (Lo) represents the olfactory area and area Vi the visceral area in Zilles's (chapter 4) cortical map. Moreover, recent evidence suggests an additional cortical area involved in taste-guided behavior—"temporal" neocortex—that is posterior to the gustatory and/or viscerotopic areas (Fitzgerald and Burton 1983) and is represented by Te3 in figure 16.1.[1] The special relationship between taste and smell in the production of flavor and the important associations between these sensory modes and visceral events (e.g., see Kiefer 1985) appear to have correspondent anatomical representation within a small cortical area roughly 4 mm long and 2 mm wide, immediately dorsal to the rhinal sulcus, which is bridged by the middle cerebral artery.

Afferent/Efferent Connections

The principal afferent nerves from the tongue, the chorda tympani branch of the facial nerve (cranial nerve VII) and the glossopharyngeal nerve (IX), project to the nucleus of the solitary tract. Although gustatory thalamocortical relationships had been delineated before 1973 (Ables and Benjamin 1960, Ganchrow and Erickson 1972), the exact pathways from the solitary tract to the forebrain were unknown. This problem was resolved by the discovery of a pontine taste area in the parabrachial nuclei (Norgren and Leonard 1973). The pontine taste area constitutes a major area of convergence for ascending taste and visceral information as well as for rostral information from various forebrain areas including olfactory, hypothalamic, cortical, and limbic structures (Travers et al. 1987).

Three routes to the GC area from the pontine taste area have been identified: (1) the classical thalamic route via the medial portion of the ventral thalamic nucleus, (2) projections via the amygdalar complex, and (3) a direct ventral route from the parabrachial area (see Lasiter and Glanzman 1983).

GC connections with gustatory thalamus, amygdala, and the parabrachial nuclei appear to be reciprocal (e.g., Saper 1982a, Shipley and Sanders 1982, Yamamoto et al. 1984a). In addition anterograde degeneration studies have revealed direct connections between insular (but not necessarily "gustatory") cortex and the caudate nucleus, the solitary tract and nucleus, and even the spinal cord in rodents (e.g., Shipley 1982, van der Kooy et al. 1982).

What may turn out to be most important with respect to an ultimate unraveling of the functional significance of the various connections with the GC is their histochemical identification. Studies directly identifying such pathways, such as the identification of somatostatinergic projections from insular cortex to the spinal cord by Shimada et al. (1985), signal the beginnings of such promising analyses. Likewise psychopharmacological studies will help identify those biochemical/neuro transmitter systems most involved in specific taste-guided behaviors; for example, the recent demonstration that noradrenergic systems do not appear to be involved in the acquisition and retention of a conditioned taste aversion helps to focus the search for anatomical and physiological correlates of associative taste processes (Jarbe et al. 1988).

Ablation Symptoms

Critical interpretations of behavioral/brain lesion studies rely on the details of often complex experimental designs. The purpose of such designs is to precisely define and uniquely characterize the effect of localized brain damage on behavioral processes. Early studies used behavioral measures as simple barometers of brain-damage–induced disruption. This was the case in the classic GC lesion studies (e.g., Benjamin and Pfaffmann 1955, Benjamin and Akert 1959), when transient and highly variable increases in detection thresholds for quinine hydrochloride were exclusively used as behavioral measures. These fragile threshold data were virtually the only kind of behavioral evidence cited for the idea of a "taste" function for GC in the 1950s and 1960s. This changed in 1972 when specifically *associative* taste processes were found to be reliably disrupted following ablations of the GC (Braun et al. 1972).

A principal strategy in our GC studies has been to "operationalize" the intended lesion to encompass tissue well beyond the area of focus: to include in the ablation everybody's reasoned idea of the location of the critical area. In the 1970s this included a very large area—about twice as large as the encircled lesion area (L) in figure 16.1. Potential variations in landmarks and conformation of cortical tissue and systematic variations as a function of age, weight, or other factors also must be taken into account. For example, Kosar and associates (1986b) noted that the apparent location of the GC moved caudally relative to bregma as a function of body weight, as did the point defining the juncture of the rhinal sulcus and the middle cerebral artery.

Slight lesion variations can profoundly influence conclusions regarding involvement of a specific brain area in a particular behavior or class of behaviors (e.g., see discussion by Braun (1989) and Frommer (1978)). In this regard Lashley (1939) had noted that a visual pattern discrimination habit could be sustained following ablation of the visual cortex with as few as 700 cells remaining in the dorsal lateral geniculate nuclei—this represented only about 2 percent of the rat's geniculostriate system. Likewise almost imperceptible sparing of a thin margin of anterolateral insular cortex results in sparing of a preoperatively instated taste habit (Kiefer et al. 1984).

Sensory-specific agnosias are among the most interesting symptoms of cortical ablation. Sensory agnosia accompanies sensory cortex ablation for a wide variety of kinds of tasks across a wide variety of species (Braun 1989). Operationally the most reliable and distinctive behavioral consequence of GC ablation is complete agnosia for learned taste aversions (Braun et al. 1981, Kiefer et al. 1984, Yamamoto et al. 1980). The agnosia effect may be used to determine whether GC lesions are complete in studies that seek to study other behavioral inclinations of rats lacking GC.

Taste agnosia following complete GC ablations is taste specific by double dissociation criteria, sparing odor aversions that had been learned under identical training conditions, and it is also a general effect across taste qualities (Kiefer et al. 1984). Taste reactivity and taste thresholds are essentially normal in rats lacking GC, and they can readily learn or relearn to discriminatively avoid sapid substances (Braun et al. 1982b), but they may use cues other than taste to do so (Braun 1983). In addition such rats appear to loose their suspiciousness of new taste cues ("neophobia"), responding to them as normal rats respond to familiar stimuli (Kiefer and Braun 1977). *With respect to their responsiveness to taste cues, naive and preoperatively experienced rats cannot be distinguished from each other after GC ablation.*

The taste agnosia effect following GC ablation cannot be accounted for on the basis of generalized damage to neocortex, as a loss of taste discriminative capacities in general, as a loss of ability to respond appropriately to the relevant unconditional stimuli, or as a loss of ability to associate tastes (or stimuli associated with tastes, such as odors) with correlated gastrointestinal events (see Braun et al. 1972, 1982b, Kiefer et al. 1984). It is a highly specific and unique effect of GC ablation that distinguishes this area of the brain from any other.

Can the symptoms accompanying GC ablation be related to a particular input pathway? At the time of our 1982 review, we noted that lesions of the amygdala had been shown to produce a constellation of symptoms highly similar to the disruptions of taste-guided behavior produced by GC ablation (e.g., Nachman and Ashe 1974). We speculated that the effects on gustatory behavior produced by amygdala ablation represented general effects not specific to taste. Some support of this view came later from the finding that only about 8 percent of amygdala units appear to be taste responsive and that the great majority of these (about 90 percent) respond also to other kinds of stimuli (tactile, thermal, acoustic) as well (Azuma et al. 1984). Using ibotenic acid lesions of GC and amygdala in a double dissociation paradigm, Dunn and Everitt (1988) recently related most of the taste effects associated with electrolytic amygdala lesions to damage sustained by fibers of passage from the parabrachial taste area (the ventral taste pathway). The bottom line regarding the amygdala issue is perhaps best conveyed by quoting the last line of the abstract in Dunn and Everitt's (1988, p. 3) lucid and thoughtful study:

We conclude that the insular cortex is involved in reactions to novelty and associative salience exclusively of taste stimuli, whereas the amygdala is probably more concerned with the reaction to more general aspects of novelty in the environment and in fear-motivated behavior.

Ablation of the gustatory thalamus also has some consequences in common with GC ablations. Both result in severe disruption of taste-aversion learning, for example (Lasiter et al. 1985b). However, although GC lesions have little or no effect on taste preference and aversion functions, at least according to intake measures (Braun et al. 1982, Lasiter et al. 1985c), gustatory thalamus lesions nearly eliminate these kinds of reactive taste functions (Lasiter 1985). Therefore the effects of

GC ablation can be much more selectively related to disruptions of associative (learning and memory) taste phenomena with sparing of more fundamental functions.

Although there are problems in defining functions of an area on the basis of residual capacities of the system when that area is missing (Braun 1978, Glassman 1978), the behavioral approach, using an operationally standardized lesion, does offer a kind of information that suggests important functional conceptual schemes, as shown below.

16.2 Function

One path to understanding the function of a central sensory area is via an empirical description of how variations of physical parameters of relevant stimulation are reflected in central processing. In this regard a difficulty with taste is the lack of clearly defined biophysical dimensions of chemicals defining the basic taste qualities (e.g., see Travers et al. 1987). Despite the stimulus problems, the typical experiment assumes four categories and employs representative stimuli from these traditionally accepted qualitative categories (e.g., NaCl, sucrose, HCl, and quinine HCl—Yamamoto et al. 1984b).

By far the most comprehensive and vigorous comparative electrophysiological research program studying the GC is that of Kawamura, Yamamoto, and colleagues of Osaka University in Japan. Their studies, among the most seminal in defining response characteristics of GC neurons, have been summarized by Yamamoto (1984) and by a series of papers in the *Journal of Neurophysiology* by Yamamoto and colleagues (1984b, 1985a,b). These papers obviate the need for a summary of this work here beyond the following two paragraphs regarding qualitative and quantitative taste coding at the neocortical level.

Two major theories of taste encoding, principally derived from peripheral recordings at the level of the chorda tympani, are the *pattern theory* and the *labeled line theory*. The pattern theory, as originally proposed by Pfaffmann (1959), assumes that qualitative encoding is based on relative patterns of neuronal firing in a population of relevant neurons. The labeled line theory (e.g., Nowlis and Frank 1981) suggests that certain neurons best register specific stimuli and that the activation of these specific neurons is the quality code. Detailed analyses of cortical neuron responses by Yamamoto and colleagues (1985a) did not favor either theory (also see Yamamoto 1984). However, a theory of their own, which they call *across-region response patterning* (Yamamoto et al. 1981), is introduced. This relatively complex theory contains elements of both the patterning theory and the labeled line theory, and it is presented as the best-available explanation of qualitative taste organization at the neocortical level (see Yamamoto 1984).[2]

Quantitative (intensity) representation appears to be quite complex and variable by electrophysiological criteria at the cortical, as compared with the brainstem, level of taste representation. Whereas the discharge of medullary taste units positively correlates with increasing concentrations of taste stimuli (e.g., Ganchrow and Erickson 1972), most of the cortical units do not (Yamamoto 1984b). Most show selective sensitivities to certain stimulus intensities (nonmonotonic), some show monotonic inhibitory responses, and others display monotonic excitatory responses. Thus, compared with brainstem units, the representation of taste intensity for most taste responsive units at the cortical level is in a direction implying greater resolution and specificity of intensity coding in individually tuned neurons. Overall, as the neuroaxis is ascended, it would appear that relevant central interneurons become tuned to increasingly specific dimensions of stimuli applied to the tongue. This implies hierarchical transformations and rerepresentations of taste information, but it says nothing about biobehavioral *function* of different levels of the taste neuroaxis.

Behavioral Dimensions of Taste Sensitivity

The qualitative and quantitative dimensions of tastes also can be defined behaviorally according to hedonic (Pfaffmann 1960, Young 1966) and other reactive criteria (see Grill and Berridge 1985). Preference and aversion responses, for example, may be measured by amounts drunk of various sapid solutions relative to the consumption of plain (usually distilled) water. Thus it is found that bitter stimuli are rejected as a function of concentration and that sucrose tends to be increasingly accepted. The response to salt is biphasic—highly preferred at low concentrations and rapidly avoided as the basic physiological concentration is exceeded (Young 1966).

Aversion and acceptance responses based on measures of amount ingested are susceptible of course to influences from postingestional factors, conditions of deprivation, and experiences with tastes. For this reason Grill and Berridge (1985) emphasize the importance of other kinds of reactive measures of taste sensitivity that are less susceptible to such influences. These measures involve assessments of patterns of facial, tongue, and other movements in time as a function of variations of taste quality and quantity.

A measure of behavioral taste sensitivity that has been largely ignored, but has special significance for an analysis of GN function, is *associative salience*. Kalat and Rozin (1970) defined *salience* essentially as the associative potential of novel flavor solutions. It was noted that this factor predicted conditionability better than CS-US contiguity and that it could be dissociated both from measures of relative palatability (Kalat and Rozin 1970) and from taste intensity (Kalat 1974). In other words salience was described as a measure of how readily specific flavor solutions acquired aversive properties when paired with toxicosis. We use the expression "associative salience" to refer to this factor, distinguishing it from what we have called *reactive salience*, which, as described previously, refers to reflexive responses to taste and flavor stimuli (Braun et al. 1982b).

Hierarchical Considerations

The gustatory system is especially amenable to hierarchical analysis (e.g., Nowlis 1977). Distinctive indications of taste involvement in behavior can be suggested for each level of the neuroaxis (e.g., Grill and Berridge 1985). Compared with, for example, auditory or visual reflexes triggered by *qualitatively* different stimuli, which in the mammal are not usually readily apparent or which quickly habituate (e.g., orientation responses to click stimuli), the gustatory reflexes are obvious and persistent.

A host of basic taste reflexes appear to be mediated at the lower brainstem level. These reflexes are perhaps best understood from the standpoint of the natural history of the animal. Basic hedonic tendencies for acceptance and rejection (Pfaffmann 1960, Nowlis 1977) provide examples of such reflexes as do the gestures, tongue movements, and other oral motor response patterns that discriminably accompany taste stimuli in decerebrated mammals (see Braun and Nowlis 1989, Braun et al. 1982b, Grill and Berridge 1985, and Steiner 1973 for discussion).

Many of these taste reflexes seem relatively easy to interpret, an example being the increased salivary output that dilutes stimuli with low pH (sour). Other unusual speculations may be suggested by analysis of the reflex pathways. For example, Braun and Nowlis (1989) point out that although the major afferent arm of the facial nerve (cranial nerve VII) is taste, from the tongue, the major *efferent* arm of this nerve supplies the muscles of facial expression. Because the patterns of facial expression for basic tastes appear to be highly similar to powerfully evocative expressions in human communication (e.g., anger, disgust, happiness), as suggested by Steiner's (1973) analyses of neonate "gustofacial" expressions, one might speculate that this taste reflex system played an important role in the evolution of human communication.

We recently outlined a hierarchical view of conditional taste aversions based on the Pavlovian (1927) idea that specific reflex capacities come to associatively serve new stimulus configurations (Braun and Nowlis 1989). Briefly stated, a capacity for forebrain modulation of the taste reflexes in the service of life experience is seen as superimposed on the brainstem taste-reflex systems—not all bitter-tasting substances are noxious, and some sweet substances may be toxic. Forebrain systems are viewed as providing an element of adaptive flexibility to otherwise stereotyped reflexes—a provision for normally rejected tastes to be accepted and vice versa—a provision especially useful for a wide-ranging omnivore such as the rat.

Further enhancing adaptive flexibility in food selection, taste stimuli associated with foods are compounded with distinctive odors; this addition of odor cues greatly increases the potential discriminative grain of learned dietary selections. Taste stimuli have been shown to actually facilitate the associative aversive significance of contiguous odor cues (Braun and Ryugo 1974, Lorden et al. 1970, Rusiniak et al. 1979). Odor stimuli serve many different kinds of biologically important aspects of an animal's life beyond ingestive decisions (i.e., reproductive, defensive, territorial, etc.). Specific olfactory cues appear to become associated with ingestion, however, on the basis of their contiguity with gustatory stimuli. This arrangement allows learned distinctions to be made, in the context of different odors, between similar taste cues that may become associated with different consequences of ingestion (i.e., malaise or homeostatic restoration). The taste learning model outlined here easily accommodates this role of olfaction in learned "taste" discrimination, and it is of interest to note that taste-facilitated learned aversions to odors do not appear to occur after ablation of GC (Lasiter et al. 1985a). Thus contiguous olfactory cues would appear to be handmaidens to taste in the service of learned food selection, and this associative recruitment of odors by tastes may depend on forebrain mechanisms.

Learned taste acceptance (Rozin and Kalat 1971) and aversion may be viewed as based on forebrain recruitment of brainstem taste reflexes by taste stimuli other than those that normally recruit the reflexes. This point of view has been discussed by others (e.g., Grill 1985, Nowlis 1977), and its principal empirical support comes from two observations: (1) The lack of conditionability of decerebrated rats to gustatory stimuli for which they display normal reactivity (Grill and Norgren 1978) and (2) the observation that the "reactive" behavioral pattern of normal rats to sucrose (normally an acceptance response) becomes essentially identical to the normal aversive pattern for quinine HCl following pairing of sucrose with chemically induced toxicosis (Grill 1975, Spector et al. 1988). Contributing further support to this view is the observation that parabrachial neurons responsive to taste were reported to change their response patterns during taste-aversion conditioning in a direction more similar to the preconditioning response patterns observed to bitter, aversive stimuli (DiLorenzo and Garcia 1983).[3]

A Pavlovian view, the foundation of the present model, asserts that taste cues and their most basic reflexes can serve different functions at different levels of representation (or "rerepresentation," to use Jackson's terminology of 1884 along the neuroaxis. Although normal taste reflexes are clearly evident in the brainstem preparation, they appear to be inflexible (Grill and Noragen 1978a,b). Therefore, by reflex criteria discriminative taste behavior is evident, yet by associative criteria it is not. What distinguishes these situations is the nature of the response that is, or becomes, tied to the taste stimulus. If reactive, regulatory, and associative functions are viewed as being based on networks of increasing complexity—reflex, reflex plus feedback, reflex plus feedback plus suppression of original reflex, respectively—then a basis for hierarchical dissociation of these functions is evident (see Flynn and Grill 1988).

Grill and Berridge (1985) thoughtfully discussed hierarchical analyses of levels of taste *reactivity* with regard to the problems of modeling the gustatory system; they make the important point that the cortex does not appear to be necessary for many, perhaps most, kinds of adaptive reactive and regulatory processes that depend to some degree on taste information. As described in more detail by Grill and Berridge (1985), this view is supported by a number of observations, such as the apparent lack of influence of neocortical ablation on either natrorectic adjustments (Wolf et al. 1970) or on certain learned responses to salt depletion (Wirsig and Grill 1982) in the rat.

The present view adds an important dimension to that elaborated by Grill and Berridge (1985). The *associative salience* of sapid stimuli is seen as a dimension distinct from "reactive" or "regulatory" salience (Braun et al 1982b), and it is this behaviorally defined stimulus dimension that highlights a principal contribution of GC to adaptive taste-guided behavior.

Associative Salience and the GC

Dissociations that may be observed between different levels of sensory-guided capacities represent fascinating general consequences of sensory neocortex lesions. Perhaps the most dramatic example of this is "blindsight" in which certain visually guided behavioral adjustments are accurately made by people with visual cortical damage to objects they claim to be unable to see (Weiskrantz et al. 1974). Conceptually similar to the blindsight example, ablation of gustatory cortex in the rat causes a distinct dissociation between associative and reactive salience to gustatory stimuli as previously described (Braun et al. 1982b). As explained in the previous section, rats lacking GC appear to lose the memorial significance of tastes that should cue learned aversions, and yet the rats continue to display essentially normal hedonic reactivity to the basic taste cues over a full range of concentrations.

The unmasking of a distinction between associative and reactive taste salience by GC ablation continues to be strongly supported (e.g., Lasiter et al. 1985c). The distinction is difficult to grasp, however, except in the context of a controlled study, because it implies selective ageusia based strictly on the psychological (associative) constraints of a behavioral situation. On the one hand rats lacking GC differentially respond to the basic taste cues in a normal fashion by reactive criteria, indicating that relevant gustatory information is available to guide behavior, as in the normal rat. However, on the other hand, rats lacking GC appear to be associatively ageusic to the very same taste cues (e.g., Braun et al. 1981). How might one account for this dissociation?

The most straightforward explanation for the associative ageusia displayed by GC-ablated rats is that they lack a key central element allowing specific taste stimuli to be tied to new patterns of behavior. Generally subscribing to Lashley's (1950) most fundamental conclusions regarding behavior-brain area relationships, we have been inclined to ignore this simple hypothesis because of its functional localization overtones.

However, it seems appropriate to reconsider a localization view. We began to do this earlier by suggesting the possibility that the GC is crucially involved in associative taste-specific processes (Kiefer et al. 1984). In this regard it is important to recognize that one need not infer functional localization of an engram in postulating loss either of critical access by a specific class of stimuli to associative processes in general or of access by such stimuli to restricted kinds of associative processes (i.e., avoidance habits, learned palatability—e.g., see Meyer 1972). A model of the brain as a matrix of nodes relevant to different kinds of possible cognitive tasks, with some nodes more critical than others for specific tasks, salvages a localization perspective without requiring that *psychologically defined* categories of behavior be localized. Such a view is evident, with regard to human brain function, in the hypothesis that "elementary operations" of various cognitive tasks may be "strictly localized" (Posner et al. 1988).

With regard to the symptoms of GC ablation in rats, it has become increasingly clear that it is not associative capacity per se that it disrupted (Kiefer et al. 1984), nor is it a capacity to discriminately react to taste cues or to relevant visceral cues (e.g., Lasiter 1983). It is the ability to associate gustatory-specific information with new behavioral patterns that appears to be lost, along with memories for the *preoperatively* learned significance of gustatory-specific cues. It is proposed that all levels of taste-behavior relation capacities are essentially intact, *except* associative salience, after the removal of the gustatory cortex. It is further suggested that the GC is *essentially* involved in all learned behaviors that are explicitly triggered by taste stimuli to the tongue.

A Hierarchy of Associative Salience

If associative taste capacities are lost after GC ablation, how then might one account for the discriminatively specific relearning of "taste"-aversion habits that is observed after the initial agnosia? A parsimonious answer to this question is that the relearning becomes based on cues that are confounded with taste information, but that are normally less salient, i.e., other kinds of sensory information allowing discrimination of sapid substances. Possible sources of such information include odor cues, postingestional cues, and differential feedback from mimetic taste reactivity (Braun and Nowlis 1989).

The principal evidence for the possibility of odor cues is the finding that although olfactory bulbectomy has by itself negligible effects on postoperative taste alacrity, it has a profound effect when combined with a localized GC ablation (Braun et al. 1982a). These results are summarized in figure 16.2.

Subtle odor cues associated with the kinds of taste stimuli used in our experiments have been shown to be discriminable by rats in a

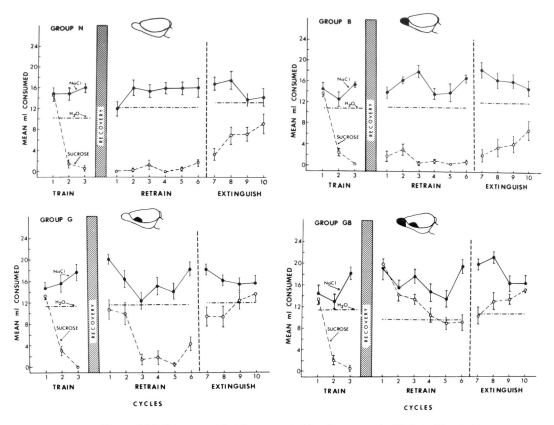

Figure 16.2 Summary of data presented by Braun et al. (1982a). Discriminative taste-aversion learning ("Train"), retention/relearning ("Retrain"), and extinction by four groups of rats (n = 12/13/group). The rats were trained to avoid 150 mM aqueous sucrose solutions, with 150 mM NaCl solutions as discriminative stimuli. The unconditional aversive stimulus was provided by intraperitoneal injections of 150 mM LiCl (15 ml/kg) that were given to rats whenever they consumed > 1 ml of sucrose solution on sucrose training or retraining trials (LiCl treatment was withdrawn during extinction). The water (H_2O) baseline is a mean of the means. The vertical lines represent standard errors.

situation restricting access to only the vapors of sapid solutions (Miller and Erickson 1966). Ordinarily these odor components are not highly salient. They appear to become so, however, when salience of the accompanying taste cues is lost. The rats lacking GC appear to base a biologically important learned discrimination on residual cues detected by an intact sensory system—in this case the olfactory system. Further evidence that olfactory cues accompanying sapid stimuli become salient following GC ablation is provided by the stimulus generalization findings of a recent study by Kiefer and colleagues (1988): Rats lacking GC no longer displayed *taste* generalization, whereas rats lacking olfactory bulbs displayed normal taste generalization after having been trained to avoid compounded taste stimuli. Rats completely lacking GC do not appear to associatively utilize gustatory information.[4]

The idea proposed here regarding the recovery of "taste" discrimination capacity following GC ablation is similar to that expressed by LeVere and LeVere (1982) in their account of recovery following ablation of the visual cortex. In a series of cleverly designed experiments, they found that certain available haptic cues in a discrimination learning situation were associatively ignored by normal rats in favor of more salient visual cues. However, following degradation of the relative salience of the visual cues by visual cortex ablation, the haptic cues readily became salient. Similarly, subtle odor cues, postingestional feedback, and even feedback from orofacial reflex responses to tastes can be viewed as sources of nontaste information that could support an apparent "taste" discrimination (Braun 1983, Braun and Nowlis 1989).

We continue to entertain the possibility of postingestional cues or taste reflex feedback cues providing a possible foundation for "taste" discriminations in the absence of both gustatory cortex and olfactory bulbs (Braun et al. 1982b, Braun and Nowlis 1989). Distinctive postingestional responses to moderate concentrations of sweet, sour, salty, or bitter stimuli are highly likely. For example, quinine hydrochloride, which is frequently used as a bitter stimulus in taste experiments, is highly active pharmacologically; Kratz and Levitsky (1978) have shown that it has enduring consequences for associated food intake even when administered intragastrically. Further supporting the idea that postingestional cues can become salient discriminants for sapid solutions is the finding that rats readily discriminate between presumably visceral consequences of cholecystokinin and lithium chloride administration and satiety (Davidson et al. 1988). Lithium chloride is the most frequently used unconditioned stimulus in taste-aversion experiments; experimental evidence of use of postingestional LiCl cues in salt discrimination was presented by Braun and colleagues (1982b, figure 10 and associated discussion).

The case for the possibility of feedback from distinctive mimetic gestures serving as a basis of taste discrimination in the absence of gustatory, olfactory, or postingestional cues is somewhat speculative at this time (Braun 1983, Braun and Nowlis 1989). The suggestion is offered as a possible ultimate potential basis for recovery of associative taste discrimination capacities after taste, olfactory, and postingestional factors have been eliminated. Such a speculation is conceptually similar to the idea that the deaf may learn to use oropharyngeal feedback in learning to speak.

The hierarchy of recovery possibility described above may explain why it is so difficult to eliminate certain apparent associative capacities, as operationally defined, by brain damage. In addition this view generally explains much of the recovery observed following the losses that accompany localized damage to the sensory neocortex (Braun 1989). In turn this account of the recovery provides a most parsimonious explanation of the initial loss following a sensory cortex lesion: It is a loss of associative access to a class of highly specific cues. Recovery through retraining is based on the use of discriminable but less salient cues that are normally ignored in favor of those that are most salient—just as the movements of the face and mouth may be ignored by people whose hearing is intact. Most important the recovery is viewed as based either on different cues (e.g., odor) or on different manifestations of the same cues (e.g., feedback from taste reflexes), but it is *not* based on relearning the associative significance of the same representations of the stimuli.

16.3   Concluding Observations

Defining boundaries of the GC can be now more precisely specified by anatomical and physiological criteria: Although longitudinal orientation and "fringe" anterior-posterior boundaries have not been specified precisely, there remains no essential disagreement concerning the focus of GC in the anterior insular cortex. In summarizing afferent and efferent connections, it is clear that modern histochemical and pharmacological studies hold an important key to ultimately understanding the cortical gustatory system.

Ablation consequences, or "symptoms," uniquely define the GC as both a cortical area and a part of the gustatory neuroaxis. The major unique consequences of GC ablation is taste-specific agnosia for preoperatively learned taste-guided behaviors. Such ablations spare odor habits that have been instated using identical training procedures, and qualitatively specific taste reflexes are also spared.

The system appears to be hierarchically organized with increasingly complex behavioral adjustments to taste stimuli being based on forebrain modulation and recruitment of basic brainstem taste reflexes.

Associative salience is a concept that characterizes a specific contribution of GC function to taste-guided behaviors, a contribution apparently similar to those of other sensory neocortical areas to learned behaviors guided by relevant sensory information. The dissociation between associative (learned) and reactive (reflexive) responses to taste cues as a function of GC ablation is based on losses of localized but unspecified functional capacities. In fact GC ablations will likely be found to severely disrupt all learned associations specifically triggered by a taste cue.

Finally, the recovery of associative "taste" discriminations following GC ablation is thought to be based on nontaste cues that become salient after GC ablation. These compensatory cues include subtle odors associated with sapid solutions, feedback from differential reactions to ingesting sapid stimuli, and, possibly, differential feedback from intact taste reflexes.

Notes

Dedicated with affection to my close friend and colleague, Ernie Lindholm, who died February 25, 1989.

This work was supported most recently by Biomedical Research Support Grant 935384 from the Graduate College at Arizona State University. The views were developed during a sabbatical leave, Spring 1988, while I enjoyed the intellectual stimulation and warm hospitality of colleagues at the Department of Psychology, Florida State University, for which I am very grateful.

1. The discovery (Fitzgerald and Burton 1983) and corroboration (Lasiter and Glanzman 1985) of the involvement in taste-aversion learning of a temporal cortical area (area 20 as defined by Krieg 1946, or area Te3 using Zilles's terminology, chapter 4) was surprising. Extensive background literature had indicated the more rostral area, the subject of this review, to be the only cortical focus markedly related to taste-guided behaviors. Benjamin and Akert (1959), for example, had originally shown single dissociation of the effects of localized ablations of the "taste nerve area" as compared to ablations of all neocortex except this area. In addition cortial lesions dorsal, rostral, or immediately caudal to the GC produced no discernible effects on taste-aversion learning (Lasiter 1982), and large control lesions of the neocortex had been shown to have no measurable effect on associative taste processes (e.g., Braun et al. 1972, Braun et al. 1981). At present conclusions regarding the nature of the effect of temporal neocortex damage on taste-guided behavior await a more sophisticated battery of behavioral testing procedures. One problem to be resolved, for example, is whether the disruption is specific to taste stimuli. Neither of the temporal cortex ablation studies cited here tested this, nor did they examine whether the effect may have been due to visceral or perirhinal cortex damage. On the basis of other work, the effect is probably based on general disruption of attentional processes (Meyer et al. 1986) and is not specific to gustatory stimuli.

2. The across-region response patterning theory is based on the observation of chemotopic organization of the GC (subareas appearing to represent dominant channels of taste information), which was quantified by partitioning the GC into a grid of sixteen rectangles each categorized by a dominant taste representation. Any plot of random dots representing a number of different categories of information in two-dimensional space (in this case, four kinds of neuronal units showing average dominant responses for particular taste stimuli) will vary greatly in its fit with a superimposed grid that is arbitrarily rotated over the plot. Certain orientations will fit well, and others will fit poorly, depending on the overall distribution of clusters of points on the grid and on the size and shape of the grid components. Statistical support for a point of view regarding distributions of clusters of units within the grid will change substantially with arbitrary manipulation of these grid parameters. Because of this problem I do not believe that support for the across-region response patterning idea has been well fashioned. A traditional factor analytic approach, without superimposition of an arbitrarily oriented and partitioned grid, might provide a more reasonable test of this interesting theory.

3. Other models have emphasized the possible importance of the emetic area (the area postrema) adjacent to the solitary tract and nucleus in the medulla in the formation of conditioned taste aversions (see Asch and Nachman 1980, Kiefer 1985), an emphasis that need not conflict with the "taste reflex" hypothesis if the view that such learning takes places at the level of the lower brainstem (e.g., Garcia et al. 1982) is discarded for lack of empirical support (Grill 1985). Forebrain systems appear to be necessary for learned taste aversions.

4. We originally believed that the apparent recovery of taste discriminations following GC ablation was based on taste-specific information. One reason for this belief was that olfaction, the most likely candidate for an alternate source of discriminative information, did not appear to be normally involved in retention. Olfactory bulbectomy did not at all disrupt preoperatively instated taste habits, while abolishing preoperatively instated *odor* habits, and GC ablation spared odor habits while abolishing taste habits (Kiefer et al. 1984). In addition we used reagent-grade chemicals dissolved in distilled water for taste stimuli, chemicals with greatly reduced potential for impurities and thus much less risk of attendant odor cues that might be salient in our training situation.

References

Ables, M. F., and Benjamin, R. M. (1960). Thalamic relay for taste in the albino rat. *Journal of Neurophysiology* 23:376–382.

Ashe, J. H., and Nachman, M. (1980). Neural mechanisms in taste aversion learning. In Sprague, J., and Epstein, A. (eds.), *Progress in psychobiology and physiological psychology, Vol. 9.* New York: Academic Press, 233–262.

Azuma, S., Yamamoto, T., and Kawamura, Y. (1984). Studies on gustatory responses of amygdaloid neurons in rats. *Experimental Brain Research* 56:12–22.

Benjamin, R. M., and Akert, K. (1959). Cortical thalamic areas involved in taste discrimination in the albino rat. *Journal of Comparative Neurology* 111:231–259.

Benjamin, R. M., and Pfaffmann, C. (1955). Cortical localization of taste in the albino rat. *Journal of Neurophysiology* 18:56–64.

Braun, J. J. (1978). Time and recovery from brain damage. In S. Finger (ed.), *Recovery from brain damage: Research and theory.* New York: Plenum Press, 165–197.

Braun, J. J. (1983). Foundations of residual associative taste salience in rats lacking gustatory neocortex. *Bulletin of the Psychonomic Society* 21:337 (abstract).

Braun, J. J. (1989). Experimental amnestic sensory agnosia: Preoperative modulation. In J. Schulkin (ed.), *Preoperative events: Their effects following brain damage.* New York: Erlbaum, 233–253.

Braun, J. J., Farber, N., and Hunt, D. (1982a). Olfactory mediated recovery from taste agnosia following gustatory neocortex ablation. *Bulletin of the Psychonomic Society* 20:156 (abstract).

Braun, J. J., Kiefer, S., and Ouellet, J. (1981). Psychic ageusia in rats lacking gustatory neocortex. *Experimental Neurology* 72:711–716.

Braun, J. J., Lasiter, P. S., and Kiefer, S. W. (1982b). The gustatory neocortex of the rat. *Physiological Psychology* 10:13–45.

Braun, J. J., and Nowlis, J. (1989). Neural pathways in learned appetitive aversions. *Nutrition* 5:121–124.

Braun, J. J., Ryugo, R. A. (1974). Taste facilitation of a learned odor aversion. *Bulletin of the Psychonomic Society* 4:253 (abstract).

Braun, J. J., Slick, T. B., and Lorden, J. S. (1972). Involvement of gustatory neocortex in the learning of taste aversions. *Physiology and Behavior* 9:637–641.

Cechetto, D. F., and Saper, C. B. (1987). Evidence for a visceroptic sensory representation in the cortex and thalamus in the rat. *The Journal of Comparative Neurology* 262:27–45.

Davidson, T. L., Flynn, F. W., and Grill, H. J. (1988). Comparison of the interoceptive sensory consequences of CCK, LiCl, and satiety in rats. *Behavioral Neuroscience* 1:134–140.

DiLorenzo, P. M., and Garcia, J. (1983). Taste responses of parabrachial units to NaCl and saccharin in rats that were pretrained to avoid Na saccharin. *Society for Neuroscience Abstracts* 9:1023.

Dunn, L. T., and Everitt, B. J. (1988). Double dissociations of the effects of amygdala and insular cortex lesions on conditioned taste aversion, passive avoidance, and neophobia in the rat using the excitotoxin ibotenic acid. *Behavioral Neuroscience* 1:3–23.

Eichenbaum, H., Shedlack, K. J., and Eckmann, K. W. (1980). Thalamocortical mechanisms in odor-guided behavior. I. Effects of lesions of the mediodorsal thalamic nucleus and frontal cortex on olfactory discrimination in the rat. *Brain, Behavior, and Evolution* 17:225–275.

Emmers, R. (1966). Separate cortical receiving areas for gustatory and tongue afferents in the rat. *Anatomical Record* 154:460.

Fitzgerald, R. E., and Burton, M. J. (1983). Neophobia and conditioned taste aversion deficits in the rat produced by undercutting temporal cortex. *Physiology and Behavior* 30:203–206.

Flynn, F. W., and Grill, H. J. (1988). Intraoral intake and taste reactivity responses elicited by sucrose and sodium chloride in chronic decerebrate rats. *Behavioral Neuroscience* 102:934–941.

Frommer, G. P. (1978). Subtotal lesions: Implications for coding and recovery of function. In S. Finger (ed.), *Recovery from brain damage.* New York: Plenum Press, 217–280.

Ganchrow, D., and Erickson, R. P. (1972). Thalamocortical relations in gustation. *Brain Research* 36:289–305.

Garcia, J., Rusiniak, K. W., Kiefer, S. W., and Bermudez-Rattoni, F. (1982). The neural integration of feeding and drinking habits. In C. D. Woody (ed.), *Conditioning: Representation of involved neural functions.* New York: Plenum Press, 567–579.

Glassman, R. B. (1978). The logic of the lesion experiment and its role in the neural sciences. In S. Finger (ed.), *Recovery from brain damage: Research and theory*. New York: Plenum Press, 4–35.

Grill, H. J. (1975). Sucrose as an aversive stimulus. *Neuroscience Abstracts* 1:525.

Grill, H. J. (1985). Introduction: Physiological mechanisms in conditioned taste aversions. *Annals of the New York Academy of Sciences* 443:67–88.

Grill, H. J., and Berridge, K. C. (1985). Taste reactivity as a measure of neural control of palatability. In J. Sprague and A. Epstein (eds.), *Progress in psychobiology and physiological psychology*, Vol. 11. New York: Academic Press, 1–61.

Grill, H. J., and Norgren, R. (1978a). Chronically decerebrate rats demonstrate satiation but not bait shyness. *Science* 210:267–269.

Grill, H. J., and Norgren, R. (1978b). The taste reactivity test: II. Mimetic responses to gustatory stimuli in chronic thalamic and chronic decerebrate rats. *Brain Research* 143:281–297.

Hall, R. D., and Lindholm, E. P. (1974). Organization of motor and somatosensory neocortex in the albino rats. *Brain Research* 66:23–38.

Halpern, B. P. (1967). Chemotopic coding for sucrose and quinine hydrochloride in the nucleus of the fasciculus solitarius. In T. Hayashi (ed.), *Olfaction and taste* (Vol. II). New York: Pergamon, 549–562.

Jackson, J. H. (1958). Evolution and dissolution of the nervous system. In J. Taylor (ed.), *Selected writings of John Hughlings Jackson* (Vol. 2). New York: Basic Books. (Originally published in 1884.)

Jarbe, T. U., Falk, U., Mohammed, A. L., and Archer, T. (1988). Acquisition and reversal of taste/tactile discrimination after forebrain noradrenaline depletion. *Behavioral Neuroscience* 102:925–933.

Kalat, J. W. (1974). Taste salience depends on novelty, not concentration, in taste-aversion learning in the rat. *Journal of Comparative and Physiological Psychology* 86:47–50.

Kalat, J. W., and Rozin, P. (1970). "Salience": A factor which can override temporal contiguity in taste-aversion learning in rats. *Journal of Comparative and Physiological Psychology* 71:192–197.

Kemble, E. D., Strudelska, D. R., and Schmidt, M. K. (1979). Effects of central amygdaloid nucleus lesions on ingestion, taste reactivity, exploration and taste aversion. *Physiology and Behavior* 22:789–793.

Kiefer, S. W. (1985). Neural mediation of conditioned food aversions. *Annals of the New York Academy of Sciences* 443:100–109.

Kiefer, S. W., and Braun, J. J. (1977). Absence of differential associative responses to novel and familiar taste stimuli in rats lacking gustatory neocortex. *Journal of Comparative and Physiological Psychology* 91:498–507.

Kiefer, S. W., Leach, L., and Braun, J. J. (1984). Taste agnosia following gustatory neocortex ablation: Dissociation from odor and generality across taste qualities. *Behavioral Neuroscience* 98:590–608.

Kiefer, S. W., Morrow, N. S., and Metzler, C. W. (1988). Alcohol aversion generalization in rats: Specific disruption of taste and odor cues with gustatory neocortex or olfactory bulb ablations. *Behavioral Neuroscience* 102:733–739.

Kosar, E., Grill, H. J., and Norgren, R. (1986a). Gustatory cortex in the rat. I. Physiological properties and cytoarchitecture. *Brain Research* 379:329–341.

Kosar, E., Grill, H. J., and Norgren, R. (1986b). Gustatory cortex in the rat. II. Thalamocortical projections. *Brain Research* 379:342–352.

Kratz, C. M., and Levitsky, D. A. (1978). Post-ingestive effects of quinine on intake of nutritive and non-nutritive substances. *Physiology and Behavior* 21:851–854.

Krieg, W. J. S. (1946). Connections of the cerebral cortex: I. The albino rat. A. Topography of the cortical areas. *Journal of Comparative Neurology* 84:221–275.

Lashley, K. S. (1939). The mechanism of vision: XVI: The functioning of small remnants of the visual cortex. *Journal of Comparative Neurology* 70:45–67.

Lashley, K. S. (1950). In search of the engram. *Symposium of the Society of Experimental Biology* 4:454–482.

Lasiter, P. S. (1982). Cortical substrates of taste aversion learning: Direct amygdalocortical projections to the gustatory neocortex do not mediate conditioned taste aversion learning. *Physiological Psychology* 10:377–383.

Lasiter, P. S. (1983). Gastrointestinal reactivity in rats lacking anterior insular neocortex. *Behavioral and Neural Biology* 39:149–154.

Lasiter, P. S. (1985). Thalamocortical relations in taste aversion learning: II. Involvement of the medial ventrobasal thalamic complex in taste aversion learning. *Behavioral Neuroscience* 3:477–495.

Lasiter, P. S., Deems, D. A., and Garcia, J. (1985a). Involvement of anterior insular gustatory neocortex in taste-potentiated odor aversion learning. *Physiology and Behavior* 34:71–77.

Lasiter, P. S., Deems, D. A., and Glanzman, D. L. (1985b). Thalamocortical relations in taste aversion learning: I. Involvement of gustatory thalamocortical projections in taste aversion learning. *Behavioral Neuroscience* 3:454–476.

Lasiter, P. S., Deems, D. A., Oetting, R. L., and Garcia, J. (1985c). Taste discriminations in rats lacking anterior insular gustatory neocortex. *Physiology and Behavior* 35:277–285.

Lasiter, P. S., and Glanzman, D. L. (1982). Cortical substrates of taste aversion learning: Dorsal prepiriform (insular) lesions disrupt taste aversion learning. *Journal of Comparative and Physiological Psychology* 96:376–392.

Lasiter, P. S., and Glanzman, D. L. (1983). Axon collaterals of pontine taste area neurons project to the posterior ventromedial thalamic nucleus and to the gustatory neocortex. *Brain Research* 258:299–304.

Lasiter, P. S., and Glanzman, D. L. (1985). Cortical substrates of taste aversion learning: Involvement of dorsolateral amygdaloid nuclei and temporal neocortex in taste aversion learning. *Behavioral Neuroscience* 99:257–276.

Leonard, C. M. (1972). The connections of the dorsomedial nuclei. *Brain, Behavior and Evolution* 6:524–541.

LeVere, T. E., and LeVere, N. D. (1982). Recovery of function after brain damage: Support for the compensation theory of the behavioral deficit. *Physiological Psychology* 10:165–174.

Lorden, J., Kenfield, M., and Braun, J. J. (1970). Response suppression to odors paired with toxicosis. *Learning and Motivation* 1:391–394.

Meyer, D. R. (1972). Access to engrams. *American Psychologist* 27:124–133.

Meyer, P. M., Meyer, D. R., and Cloud, M. D. (1986). Temporal neocortical injuries in rats impair attending but not complex visual processing. *Behavioral Neuroscience* 100:845–851.

Miller, S. D., and Erickson, R. P. (1966). The odor of taste solutions. *Physiology and Behavior* 1:145–146.

Nachman, M., and Ashe, J. H. (1974). Effects of basolateral amygdala lesions on neophobia, learned taste aversions, and sodium appetite in rats. *Journal of Comparative and Physiological Psychology* 87:622–643.

Norgren, R., and Leonard, C. M. (1973). Ascending central gustatory connections. *Journal of Comparative Neurology* 150:217–238.

Nowlis, G. H. (1977). From reflex to representation: Taste-elicited tongue movements in the human newborn. In J. M. Weiffenbach (ed.), *Taste and development: The genesis of sweet preference* (Department of Health, Education, and Welfare Publication No. NIH 77-1068). Washington, D.C.: U.S. Government Printing Office.

Nowlis, G. H., and Frank, M. (1981). Quality coding in gustatory systems of rats and hamsters. In D. M. Norris (ed.), *Perception of behavioral chemicals*. Amsterdam: Elsevier/North Holland, 59–80.

Pavlov, I. P. (1960). *Conditioned reflexes*. New York: Dover. (Originally published in 1927.)

Pfaffmann, C. (1959). The sense of taste. In J. Field, H. W. Magoun, and V. E. Hall (eds.), *Handbook of physiology* (Vol. 1). Washington, D.C.: American Physiological Society.

Pfaffmann, C. (1960). The pleasures of sensation. *Psychological Review* 67:253–268.

Posner, M. I., Petersen, S. E., Fox, P. T., and Raichle, M. E. (1988). Localization of cognitive operations in the human brain. *Science* 240:1627–1631.

Rozin, P., and Kalat, J. W. (1971). Specific hungers and poison avoidance as adaptive specializations of learning. *Psychological Review* 78:459–486.

Rusiniak, K. W., Hankins, W. G., Garcia, J., and Brett, L. P. (1979). Flavor-illness aversions: Potentiation of odor by taste in rats. *Behavioral and Neural Biology* 25:1–17.

Saper, S. B. (1982a). Reciprocal parabrachial-cortical connections in the rat. *Brain Research* 242:33–40.

Saper, S. B. (1982b). Convergence of autonomic and limbic projections in the insular cortex of the rat. *Journal of Comparative Neurology* 210:163–173.

Shimada, S., Shiosaka, S., Takami, K., Yamano, M., and Tohyama, M. (1985). Somatostatinergic neurons in the insular cortex project to the spinal cord: Combined retrograde axonal transport and immunohistochemical study. *Brain Research* 326:197–200.

Shipley, M. T. (1982). Insular cortex projection to the nucleus of the solitary tract and brainstem visceromotor regions in the mouse. *Brain Research Bulletin* 8:139–148.

Shipley, M. T., and Sanders, M. S. (1982). Special senses are really special: Evidence for a reciprocal, bilateral pathway between insular cortex and nucleus parabrachialis. *Brain Research Bulletin* 8:493–501.

Spector, A. C., Breslin, P., and Grill, H. J. (1988). Taste reactivity as a dependent measure of the rapid formation of conditioned taste aversion: A tool for the neural analysis of taste-visceral associations. *Behavioral Neuroscience* 102:942–952.

Steiner, J. E. (1973). The human gustofacial response. In J. F. Bosma (ed.), *Fourth symposium on oral sensation and perception: Development in the fetus and infant* (Department of Health, Education, and Welfare Publication No. NIH 73-546). Washington, D.C.: U.S. Government Printing Office.

Travers, J. B., Travers, S. P., and Norgren, R. (1987). Gustatory neural processing in the hindbrain. *Annual Review Neuroscience* 10:595–632.

van der Kooy, D., Mcginty, J. F., Koda, L., Gerfen, C. R., and Bloom, F. E. (1982). Visceral cortex: A direct connection from prefrontal cortex to the solitary nucleus in the rat. *Neuroscience Letters* 33:123–127.

Welker, C. (1971). Microelectrode delineation of fine grain somatotopic organization of Sml cerebral neocortex in albino rat. *Brain Research* 26:259–275.

Weiskrantz, L., Warrington, E. K., Sanders, M. D., and Marshall, J. C. (1974). Visual capacity in the hemianopic field following a restricted occipital ablation. *Brain* 97:709–728.

Wirsig, C. R., and Grill, H. J. (1982). Contribution of the rat's neocortex to ingestive control: I. Latent learning for the taste of sodium chloride. *Journal of Comparative and Physiological Psychology* 96:615–627.

Wolf, G., DiCara, L., and Braun, J. (1970). Sodium appetite in rats after neocortical ablation. *Physiology & Behavior* 5:1265–1269.

Woolsey, C. N. (1958). Organization of somatic sensory and motor areas of the cerebral cortex. In H. F. Harlow and C. N. Woolsey (eds.), *Biological and biochemical bases of behavior*. Madison: University of Wisconsin Press, 63–81.

Yamamoto, T. (1984). Taste responses of cortical neurons. *Progress in Neurobiology* 23:273–315.

Yamamoto, T., Azuma, S., and Kawamura, Y. (1984a). Functional relations between the cortical gustatory area and the amygdala: Electrophysiological and behavioral studies in rats. *Experimental Brain Research* 56:23–31.

Yamamoto, T., Matsuo, R., and Kawamura, Y. (1980). Localization of the cortical gustatory area in rats and its role in taste discrimination. *Journal of Neurophysiology* 44:440–454.

Yamamoto, T., Yuyama, N., Kato, T., and Kawamura, Y. (1984b). Gustatory responses of cortical neurons in rats. I. Response characteristics. *Journal of Neurophysiology* 51:616–635.

Yamamoto, T., Yuyama, N., Kato, T., and Kawamura, Y. (1985a). Gustatory responses of cortical neurons in rats. II. Information processing of taste quality. *Journal of Neurophysiology* 53:1356–1369.

Yamamoto, T., Yuyama, N., Kato, T., and Kawamura, Y. (1985b). Gustatory responses of cortical neurons in rats. III. Neural and behavioral measures compared. *Journal of Neurophysiology* 6:1370–1386.

Yamamoto, T., Yuyama, N., and Kawamura, Y. (1981). Cortical neurons responding to tactile, thermal and taste stimulations of the rat's tongue. *Brain Research* 221:202–206.

Young, P. T. (1966). Hedonic organization and regulation of behavior. *Psychological Review* 37:60–70.

V   Association Cortex

17 Association Cortex in the Rat

Bryan Kolb

The term *association cortex* is a relic from the era of the British associationists of the 1800s. In the early 1900s physiologists picked up the term because they viewed the brain as something akin to a switchboard. The implication of their use was that messages from different senses became associated in the large areas of neocortex outside the traditional primary sensory regions. With further neurophysiological research over the ensuing decades, the size of cortical areas viewed as "association" shrank drastically because there turned out to be very little tissue that actually received inputs from more than one sensory modality. Nonetheless the term association cortex remains and is generally used with respect to the primate brain to refer to prefrontal, posterior parietal, and the anterior temporal cortex, which includes the tissue lying at the depths of the superior temporal sulcus.

Progress in the study of association cortex in nonprimate species has been slow for at least two reasons: First, it is widely assumed that any major variations in the neocortex of different mammalian species would be in the association cortex. For example, in their series of volumes on the cortex, Peters and Jones (1985, p. ix) have suggested, ". . . it is the development of the association areas that accounts for the greatest difference between the brains of primate and nonprimate species, and these areas have long been viewed as crucial in the formation of higher cognitive and behavioral functions." In other words, because primates have large association areas and are superior in intellect to other species, it is likely that the association areas are responsible for this. It follows directly that animals with modest intellectual capacities will have small, or nonexistent, association areas. Thus it would not be worth anyone's while to study the association cortex in species such as the rat.

Second, it has proved difficult to agree on how to define what would be prefrontal, posterior parietal, or temporal association cortex in non-primates, including rodents. Krieg (1946) identified cortical areas that he believed to be equivalent to prefrontal (Krieg's areas 8, 10) and posterior parietal cortex (Krieg's area 7, 39), but subsequent workers have disagreed with Krieg's conclusions (see chapter 4 by Zilles), in part because details of cytoarchitecture are significantly different in these regions in monkeys and rats. Furthermore, although there has been extensive research on the sensory regions of the cat brain, there has been virtually no work on the prefrontal cortex (see Warren, Warren, and Akert 1972) or the posterior parietal function in the cat (but see an anatomical study by Olson and Lawler (1987). In fact there is little help provided in using cytoarchitectonic criteria from work done in any other nonprimate species. As a result we must consider other criteria to help us define the association regions in the rat.

McCulloch (1944) proposed that cortical afferents from thalamic nuclei could provide an alternative basis for identifying cortical subdivisions. On this basis the areas innervated by the mediodorsal nucleus (MD) and lateral complex of the thalamus could define the prefrontal and posterior parietal regions, respectively. However, this has also proved problematic. Although there is a clear region of MD-projection cortex in the rat, it is now apparent that there is considerable overlap in thalamic projections. Furthermore the posterior thalamic complex of rodents is far simpler than that of primates, being composed of only a large lateral posterior (LP) nucleus. If this area is taken as equivalent to the LP/pulvinar of the primate, as has been suggested by Jones (1985), then there are grounds for identifying cortical regions in the rat that could be equivalent to the posterior parietal cortex of the monkey, but at the same time this tissue could be considered secondary visual cortex (see chapter 12 by Dean).

Another basis for identifying association areas in the rat is to consider not only the thalamic connections but also the cortico-cortical connections. One difficulty in this type of analysis, however, is that we have seen already that there are major differences in the number of sensory representations in different species (chapter 1). Nonetheless I argue in chapter 19 that it is possible to use a combination of thalamic and cortico-cortical connections to identify regions in the rat that likely correspond to the prefrontal and posterior parietal cortex in the monkey and that there is at least suggestive evidence of a form of temporal association cortex as well.

If the associational regions of the rat are to be useful as models of mammalian association cortex function, then it is necessary to demonstrate that the functions of these areas in the rat are similar to those in other species. In chapters 18 and 19 I consider this problem for the prefrontal and the posterior parietal and temporal regions, respectively, and make the point that there are important parallels in the function of the associative areas, although there are differences in details. In particular there is growing evidence that the prefrontal cortex of the rat plays a major role in the organization of behavior in time (that is, the temporal organization of behavior) in addition to a role in affective behavior (e.g., Kolb 1984). Similarly evidence is accumulating to implicate the posterior parietal region of the rat in visuospatial guidance and cross-modal matching as well as the temporal region in object recognition. These functions of the association areas of rats are reminiscent of the claims about the organization of the association regions in primates (see Kolb and Whishaw 1990 for a review) and imply that there may be continuity across the mammalian brain, even in the fundamental organization of the associative areas. Nonetheless, as I point out in chapter 18, there are differences too, and the differences may prove as interesting as the similarities in understanding the organization of the mammalian association cortex.

References

Kolb, B. (1984). Functions of the frontal cortex of the rat: A comparative review. *Brain Research Reviews* 8:65–98.

Kolb, B., and Whishaw, I. Q. (1990). *Fundamentals of Human Neuropsychology.* 3rd ed. New York: Freeman & Co.

Krieg, W. J. S. (1946). Connections of the cerebral cortex. I. The albino rat. B. Structure of the cortical areas. *Journal of Comparative Neurology* 84:277–321.

Jones, E. G. (1985). *The Thalamus.* New York: Plenum.

McCulloch, W. S. (1944). The functional organization of the cerebral cortex. *Physiological Reviews* 24:390–407.

Olson, C. R., and Lawler, K. (1987). Cortical and subcortical afferent connections of a posterior division of feline area 7 (area 7p). *Journal of Comparative Neurology* 259:13–30.

Peters, A., and Jones, E. J. (1985). *Cerebral Cortex. Volume 4: Association and Auditory Cortices.* New York: Plenum Press.

Warren, J. M., Warren, H. B., and Akert, K. (1972). The behavior of chronic cats with lesions in the frontal association cortex. *Acta Neurobiologiae Experimentalis* 32:345–392.

18 Prefrontal Cortex

Bryan Kolb

It was widely assumed before the 1960s that the rat did not have cortex that could be considered analogous to the prefrontal cortex of primates. Two studies were particularly influential in changing this view: First, Leonard (1969) showed that the dorsal medial thalamic nucleus of the rat projected to two distinct regions of frontal cortex in the rat and that, according to the definition of Rose and Woolsey (1948), this could be considered prefrontal cortex. Leonard's experiment was important because (1) it suggested that previous lesion studies focusing on the frontal polar cortex as a prefrontal analog were not removing the appropriate tissue, and (2) it allowed a reinterpretation of a small literature on the effects of "anterior cingulate" lesions on the behavior of rats. Second, Divac (1971) was the first to show that removal of one of these putative prefrontal regions in the rat led to a deficit in spatial reversal learning, which was believed by many at that time to be one of the most consistent effects of prefrontal lesions in primates and carnivores. Divac's experiment led to several more extensive examinations of the effect of lesions of the prefrontal regions in rats (e.g., Wikmark et al. 1973, Kolb et al. 1974). In the two decades since the initial studies of Leonard and Divac, we have come a long way in our understanding of the structure and functional organization of the prefrontal cortex of the rat, and it is the purpose of this chapter to review this research. I begin with a consideration of the structure and connections of the prefrontal cortex before reviewing the behavioral effects of lesions to the prefrontal cortex.

18.1 Structural Organization

Unlike the posterior and temporal regions of the neocortex, the cortex of the frontal pole of mammals is not easily defined by its sensory inputs. This has led to a long-standing disagreement over what constitutes equivalent frontal cortical areas in different species. Krieg's classical map of the rat cortex borrowed the terminology of Brodmann and led to what we now know is an erroneous belief that the frontal pole constituted the areas that could be considered equivalent to the prefrontal regions of the primate. To define the prefrontal areas of the rat, we need to consider the cytoarchitectonics, thalamocortical projections, other subcortical projections, and cortico-cortical projections.

Cytoarchitectonics

If we use Rose and Woolsey's (1948) definition of prefrontal cortex as that cortex receiving afferents from medialis dorsalis of the thalamus (MD), then we can identify several distinct frontal cortical regions in the rat (Krettek and Price 1977b, van Eden and Uylings 1985). These include (1) an anterior cingulate area (Zilles's Cg1, Cg2, Cg3), (2) an infralimbic area (IL), (3) an orbital area (LO, VLO, VO, MO), (4) an agranular insular area, which can be subdivided into a ventral and dorsal component (AIV, AID), and (5) a small strip of precentral cortex (Fr2), which is probably equivalent to the frontal eye fields of primates (figure 18.1; see also figure 4.4). On the medial aspect of the hemisphere, the Cg areas are distinguished by being thicker than the underlying PL and IL areas, in part because of a distinctly broader layer V. In the PL region layer V is clear, but the cells are more tightly packed than in Cg. There is a clear change in IL, where the lamination becomes indistinct and the cortex is markedly thinner. On the lateral aspect of the hemisphere the insular areas are easily distinguished from the adjacent cortex because of the lack of the granular layer IV in the insular cortex. The dorsal and ventral insular areas are distinguished by the clear reduction in cortical thickness in the ventral region. The four orbital regions are homogeneous in architecture, but can be distinguished by their thalamic inputs.

Thalamocortical Connections

As in other species there is a topographic organization of the projections from MD that appears to respect the different cortical subfields (e.g., Divac et al. 1978, Groenewegen 1988) (figure 18.2). Further the different subregions of MD have distinctive inputs, which presumably influence prefrontal function (figure 18.2). MD is not the only thalamic afferent to the rat prefrontal cortex, however, as part of the medial MD-projection cortex receives overlapping projections from the medial anterior nucleus (AM), the ventral nucleus (V), or the paratenial nucleus (PT), as well as the lateral posterior nucleus (LP), as illustrated in figure 18.2 (Divac et al. 1978). (A parallel arrangement of converging thalamic connections can be seen in other species as well, including monkeys (e.g., Goldman-Rakic and Porrino 1985).)

Other Subcortical Connections

In addition to the thalamocortical connections, there are extensive connections to and from other subcortical areas. Thus different regions of the prefrontal cortex receive projections from the substantia nigra and ventral tegmentum (see below), amygdala (e.g., Cassell et al. 1989,

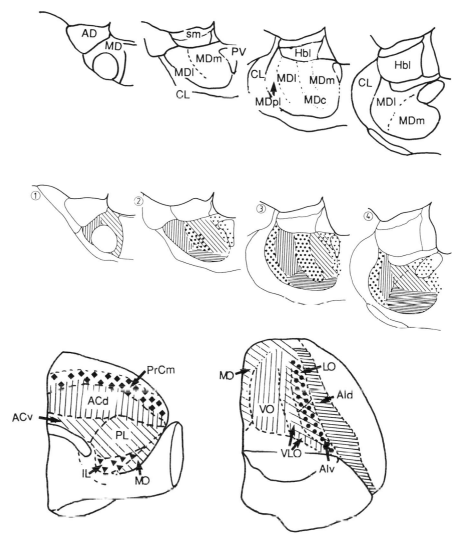

Figure 18.1 Illustration of the subregions of the frontal pole of the rat and the projections from the nucleus medialis dorsalis (MD). (A) Parcellation of MD. (B) Summary of the pattern of MD-cortical connections. (C) Parcellation of frontal cortex. (Adapted from Groenewegen 1988.)

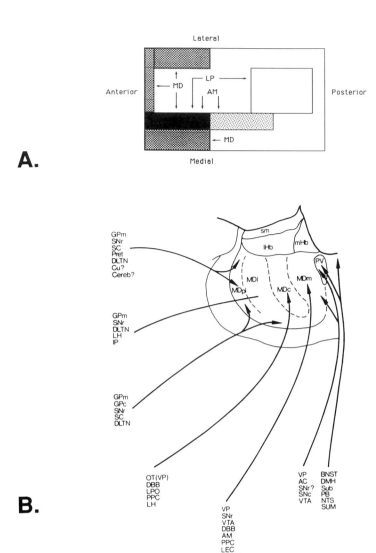

Figure 18.2 (A) Schematic illustrations of the types of overlap of thalamic projections to the prefrontal cortex of the rat. The largest rectangle represents the folded-out neocortex of the right hemisphere, with the frontal pole at the top. The gray area represents the area receiving projections from medialis dorsalis (MD), ventral tegmentum, and basolateral amygdala; the stippled area represents the area receiving projections from only medialis anterior (AM); the black area represents the area receiving projections from MD, AM, posterior lateralis posterior (LP), basolateral amygdala, and ventral tegmentum. (Adapted from Divac et al. 1978b.) (B) Summary of afferents of MD. (Adapted from Groenewegen 1988.) AC = nucleus accumbens; AM = amygdala; BNST = bednucleus of stria terminalis; DBB = nucleus of the diagonal band of Broca; DLTN = dorsolateral tegmental nucleus; DMH = dorsomedial hypothalamus; GPc = globus pallidus, caudal part; GPm = globus pallidus, medial part; IP = interpeduncular nucleus; LEC = lateral entorhinal cortex; LH = lateral hypothalamus; LPO = lateral preoptic area; NTS = nucleus of the solitary tract; OT = olfactory tubercle; PB = parabrachial nuclei; PPC = prepiriform cortex; Pret = pretectum; SC = superior colliculus; SNc = substantia nigra, pars compacta; SNr = substantia nigra, pars reticulata; Sub = subiculum; SUM = supramammillary nuclei; VP = ventral pallidum; VTA = ventral tegmental area of Tsai.

Krettek and Price 1977b, 1978), claustrum (e.g., Divac et al. 1978), lateral hypothalamus (e.g., Divac 1979, Leonard 1969), and CA1 of the hippocampus (e.g., Ferino et al. 1987, Swanson 1981). Similarly there are prefrontal projections to MD (Cornwall and Phillipson 1988, Krettek and Price 1977a), the striatum (Donoghue and Herkenham 1986, Ferino et al. 1987, Veening et al. 1980), nucleus accumbens (Beckstead 1979), amygdala (Beckstead 1979, Krettek and Price 1977b), lateral septum (Beckstead 1979), midbrain (Hardy 1986), mesencephalon and pons (Beckstead 1979), as well as direct projections to autonomic regions of the brainstem (e.g., Terreberry and Neafsey 1987). The dopaminergic and amygdaloid projections are particularly intriguing because they appear to overlap and to be coextensive with the MD projections (figure 18.3). Indeed since the first demonstration of dopaminergic innervation to the PFC by Thierry and colleagues (1973), there has been considerable elaboration of these connections (e.g., Berger 1976, Divac et al. 1978, Emson and Koob 1978, Lindvall et al. 1978) and interest both in the stimulation of this region (see below) as well as in sensitization of these dopaminergic neurons (e.g., Eichler and Antelman 1979, Robinson et al. 1985). Curiously it appears that the turnover of dopamine in PFC is especially high in comparison with striatal turnover, even though the concentration of dopamine is substantially lower in the PFC than in the striatum (Jones et al. 1986). This high turnover suggests that the PFC may be an ideal region for studies using in vivo dialysis techniques to correlate catecholamine activity with behavior.

Cortico-cortical Connections
The prefrontal cortex receives two types of cortico-cortical projections: those from sensory regions and those from the posterior parietal area. Figures 2.1 and 19.2 summarize these connections and show that although there are projections from visual, somatosensory, and auditory areas, the connections are most extensive from the visual areas. There is some debate regarding the nature and position of the posterior par-

Dopamine   Amygdala

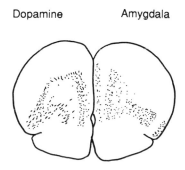

Figure 18.3 (A) Pattern of noradrenergic and dopaminergic projections to the frontal cortex of the rat. (Adapted from Lindvall et al. 1978.) (B) Pattern of amygdala projections to the frontal cortex of the rat. (Adapted from Krettek and Price 1977a.)

ietal cortex of the rat, but on the basis of its cytoarchitecture, thalamic connections, cortico-cortical connections, and behavioral changes after lesions, Krieg's area 7 is a likely candidate (see chapter 19). This region receives projections from visual and somatosensory regions and sends projections to MD-projection areas, the heaviest projections being to the orbital region and the frontal eye fields.

18.2   Effects of Lesions of the Prefrontal Cortex

It is evident from the anatomical work discussed above that the prefrontal cortex of the rat is made up of several subregions that are likely to be functionally distinct. Unfortunately no studies have made discrete lesions of each of these regions and then compared the subsequent behavioral changes. Nonetheless it is clear from lesion studies that there are at least three distinct prefrontal regions, including (1) a medial frontal region (MF), which is made up of several regions that are probably functionally distinct (Cg1 to CgIL), (2) an orbital frontal region (OF), which is also made up of several regions that are probably functionally distinct (LO, VO, VLO, MO, AI), and (3) a region that is likely analogous to the frontal eye fields of primates (Fr2). I shall treat these three regions as single functional entities, although in view of the distinct connections of subregions of both the MF and OF cortex, this is certainly an oversimplification. To simplify the discussion of the effects of PFC lesions, I have reduced (somewhat arbitrarily) the symptoms of PFC damage into five different classes of behavioral change. My review is selective because it would be impractical to try to consider every published study on the effects of prefrontal lesions in rats. (For a discussion of the effects of neonatal PFC lesions, see chapter 23.)

Temporary Memory
Rats with medial frontal, but not orbital frontal, lesions are impaired at a variety of delay-type tests including delayed response, delayed alternation, and delayed nonmatching to sample (see tables 18.1 and 18.2). These deficits are large because the animals can neither acquire nor postoperatively retain the ability to perform these tasks with any significant delays.

   The source of the deficits on delay tasks is uncertain, although it seems likely that MF lesions interfere with some sort of memory process that normally functions to hold sensory information "on line" for some temporal interval until a behavior is produced or a decision reached. This process has been characterized in many ways, including terms like working memory, short-term memory, representational memory, and a temporary memory buffer, but the essential idea is that there is a memory process that provides a temporary neural record of stimulus or motor events that occur over time. This allows animals to respond to sensory information after some delay and in the absence of the original

Table 18.1 Summary of Species-Specific Behavior of Rats with Prefrontal Lesions

Behavioral Test	Medial Frontal	Orbital Frontal	Basic Reference
Maternal behavior	impaired	normal	Stamm 1955, Wilsoncroft 1963
Nest building	impaired	normal	Kolb and Whishaw 1983b
Male social behavior	abnormal	abnormal	Kolb 1974c, de Bruin et al. 1983
Female social behavior	?	abnormal	Ferreira et al. 1987
Male sexual behavior	abnormal	?	Larsson 1970, Michel 1973
Female sex behavior	?	?	—
Activity and rhythms	normal	increased activity	Kolb 1974b
Swimming	abnormal	abnormal	Kolb and Whishaw 1983b
Grooming	normal	transient abnormal	Kolb and Whishaw 1983b
Food hoarding	abnormal	normal	Kolb 1974a
Neophobia	normal	normal	Divac et al. 1975
Taste aversion	normal	normal	Kolb et al. 1977
Defensive burying	abnormal	?	Kolb and Whishaw 1981

For further references, see text.

stimuli. I shall call this temporary memory. Importantly, rats with MF lesions are not amnesic for other types of tasks, such as the Morris water maze, which suggests that the deficits on delay tasks are unlike those observed after hippocampal lesions.

Although deficits in temporary memory are easily demonstrated in delay-type tasks, temporary memory deficits do occur in a variety of other behavioral tasks after MF lesions. For example, Kesner and his colleagues have devised two interesting memory tests that utilize the radial arm maze. In one test animals must keep track of the order in which they enter different arms so that when they are given a choice of two previously visited arms, they must choose the arm visited most recently (Kesner and Holbrook 1987). In the other test the animals must choose between a novel arm and one of several that they have just visited (Kesner 1989). Rats with MF lesions are impaired severely at both of these tests, and although there is not an explicit delay in the procedure, there is certainly a delay between entering an arm in the initial phase of testing and choosing an arm in the probe test. Similarly rats with MF lesions show a retarded habituation to novel stimuli in a variety of settings (Kolb 1974b). Again the deficit can be interpreted as an inability to keep track of sensory events over time.

One of the important characteristics of most delay-type tasks is that they have a spatial component to them, and at one time it was believed that temporary memory deficits after PFC lesions might be restricted to spatial tasks (e.g., Goldman and Rosvold 1970). This now seems un-

Table 18.2 Summary of Performance of Learning Tasks of Rats with Prefrontal Lesions

Type of Test	Medial Frontal	Orbital Frontal	Basic Reference
Habituation			
Heart rate	poor	?	Glaser and Griffin 1962
Flexor reflex	poor	?	Griffin and Pearson 1967
Headshake	poor	?	Roydes 1970
Activity	poor	normal	Kolb 1974d
Head poke	poor	normal	Kolb 1974d
Motor learning			
latch puzzles	poor	poor	Kolb and Whishaw 1983b
bar pressing	normal	normal	Kolb et al. 1974
Delayed reaction			
Delayed response	poor	normal	Kolb et al. 1974
Delayed alternate	poor	normal	Larsen and Divac 1978, van Haaren et al. 1985
Spontaneous alternate	fail	normal	Divac et al. 1975
Delayed nonmatch to sample	fail	?	Kolb et al. 1989
Spatial			
Lashley III	poor	normal	Thomas and Weir 1975
Morris water	poor	poor	Kolb et al. 1983
Olton radial arm	poor	very poor	Becker et al. 1980
Kesner radial	poor	?	Kesner and Holbrook 1987
Maier maze	poor	?	Hermann et al. 1985
Discrimination reversal			
Tactile	poor	?	Gabriel et al. 1979
Object	poor	?	Becker et al. 1980
Spatial	poor	normal	Divac 1971
Aversive			
Passive avoid	normal	normal	Kolb and Whishaw 1981
One-way avoid	poor	normal	Kolb and Nonneman 1978
Two-way avoid	poor	normal	Kolb and Nonneman 1978
Scheduled reinforcement			
DRL	poor	normal	Nonneman et al. 1974
	normal	poor	Kolb et al. 1974
FR	normal	?	Numan and Grant 1980
FI	abnormal		Olton 1989
Bar press extinction	normal	poor	Kolb et al. 1974

For further references, see text.

likely, however, because animals are also impaired at nonspatial memory tasks such as delayed nonmatching to sample (e.g., Mishkin and Appenzeller 1987). It is likely, however, that the spatial and nonspatial temporary memory deficits can be dissociated in the rat as has recently been done in the monkey (see Kolb and Whishaw 1990, ch. 19, for an extensive discussion). On the basis of the work on the monkey, it is likely that more dorsal MF lesions, which include the frontal eye fields, will disrupt spatial memory tasks, whereas lesions of the MO and/or IL regions will disrupt nonspatial temporal memory tasks.

Spatial Orientation

Rats with MF lesions are impaired at the acquisition of every spatial maze task in which they have been tested (e.g., Becker et al. 1980, Herrmann et al. 1985, Kolb et al. 1983). It is thus tempting to compare this result with the effects of hippocampal lesions, which have a similar effect (e.g., O'Keefe and Nadel 1978). There are several reasons to question such a comparison, however.

First, although MF lesions impair the acquisition of spatial mazes, the animals usually eventually learn the maze, which suggests that they are able to use spatial information to guide behavior. Second, animals with MF lesions are frequently not impaired at the retention of spatial mazes. For example, rats trained in the Morris water maze before operation are indistinguishable from control animals postoperatively (Sutherland 1985). Thus they are clearly able to navigate to the correct spatial location in the absence of the PFC, which implies either that the PFC is not crucial to the determination of spatial location or that it is only involved in the initial learning of spatial location. This would seem to be different from the role of the hippocampus, although there is one intriguing similarity: Sutherland and Arnold (1987) showed that although rats with hippocampal lesions showed amnesia for spatial information if the lesion was inflicted soon after training, there was a temporally graded reduction in memory loss such that if the lesions were made three months after initial learning; the animals retained the ability to perform the preoperatively acquired Morris water maze task nearly as well as did normal control animals. In other words, although the temporal details are different, it appears that animals can retain spatial information and navigate to spatial locations in the absence of the PFC or hippocampus. It is thus not at all clear how the animals are solving the problems or what role either of these structures actually plays in spatial navigation.

Sequential Behavior

Rats with PFC lesions are consistently impaired at behavioral tasks in which they are required to make a series of behavioral responses in a particular sequence. This includes "natural" behaviors such as nest building or food hoarding in which materials must be moved and manipulated in an organized sequence (e.g., Kolb and Whishaw 1983a) as well as in learned behaviors such as the opening of puzzle latches (e.g., Kolb and Whishaw 1983b). There is reason to suspect that the focus for this effect is the more ventral medial frontal cortex, possibly including regions VO, MO, and/or IL. Mogensen and Divac (1984) found that animals with OF lesions that included VO and MO were impaired when they had to learn that a lever press was only rewarded if a rod was pushed previously in the presence of a cue light. Medial lesions that spared MO and VO did not produce a deficit. Similarly I have repeatedly observed that rats with shallow MF lesions are not impaired at food hoarding, whereas animals with more ventrally extending lesions that include IL and MO often have a nearly total abolition of successful food hoarding (Kolb 1973). Similarly, large OF lesions that include VO and MO reduce food hoarding as well.

Behavioral Flexibility

In contrast to lower vertebrates mammals have evolved remarkable behavioral plasticity as characterized by the ability to adopt new strategies for problem solving when environmental contingencies change. Rats with PFC lesions are particularly poor at showing this behavioral flexibility. Perhaps the best example is reversal learning. Rats with MF lesions usually learn the initial correct responses as quickly as normal animals do, but when there is a shift in the correct response to another object or place, they tend to perseverate on the initially correct solution (table 18.2). Moreover rats with PFC lesions are often slower to adopt the correct strategy to solve a variety of tasks, but once they do, they appear to learn as quickly as normal animals. For example, in our studies on forepaw reaching in rats with MF lesions, we have been struck by the rats' slowness to learn that they cannot reach the food with their mouth or tongue. Normal animals quickly abandon this strategy, whereas some rats with PFC damage persist indefinitely and do not spontaneously switch to paw use without extensive shaping. Similarly when OF rats are placed in a large swimming pool, they are very slow to abandon trying to climb up the walls, which again is a prepotent response for normal animals, but once they do so, they acquire problems such as the Morris water maze as quickly as do normal animals. Finally, in a study of play behavior in rats having received frontal lesions as infants, Kolb and Gorney (in preparation) found that although frontal animals were at least as active as control animals, they virtually never initiated play behavior. Once initiated by a normal animal, however, they did show all the normal components of play behavior, although again it was less frequent than normal. Taken together, these behavioral symptoms suggest that PFC lesions reduce the spontaneity and variability of behavior. A similar conclusion has been reached by Milner and colleagues (1985) in their analysis of the behavior of human frontal lobe patients.

Social and Sexual Behavior

PFC lesions have been shown to alter both sexual and social behavior in rats, the effects being somewhat different after OF and MF lesions (de Bruin, in press, de Bruin et al. 1983, Holson, 1986a,b,c, Kolb 1974c, Kolb and Nonneman 1974, Larsson 1970, Lubar et al. 1973, Michal 1973). Thus OF lesions increase aggressiveness in male rats, whereas MF lesions seem to increase timidity. In addition MF lesions alter the normal pattern of sexual behavior in male rats, rendering them less likely to mate successfully. The cause of these changes in social and sexual behavior has not been identified, but there are at least three likely explanations: First, many of these behaviors require that the animals perform a sequence of behaviors in a particular order, and rats with PFC lesions are impaired at this (see above). Second, both sexual and social behavior in rodents depends highly on olfactory input, and the orbital cortex receives olfactory inputs (as do the amygdala and MD, both of which have extensive connections to the PFC), and OF lesions have been shown to disrupt olfactorily guided behavior (Eichenbaum et al. 1980, Ferreira et al. 1987). Third, both the amygdala and meso-cortical dopaminergic systems have been implicated in affective behavior, and both of these regions project to the PFC (figure 18.3).

Summary

Damage to the PFC leads to a wider variety of behavioral changes than does damage to any other neocortical region in the rat. Virtually every species-typical behavior is disrupted, and the performance of a wide variety of learning tasks is impaired. At least three conclusions can be drawn from these studies: First, although PFC lesions disrupt species-typical behaviors, most of the components of these behaviors remain. Moreover it appears that even decorticated rats are able to produce most of the components of even complex species-typical behavioral patterns, such as sexual or maternal behavior, under at least a restricted range of circumstances (see chapter 10 by Whishaw). Thus PFC lesions affect the organization of these behaviors rather than the production of their components. One exception to this generalization is the effect of OF lesions on behaviors that have a significant olfactory component. The insular cortex almost certainly plays a central role in olfactory processing, which is likely mediated by a pyriform-amygdala-MD-OF circuit. Second, the poor performance on the variety of learning may be reduced in large part to two behavioral changes: an impairment in temporary memory and a reduction in behavioral flexibility. This does not rule out other deficits, however, but to date there is little compelling evidence of other changes (cf. Kesner 1989, Kolb et al. 1989). Third, there is clear evidence for a functional dissociation of at least the medial and orbital regions of the rat PFC (Kolb 1984) and at least hints at further dissociations within these regions.

18.3 Electrophysiological Studies

There have been surprisingly few electrophysiological recording studies of the activity of cells in the rat prefrontal cortex, and it is difficult to relate most of those that are available to the results of lesion studies (e.g., Kanki et al. 1983, Mora et al. 1976, Peterson 1986, Rolls and Cooper 1973, Stern et al. 1984, 1985). One series of studies is especially intriguing, however, because Sakurai and his colleagues have reported several experiments in which they have shown unique patterns of multiunit activity in the medial frontal cortex of rats trained in delay-type tasks (e.g., Sakurai and Sugimoto 1986). These units were activated vigorously during the delay before responses and the increased firing ending with the response. Parallel results have been shown for units in the monkey prefrontal cortex and have led to the suggestion that the prefrontal cortex plays a role in temporal memory—a conclusion that is in accord with the results of lesion studies.

In dozens of studies the prefrontal regions have been electrically stimulated, both to observe elicited behavior as well as to study the reinforcing effects of such stimulation. The results show that (1) rats will self-stimulate in the medial and orbital regions, which has been taken as evidence of some role of the prefrontal cortex (possibly the dopaminergic-rich regions of PFC) in reward (e.g., Cobo et al. 1989, Robertson et al. 1986, Rolls and Cooper 1974), (2) medial frontal stimulation can either suppress or induce different behaviors, depending on the context (e.g., Corbett and Stellar 1983, Sinnamon and Galer 1984, Wilcott 1981), and (3) both medial and orbital stimulation can affect cardiovascular function (see below). In each of these cases there is reason to believe that the effects are unique to the prefrontal cortex and do not occur from stimulation in other neocortical sites.

At present it is difficult to reach general conclusions from the available electrophysiological studies of the prefrontal cortex of rats. It does appear, however, that prefrontal unit activity is distinctive during delays, which suggests a role of the prefrontal cortex in temporary memory, and that prefrontal stimulation is rewarding, which suggests a role of the prefrontal cortex in the neural circuit underlying reinforcement, possibly including the amygdala and dopaminergic systems.

18.4 Sex Differences in PFC Function

There have been few direct studies of sex differences in PFC function, but evidence is accumulating in support of this notion. First, there is considerable evidence that gonadal hormones differentially influence cortical structure (for review, see chapter 21 by Juraska). Second, there is accumulating evidence that there is a sex difference in the structure of the PFC. Thus van Eden and colleagues (1984) showed sex-related differences in the development of the PFC and Kolb and Stewart (in preparation) have shown sex differences in the dendritic arbor of cells in Cg1, Cg3, and AID of adult animals. Moreover in the latter study the sex differences were blocked by neonatal castration. In addition in a related study Kolb and Fantie (in preparation) have found that frontal cortical grafts from either male or female donors are differentially affected by the gonadal state of the host: There is a greater growth of dendritic arbor in the grafts placed in male versus female animals. Third, several studies have shown sex differences in the effects of PFC lesions. For example, it appears that whereas OF lesions increase aggression in male rats (Kolb 1974c, de Bruin et al. 1983), similar lesions reduce aggression in female rats (Ferreira et al. 1987). Similarly OF lesions produce truly massive changes in wheel running activity in female rats, but rather small changes in male rats (Kolb 1974a). Studies of maze learning have also shown sex differences because MF lesions in females reliably produce larger deficits in the Morris water maze and a version of the radial arm maze (Kolb 1988). Curiously the reverse is true in a "landmark" task in which animals must learn the relation between a goal and a spatially discontiguous cue (Kolb 1988). Finally, there appears to be a variety of complex interactions between sex and the behavioral effects of neonatal frontal lesions in rats (e.g., Kolb 1987). Taken together, both the anatomical and behavioral studies suggest that gonadal hormones influence both the structure and function of the PFC as well as the hippocampus and other subcortical structures. The mechanism of action remains to be determined.

18.5 Asymmetry in PFC Function

R. G. Robinson and his colleagues were the first to show in a series of studies that whereas right frontal lesions in rats increased wheel running activity postoperatively, there was no corresponding effect of left frontal lesions (e.g., Robinson and Coyle 1980). This asymmetrical effect occurs regardless of whether the lesion is produced by suction, kainic acid, 6-hydroxydopamine, ischemia, or knife cut. More important, however, the lesion need not be confined to the PFC to produce the behavioral asymmetry, which Robinson and Coyle propose is related to asymmetrical catecholaminergic effects of the lesions because it may be located in adjacent tissue. Further evidence of PFC asymmetry comes from studies showing that although removal of the dorsomedial MD-projection cortex (largely Fr2 in figure 18.1) from either hemisphere produces contralateral neglect, the details of behavioral change vary considerably between left and right hemisphere lesions (Vargo et al. 1988). These asymmetrical behavioral differences are difficult to explain, but are consistent with the general idea of an asymmetry in the PFC of rats.

18.6 Autonomic Functions of the PFC

Although less studied than other aspects of PFC function, it has been known for at least 100 years that the PFC exerts control over the autonomic nervous system (Neafsey, in press). Over the past decade evidence has accumulated to show that two medial regions (IL, PL) and one orbital region (AI) have extensive connections with structures involved in autonomic function. In particular these PFC regions (particularly IL and AI) project to the lateral dorsal tegmental nucleus (LDT) of the dorsal pons as well as various subnuclei of the solitary nucleus (SNM) of the dorsal medulla. The LDT is involved in micturition, and the SNM receives inputs from the heart, baroreceptors, lungs, and gut (e.g., Ruggiero et al. 1987, Satoh and Fibiger 1986, Terreberry and Neafsey 1987, van der Kooy et al. 1984). Furthermore the AI receives projections, both directly and indirectly, from the SNM and the olfactory system, and the AI lies adjacent to the gustatory cortex and may even include neurons sensitive to tastes (Cechetto and Saper 1987). Evidence from both stimulation and lesion studies supports the anatomical results. For example, low-level stimulation of both IL and AI elicits changes in both cardiovascular and gastric responses (e.g., Burns and Wyss 1985, Hurley-Gius and Neafsey 1986, Ruggiero et al. 1987), and lesions of the midline cortex alter the normal autonomic responses to conditioned emotional stimuli (Neafsey, in press). Similarly damage to the orbital regions alters chronic body weight in male (but not female) rats (e.g., Kolb et al. 1977).

Although little is known of the details of PFC involvement in autonomic function, the results to date lead Terreberry and Neafsey (1987) to propose that the midline regions (PL, IL) are involved in "motor" aspects of visceral control, whereas the insular region is involved in "sensory" aspects. This idea is provocative and awaits further elaboration. Another intriguing aspect of the prefrontal role in autonomic function comes from evidence of a prefrontal role in stress responses. For example, it has been reported that there is a selective activation of the mesocortical dopamine system by stress (Thierry et al. 1976) and that removal of the MF region reduces gastric pathology produced by stress (Sullivan and Henke 1986). Furthermore multiunit activity in the midline PFC is altered by stress and by benzodiazepines (Henke 1984).

18.7 Summary

Three general conclusions can be drawn from the anatomical and behavioral studies of the rat's prefrontal cortex: First, there are several distinct anatomical regions in the prefrontal cortex, each of which has dissociable cytoarchitecture as well as thalamocortical, cortico-cortical, and subcortical connections. Second, although there are no studies functionally dissociating all of these areas, there is good evidence that the midline and orbital regions can be functionally dissociated. Third, a comparison of prefrontal anatomy and the effects of prefrontal lesions in rodents and primates reveals striking similarities (Kolb 1984) as well as clear differences (Kolb, in press). Both species have a frontal cortical region with connections to MD and a striking parallel in subcortical connections. Further the general effects of lesions and the general characteristics of electrophysiological activity reveal important and striking similarities. There are significant differences, however, in the general features of cortico-cortical connectivity as well as in the details of behavioral change following lesions. One key to understanding the details of prefrontal organization in mammals may be found in the study of both the cortico-cortical inputs to different prefrontal areas as well as in the study of the differences in behavioral patterns of different mammalian species. These behavioral patterns have evolved in response to specific ecological pressures, and the unique pattern of cortical development in different species will likely reflect the different neural requirements for particular species-typical behaviors. The apparent general similarity in prefrontal function across mammals may reflect the similarity in general requirements of mammalian behavioral patterns, whereas the differences in the details of prefrontal organization in mammals may reflect interspecies variability and the adaptedness of behavior. It is now clear that there are general similarities in prefrontal function and organization across mammals and that rats may provide a useful model to study general functions of the PFC. In addition, however, neuroscientists should now be able to effectively study prefrontal function by taking advantage of the differences in behavior and prefrontal structure in different mammals. Thus, just as studies of the rat PFC have provided evidence of unity of prefrontal function in mammals, they should also promise evidence of the diversity of prefrontal function.

References

Becker, J. T., Walker, J. A., and Olton, D. S. (1980). Object discrimination by rats: the role of frontal and hippocampal systems in retention and reversal. *Physiology and Behavior* 24:33–38.

Beckstead, R. M. (1979). An autoradiographic examination of corticocortical and subcortical projections of the mediodorsal-projection (prefrontal) cortex in the rat. *Journal of Comparative Neurology* 184:43–61.

Berger, B., Thierry, A. M., Tassin, J. P., and Moyne, M. A. (1976). Dopaminergic innervation of the rat prefrontal cortex: A fluorescence histochemical study. *Brain Research* 106:133–145.

Burns, S. M., and Wyss, J. M. (1985). The involvement of the anterior cingulate cortex in blood pressure control. *Brain Research* 340:71–77.

Cassell, M. D., Chitick, C. A., Siegel, M. A., and Wright, D. J. (1989). Collateralization of the amygdaloid projections of the rat prelimbic and infralimbic cortices. *Journal of Comparative Neurology* 279:235–248.

Cechetto, D. F., and Saper, C. B. (1987). Evidence for a viscerotopic sensory representation in the cortex and thalamus in the rat. *Journal of Comparative Neurology* 262:27–45.

Cobo, M., Ferrer, J. M. R., and Mora, F. (1989). The role of the lateral cortico-cortical prefrontal pathway in self-stimulation of the medial prefrontal cortex in the rat. *Behavioural Brain Research* 31:257–265.

Corbett, D., and Stellar, J. R. (1983). Neurological reactivity during medial prefrontal cortex stimulation: Effects of self-stimulation experience. *Physiology and Behavior* 31:771–776.

Cornwall, J., and Phillipson, O. T. (1988). Afferent projections to the dorsal thalamus of the rat as shown by retrograde lectin transport. I. The mediodorsal nucleus. *Neuroscience* 24:1035–1049.

de Bruin, J. P. C. (In press). Social behavior and the prefrontal cortex. *Progress in Brain Research.*

de Bruin, J. P. C., van Oyen, H. G. M., and van de Poll, N. (1983). Behavioural changes following lesions of the orbital prefrontal cortex in male rats. *Behavioural Brain Research* 10:209–232.

Divac, I. (1971). Frontal lobe system and spatial reversal in the rat. *Neuropsychologia* 9:171–183.

Divac, I. (1979). Patterns of subcortico-cortical projections as revealed by somatopetal horseradish peroxidase tracing. *Neuroscience* 4:455–461.

Divac, I. (1979). Patterns of subcortico-cortical projections as revealed by somatopetal horseradish peroxidase tracing. *Neuroscience* 4:455–461.

Divac, I., Björklund, A., Lindvall, O., and Passingham, R. E. (1978a). Converging projections from the mediodorsal thalamic nucleus and mesencephalic dopaminergic neurons to the necortex in three species. *Journal of Comparative Neurology* 180:59–71.

Divac, I., Gade, A., and Wikmark, R. E. G. (1975). Taste aversion in rats with lesions in the frontal lobes: no evidence for interoceptive agnosia. *Physiological Psychology* 3:43–46.

Divac, I., Kosmal, A., Björklund, A., and Lindvall, O. (1976). Subcortical projections to the prefrontal cortex in the rat as revealed by the horseradish peroxidase technique. *Neuroscience* 3:785–796.

Divac, I., Mogensen, J., Blanchard, R. J., and Blanchard, D. C. (1984). Medial cortical lesions and fear behavior in the wild rat. *Physiological Psychology* 12:271–274.

Divac, I., Wikmark, R. G. E., and Gade, A. (1975). Spontaneous alternation in rats with lesions in the frontal lobes. An extension of the frontal lobe syndrome. *Physiological Psychology* 3:39–42.

Donoghue, J. P., and Herkenham, M. (1986). Neostriatal projections from individual cortical fields conform to histochemically distinct striatal compartments in the rat. *Brain Research* 365:397–403.

Eichenbaum, H., Shedlack, K. J., and Eckmann, K. W. (1980). Thalamocortical mechanisms in odor-guided behavior. I. Effects of lesions of the mediodorsal thalamic nucleus and frontal cortex on olfactory discrimination in the rat. *Brain, Behavior, and Evolution* 17:255–275.

Eichler, A. J., and Antelman, S. M. (1979). Sensitization to amphetamine and stress may involve nucleus accumbens and medial frontal cortex. *Brain Research* 176:412–416.

Emson, P. C., and Koob, G. F. (1978). The origin and distribution of dopamine-containing afferents to the rat prefrontal cortex. *Brain Research* 142:249–267.

Ferino, F., Thierry, A. M., and Glowinski, J. (1987). Anatomical and electrophysiological evidence for a direct projection from Ammon's horn to the medial prefrontal cortex in the rat. *Experimental Brain Research* 65:421–426.

Ferreira, A., Dahlof, L.-G., and Hansen, S. (1987). Olfactory mechanisms in the control of maternal aggression, appetite, and fearfulness: Effects of lesions to olfactory receptors, mediodorsal thalamic nucleus, and insular prefrontal cortex. *Behavioral Neuroscience* 101:709–717.

Gabriel, S., Freer, B., and Finger, S. (1979). Brain damage and overlearning reversal effect. *Physiological Psychology* 7:327–332.

Glaser, E. M., and Griffin, J. P. (1962). Influence of cerebral cortex on habituation. *Journal of Physiology* 160:429–445.

Goldman-Rakic, P. S., and Porrino, L. J. (1985). The primate mediodorsal (MD) nucleus and its projections to the frontal lobe. *Journal of Comparative Neurology* 242:535–560.

Goldman, P. S., and Rosvold, H. (1970). Localization of function within the dorsolateral prefrontal cortex of the rhesus monkey. *Experimental Neurology* 27:291–304.

Griffin, J. A., and Pearson, J. A. (1967). Habituation of the flexor reflex in spinal rats, and in rats with frontal cortex lesions followed by spinal transection. *Brain Research* 6:777–780.

Groenewegen, H. J. (1988). Organization of the afferent connections of the mediodorsal thalamic nucleus in the rat, related to the mediodorsal-prefrontal topography. *Neuroscience* 24:379–431.

Hardy, S. G. P. (1986). Projections to the midbrain from the medial versus lateral prefrontal cortices of the rat. *Neuroscience Letters* 63:159–164.

Henke, P. G. (1984). The anterior cingulate cortex and stress: Effects of chlordiazepoxide on unit-activity and stimulation-induced gastric pathology in rats. *International Journal of Psychophysiology* 2:23–32.

Herrmann, T., Poucet, B., and Ellen, P. (1985). Spatial problem solving in the rat following medial frontal lesions. *Physiological Psychology* 13:21–25.

Holson, R. R. (1986a). Medial prefrontal cortical lesions and timidity in rats. I. Reactivity to aversive stimuli. *Physiology and Behavior* 37:221–230.

Holson, R. R., and Walker, C. (1986b). Medial prefrontal cortical lesions and timidity in rats. II. Reactivity to novel stimuli. *Physiology and Behavior* 37:221–230.

Holson, R. R. (1986c). Medial prefrontal cortical lesions and timidity in rats. III. Behavior in a semi-natural environment. *Physiology and Behavior* 37:239–247.

Hurley-Gius, K. M., and Neafsey, E. J. (1986). The medial frontal cortex and gastric motility: Microstimulation results and their possible significance for the overall pattern of organization of rat frontal and parietal cortex. *Brain Research* 365:241–248.

Jones, M. W., Kilpatrick, I. C., and Phillipson, O. T. (1986). The agranular insular cortex: a site of unusually high dopamine utilisation. *Neuroscience Letters* 72:330–334.

Kanki, J. P., Martin, T. L., and Sinnamon, H. M. (1983). Activity of neurons in the anteromedial cortex during rewarding brain stimulation, saccharin consumption, and orienting behavior. *Behavioural Brain Research* 8:69–84.

Kesner, R. (1989). Retrospective and prospective coding of information: role of the medial prefrontal cortex. *Experimental Brain Research* 74:163–167.

Kesner, R. P., and Holbrook, T. (1987). Dissociation of item and order spatial memory in rats following medial prefrontal cortex lesions. *Neuropsychologia* 25:653–664.

Kolb, B. (1973). The behavior of rats with chronic lesions in MD-projection cortex. Unpublished doctoral thesis, Pennsylvania State University, University Park, PA.

Kolb, B. (1974a). Dissociation of the effects of lesions of the orbital or medial aspect of the prefrontal cortex of the rat with respect to activity. *Behavioral Biology* 10:329–343.

Kolb, B. (1974b). Some tests of response habituation in rats with prefrontal lesions. *Canadian Journal of Psychology* 12:466–474.

Kolb, B. (1974c). Social behavior of rats with chronic prefrontal lesions. *Physiological Psychology* 87:466–474.

Kolb, B. (1974d). Prefrontal lesions alter eating and hoarding behavior in rats. *Physiology and Behavior* 12:507–511.

Kolb, B. (1984). Functions of the frontal cortex of the rat: a comparative review. *Brain Research Reviews* 8:65–98.

Kolb, B. (1987). Recovery from early cortical damage in rats. I. Differential behavioral and anatomical effects of frontal lesions at different ages of neural maturation. *Behavioural Brain Research* 25:205–220.

Kolb, B. (1988). Gonadal hormones affect cortical development, organization and function in rats. *Society for Neuroscience Abstracts* 14:595.

Kolb, B. (In press). Animal models for human PFC-related disorders. *Progress in Brain Research*.

Kolb, B., Buhrman, K., and McDonald, R. (1989). Dissociation of prefrontal, posterior parietal, and temporal cortical regions to spatial navigation and recognition memory in the rat. *Society for Neuroscience Abstracts* 15:607.

Kolb, B., and Gorney, B. (In preparation). *Neonatal frontal lesions alter play behavior in the rat.*

Kolb, B., and Nonneman, A. J. (1974). Frontolimbic lesions and social behavior in the rat. *Physiology and Behavior* 13:637–643.

Kolb, B., and Nonneman, A. J. (1978). Sparing of function in rats with early prefrontal cortex lesions. *Brain Research* 151:135–148.

Kolb, B., Nonneman, A. J., and Singh, R. K. (1974). Double dissociation of spatial impairments and perseveration following selective prefrontal lesions in rats. *Journal of Comparative and Physiological Psychology* 87:772–780.

Kolb, B., Sutherland, R. J., and Whishaw, I. Q. (1983). A comparison of the contributions of the frontal and parietal association cortex to spatial localization in rats. *Behavioral Neuroscience* 97:13–27.

Kolb, B., and Whishaw, I. Q. (1981). Neonatal frontal lesions in the rat: sparing of learned but not species-typical behavior in the presence of reduced brain weight and cortical thickness. *Journal of Comparative and Physiological Psychology* 95:863–879.

Kolb, B., and Whishaw, I. Q. (1983a). Problems and principles in cross-species generalizations. In T. E. Robinson (ed.), *Behavioural Approaches to Brain Research.* New York: Oxford University Press.

Kolb, B., and Whishaw, I. Q. (1983b). Dissociation of the contributions of the prefrontal, motor, and parietal cortex to the control of movement in the rat. *Canadian Journal of Psychology* 37:211–232.

Kolb, B., and Whishaw, I. Q. (1990). *Fundamentals of Human Neuropsychology, Third Edition.* New York: W. H. Freeman & Co.

Kolb, B., Whishaw, I. Q., and Schallert, T. (1977). Aphagia, behavior sequencing, and body weight set point following orbital frontal lesions in rats. *Physiology and Behavior* 19:93–103.

Krettek, J. E., and Price, J. L. (1977a). Projections from the amygdaloid complex to the cerebral cortex and thalamus in the rat and cat. *Journal of Comparative Neurology* 172:687–722.

Krettek, J. E., and Price, J. L. (1977b). The cortical projections of the mediodorsal nucleus and adjacent thalamic neuclei in the rat. *Journal of Comparative Neurology* 171:157–192.

Larsen, J. K., and Divac, I. (1978). Selective ablations within the prefrontal cortex of the rat and performance of delayed alternation. *Physiological Psychology* 6:15–17.

Larsson, L. (1970). Mating behavior in the male rat. In L. R. Aronson, E. Tobach, D. S. Lehrman, and J. S. Rosenblatt (eds.), *Development and Evolution of Behavior.* San Francisco: W. H. Freeman & Co.

Leonard, C. M. (1969). The prefrontal cortex of the rat. I. Cortical projections of the mediodorsal nucleus. II. Efferent connections. *Brain Research* 12:321–343.

Lindvall, O., Björklund, A., and Divac, I. (1978). Organization of catecholamine neurons projecting to the frontal cortex in the rat. *Brain Research* 142:1–24.

Lubar, J. F., Herrmann, T. J., Moore, D. R., and Shouse, M. N. (1973). Effect of septal and frontal ablations on species typical behavior in the rat. *Journal of Comparative and Physiological Psychology* 83:260–270.

Michal, E. K. (1973). Effects of limbic lesions on behavior sequences and courtship behavior of male rats (*Rattus norvegicus*). *Behaviour* 44:264–285.

Milner, B., Petrides, M., and Smith, M. L. (1985). Frontal lobes and the temporal organization of memory. *Human Neurobiology* 4:137–142.

Mishkin, M., and Appenzeller, T. (1987). The anatomy of memory. *Scientific American* 256:80–89.

Mogensen, J., and Divac, I. (1984). Sequential behavior after modified prefrontal lesions in the rat. *Physiological Psychology* 12:41–44.

Mora, F., Sweeney, K. F., Rolls, E. T., and Sanguinetti, A. M. (1976). Spontaneous firing rate of neurones in the prefrontal cortex of the rat: Evidence for a dopaminergic inhibition. *Brain Research* 116:516–522.

Neafsey, E. J. (In press). Prefrontal cortical control of the autonomic nervous system: Anatomical and physiological observations. *Progress in Brain Research.*

Nonneman, A. J., Voigt, J., and Kolb, B. (1974). Comparisons of behavioral effects of hippocampal and prefrontal cortex lesions in the rat. *Journal of Comparative and Physiological Psychology* 87:249–260.

Numan, R., and Grant, K. A. (1980). Lateral, but not medial, frontal lesions impair fixed ratio performance in rats. *Physiology and Behavior* 24:625–627.

O'Keefe, J., and Nadel, L. (1978). *The Hippocampus as a Cognitive Map.* New York: Oxford University Press.

Olton, D. S. (1989). Frontal cortex, timing and memory. *Neuropsychologia* 27:121–130.

Peterson, S. L. (1986). Prefrontal cortex neuron activity during discriminative conditioning paradigm in unanesthetized rats. *International Journal of Neuroscience* 29:245–254.

Robertson, A., Laferriere, A., and Milner, P. M. (1986). The role of corticocortical projections in self-stimulation of the prelimbic and sulcal prefrontal cortex in rats. *Behavioural Brain Research* 21:129–142.

Robinson, R. G., and Coyle, J. T. (1980). The differential effect of right versus left hemispheric cerebral infarction on catecholamines and behavior in the rat. *Brain Research* 188:63–67.

Robinson, T. E., Becker, J. B., Moore, C. J., Castaneda, E., and Mittleman, G. (1985). Enduring enhancement in frontal cortex dopamine utilization in an animal model of amphetamine psychosis. *Brain Research* 343:374–377.

Rolls, E. T., and Cooper, S. J. (1974). Anesthetization and stimulation of the sulcal prefrontal cortex and brain-stimulation reward. *Physiology and Behavior* 12:563–571.

Rolls, E. T., and Cooper, S. J. (1973). Activation of neurones in the prefrontal cortex by brain stimulation reward in the rat. *Brain Research* 60:351–368.

Rose, J. E., and Woolsey, C. N. (1948). The orbitofrontal cortex and its connections with the mediodorsal nucleus in rabbit, sheep and cat. *Research Publications of the Association of Nervous and Mental Disease* 27:210–232.

Roydes, R. L. (1970). Frontal lesions impair habituation of the headshake response in rats. *Physiology and Behavior* 5:1133–1137.

Ruggiero, D. A., Mraovitch, S., Granata, A. R., Anwar, M., and Reis, D. J. (1987). A role of insular cortex in cardiovascular function. *Journal of Comparative Neurology* 257:189–207.

Sakurai, Y., and Sugimoto, S. (1986). Multiple unit activity of prefrontal cortex and dorsomedial thalamus during delayed go/no-go alternation in the rat. *Behavioural Brain Research* 20:295–301.

Satoh, K., and Fibiger, H. C. (1986). Cholinergic neurons of the laterodorsal tegmental nucleus: efferent and afferent connections. *Journal of Comparative Neurology* 253:277–302.

Sinnamon, H. M., and Galer, B. S. (1984). Head movements elicited by electrical stimulation of the anteromedial cortex of the rat. *Physiology and Behavior* 33:185–190.

Stamm, J. S. (1955). The function of the median cerebral cortex in maternal behavior of rats. *Journal of Comparative and Physiological Psychology* 48:347–356.

Stern, W. C., Pugh, W. W., and Morgane, P. J. (1985). Single unit activity in frontal cortex and caudate nucleus of young and old rats. *Neurobiology of Aging* 6:245–248.

Stern, W. C., Pugh, W. W., Resnick, O., and Morgane, P. J. (1984). Developmental protein malnutrition in the rat: Effects on single-unit activity in the frontal cortex. *Brain Research* 306:227–234.

Sullivan, R. M., and Henke, P. G. (1986). The anterior midline cortex and adaptation to stress ulcers in rats. *Brain Research Bulletin* 17:493–496.

Sutherland, R. J. (1985). The navigating hippocampus: An individual medley of space, memory and movement. In G. Bujzsaki and C. H. Vanderwolf (eds.), *Electrical Activity of the Archicortex*. Budapest: Hungarian Academy of Sciences.

Sutherland, R. J., and Arnold, K. (1987). Temporally graded loss of place memory after hippocampal damage. *Neuroscience* 22:S175.

Swanson, L. W. (1981). A direct projection from Ammon's horn to prefrontal cortex in the rat. *Brain Research* 217:150–154.

Terreberry, R. R., and Neafsey, E. J. (1987). The rat medial frontal cortex projects directly to autonomic regions of the brainstem. *Brain Research Bulletin* 19:639–649.

Theirry, A. M., Blanc, G., Sobel, A., Stinus, L., and Glowinski, J. (1973). Dopaminergic terminals in the rat cortex. *Science* 182:499–501.

Thierry, A. M., Tassin, J. P., Blanc, A., and Glowinski, J. (1976). Selective activation of the mesocortical DA system by stress. *Nature* 263:242–244.

Thomas, R. K., and Weir, V. K. (1975). The effects of lesions in the frontal or posterior association cortex of rats on maze III. *Physiological Psychology* 3:210–214.

van der Kooy, D., Koda, L. Y., McGinty, J. F., Gerfen, C. R., and Bloom, F. E. (1984). The organization of projections from the cortex, amygdala, and hypothalamus to the nucleus of the solitary tract in rat. *Journal of Comparative Neurology* 224:1–24.

van Eden, C. G., and Uylings, H. B. M. (1985). Cytoarchitectonic development of the prefrontal cortex in the rat. *Journal of Comparative Neurology* 241:253–267.

van Eden, C. G., Uylings, H. B. M., and van Pelt, J. (1984). Sex-difference and left-right asymmetries in the prefrontal cortex during postnatal development in the rat. *Developmental Brain Research* 12:146–153.

van Haaren, F., de Bruin, J. P. C., Heinsbroek, R. P. W., and van de Poll, N. E. (1985). Delayed spatial response alternation: Effects of delay-interval duration and lesions of the medial prefrontal cortex on response accuracy of male and female Wistar rats. *Behavioural Brain Research* 18:41–49.

Vargo, J. M., Corwin, J. V., King, V., and Reep, R. L. (1988). Hemispheric asymmetry in neglect produced by unilateral lesions of dorsomedial prefrontal cortex in rats. *Experimental Neurology* 102:199–209.

Veening, J. G., Cornelissen, F. M., and Lieven, P. A. J. M. (1980). The topical organization of the afferents to the caudatoputamen of the rat. A horseradish peroxidase study. *Neuroscience* 5:1253–1268.

Wikmark, R. G. E., Divac, I., and Weiss, R. (1973). Delayed alternation in rats with lesions of the frontal lobes: implications for a comparative neuropsychology of the prefrontal system. *Brain, Behaviour, and Evolution* 8:329–339.

Wilcott, R. C. (1981). Medial and orbital cortex and the suppression of behavior in the rat. *Physiology and Behavior* 27:237–241.

Wilsoncroft, W. E. (1963). Effects of medial cortex lesions on the maternal behavior of the rat. *Psychological Reports* 13:835–838.

19 Posterior Parietal and Temporal Association Cortex

Bryan Kolb

The purpose of this chapter is to review the evidence regarding the presence, structure, organization, and function of the posterior associative neocortex of the rat. It begins with a discussion of the anatomical organization of the posterior parietal region, a consideration of the limited literature on the effects of selective lesions, and then reviews the literature with respect to the temporal cortex. The chapter is brief, which is largely because of the limited work on the posterior association cortex of rats. Indeed there is a striking contrast in the extent of work on the visual, somatosensory, and motor cortex of the rat and the posterior association cortex of the rat.

19.1 Identifying the Posterior Parietal Cortex

There are three principal ways that one could try to identify a posterior parietal region: (1) cytoarchitecture and myeloarchitecture, (2) thalamocortical connections, and (3) cortico-cortical connections.

Cyto- and Myeloarchitecture

Krieg (1946) identified three regions between the somatosensory cortex and the visual cortex, which he labeled areas 7, 39, and 40. Krieg characterized this cortex as being significantly thinner than the somatosensory cortex (Par1) as layers II and III become thin and closely packed and layer IV is reduced relative to the parietal cortex anterior to it, but still can be seen as a separate layer. Myeloarchitectonically Krieg's area 7 has noticeably fewer fibers than the primary somatosensory cortex has, and at the boundary to Krieg's area 18b, there are no virtually no fibers visible, especially in the upper layers.

One question about the identification of the posterior parietal cortex (PPC) of the rat arises from Zilles's atlas of the rat cortex. Zilles does not show any difference between the putative PPC of Krieg and his areas Oc2M and Oc2L, although he does concede the possibility that a separate PPC may be distinguishable (see chapter 4 by Zilles). In my own material I too find it very difficult to see a change in Nissl-stained material, but the myelin material does appear to agree with Krieg, at least with respect to what he calls area 7. There is a region from about −4 mm to −6 mm from the bregma in which the myelin is reduced from somatosensory cortex and heavier than in most of area Oc2M. (For the remainder of this chapter, I call this area of intermediate myelin the posterior parietal cortex, or PPC.) Similarly there appears to be a reduction in acetylcholinesterase staining of layer IV in the PPC before increasing again in Oc2M. Perhaps results from other stains, especially immunohistochemical stains, will clarify this question.

Finally, one interesting aspect of this PPC area is that it would appear to overlap with a region that has a retinotopic map (area AM of Olavarria and Monterro 1981) as well as connections with the superior colliculus (Espinoza and Thomas 1983, Olavarria and van Sluyters 1982).

Thalamo-cortical Connections

The lateral posterior nucleus (LP), which is probably the rodent analog of the posterior complex of the primate (Jones 1985), projects to a wide region of neocortex including Oc1, Oc2M, and Oc2L (e.g., chapter 12 by Dean), which includes PPC, as well as projecting to the medial part of MD-projection cortex (Divac et al. 1978), corresponding to Zilles Cg1, Cg2, and Cg3. This overlapping projection with MD-projection cortex resembles the projection from the pulvinar to the prefrontal cortex of the monkey, giving further credence to the parallel between the PPC of the rat and the PPC of the monkey. Furthermore the extensive projections of the LP with the prefrontal cortex, PPC, visual areas, and the posterior cingulate cortex are consistent with the idea that the LP/pulvinar complex may be central to a network of connections that link many structures in the analysis of visuospatial information (Goldman-Rakic 1987).

One difficulty with the thalamocortical definition of PPC in the rat is that its LP projects to such a wide area of cortex, including both peristriate areas Oc2M and Oc2L. There needs to be a careful study of the LP projections to see if there are subdivisions within this nucleus with regard to posterior cortical projections, as well as with frontal projections. One might predict that if the LP projection to frontal cortex is analogous to the pulvinar projection in the monkey, then there would be a discrete region projecting to PPC and prefrontal cortex, and this region should be dissociable from that projecting to Oc1 and Oc2L.

Cortico-cortical Connections

Before considering the cortico-cortical connections of the putative PPC cortex, it is necessary to consider what pattern of connections might be taken as being analogous to that of the primate. To simplify this problem, I have drawn a hypothetical map of cortico-cortical connections in the putative protypical mammal (figure 19.1A). In this schema there are two major interconnected association regions—the prefrontal and posterior parietal cortices—both of which receive "sensory" inputs. Figure

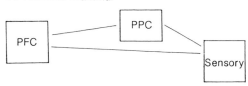

A. Primitive mammal

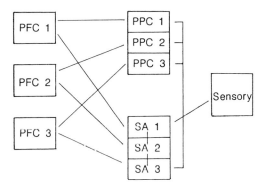

B. Advanced mammal

Figure 19.1 (A) Hypothetical general pattern of long cortico-cortical connections from the primary sensory regions to the prefrontal cortex (defined as MD-projection cortex) and the posterior parietal cortex in a simple mammalian brain. (B) Hypothetical pattern of long cortico-cortical connections from the primary sensory to the sensory association, prefrontal, and posterior parietal regions in an advanced mammalian brain.

19.1B illustrates an elaboration of this basic plan in which it is further hypothesized that as the sensory areas develop in mammalian evolution, both the posterior parietal and prefrontal regions correspondingly expand. Thus the size of both of the association zones is directly related to the development of the secondary sensory zones. Presumably as new sensory abilities develop in the expanding sensory association regions, there is a corresponding increase in the extent of associated prefrontal and posterior parietal areas, with which they are connected (for an elaboration of this idea, see Petrides and Pandya 1988).

If we now apply the general plan of cortical connectivity to the cortex of the rat, it is possible to identify a parallel pattern of cortico-cortical connectivity, which is summarized in figure 19.2. The tissue between Par1 and Oc1 receives projections from Oc2L, Oc2M, Oc1, Te1, and Par1, and it subsequently sends projections to most regions of prefrontal cortex (e.g., Miller and Vogt 1984, Torrealba, Olavarria, and Carrasco 1984, Olavarria and Montero 1984, Kolb and Walkey 1987). This pattern of connections is similar in general plan to that of the monkey, but still there are some identifiable differences. For example, there are direct projections from auditory and somatosensory areas in the rat rather than having projections from a series of secondary sensory areas into

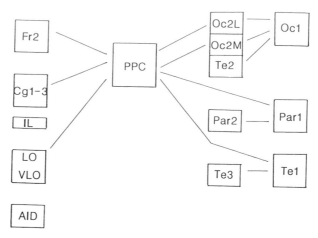

Figure 19.2 Long cortico-cortical connections of the primary and secondary sensory regions to the putative posterior parietal cortex (PPC) in the rat. (See chapter 4 by Zilles for abbreviations.)

the PPC. This parallels the difference in perirhinal connections in the two species as the perirhinal region receives direct primary sensory projections in the rat (Deacon et al. 1983), but in the monkey the connections are exclusively from secondary sensory cortex (Pandya and Yeterian 1985). It is difficult to guess what the more direct sensory projections to association areas might imply about the PPC. It may reflect the less advanced development of secondary sensory areas in the rat, which has a pattern of cortico-cortical connections that is more like the primitive type illustrated in figure 19.1. In any event there appears to be a region of posterior cortex that receives inputs from visual, auditory, and somatosensory regions and that has reciprocal connections with the prefrontal cortex.

A final feature of cortical connectivity, which is not shown in the figures, is the relationship between PPC and the cingulate cortex. There is a large projection from both the PFC and the PPC to cingulate cortex of the monkey, and this is also true of the rat (Vogt 1985).

In summary, on the basis of various anatomical criteria, it can be argued that there is an area in the rat cortex that lies in the cortex between Zilles's Par1 and Oc1 is an analog of the posterior parietal cortex of the monkey.

Effects of Lesions to the PPC
There are relatively few studies that have been designed specifically to study the effects of PPC lesions in rats and the review of this literature is necessarily limited (but see also Thompson et al. 1986). It should also be noted parenthetically that at least part of the PPC is often removed to produce a "lesion control" group in studies of hippocampal function, so a review of this literature might be helpful.

Rats with PPC lesions have been studied on three basic types of tasks: (1) visual discriminations, (2) conditional visual-somatic associations, and (3) spatial mazes (table 19.1).

Visual Discrimination Tests Overall the behavioral data show that rats with PPC generally do not have deficits on tests of either simple or complex visual discriminations, although some studies have found mild deficits in complex visual discrimination tasks. Even in these studies, however, the animals have been able to acquire the discriminations, there are simply slower than normal animals. Furthermore, in a study by Kolb, Buhrman, and McDonald (1989), rats with PPC lesions performed as well as controls on a visual matching to sample task (Aggleton 1985) in which the animals were exposed to one visual stimulus (e.g., stripes) and were then presented with the same stimulus and a novel stimulus (e.g., dots). The animals' task was to choose the novel stimulus and even when a 20-s delay was imposed between the initial stimulus and the subsequent choice, the animals performed as well as control animals (figure 19.3). This task is typically referred to as a delayed nonmatching to sample task.

Somatic-Visual Conditional Task In contrast to the performance on visual discrimination tests, rats with PPC lesions are impaired on a task in which they must learn to match a tactile cue (roughness of the floor) with a visual cue. Thus a smooth floor is associated with reward at one visual stimulus, whereas a rougher floor is associated with reward at another. Rats with PPC lesions performed poorly at this task, and several animals could not acquire the task. Rats with lesions in Oc1, Oc2L, or Te1 were unimpaired at the task. This task is intriguing because the PPC receives both visual and somatic inputs (see above), and both visual and somatic evoked potentials have been recorded from the same PPC sites in mice (Wagner, Mangini, and Pearlman 1980). The PPC therefore may function to associate stimuli from at least somatic and visual modalities, as has been suggested for the primate (see Kolb and Whishaw 1990, ch. 17, for a review).

Visual-Spatial Tasks Rats with PPC lesions have been tested on a wide range of maze tests, and they appear to be impaired at virtually every type of maze test normally given to rats (table 19.1). The deficits vary considerably in severity, with the largest deficits on tests such as the Hebb-Williams and Lashley III mazes. The overall conclusion from all of the maze studies must be that the PPC plays some role in visual navigation in rats. This is important because perhaps the most striking behavioral effect of PPC lesions in both human and nonhuman primates is the impairment in visuospatial abilities (e.g., Kolb and Whishaw 1990). Mishkin and his colleagues have argued that the visual system has two major outflows: one to the PPC carrying spatial data and one

Table 19.1 Summary of the Effects of Lesions of the PPC of Rats

Behavior	Status	Reference
Visual learning		
1. Black/white discrimination	OK	Boyd and Thomas 1977
	X	McDaniel and Wall 1988
Black/white reversal	OK	Boyd and Thomas 1977
2. Pattern discrimination	OK	McDaniel and Braucht 1984
		McDaniel and Wall 1988
		McDaniel et al. 1979
		Kolb et al. 1989
	X	Boyd and Thomas 1977
		McDaniel and Wall 1988
3. Swim to black platform	OK	Kolb and Walkey 1987
Cross modal learning		
1. Visual/somatic association	X	Pinto-Hamuy et al. 1987
Spatial learning		
1. Lashley III maze	X	Thomas and Weir 1975
2. Hebb-Willams maze	X	Boyd and Thomas 1977
3. Spatial reversals	X	McDaniel and Thomas 1978
		Kolb et al. 1983
4. Morris water maze	X	Kolb et al. 1983, 1987
		Kolb and Whishaw 1985
		Kolb and Walkey 1987
		DiMattia and Kesner 1988a,b
5. Place learning set	X	Whishaw 1987
6. Radial arm maze	X	Kolb et al. 1983
		Kolb and Whishaw 1985
7. Landmark task	X	Kolb and Walkey 1987
8. Spatial list learning	X	DiMattia and Kesner 1988a,b
		Kametani and Kesner 1989

X = significant impairment; OK = impairment.

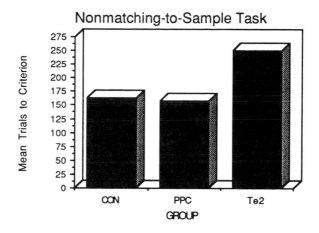

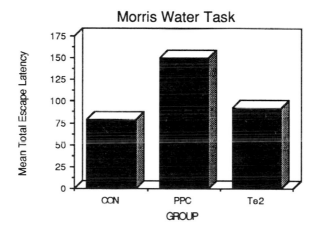

Figure 19.3 Summary of the performance normal (CON), posterior parietal (PPC), and Te2-ablated rats on the Morris water maze and a nonmatching to sample task. The PPC rats are impaired at the former task, and the Te2 rats are impaired at the latter task.

Kolb: Posterior Parietal and Temporal Association Cortex

to the inferotemporal cortex carrying data pertaining to object recognition (e.g., Mishkin and Ungerleider 1982). The data from PPC lesions in rats imply that the visuospatial route through the parietal cortex may be found generally in mammals.

The evidence of spatial navigation deficits in rats with PPC lesions is consistent with observations by McNaughton and his colleagues, who have found cells in PPC that could be involved in spatial representation (Chen and McNaughton 1988, McNaughton, Green and Mizumori 1986). In these studies most of the cells they recorded fired during a particular state of motion (e.g., left turn, right turn) or in response to visual stimulation (e.g., light one), but a small number of visually sensitive cells showed location selectivity reminiscent of hippocampal place cells. That is, the cells fired only when the animal was in a particular location in the visual world.

Finally, it is worth noting here that Kesner has suggested that the PPC of rats might function in forming a memory store for spatial location (Kesner 1989, Kametani and Kesner 1989). This is an interesting idea, but Kesner has yet not presented compelling data in support of his case, in large part because his rats' lesions are not confined to the PPC, and he finds his largest effects when the lesions include large areas of primary somatosensory cortex (Par1). Nevertheless, although Kesner's hypothesis can be seen as only tentative, it is consistent with the general role of the PPC in spatial guidance outlined in this chapter.

The nature of the spatial impairment in rats with PPC lesions remains controversial. Although rats with PPC lesions are impaired at spatial learning tasks, they are not as impaired as are rats with hippocampal, prefrontal, or posterior cingulate lesions (e.g., Sutherland, Whishaw, and Kolb 1988). The spatial navigation behavior of rats with PPC lesions is consistent in one aspect, however: the animals are always poor at their trajectories to places, and even with extended training or pretraining this deficit persists. The most likely explanation of this deficit appears to be one of a deficit in perceiving the spatial relations between objects, such that the animals do not orient themselves accurately with respect to spatial information. Normal animals may be able to look around in space and to determine, on the basis of only a few cues, the spatial location of a target. In contrast rats with PPC lesions are poor at orienting to these cues and thus cannot perceive the spatial relations between objects. This deficit is reminiscent of similar deficits in humans and nonhuman primates (for a review, see Kolb and Whishaw 1990, ch. 23). The posterior parietal deficit is likely dissociable from frontal or hippocampal deficits in that there is no additional memory deficit after PPC lesions, whereas there may be after prefrontal or hippocampal lesions. Hence animals with PPC lesions perform normally on tests such as delayed nonmatching to sample, whereas animals with hippocampal or prefrontal lesions do not (e.g., Kolb et al. 1989).

One puzzling aspect of spatial orientation deficits in different species is that the deficits observed in humans appear to be far greater than those seen in either monkeys or rats because there is no compelling evidence in nonhumans for a topographic agnosia similar to that found in humans with large parietal lesions. This difference is curious because nonhuman species often appear to have spatial orientation skills that are superior to those of humans! One possibility for this apparent difference may be that comparable functions have not been studied in humans and nonhumans. Another is that the larger posterior parietal region of humans has developed an ability to perform more cognitive spatial functions (such as spatial rotations), and it is the loss of this ability that humans find so debilitating.

19.2 Identifying the Temporal Association Cortex

There is a zone in the lateral posterior cortex of the rat (Krieg's area 36, Zilles's area Te2) that has some resemblance to inferotemporal cortex of the monkey. This region receives projections from LP (Mason and Gross 1981) as well as from visual cortical areas Oc1, Oc2L, and Oc2M (Miller and Vogt 1984). Finally, it projects to the perirhinal region (Deacon et al. 1983) and receives projections from the entorhinal cortex (Kosel et al. 1982). These connections are similar to those of the monkey (e.g., Pandya and Yeterian 1985), with the exception of the direct projection from Oc1.

Effects of Lesions to Te2

There appears to be only two studies in which the effects of selective lesions restricted to Te2 have been examined. In the first, Williams and colleagues (1986) found that rats with Te2 lesions were mildly impaired at the postoperative retention of a visual pattern discrimination, but not in the retention of a spatial alternation task. In the second study, Kolb, Buhrman, and McDonald (1989) found that rats with Te2 lesions were completely unable to learn a visual matching to sample task, even with no delay (figure 19.3), although they were able to acquire a simple horizontal/vertical stripes discrimination. The same animals were subsequently able to learn a spatial navigation task (Morris water maze) as quickly as were controls. Thus, on the basis of these studies, rats with area Te2 lesions appear to have a deficit in learning complex visual discriminations, but are not impaired at learning two forms of visual spatial tests or at learning simple discriminations.

The results of these two experiments lead to two conclusions: First, the temporal cortex of the rat probably has some function in the discrimination of complex visual information, such as would be required in object discrimination. This function is reminiscent of the effects of inferotemporal lesions in monkeys. Second, the contrast between the performance of rats with PPC lesions and Te2 lesions on tests of visual discrimination learning and spatial learning is striking and suggests two distinct visual processing routes in the rat: one for spatial guidance and one for the kind of visual analysis required for object recognition. This distinction is precisely what Mishkin and Ungerleider (1982) proposed for the monkey. Should future studies with the rat support this hypothesis, it would imply that Mishkin's two cortical visual systems may be a basic feature of cortical organization in mammals.

19.3 Conclusions

In summary, the posterior cortex of the rat may exemplify a basic form of mammalian neocortical organization in which there are two dissociable regions of association cortex that are analogs of the posterior parietal and inferotemporal cortex of nonhuman primates. There is reason to believe that the PPC region of the rat is involved in visual spatial guidance and cross-modality matching and that it is functionally related to the prefrontal cortex. In contrast the temporal cortex appears to be involved in visual object recognition.

The identification of a PPC that appears to be involved in visuospatial guidance may prove particularly useful because rats have excellent spatial skills and are well suited to studies in which they must move around in space. This contrasts with primates that are large and not easily studied in tasks in which they must move about in the world. Dean points out (chapter 12) that the tectocortical visual system in the rat is likely to be more important relative to the geniculostriate system, which presumably feeds into the temporal association cortex. This may well be true, especially in view of the relatively modest acuity of the rat, and the absence of color perception. Nonetheless the temporal association region is large in the rat, especially relative to the PPC, and should be suitable for considerably more study than there has been to date.

References

Aggleton, J. (1985). One trial object recognition by rats. *Quarterly Journal of Experimental Psychology* 37B:279–294.

Boyd, M. G., and Thomas, R. K. (1977). Posterior association cortex lesions in rats: Mazes, pattern discrimination, and reversal learning. *Physiological Psychology* 5:455–461.

Chen, L. L., and McNaughton, B. L. (1988). Spatially selective discharge of vision and movement modulated posterior parietal neurons in the rat. *Society for Neuroscience Abstracts* 14:818.

Deacon, T. W., Eichenbaum, H., Rosenberg, P., and Eckmann, K. W. (1983). Afferent connections of the perirhinal cortex in the rat. *The Journal of Comparative Neurology* 220:168–190.

DiMattia, B. V., and Kesner, R. P. (1988a). Role of the posterior parietal association cortex in the processing of spatial event information. *Behavioral Neuroscience* 102:397–403.

DiMattia, B. V., and Kesner, R. P. (1988b). Spatial cognitive maps: Differential role of parietal cortex and hippocampal formation. *Behavioral Neuroscience* 102:471–480.

Divac, I., Kosmal, A., Bjorklund, A., and Lindvall, O. (1978). Subcortical projections to the prefrontal cortex in the rat as revealed by the horseradish peroxidase technique. *Neuroscience* 3:785–796.

Espinoza, S. G., and Thomas, H. C. (1983). Retinotopic organization of striate and extrastriate visual cortex in the hooded rat. *Brain Research* 272:137–144.

Goldman-Rakic, P. S. (1987). Circuitry of primate prefrontal cortex and regulation of behavior by representational memory. *Handbook of Physiology: The Nervous System V.* Washington: American Physiological Society, pp. 373–417.

Jones, E. G. (1985). *The Thalamus.* New York: Plenum.

Kametani, H., and Kesner, R. P. (1989). Retrospective and prospective coding of information: Dissociation of parietal cortex and hippocampal formation. *Behavioral Neuroscience* 103:84–89.

Kesner, R. P. (1989). Retrospective and prospective coding of information: Role of the medial prefrontal cortex. *Experimental Brain Research* 74:163–167.

Kolb, B., Buhrman, K., and McDonald, R. (1989). Dissociation of prefrontal, posterior parietal, and temporal cortical regions to spatial navigation and recognition memory in the rat. *Society for Neuroscience Abstracts* 15:607.

Kolb, B., Holmes, C., and Whishaw, I. Q. (1987). Recovery from early cortical lesions in rats. III. Neonatal removal of posterior parietal cortex has greater behavioral and anatomical effects than similar removals in adulthood. *Behavioral Brain Research* 26:119–137.

Kolb, B., Sutherland, R. J., and Whishaw, I. Q. (1983). A comparison of the contributions of the frontal and parietal association cortex to spatial localization in rats. *Behavioral Neuroscience* 97:13–27.

Kolb, B., and Walkey, J. (1987). Behavioural and anatomical studies of the posterior parietal cortex in the rat. *Behavioural Brain Research* 23:127–145.

Kolb, B., and Whishaw, I. Q. (1985). Earlier is not always better: Behavioral dysfunction and abnormal cerebral morphogenesis following neonatal cortical lesions in the rat. *Behavioural Brain Research* 17:25–43.

Kolb, B., and Whishaw, I. Q. (1990). *Fundamentals of Human Neuropsychology.* 3rd ed. New York: Freeman & Co.

Kosel, K. C., van Hoesen, G. W., and Rosene, D. L. (1982). Non-hippocampal cortical projections from the entorhinal cortex in the rat and rhesus monkey. *Brain Research* 244:201–213.

Krieg, W. J. S. (1946). Connections of the cerebral cortex. *Journal of Comparative Neurology* 84:277–321.

Mason, R., and Gross, G. A. (1981). Cortico-recipient and tecto-recipient visual zones in the rat's lateral posterior (pulvinar) nucleus: an anatomical study. *Neuroscience Letters* 25:107–112.

McDaniel, W. F., and Braucht, G. S. (1984). Pattern discrimination acquisition and performance following regionally limited posterior neocortical ablations. *IRCS Medical Science* 12:1086–1087.

McDaniel, W. F., and Thomas, R. K. (1978). Temporal and parietal association cortex lesions and spatial and black-white reversal learning in the rat. *Physiological Psychology* 6:300–305.

McDaniel, W. F., Wildman, L. D., and Spears, R. H. (1979). Posterior association cortex and visual pattern discrimination in the rat. *Physiological Psychology* 7:241–244.

McDaniel, W. F., and Wall, T. T. (1988). Visuospatial functions in the rat following injuries to striate, peristriate, and parietal neocortical sites. *Psychobiology* 16:251–260.

McNaughton, B. L., Green E. J., and Mizumori, S. J. Y. (1986). Representation of body-motion trajectory by rat sensory-motor cortex neurons. *Society for Neuroscience Abstracts* 12:260.

Miller, M. W., and Vogt, B. A. (1984). Direct connections of rat visual cortex with sensory, motor, and association cortices. *The Journal of Comparative Neurology* 226:184–202.

Mishkin, M., and Ungerleider, L. (1982). Contributions of striate inputs to the visuospatial functions of parieto-preocciptal cortex in monkeys. *Behavioural Brain Research* 6:57–77.

Olavarria, J., and Montero, V. M. (1981). Reciprocal connections between the striate cortex and extrastriate cortical visual areas in the rat. *Brain Research* 217:358–363.

Olavarria, J., and Montero, V. M. (1984). Relation of callosal and striate-extrastriate cortical connections in the rat: morphological definition of extrastriate visual areas. *Experimental Brain Research* 54:240–252.

Olavarria, J., and van Sluyters, R. C. (1982). The projection from striate and extrastriate cortical areas to the superior colliculus in the rat. *Brain Research* 242:332–336.

Pandya, D., and Yeterian, E. H. (1985). Architecture and connections of cortical association areas. In A. Peters and E. G. Jones (eds.), *Cerebral Cortex, 4: Association and Auditory Cortices*, pp. 3–61. New York: Plenum.

Petrides, M., and Pandya, D. N. (1988). Association fiber pathways to the frontal cortex from the superior temporal region in the rhesus monkey. *Journal of Comparative Neurology* 273:52–66.

Pinto-Hamuy, T., Olavarria, J., Guic-Robles, E., et al. (1987). Rats with lesions in anteromedial extrastriate cortex fail to learn a visuosomatic conditional response. *Behavioural Brain Research* 25:221–231.

Reep, R. L., Corwin, J. V., Hashimoto, A., and Watson, R. T. (1984). Afferent connections of medial precentral cortex in the rat. *Neuroscience Letters* 44:247–252.

Sutherland, R. J., Whishaw, I. Q., and Kolb, B. (1988). Contributions of cingulate cortex to two forms of spatial learning and memory. *Journal of Neuroscience* 8:1863–1872.

Thomas, P. K., and Weir, V. R. (1975). The effects of lesions in the frontal or posterior association cortex of rats on maze III. *Physiological Psychology* 3:210–214.

Thompson, R., Huestis, P. W., Crinella, F. M., and Yu, J. (1986). The neuroanatomy of mental retardation in the white rat. *Neuroscience and Biobehavioral Reviews* 10:317–338.

Torrealba, F., Oavarria, J., and Carrasco, M. A. (1984). Cortical connections of the anteromeidal extrastriate visual cortex in the rat. *Experimental Brain Research* 56:543–549.

Vogt, B. A. (1985). Cingulate cortex. In A. Peters and E. G. Jones (eds.), *Cerebral Cortex, 4: Association and Auditory Cortices*, pp. 89–149. New York: Plenum.

Vogt, B. A., and Miller, M. W. (1983). Cortical connections between rat cingulate cortex and visual, motor, and postsubicular cortices. *The Journal of Comparative Neurology* 216:192–210.

Wagner, E., Mangini, N. J., and Pearlman, A. L. (1980). Retinotopic organization of striate and extrastriate visual cortex in the mouse. *Journal of Comparative Neurology* 193:187–202.

Whishaw, I. Q. (1987). Hippocampal, granule cell and CA3-4 lesions impair formation of a place learning-set in the rat and induce reflex epilepsy. *Behavioural Brain Research* 24:59–72.

Williams, G., Mogensen, J., Lindvall, O., Bjorklund, A., and Divac, I. (1986). *Behavioral and Biochemical Evidence for a Visual Association Cortical Area in the Rat*. Paper presented at the EBBS meeting, Marseille.

VI Plasticity

20   Plasticity and Change

Richard C. Tees

Plasticity is a term with a long history. In current usage plasticity can refer to virtually any form of change in the nervous system or behavior ranging from changes in axon spouting after peripheral lesions to experience-dependent information storage. Lund (1978) reminded us that "predictability" of the brain's form and its connections is identified as *neural specificity*; exceptions to this predictable pattern in particular circumstances represent *neural plasticity*. It is good to keep in mind that these terms are simply descriptive and not explanatory with respect to any phenomena, and often their use is affected by and bound to the techniques used to demonstrate their existence.

The purpose of the next five chapters is to outline what degree of plasticity there is in specific circumstances with respect to important brain-behavior relationships involving the rat's cortex. It is clear from these as well as earlier chapters that there seems to be a common mammalian response to environmental enrichment and deprivation, transplant, lesions, etc. Two prime questions addressed are: What role does experience or function play in defining and establishing a particular set of interconnected cortical neurons and related behavioral competence(s)? and How stable are the neuronal patterns in adult intact or brain-damaged animals? It is interesting to remember that, although the notion that function required to *maintain* the integrity of the immature system is fairly well documented and accepted, possible *inductive* or *facilitative* roles for experience before complete neural maturation or later have not been appreciated until recently.

Perhaps the most dramatic and explicit statement of the predetermined point of view concerning the nonparticipation of behavior and stimulation history in the maturation of the nervous system is the following:

The architecture of the nervous system and the concomitant behavior patterns result from self-generating growth and maturation processes that are determined entirely by inherited, intrinsic factors, to exclusion of functional adjustment, exercise, or anything else akin to learning. (Hamburger 1962)

Equally extreme and farfetched statements have been made by supporters on the other side of the theoretical fence:

John Locke's doctrine of the tabula rasa rests on solid embryological as well as psychological grounds. If [the nervous system] allows afferent impulses to diffuse or spread so widely that the possibility is open for any sensory organ to acquire functional connections with any muscle. (Holt 1931)

In introducing changes that take place when the cortex is damaged in rodents, Kolb (chapter 23) attempts to distinguish between the behavioral changes that follow cortical injury, which he refers to as *recovery* or *sparing of function,* and the changes in anatomy and physiology of the remaining brain, which he calls *plasticity.* Although I think it is important to distinguish between recovery and sparing of function, let me raise a somewhat different issue of concern about the term plasticity itself, which could be viewed as misleading. In conventional speech, when we think of something as plastic, we think of it as being molded into virtually any new configuration, which then would remain stable until some further modifying event occurred. There are examples (particularly from the controlled rearing literature) that would suggest that a return to a normal state after a period of abnormal experiential input is a more probable event in the remolding process. An alternative to the term plasticity that Aslin (1981) has offered is the term *elasticity,* which also implies modifiability but with the additional property of a potential return to the previous state. Perhaps it is easier with the term elasticity to keep in mind the assumption that there may well be a genetically specified range of acceptable environmental inputs that fulfill certain basic requirements for influencing the developing organism. For instance, Aslin's own unified model reiterated the concept of a sensitive period that embodies both a delimited age range of enhanced sensitivity to experiential inputs and a *selectivity* for those inputs that can modify the brain and competence during this age range. Singer (e.g., 1986) has emphasized modification rules that not only include the activation of postsynaptic cells as a necessary prerequisite for the induction of the experience-dependent modification (and, obviously, sensory input), but also the operation of several independent gating systems that reflect the central state of the system. In simple terms Singer is making the point that rats need to be aroused or to pay attention to potentially influential signals and probably use them in the control of their behavior if such stimuli are to have a sizable impact on the development of cortical functions. (We have referred to the necessity of "behavioral demand" of any environmental exposure in chapter 22.) Endogenous and exogenous agents of arousal may be thought of as "enabling stimuli" that facilitate the emergence of enduring effects of the stimuli that accompany them (Rauschecker and Marler 1987). In reading these five chapters, you will be able to see the authors coming to grips with what the "rules" are.

In the first chapter Janice Juraska reviews the information that exposure to different environments alters synaptogenesis in respect of several cortical areas. Cortical areas (particularly Oc1) show increases in thickness with complex rearing and decreases with sensory deprivation. Complex rearing leaves animals with more synapses, more dendrites, and more spines in comparison with animals reared under isolated or restricted conditions. These changes seemed to correlate reasonably well with changes or differences in certain behavioral competences, particularly those related to spatial ability. In addition Juraska's review provides important new information that there are in fact sex differences in response to environmental conditions. That is to say, the changes in synapses per neuron seem to be differentially affected in male and female rats reared under complex environmental conditions.

Chapter 22 by Tees outlines another proposition—that some abilities are more or less affected by controlled rearing (both restricted and complex). Those competences most affected by controlled rearing seem to reflect the operation of areas of cortex beyond primary projection areas. It is made clear that the impact of experience (as reflected in the outcome of controlled rearing) appears to be much more diffused than that observed with specific cortical lesions (see part II). In the case of certain competences, the impact is less than that produced by specific cortical lesions, and in other cases it is greater. The point is that it is different. Two notions are contrasted about the impact of manipulations of stimulation history utilizing a modular approach to analysis of the evidence. Some modules may be more affected than others by manipulations of experience. Those modules apparently involve competences whose operations require more information and integration, are more influenced by both global and selective attentional processes, and seen to be more vulnerable to changes than early stimulation history. An alternative view holds that controlled rearing affects every operation somewhat equally. The more operations there are, the more modules are required to perform a task successfully and the greater is the impact of controlled rearing. Thus the small but real effects on the rat's ability to resolve details, to orient, and to remember produce cumulative and sizable effects on those cortically dependent behaviors that rely on many of these operations.

The next three chapters in this part focus on savings and recovery after traumatic brain damage. Although these reviews again illustrate that brain lesions and sensory deprivation have very different outcomes, there is a way of linking the evidence provided by research in the two areas. One can argue that the reorganizational changes sometimes found after brain damage represent the continuation or acceleration of developmental neuronal growth processes. Historically researchers interested in recovery were concerned only with whether it took place or not. Then it appeared that recovery may be more likely to emerge under certain conditions. Investigators then examined the issue of how observed recovery might be mediated, focusing on reactive synaptogenesis, the rerouting of axons, and the failure of axons to retract on schedule.

Finger and Almli (1985) have argued that the idea that dynamic neuronal events of any sort have become an established part of the gene pool because they are able to serve as recovery or healing mechanisms makes little sense. In any event, although axon growth and synaptogenesis may be more apparent early in life, it is not restricted to early developmental time periods, as was previously thought. The evidence for continuous synaptic modification and turnover has achieved considerable acceptance (e.g., Greenough 1986). If circuit changes observed in response to neural injury are really developmental growth processes, it might be expected that each of these processes might be more "operational" and extensive when injuries are sustained during periods of relatively rapid brain growth and development. To some extent the literature that Kolb outlines supports this expectation. Kolb's studies examining behavioral recovery after lesions at ten days of age (vs. earlier or later) make it clear that the growth of dendrites and synapses in the remaining cortex is closely related to any evidence of saving or recovery. The hypothesis that neural changes associated with cortical injury are fundamentally related to normal developmental growth mechanisms requires that two associated issues be considered: first, how these might be triggered on injury, and second, if they are triggered, whether these reactive events are random or regulated processes. As Castro makes evident in chapter 24, these processes do follow a set of developmental rules. Normal unilateral corticotectal projections are "replaced" by bilateral projections in response to neonatal removal of contralateral cortex in the rat. Bilateral retinotectal inputs in the rat that represent an earlier stage of development can be maintained later in life by damaging the projections from one eye before they would normally retract.

If injury-induced neural organization is regulated within developmental constraints, it is not difficult to understand why it may lead to recovery, neurological dysfunction, or perhaps little noticeable behavior outcome under different injury conditions. An examination of the research literatures (e.g., Kolb, Castro, and Dunnett—chapters 23, 24, and 25, respectively) documents the fact that the association between these reorganizational events and the recovery of functions is inconsistent. The contribution of these developmental growth processes to recovery must be inconsistent because the growth processes are occurring against the backdrop of a damaged brain and thus may make connections different from those ordinarily seen. The processes are coming out of order with any kind of program for normal development. This may make it easier to understand why lesions at day 1 or day 2 may have more serious (and different) consequences than those occurring at day 10 in the life of the rodent.

Other observations in Dunnett's chapter make it evident that although cortical graft tissue may come to form connections with host brain, those connections do not necessarily underlie the functional recovery that is observed. Rather the rapid emergence of behavioral changes indicates that the graft stimulates or secretes neurotrophic factors that promote functional recovery in the host brain. This suggests that a similar pattern of recovery would be induced by the implantation of astrocytes or adult tissue grafts predominantly comprised of glia. Dunnett also makes clear that functional deficits over and above those induced by the lesions may well be observed once the embryonic grafts have established connections. Although the work to date cannot resolve why these impairments occur, it does underline the fact that the presence of these events (grafts) and developmentally triggered growth processes by then can have deleterious effects. Castro's chapter focuses on unilateral lesions involving the sensorimotor cortex of the newborn rat, and it is clear that one ends up with a widespan "remodeling" or reorganization of several cortical projections that originate from the opposite unablated hemisphere. In general the evidence suggests that the lesion-induced, cortical efferent plasticity observed represents a less dense but topographical mirror image of the normal projections and reflects normal growth of axons in the areas deprived of their normal afferent inputs. In many cases these projections demonstrate topographical distributions comparable to normal pathways and from synaptic contacts that appear to be functional physiologically.

In Kolb's chapter there is an outline of factors that influence recovery or sparing, as well as anatomical and physiological plasticity. Factors such as age of lesion and differences between kind or size of lesion all have an influence on the outcome. For example, with respect to location, Whishaw and Kolb (chapters 10 and 23, respectively) reported that rats with extensive preoperative training in reaching tasks showed complete recovery after adult motor cortex lesions, whereas the impact of pre- or postoperative training on recovery from primary sensory lesions (e.g., Tees 1975) is clearly very much different.

Interestingly Kolb attempts to list and describe the characteristics of postlesion outcomes relating to plasticity, recovery, and sparing in much the same way that Tees (chapter 22) attempts to list outcomes relating to the impact of controlled rearing.

Kolb also makes the case very persuasively that it is extremely important to collect information about brain and behavior relations at several levels of analysis, including behavioral. As far as behavioral evidence is concerned, several observations from all of the chapters need to be underlined. One is the importance of a broad and judicial choice of a battery of behavioral tests. Clearly, with respect to the emerging impact of controlled rearing or lesions, the ideal design involves the administration of a battery of tests to subjects with different lesions and/or with different (complex vs. restricted) stimulation histories. To make statements regarding the specificity of brain and behavior relations, one needs to be sure that different manipulations produced nonglobal impairments or changes. There is another aspect to choosing behavioral tasks, which has to do with the value of choosing several measures of what you believe to be a specific competence. As Kolb and his coworkers found out, in examining the impact of neonatal parietal and frontal lesions on spatial behavior in rats, the utilization of three different behavioral tests (Morris water maze, radial arm maze, and spatial reversal task) yielded a very much more complex picture of both the function of different cortical areas well as the extent of recovery after early lesions. One point touched on by Kolb's chapter and several others is the distinction between efficiency in solving a given task or problem and the heuristics involved. For instance, it is clear that blind complex-reared rodents are more effective spatially on certain tests than blind normally reared subjects, who in turn are more effective in some instances than blind restrictively reared rodents. What do these differences in efficiency reflect? For instance, if dark-reared blind animals are using a movement-based or body-centered coding system to solve spatial problems, they are likely to be more error prone than if they used geometric heuristics in such problems. Errors are not necessary consequences of strategy; it is possible to reach correct solutions in spatial tasks using body-centered spatial strategies, and in fact blind dark-reared animals can and do solve spatial problems. Clearly it is very important to use different kinds of tests of spatial ability to try to zero in on whether different animals recovering from specific lesions or controlled rearing are in fact using different strategies.

One final observation about behavioral testing has to do with whether the test is a sensitive measure of the particular kind of behavior being tested, that is to say, whether we are testing at the limits of a normal animal's ability. Paradiso (1988) has indicated that the "performance" of networks of cells depends to a great extent on the number of cells used in the network. For example, although the orientation tuning properties of cortical neurons change little with decreasing contrast, they do, however, reduce the number of responsive cells and a proportion of cells activated in the intact network by a stimulus such as an oriented line. In a large network this reduction may have little effect because the number of cells activated would still be very large. If for some reason, however, the number of cells available in the network is already reduced because of impact for restrictive controlled rearing or lesion, the number of cells activated by a visual stimulus (e.g., a geometric pattern at low contrast or presented in noise) may fall into a range where this is very critical for discrimination. Consequently, significant changes in discriminative performance would be observed by such "sensitive" tests, and our conclusions about recovery or savings would be altered.

References

Aslin, R. N. (1981). Experiential influences and sensitive periods in perceptual development: A unified model. In R. N. Aslin, J. R. Alberts, and M. R. Peterson (eds.), *Development of perception: Vol. 2. The visual system* (pp. 45–110). New York: Academic Press.

Finger, S., and Almli, C. R. (1985). Brain damage and neuroplasticity: Mechanisms of recovery or development? *Brain Research Reviews* 10:177–186.

Greenough, W. T. (1986). What's special about development? Thoughts on the bases of experience-sensitive synaptic plasticity. In W. T. Greenough and J. M. Juraska (eds.), *Developmental neuropsychobiology* (pp. 387–407). Orlando, FL: Academic Press.

Hamburger, V. (1962). Ontogeny of behaviour and its structural basis. In D. Richter (ed.), *Comparative neurochemistry* (pp. 21–43). Oxford: Pergamon.

Holt, E. B. (1931). *Animal drive and the learning process.* New York: Holt.

Lund, R. D. (1978). *Development and plasticity of the brain.* New York: Oxford University Press.

Singer, W. (1986). Neural activity as a shaping factor in postnatal development of visual cortex. In W. T. Greenough and J. M. Juraska (eds.), *Developmental neuropsychobiology* (pp. 271–293). Orlando, FL: Academic Press.

Paradiso, M. A. (1988). A theory for the use of visual orientation information which exploits the columnar structure of striate cortex. *Biological Cybernetics* 58:35–49.

Rauschecker, J. P., and Marler, P. (1987). Cortical plasticity and imprinting: Behavioral and physiological contrasts and parallels. In J. P. Rauschecker and P. Marler (eds.), *Imprinting and cortical plasticity: Comparative aspects of sensitive periods* (Vol. 1, pp. 349–366). New York: Wiley.

Tees, R. C. (1975). The effects of neonatal striate lesions and visual experience on form discrimination in the rat. *Canadian Journal of Psychology* 29:66–85.

21 The Structure of the Rat Cerebral Cortex: Effects of Gender and the Environment

Janice M. Juraska

Reports of a clearly discernible sex difference in the midsagittal size of the human corpus callosum have generated considerable interest (de Lacoste-Utamsing and Holloway 1982, Holloway and de Lacoste 1986), and a large number of studies have attempted to confirm the finding of a larger splenium in females. To date, published reports by other investigators have not been successful (Bell and Variend 1985, Bleier et al. 1986, Clarke et al. 1989, Demeter et al. 1988, Kertesz et al. 1987, Weber and Weis 1986, Witelson 1985) in detecting such a sex difference, but some investigators have noted the considerable variability in the size and shape of the human corpus callosum (Bleier et al. 1986, Weber and Weis 1986). It would be difficult to disentangle all of the factors that could contribute to variability in the gross size of the human corpus callosum, but it is not surprising that the cortical anatomy of the human is variable. Even in the rat (a species with a "simpler" cortex that most would agree could be less plastic in response to the environment than the human cortex), the anatomy of the cerebral cortex varies not only with gender but also with the complexity of the rearing environment. Both gender and environmentally induced alterations in cortical structure in the rat are examined here. The literature on the effects of environmental stimulation on the cortex has been reviewed many times (e.g., Greenough 1976, Rosenzweig and Bennett 1978, Renner and Rosenzweig 1987, Greenough and Chang 1988), and this chapter summarizes only selected findings. The indications that the effects of gender and the environment interact have implications beyond the cortex of the rat, and they are also discussed in this review.

21.1 Environmental Plasticity

Differential Environments

Hebb (1947) initiated examination of the effects of the environment on ability by testing rats raised in his home. He reported that this experience increased the learning ability of these rats relative to laboratory-reared rats. This led to work, first by Hebb's students, and later by others on the behavioral effects of stimulating laboratory environments.

The vast majority of studies have indicated that rats from a stimulating environment outperformed less stimulated rats on tasks such as mazes (Forgays and Forgays 1952, Hymovitch 1952, Brown 1968, Greenough et al. 1972, Juraska et al. 1984), discrimination reversals (Krech et al. 1962), and sequential alternations (Nyman 1967). One interesting note is that rats from a more stimulating environment appear to be quite flexible in their choice of cues for solving a task. For example, it has been demonstrated through maze rotation that the superiority of more stimulated rats on the Hebb-Williams maze is a result of their use of cues from outside the maze (Forgays and Forgays 1952, Hymovitch 1952, Brown 1968). One might assume that most of the maze superiority of stimulated rats stems from the use of distal, spatial cues. In contrast, we have found that in the seventeen-arm radial maze, the more stimulated rats were more likely to use a nonspatial strategy, visiting each adjacent arm in turn, than were rats reared in isolation (Juraska et al. 1984). Thus a stimulating environment affects more than spatial abilities. Easier tasks, such as simple visual discriminations, often do not result in differences, possibly because of floor effects (Krech et al. 1962, Nyman 1967). (Related behavioral effects of early visual deprivation are reviewed by Tees in chapter 22.) Despite the behavioral differences that were beginning to be documented during the 1950s, no one suspected that the brain would show observable changes following exposure to stimulating environments.

A group at Berkeley (i.e., Rosenzweig et al. 1962) standardized the environments with the enriched condition (EC) consisting of a large cage that housed a group of rats and a changing set of objects or toys. The effects of that environment were compared with those engendered by a social condition (SC), in which several rats were simply housed together, or an impoverished condition (IC), in which rats were housed alone. The terms *enriched* and *impoverished* have more recently given way in many laboratories to the more neutral terms *complex* and *isolated*. Although the effects of the extreme environments EC and IC are more commonly compared, when an SC environment has been included in an investigation, the behavioral and neural effects of SC are found to be intermediate to those of EC and IC conditions. In any event the EC-IC differences are the primary focus of this review.

The Berkeley group discovered that the cortices of EC rats weighed more and were thicker than those of IC rats (Rosenzweig et al. 1962). The occipital area showed the largest and most consistent differences regardless of the age at which the differential environments were first introduced and of the length of exposure to the environments. Virtually all of these studies involve only male rats; the few exceptions are discussed later.) Recently the list of differences has been augmented by reports of a greater splenial area of the corpus callosum in EC than IC rats of both sexes (Juraska and Kopcik 1988). The splenium carries axons from neurons of the occipital and temporal cortex. One question that could be posed is why is it that the occipital cortex is the most influenced by these environments. It would seem that many of the tasks at which EC rats show considerable superiority—for example, mazes, reversals—are sensitive to hippocampal function (O'Keefe and Nadel 1978).

There have been contradictory findings on the response of the hippocampus to the differential environments. One problem is that the measurement of the size of the hippocampus is not as readily accomplished as in the cortex because the hippocampus changes shape rapidly across successive tissue sections. The cell populations are also diverse (Green and Juraska 1985, Fitch et al. 1989), and this can confound the differences between groups. The bulk of the evidence indicates that hippocampal thickness (Diamond et al. 1976, Jones and Smith 1980) and the dendritic branching in the dentate gyrus and CA3 area (Juraska et al. 1985, Juraska et al. 1989) do not show major EC-IC differences (at least in the male rat).

Although considerable research effort has been directed toward understanding the cognitive map and spatial functions of the hippocampus, it is clear that the posterior cerebral cortex is also important for spatial competence, as reflected in performance on tasks such as mazes (see chapter 19 by Kolb). For example, selective lesions of the occipital cortex disrupt performance on the radial maze more than does blinding (Goodale and Dale 1981). In addition the EC-IC differences in the size of the occipital cortex have been found in both blinded rats (Krech et al. 1963) and in rats raised in these environments in the dark (Rosenzweig et al. 1969). Such findings make it clear that the occipital cortex is not simply an area involved in visual processing in the rat. This, along with its role in vision, helps to explain its plasticity in response to the differential environments.

The influence of the differential environments on the weight and thickness of the occipital cortex has been the impetus for finer examination of this area. The hope has been that the types of plasticity found in response to these very diverse environments would serve as a model for what could be found in more subtle manipulations (i.e., specific training paradigms). Table 21.1 lists the major cellular changes that underlie the size differences in the occipital cortex. The studies cited were not always the first to investigate a particular anatomical measure. Many of the older studies are inaccurate because they did not use stereological corrections for size differences in the structures measured. When a relatively thin section is made through a three-dimensional structure such as a cell body or synapse, larger structures are more likely to appear in more sections and thus inflate density counts. In other words, the density and size of any three-dimensional entity are confounded. There are mathematical corrections that can be made to separate size and density, although this becomes more technically dif-

Table 21.1 The Principal Cellular Differences in the Occipital Cortex between Rats Raised in Enriched Condition (EC) and Impoverished Condition (IC)

Cellular Variable	Environment	Reference
Neuron size	EC > IC	Diamond et al. 1967
Neuron density	IC > EC	Turner and Greenough 1985
Dendritic branching	EC > IC	Volkmar and Greenough 1972
Dendritic spine density	EC > IC	Globus et al. 1973
Number of unmyelinated axons in splenial corpus callosum	EC > IC	Juraska and Kopcik 1988
Size of unmyelinated axons in splenial corpus callosum	EC > IC	Juraska and Kopcik 1988
Number of synapses per neuron	EC > IC	Turner and Greenough 1983
Size of synaptic contact	EC > IC	West and Greenough 1972
Synaptic plate perforations	EC > IC	Greenough et al. 1978
Percentage of total tissue volume	EC > IC	Black et al 1987
Capillary vessels		
Astrocytic nuclei	EC > IC	Sirevaag and Greenough 1987
Oligodendrocytic nuclei	EC > IC	Sirevaag and Greenough 1987
Mitochondria	EC > IC	Sirevaag and Greenough 1987

ficult for highly irregular structures such as glial cell nuclei and capillaries (Weibel 1979). Only recently have stereological considerations and corrections been widely (but unfortunately not always) adopted.

As can be seen in table 21.1, the differential environments have profound effects on the structure of the cortex. It is clear that the number of synapses and the supporting metabolic systems show considerable plasticity. Most of the cellular changes are not restricted to a "critical period," as evidenced by the fact that rats first placed in the environments as adults also display EC-IC differences in dendritic length (Uylings et al. 1978, Juraska et al. 1980), in the number of synapses per neuron (Hwang and Greenough 1986), and in the amount of capillary vessels (Black et al. 1988). Although these studies indicate that an array of changes can occur in adult rats in response to the differential environments, the differences tend to be not as large as those found when the environments are imposed at weaning.

It should be noted that many of the same cellular indices in the occipital cortex that vary with the differential environments also are affected by visual deprivation (for reviews, see Globus 1975, Boothe et al. 1986). For example, monocular deprivation results in a thinner and more cell-dense cortex contralateral to the deprived eye (Fifkova and Hassler 1969), as well as fewer dendritic spines on pyramidal neurons in the deprived cortex (Fifkova 1968). Dark rearing also affects dendritic spine numbers (Valverde 1971) and the density of synapses per unit volume (Gabbott and Stewart 1987). Although there is evidence for a sensitive period for the effects of monocular deprivation on spine numbers (Rothblat and Schwartz 1979), many of the effects of dark rearing are *partially* reversible after early development. For example, some reversible effects occur in spine numbers (in mice) (Valverde 1971), the number of synapses, especially symmetrical synapses (Gabbott and Stewart 1987), and the number of glial cells (Gabbott et al. 1986). Clearly the cortex of the adult rat retains some plasticity in response to environmental conditions.

Training Paradigms

Given the magnitude and pervasiveness of the plasticity of the rat cortex to the differential environments, the question arose as to whether formal training in standard learning paradigms might produce observable cortical changes. The evidence is clear—it does. Extensive maze experience (30 days) increased both the weight of the whole and the occipital cortex in rats (Bennett et al. 1979). Training for 26 days in the Hebb-Williams maze also induced dendritic changes in the occipital cortex, although these changes did not involve the entire dendritic tree (as did the changes produced by differential environments) but rather were restricted to the apical branches (Greenough et al. 1979). Maze training provides several types of environmental stimulation (as does the complex environment), and it is difficult to determine whether particular neural changes are due to differences in learning per se. To try to examine this, Chang and Greenough (1982) cut the posterior corpus callosum and blocked vision in one eye with an opaque contact lens. This resulted in one visually "trained" and one "untrained" cortex within the same animal, whereas the effects of many other variables (e.g., motor movement, motivation, stress) were equivalent with respect to the two hemispheres. As was the case when both hemispheres were trained, the isolated trained hemisphere had greater branch length of apical oblique dendrites than the untrained. Although the specific influence of learning was not disentangled from visual stimulation, this experiment demonstrated that the neural changes found after maze training were not due to nonspecific metabolic or hormonal processes.

Surprisingly, the changes described above in the apical dendritic tree were evident in other training situations. Greenough and colleagues (1985) found that training rats to reach for food with either their preferred or nonpreferred paw resulted in a greater length of apical dendritic branches in the motor cortex opposite to the trained paw. There was some tendency for the rats using the nonpreferred paw to show larger training differences between the hemispheres than rats that used only their preferred paw in the task. However, the principal finding was that the use of the neurons opposite the trained paw, regardless of the paw's initial preferability, appeared to induce the apical dendritic differences.

None of these dendritic changes are thought to be the "engram" because many parts of the brain are undoubtedly involved in these tasks. They demonstrate that increases in dendrites are observable in association with learning in the cortex. This is compatible with the view that the anatomical plasticity following experience in the differential environments is also due to differential learning experience. At the very least, it is apparent that the structure of the cortex is plastic both during development and adulthood.

21.2 Sex Differences

Environmental rearing conditions and training are not the only factors that can influence the size and structure of the rat cerebral cortex. Gender also has an important influence on cortical structure in the rat, and it has not been as thoroughly explored.

Cortical Size

Pfaff (1966) published a short report in which he found that the cross-sectional area of several brain regions, including the neocortex, was larger in adult male rats. Because neither cell counts nor measures of nuclear size revealed any sex differences in the cortex, the basis for the size differences was unclear. In this brief report important details were not specified, including which areas of the cortex were examined. Virtually no additional work was done for years on this topic. In 1975 Gregory reported that male rats had larger layer V pyramidal neurons in the somatosensory cortex than did female rats. However, the rats were only thirty-six days old, so it was not clear whether the differences due to sex reflected differences in rate of maturation or adult differences in neuronal size that appear at a young age. Subsequently Yanai (1979), by measuring the cortex in one sagittal plane, confirmed the adult sex difference in overall cortical size and neuron size. He found that the packing density of cells in the female rat was higher, and thus the total number of cells was probably comparable for males and females. One problem with Yanai's study is that both the counts and size measurements probably included glial cells as well as neurons. (This was evident from the small cell diameters reported and the low magnification used for the counting of cells.) Together the studies by Pfaff and Yanai seemed to indicate that males have a thicker cortex than females. The basis for this was unclear: The cell size measurements were inconsistent, and in neither study had stereological techniques been used in making the cell counts.

One necessary step in understanding the basis for cortical sex differences is the delineation of the extent of the differences. Are there size differences in every cortical area and in every layer? Silvia Reid and I have started to address these questions. The overall thickness of the cortex has been measured in ten littermate pairs of socially housed male and female rats at 90 days of age. Five coronal planes of section have been examined that include all major cortical areas (i.e., frontal, parietal, temporal, occipital), and five thickness measurements have been taken at each plane (figure 21.1). Of the 25 measurements, 16 showed significant ($p < .05$) differences, with males having a thicker cortex than females. In fact in 24 of 25 measurements, the mean thickness of the male cortex exceeded that of the female, so it can be concluded that sex differences are pervasive in the thickness of the rat cortex. Preliminary measurements of cortical layers indicate that not all layers show significant dimorphism. In the parietal cortex (FL according to Zilles (1985)), the sex differences are centered in layer VI, the only layer that was significantly different in size (8.9 percent $p < .0001$). In contrast, in the binocular area of the occipital cortex (Oc1B) males had thicker layers II through III (8.0 percent, $p < .02$) and layer VI (6.6 percent, $p < .04$). Cortical thickness differences could of course indicate a difference in the shape of the cortex between the sexes. We found however, that both the length and width (measured at the widest point) of the cortex were significantly larger in males. This implies a sex difference in cortical volume.

The hormonal events that could be responsible for the size differences in the cortex also have not been thoroughly explored. Pfaff (1966) reported that the nuclear and nucleolar diameters of cortical neurons were altered by neonatal gonadectomy of males, but circulating steroids are known to influence these measures in the hypothalamus (Lisk and Newlon 1963, Ifft 1964). On the other hand Diamond and colleagues (1979) found that neonatal ovariectomy resulted in increased cortical thickness in adult females, whereas neonatal gonadectomy had no effect on the thickness of the cortex in males. These effects occurred, however, despite a lack of sex differences in cortical size (Diamond et al. 1979). This contrasts with Stewart and Kolb's (1988) findings that neonatal gonadectomy of male rats resulted in a thicker cortex overall, due to an increase in the size of the left side (see below), whereas in females neonatal ovariectomy did not alter cortical size.

Sex differences in parts of the nervous system associated with reproduction, such as the medial preoptic area and spinal nucleus of the bulbocavernosus, are almost entirely determined by developmental androgens (reviewed by Arnold and Gorski 1984). It is parsimonious to expect that similar hormonal influences occur in the cerebral cortex as well. In the rat brain, most sexual differentiation appears to be due to the aromatization of testosterone to estrogen (Goy and McEwen 1980). Estrogen receptors have been found in the developing cortex of the rat, but they disappear by adulthood (MacLusky et al. 1979, Sheridan 1979, Gerlach et al. 1983). More recently aromatizing enzyme has been found in the cortex (MacLusky et al. 1986), which indicates that developmental

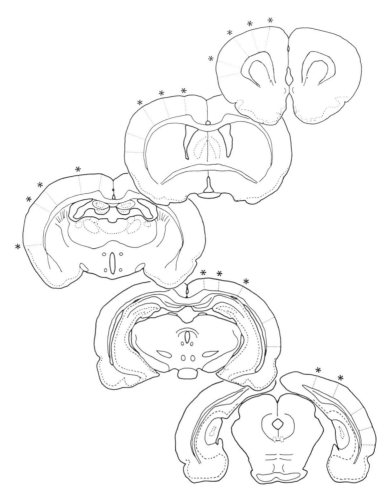

Figure 21.1 The five coronal section planes at which cortical thickness was measured. Dotted lines indicate the locations at which measurements were taken from both hemispheres. Asterisks mark the locations where significant differences ($p < .05$) in thickness were found between the sexes.

androgens can interact directly with cortical cells. Indirect effects of hormones through dimorphic afferents have not been directly demonstrated in the cortex (or any other brain area), but cannot be discounted. Also, less conventional hormonal influences could play a role. For example, the rat cerebral cortex contains progesterone receptors in both the neonate and adult (MacLusky and McEwen 1978, Kato and Onouchi 1981), and exposure to an excess of progesterone prenatally increases cortical dendritic branching (Menzies et al. 1982). Further exploration of the hormonal basis for the sexual differentiation of the cortex is clearly needed.

Model for Dyslexia?

Human males and females differ in the incidence of many disorders and diseases. It has been hypothesized that the presence of testosterone while the cortex is developing could render the male relatively more susceptible to cortical malformation (Geschwind and Behan 1982). One outcome of this susceptibility may be developmental dyslexia, a disorder that manifests itself in an impairment in learning to read despite adequate intelligence and opportunity. Males are much more prone to this disorder than are females (by three to ten times) (Maccoby and Jacklin 1974, Vellutino 1978), and consequently the elevated levels of testosterone during prenatal development in males are likely to play a role in the etiology of the syndrome. Geschwind and Behan (1982) have hypothesized that developmental testosterone could slow the development of the left hemisphere in human males, sometimes enough to interfere with the normal patterns of neuronal migration. This could result in the ectopias (neurons in the wrong location) that have been observed in the cortex of young dyslexics and are especially numerous in the left cortex (Kemper 1984, Sherman and Galaburda 1985). Thus testosterone could predispose the cortex to defects in neuronal migration. Why then wouldn't all males be dyslexic? One possibility is that a small subset of males experience developmental testosterone titers that are higher or more prolonged than average. This is difficult to test in humans. However, the rat provides an excellent model system to examine this possibility because much of its surge of developmental testosterone occurs postnatally and cortical neurons are still migrating during the first postnatal week of life (Raedler and Sievers 1975).

Jan Kim, Silvia Reid, and I have tested this hypothesis by assessing the disruption produced in the development of the rat cortex by the administration of testosterone proprionate (500 μg in oil) in a series of injections to intact male rat pups at 3, 5, and 7 days of age. (Male littermate controls were oil injected at the same ages.) The rats were killed at weaning age (25 days) because dyslexia is first detected before puberty in humans. To date, measurements of cortical thickness, layer thickness, and the proportion of layer thickness to overall cortical thickness have been made in area Fr1 (primary frontal cortex), Oc1M (monocular visual cortex), Oc1B (binocular visual cortex), and Te1 (primary auditory cortex) (6 to 9 animals per group). The excess testosterone had no discernable effects on these cortical measures. Similar to the adult study of sex differences described in the preceding section, there were no differences between the hemispheres nor interactions between hemisphere and hormonal condition. We also failed to find any obvious abnormalities such as ectopias in the males treated with excess testosterone. Thus testosterone given at this dosage and time schedule does not grossly disrupt cortical development. Of course more subtle effects of testosterone on the cellular level are still possible. Effects could also occur if testosterone were given on a different schedule. Still these results make it less likely that perturbations of testosterone in the developing rat can serve as a model for the etiology of cortical malformations apparently associated with dyslexia.

Asymmetries

Another form of sexual dimorphism in the rat cortex involves asymmetries. The right cortex of male rats has been reported to be thicker than the left, whereas no such asymmetry has been observed in the cortex of female rats (Diamond et al. 1981, Diamond et al. 1983, Stewart and Kolb 1988); similar findings have been documented in cortical volume (although the difference is quite small—1.5 percent difference between the hemispheres in males) (Sherman and Galaburda 1985). However, population asymmetries have not always been found in male rats (Galaburda et al. 1986). In one case both male and female rats have been reported to have a R > L asymmetry at 15 days of age (Kolb et al. 1982), although other investigators have observed sex differences in asymmetry that varied considerably at different ages (Van Eden et al. 1984).

We found almost no indications of consistent asymmetries in our measurement of cortical size. In both sexes the right hemisphere was significantly wider, but the left was significantly longer. Only 3 of the 25 thickness measurements showed a significant effect of hemisphere, and they were not all in the same direction. These differences are probably due to chance. In any event, the measurements of thickness showed no consistent direction due to hemisphere, nor were there any indications of interactions between sex and hemisphere.

Thus in our sample there were reliable sex differences in the thickness of the cortex, but little to indicate asymmetries in gross thickness or sex differences in such asymmetries. Other studies have demonstrated that prenatal stress to male rats results in a lack of cortical asymmetry as adults (Fleming et al. 1986, Stewart and Kolb 1988), which could be due to the decrease in testosterone secretion that accompanies such stress (Ward and Weisz 1980). Also Stewart and Kolb (1988) failed to find any sex differences in the thickness of the cortex of prenatally stressed rats of several strains including the same strain, Long-Evans, that we used.

Thus Stewart and Kolb found that prenatally stressed rats lacked cortical asymmetries and cortical sex differences. The rats we sampled were conceived and born in our departmental colony, and we have no reason to believe that they were stressed at any time. The sex differences in cortical thickness that we observed also make it unlikely that the lack of asymmetries in our study arose from early stress. The lack of asymmetries in cortical thickness do not, of course, preclude the possibility of asymmetries on a cellular level.

The hormonal basis of asymmetries has also been a source of some controversy. Diamond and colleagues (1981) found that neonatal ovariectomy of female rats resulted in the male pattern (R > L) of asymmetry in the occipital cortex. Neonatal gonadectomy of male rats had no effect. This is in contrast to the results of a study by Stewart and Kolb (1988), that neonatal gonadectomy of male, but not female, rats altered the sex-specific pattern of hemispheric asymmetries throughout the cortex.

Fine Structure

The cellular basis for the sexual dimorphism in cortical size (and when found, asymmetries) is unknown. Male rats have more neurons in other dimorphic areas of the CNS such as the sexually dimorphic nucleus of the POA and the spinal nucleus of bulbocavernosus (Arnold and Gorski 1984). Thus there is some reason to suspect that cortical sex differences could be due, in part, to differences in neuron number. The final story of what underlies the sex difference in cortical thickness is likely to be as complex as is the case for the thickness differences between the cortices of EC and IC rats.

In addition to neuron number, another characteristic that could account for the thickness difference between the sexes is the size and complexity of the dendritic tree. One problem is that, unlike neuron number, the dendritic tree can be altered by the environment (see table 21.1), at least in male rats. Would the dendritic fields of female rats be comparably affected by the differential environments? Would the relative differences between males and females be expanded or contracted by the environmental conditions? There have been indications that the sexes might show differences in plasticity to the differential environments. Diamond and colleagues (Diamond et al. 1971, Hamilton et al. 1977) examined cortical thickness in female rats housed in the differential environments from early adulthood (60 days). They found that there were significant differences in cortical thickness between females in EC and IC that were smaller in percentage terms than the differences in males. Unfortunately no statistical comparisons were made between the sexes, which makes drawing conclusions difficult.

I have investigated the possibility that there may be sex differences in the dendritic tree and that the environment may affect such differences. Three populations of neurons were examined from the occipital cortex (Oc1) of male and female rats raised in EC and IC from weaning to 55 days of age (Juraska 1984). Figure 21.2 illustrates the total dendritic length of these three neuronal populations. Layer V basilar (and apical) dendrites did not differ as a function of sex either in terms of environmental plasticity or in respect to comparisons within each environment. Layer IV stellate neurons showed sex differences both in plasticity (males had EC-IC dendritic differences) and within EC (males had more dendritic material than females). Similar to layer IV stellate neurons, layer III pyramidal neurons showed greater differences between the environments in males and sex differences in the EC rats (males > females). Thus the environment had a profound influence on the sex differences in dendritic branching. No sex differences were evident in rats from the IC environment, yet prominent sex differences were found in two out of three cell populations in the EC rats.

One might conclude from these data that male rats benefit more from the complex environment than do female rats, possibly because of a greater tendency to explore or play. There are two reasons why we do not believe that this is true: First, we have performed systematic observations of the social and object interactions performed by both sexes in the complex environment and found only few and very small sex differences (Juraska and Meyer 1986). Second, we have found that sex differences in dendritic branching in the hippocampal dentate gyrus and CA3 area often favor the females from the complex environments over their male littermates. In these studies we have also found that,

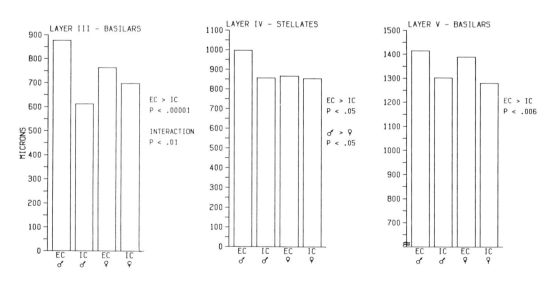

Figure 21.2 The total dendritic length for basilar dendrites of layer III pyramidal neurons, layer IV stellate dendrites and basilar dendrites of layer V pyramidal neurons. (From Juraska 1984. Used with permission from Elsevier.)

similar to the cortex, sex differences are more likely to exist or be larger in the hippocampus of EC than of IC rats (Juraska et al. 1985, 1989).

This startling phenomenon—that sex differences can vary with the environment—has implications beyond these particular environments. Any brain area that can be altered by environmental stimulation, learning, stress, and so on may also show sex differences that vary with the situation. One cannot draw conclusions about sex differences beyond the environmental conditions that were used. This is true even when no environmental manipulations are deliberately performed. Conversely the diverse environments in which, for example, humans live are likely to make sex differences more difficult to document. A neural sex difference present in one environment could be easily obscured by the variability in sex differences due to other environments. This increased variability would also make it more probable that spurious sex differences could be reported if the sample were small.

The controversy surrounding the report of sex differences in the size and shape of the human corpus callosum described at the beginning of this chapter spurred our interest in sex differences in the rat corpus callosum (Juraska and Kopcik 1988). We raised male and female rats in the differential environments from weaning to fifty-five days of age. Both the midsagittal size and underlying composition of the corpus callosum were examined. The midsagittal length of the corpus callosum was divided into thirds, and the area of each third was measured (see figure 21.3). No sex differences were found in the area of the splenium (posterior third) or in the other thirds. There was a large effect of environment in each third, with a significant interaction in the anterior two-thirds, which indicated that the corpus callosum of females had more plasticity in the nonsplenial areas.

There has been a report of a sex difference (male > female) in the size of the rat corpus callosum (Berrebi et al. 1988). The measurements were made 50 μm to 100 μm lateral to the midsagittal plane, which could indicate a sex difference in the splaying out of the pathway as it runs laterally. Also there were statistically significant interactions between sex and early handling for the majority of measures such that most of the sex differences appeared in the rats that had been handled during infancy. This study again illustrates that the environment can alter the size of the corpus callosum.

The lack of sex differences in the rat corpus callosum does not deal directly with the issue of whether there are sex differences in the splenial area of the corpus callosum of humans. The magnitude of the change in size in the rat corpus callosum following exposure to differential environments, however, casts a new light on the controversy in humans. Humans are raised in varied environments, and it would be logical to believe that the size of the corpus callosum is as plastic in humans as in rats. The environment could increase variability so that

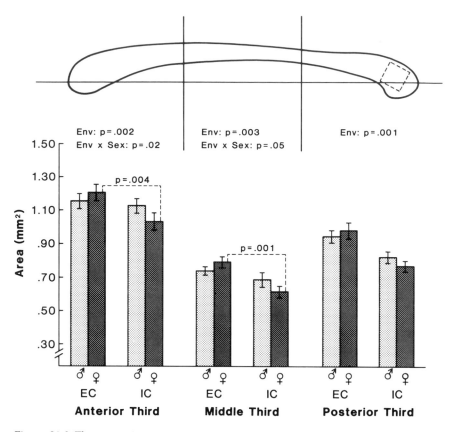

Figure 21.3 The gross size measurements of the midsagittal corpus callosum at 55 days of age. The upper portion of the figure illustrates the method for dividing the corpus callosum into thirds perpendicular to its longest axis, which is represented by the horizontal line. The dashed area indicates the sampling region for electron microscopy. The lower portion is a graph of the measurements of area (mm²) of each third (From Juraska and Kopcik 1988. Used with permission from Elsevier.)

sex differences could be obscured or could appear by chance if small numbers of subjects are examined. The search for human sex differences may need to take environmental conditions into account.

Despite the lack of sex differences in the size of the corpus callosum, it remained possible that the underlying axonal morphology could be dimorphic. We counted axons from electron micrographs taken in the splenium. Unmyelinated axons were more numerous in females from both environments (figure 21.4a), whereas myelinated axons were more numerous in females than males from EC (figure 21.4b). Because the small, unmyelinated axons outnumber the larger, myelinated fibers by ten to one, females from both environments have more axons than their male counterparts.

Males from EC, on the other hand, have larger axons than do females from EC (figure 21.5b). Both sexes from EC have larger and more unmyelinated axons in comparison with IC rats (figure 21.5a).

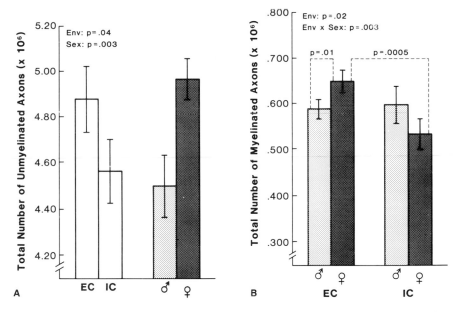

Figure 21.4 The total number of unmyelinated (A) and myelinated (B) axons in the posterior fifth of the corpus callosum. The group differences that contributed to the interaction between the sex and environment factors are indicated by dashed lines on graph B. (From Juraska and Kopcik 1988. Used with permission from Elsevier.)

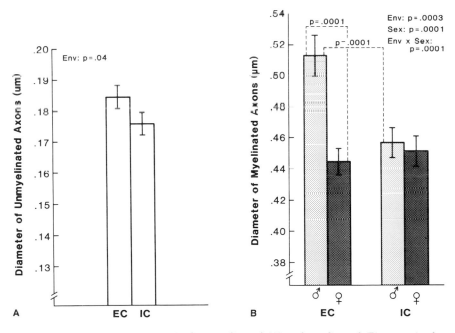

Figure 21.5 The diameter (in μm) of unmyelinated (A) and myelinated (B) axons in the splenium of the corpus callosum. The group differences that contributed to the interaction between the sex and environment factors are indicated by dashed lines on graph B. (From Juraska and Kopcik 1988. Used with permission from Elsevier.)

Juraska: Effects of Gender and Environment

Although changes in axon size could occur at any time in the lifespan, changes in axon number are less obvious. Axons first cross the midline at embryonic day 18 in the sensorimotor cortex, and the adult anterior-posterior length is achieved by the second postnatal week (Valentino and Jones 1982). It is generally believed that axons have finished crossing well before weaning (25 days). In addition to crossing, axons are also pruned during development, and the projecting neurons reach an adult distribution by postnatal day 15 (Olavarria and van Sluyters 1985). It is not known, however, when the pruning actually stops. Our data indicate that pruning is likely to occur after weaning and that it is influenced by both gender and rearing environment.

The dissociation between the size of the corpus callosum and the axonal sex differences points to the inadequacy of gross size as anything but a first measure. The underlying organizational differences are the essence of sex (and plasticity) effects. Although male rats have a larger cortex than females have, the cellular differences between the sexes are more complicated than the size difference indicates. We have only begun to explore these differences.

21.3 Conclusions

The list of cortical differences due to the differential environments appears to offer a coherent picture: increased cortical thickness, more dendrites, more synapses per neuron, and more capillaries all accompany exposure to more complex environments. Sex differences in the cortex have not been as well described, and the existing evidence suggests that the story may not turn out to be as simple. Certainly at this point we know too little to make generalizations about sex differences in a higher-order region of the brain such as the cortex.

To summarize what we do know about sex differences in the rat cortex: (1) the male cortex is larger than the female cortex, sometimes there is also asymmetry of cortical size in the male (R > L), but not in the female; (2) not every cortical layer contributes to the dimorphism in cortical size; (3) there are indications that males have somewhat larger neurons than females have, but it is unclear whether this is the rule or involves a more selective difference; (4) males can have larger dendritic trees than do females, but this varies with the environment and the neuronal population; (6) females have more axons in the splenium of the corpus callosum, whereas males tend toward larger axons. In sum the female rat cortex is not a miniature version of the male cortex, but rather is organized differently.

Acknowledgments

The unpublished work as supported by NSF BNS 8519681 and MH41728. I thank Silvia Reid for figure 21.1 and Jan Kim for comments on the manuscript.

References

Arnold, A. P., and Gorski, R. A. (1984). Gonadal steroid induction of structural sex differences in the central nervous system. *Annual Review of Neuroscience* 7:413–442.

Bell, A. D., and Variend, S. (1985). Failure to demonstrate sexual dimorphism of the corpus callosum in childhood. *Journal of Anatomy* 143:143–147.

Bennett, E. L., Rosenzweig, M. R., Morimoto, H., and Hebert, M. (1979). Maze training alters brain weights and cortical RNA/DNA ratios. *Behavioral and Neural Biology* 26:1–22.

Berrebi, A. S., Fitch, R. H., Ralphe, D. L., Denenberg, J. O., Friedrich, V. L., Jr., and Denenberg, V. H. (1988). Corpus callosum: region-specific effects of sex, early experience and age. *Brain Research* 438:216–224.

Black, J. E., Sirevaag, A. M., and Greenough, W. T. (1987). Complex experience promotes capillary formation in young rat visual cortex. *Neuroscience Letters* 83:351–355.

Black, J. E., Zelazny, A. M., and Greenough, W. T. (1988). Complex experience induces capillaries in visual cortex of adult rats. *Society for Neuroscience Abstracts* 14:1135.

Bleier, R., Houston, L., and Byne, W. (1986). Can the corpus callosum predict gender, age, handedness, or cognitive differences? *Trends in Neuroscience* 9:391–394.

Boothe, R. G., Vassdal, E., and Schneck, M. (1986). Experience and development in the visual system: anatomical studies. In W. T. Greenough and J. M. Juraska (eds.), *Developmental NeuroPsychobiology.* Orlando, FL: Academic Press, 296–315.

Brown, R. T. (1968). Early experience and problem-solving ability. *Journal of Comparative and Physiological Psychology* 65:433–440.

Chang, F.-L. F., and Greenough, W. T. (1982). Lateralized effects of monocular training on dendritic branching in adult split-brain rats. *Brain Research* 232:283–292.

Clarke, S., Kraftsik, R., van der Loos, H., and Innocenti, G. M. (1989). Forms and measures of adult and developing human corpus callosum: Is there sexual dimorphism? *Journal of Comparative Neurology* 280:213–230.

de Lacoste-Utamsing, C., and Holloway, R. L. (1982). Sexual dimorphism in the human corpus callosum, *Science* 216:1431–1432.

Demeter, S., Ringo, J. L., and Doty, R. W. (1988). Morphometric analysis of the human corpus callosum and anterior commissure. *Human Neurobiology* 6:219–226.

Diamond, M. C., Dowling, G. A., and Johnson, R. E. (1981). Morphologic cerebral cortical asymmetry in male and female rats. *Experimental Neurology* 71:261–268.

Diamond, M. C., Ingham, C. A., Johnson, R. E., Bennett, E. L., and Rosenzweig, M. R. (1976). Effects of environment of morphology of rat cerebral cortex and hippocampus. *Journal of Neurobiology* 7:75–85.

Diamond, M. C., Johnson, R. E., and Ehlert, J. (1979). A comparison of cortical thickness in male and female rats—normal and gonadectomized, young and adult. *Behavioral and Neural Biology* 26:485–491.

Diamond, M. C., Johnson, R. E., and Ingham, C. (1971). Brain plasticity induced by environment and pregnancy. *International Journal of Neuroscience* 2:171–178.

Diamond, M. C., Johnson, R. E., Young, D., and Singh, S. S. (1983). Age-related morphologic differences in the rat cerebral cortex and hippocampus: male-female, right-left. *Experimental Neurology* 81:1–13.

Diamond, M. C., Lindner, B., and Raymond, A. (1967). Extensive cortical depth measurements and neuron size increases in the cortex of environmentally enriched rats. *Journal of Comparative Neurology* 131:357–364.

Fifkova, E. (1968). Changes in the visual cortex of rats after unilateral deprivation. *Nature* 220:379–381.

Fifkova, E., and Hassler, R. (1969). Quantitative morphological changes in visual centers in rats after unilateral deprivation. *Journal of Comparative Neurology* 135:167–178.

Fitch, J. M., Juraska, J. M., and Washington, L. W. (1989). The dendritic morphology of pyramidal neurons in the rat hippocampal CA3 area. I. Cell types. *Brain Research* 479:105–114.

Fleming, D. E., Anderson, R. H., Rhees, R. W., Kinghorn, E., and Bakaitis, J. (1986). Effects of prenatal stress on sexually dimorphic asymmetries in the cerebral cortex of the male rat. *Brain Research Bulletin* 16:395–398.

Forgays, D. G., and Forgays, J. W. (1952). The nature of the effect of free-environmental experience in the rat. *Journal of Comparative and Physiological Psychology* 45:322–329.

Gabbott, P. L. A., and Stewart, M. G. (1987). Quantitative morphological effects of dark-rearing and light exposure on the synaptic connectivity of layer 4 in the rat visual cortex (area 17). *Experimental Brain Research* 68:103–114.

Gabbott, P. L. A., Stewart, M. G., and Rose, S. P. R. (1986). The quantitative effects of dark-rearing and light exposure on the laminar composition and depth distribution of neurons and glia in the visual cortex (area 17) of the rat. *Experimental Brain Research* 64:225–232.

Galaburda, A. M., Aboitiz, F., Rosen, G. D., and Sherman, G. F. (1986). Histological asymmetry in the primary visual cortex of the rat: Implications for mechanisms of cerebral asymmetry. *Cortex* 22:151–160.

Gerlach, J. L., McEwen, B. S., Toran-Allerand, C. D., and Friedman, W. J. (1983). Perinatal development of estrogen receptors in mouse brain assessed by radioautography, nuclear isolation, and receptor assay. *Developmental Brain Research* 11:7–18.

Geschwind, N., and Behan, P. (1982). Left-handedness: Association with immune disease, migraine and developmental learning disorder. *Proceedings of the National Academy* 79:5097–5100.

Globus, A. (1975). Brain morphology as a function of presynaptic morphology and activity. In A. H. Riesen (ed.), *The Developmental Neuropsychology of Sensory Deprivation*. New York: Academic Press, 9–91.

Globus, A., Rosenzweig, M. R., Bennett, E. L., and Diamond, M. C. (1973). Effects of differential experience on dendritic spine counts in rat cerebral cortex. *Journal of Comparative and Physiological Psychology* 82:175–181.

Goodale, M. A., and Dale, R. H. I. (1981). Radial-maze performance in the rat following lesions of posterior neocortex. *Behavioral Brain Research* 3:273–288.

Goy, R. W., and McEwen, B. S. (1980). *Sexual Differentiation of the Brain.* Cambridge, MA: MIT Press.

Green, E. J., and Juraska, J. M. (1985). The dendritic morphology of hippocampal dentate granule cells varies with their position in the granule cell layer: A quantitative Golgi study. *Experimental Brain Research* 59:582–586.

Greenough, W. T. (1976). Enduring brain effects of differential experience and training. In M. R. Rosenzweig and E. L. Bennett (eds.), *Neural Mechanisms of Learning and Memory.* Cambridge, MA: MIT Press, 255–278.

Greenough, W. T., and Chang, F.-L. F. (1988). Plasticity of synapse structure and pattern in the cerebral cortex. In A. Peters and E. G. Jones (eds.), *Cerebral Cortex, Vol. 7.* New York: Plenum, 391–440.

Greenough, W. T., Juraska, J. M., and Volkmar, F. R. (1979). Maze training effects on dendritic branching in occipital cortex of adult rats. *Behavioral and Neural Biology* 26:287–297.

Greenough, W. T., Larson, J. R., and Withers, G. S. (1985). Effects of unilateral and bilateral training in a reaching task on dendritic branching of neurons in the rat motor-sensory forelimb cortex. *Behavioral and Neural Biology* 44:301–314.

Greenough, W. T., Madden, T. C., and Fleischmann, T. B. (1972). Effects of isolation, daily handling, and enriched rearing on maze learning. *Psychonomic Science* 27:279–280.

Greenough, W. T., West, R. W., and DeVoogd, T. J. (1978). Sub synaptic plate perfora tions: changes with age and experience in the rat. *Science* 202:1096–1098.

Gregory, E. (1975). Comparison of postnatal CNS development between male and female rats. *Brain Research* 99:152–156.

Hamilton, W. L., Diamond, M. C., Johnson, R. E., and Ingham, C. A. (1977). Effects of pregnancy and differential environments on rat cerebral cortical depth. *Behavioral Biology* 19:333–340.

Hebb, D. O. (1974). The effects of early experience on problem solving at maturity. *American Psychologist* 2:737–745.

Holloway, R. L., and de Lacoste, M. C. (1986). Sexual dimorphism in the human corpus callosum: an extension and replication study. *Human Neurobiology* 5:87–91.

Hwang, H. M., and Greenough, W. T. (1986). Spine formation and synaptogenesis in rat visual cortex: A series section developmental study. *Society for Neuroscience Abstracts* 10:579.

Hymovitch, B. (1952). The effects of experimental variations on problem solving the rat. *Journal of Comparative and Physiological Psychology* 45:313–321.

Ifft, J. D. (1964). The effect of endocrine gland extirpations on the size of nucleoli in rat hypothalamic neurons. *Anatomical Record* 202:88A.

Jones, D. G., and Smith, B. J. (1980). Morphological analysis of the hippocampus following differential rearing in environments of varying social and physical complexity. *Behavioral and Neural Biology* 30:135–147.

Juraska, J. M. (1984). Sex differences in dendritic response to differential experience in the rat visual cortex. *Brain Research* 295:27–34.

Juraska, J. M., Fitch, J., Henderson, C., and Rivers, N. (1985). Sex differences in the dendritic branching of dentate granule cells following differential experience. *Brain Research* 333:73–80.

Juraska, J. M., Fitch, J. M., and Washburne, D. L. (1989). The dendritic morphology of pyramidal neurons in the rat hippocampal CA3 area. II. Effects of gender and experience. *Brain Research* 79:115–121.

Juraska, J. M., Greenough, W. T., Elliott, C., Mack, K., and Berkowitz, R. (1980). Plasticity in adult rat visual cortex: An examination of several cell populations after differential experience. *Behavioral and Neural Biology* 29:157–167.

Juraska, J. M., Henderson, C., and Muller, J. (1984). Differential rearing experience, gender and radial maze performance. *Developmental Psychobiology* 17:209–215.

Juraska, J. M., and Kopcik, J. R. (1988). Sex and environmental influences on the size and ultrastructure of the rat corpus callosum. *Brain Research* 450:1–8.

Juraska, J. M., and Meyer, M. (1986). Behavioral interactions of postweaning male and female rats with a complex environment. *Developmental Psychobiology* 19:493–500.

Kato, J., and Onouchi, T. (1981). Progesterone receptors in the cerebral cortex of neonatal female rats. *Developmental Neuroscience* 4:427–432.

Kemper, T. L. (1984). Asymmetrical lesions in dyslexia. In N. Geschwind and A. M. Galaburda (eds.), *Cerebral Dominance. The Biological Foundations.* Cambridge, MA: Harvard University Press, 75–89.

Kertesz, A., Polk, M., Howell, J., and Black, S. E. (1987). Cerebral dominance, sex, and callosal size in MRI. *Neurology* 37:1385–1388.

Kolb, B., Sutherland, R. J., Nonneman, A. J., and Whishaw, I. Q. (1982). Asymmetry in the cerebral hemispheres of the rat, mouse, rabbit, and cat: The right hemisphere is larger. *Experimental Neurology* 78:348–359.

Krech, D., Rosenzweig, M. R., and Bennett, E. L. (1962). Relations between brain chemistry and problem-solving among rats raised in enriched and impoverished environments. *Journal of Comparative and Physiological Psychology* 55:801–807.

Krech, D., Rosenzweig, M. R., and Bennett, E. L. (1963). Effects of complex environment and blindness on rat brain. *Archives of Neurology* 8:403–412.

Lisk, R. D., and Newlon, M. (1963). Estradiol: Evidence for its direct effect on hypothalamic neurons. *Science* 139:223–224.

Maccoby, E. E., and Jacklin, C. N. (1974). *The Psychology of Sex Differences*. New York: Freeman.

MacLusky, N. J., Chaptal, C., and McEwen, B. S. (1979). The development of estrogen receptor systems in the rat brain and pituitary: postnatal development. *Brain Research* 178:143–160.

MacLusky, N. J., Clark, A. S., and Toran-Allerand, C. D. (1986). Aromatase activity in explant cultures of the developing mouse brain: Is the rodent cerebral cortex a target for locally-synthesized estrogen? *Society for Neuroscience Abstracts* 12:1217.

MacLusky, N. J., and McEwen, B. S. (1978). Oestrogen modulates progestin receptor concentrations in some rat brain regions but not in others. *Nature* 274:276–278.

Menzies, K. D., Drysdale, D. B., and Waite, P. M. E. (1982). Effects of prenatal progesterone on the development of pyramidal cells in rat cerebral cortex. *Experimental Neurology* 77:654–667.

Nyman, A. J. (1967). Problem solving in rats as a function of experience at different ages. *Journal of Genetic Psychology* 110:31–39.

O'Keefe, J., and Nadel, L. (1978). *The Hippocampus as a Cognitive Map*. Oxford: Clarendon Press.

Olavarria, J., and van Sluyters, R. C. (1985). Organization and postnatal development of callosal connection in the visual cortex of the rat. *Journal of Comparative Neurology* 239:1–26.

Pfaff, D. W. (1966). Morphological changes in the brains of adult male rats after neonatal castration. *Journal of Endocrinology* 36:415–416.

Raedler, A., and Sievers, J. (1975). The development of the visual system of the albino rat. *Advances in Anatomy, Embryology and Cell Biology* 50:fasc. 3.

Renner, M. J., and Rosenzweig, M. R. (1987). *Enriched and Impoverished Environments*. New York: Springer Verlag.

Rosenzweig, M. R., Krech, D., Bennett, E. L., and Diamond, M. (1962). Effects of environmental complexity and training on brain chemistry and anatomy: A replication and extension. *Journal of Comparative and Physiological Psychology* 55:429–437.

Rosenzweig, M. R., and Bennett, E. L. (1978). Experiential influences on brain anatomy and brain chemistry in rodents. In G. Gottlieb (ed.), *Studies on the Development of Behavior and the Nervous System*. New York: Academic Press, 289–387.

Rosenzweig, M. R., Bennett, E. L., Diamond, M. C., Wu, S.-Y., Slagle, R. W., and Saffran, E. (1969). Influences of environmental complexity and visual stimulation on development of occipital cortex in rat. *Brain Research* 14:427–445.

Rothblat, L. A., and Schwartz, M. L. (1979). The effect of monocular deprivation on dendritic spines in visual cortex of young and adult albino rats: evidence for a sensitive period. *Brain Research* 161:156–161.

Sheridan, P. J. (1979). Estrogen binding in the neonatal neocortex. *Brain Research* 178:201–206.

Sherman, G. F., and Galaburda, A. M. (1985). Asymmetries in anatomy and pathology in the rodent brain. In S. D. Glick (ed.), *Cerebral lateralization in nonhuman species.* New York: Academic Press, 89–107.

Sirevaag, A. M., and Greenough, W. T. (1987). Differential rearing effects on rat visual cortex synapses. III. Neuronal and glial nuclei, boutons, dendrites, and capillaries. *Brain Research* 424:320–332.

Stewart, J., and Kolb, B. (1988). The effects of neonatal gonadectomy and prenatal stress on cortical thickness and asymmetry in rats. *Behavioral and Neural Biology* 49:344–360.

Turner, A. M., and Greenough, W. T. (1983). Synapses per neuron and synaptic dimensions in occipital cortex of rats reared in complex, social, or isolation housing. *Acta Stereologica* 2 (supplement 1):239–244.

Turner, A. M., and Greenough, W. T. (1985). Differential rearing effects on rat visual cortex synapses. I. Synaptic and neuronal density and synapses per neuron. *Brain Research* 329:195–203.

Uylings, H. B. M., Kuypers, K., and Veltman, W. A. M. (1978). Environmental influences on neocortex in later life. *Progress in Brain Research* 48:261–274.

Valentino, K. L., and Jones, E. G. (1982). The early formation of the corpus callosum: a light and electron microscopic study in foetal and neonatal rats. *Journal of Neurocytology* 11:583–609.

Valverde, F. (1971). Rate and extent of recovery from dark rearing in the visual cortex of the mouse. *Brain Research* 33:1–11.

Van Eden, C. G., Uylings, H. B. M., and Van Pelt, J. (1984). Sex-difference and left-right asymmetries in the prefrontal cortex during postnatal development in the rat. *Developmental Brain Research* 12:146–153.

Vellutino, F. R. (1978). Toward an understanding of dyslexia: Psychological factors in specific reading disability. In A. L. Benton and D. Pearl (eds.), *Dyslexia—An Appraisal of Current Knowledge.* New York: Oxford University Press, 61–112.

Volkmar, F. R., and Greenough, W. T. (1972). Rearing complexity affects branching of dendrites in the visual cortex of the rat. *Science* 176:1445–1447.

Ward, I. L., and Weisz, J. (1980). Maternal stress alters plasma testosterone in fetal males. *Science* 207:328–329.

Weber, G., and Weis, S. (1986). Morphometric analysis of the human corpus callosum fails to reveal sex-related differences. *Journal für Hirnforschung* 27:237–240.

Weibel, E. R. (1979). *Stereological Methods, Vol. 1. Practical Methods for Biological Morphometry.* London: Academic Press.

West, R. W., and Greenough, W. T. (1972). Effect on environmental complexity on cortical synapses of rats. *Behavioral Biology* 7:279–284.

Witelson, S. F. (1985). The brain connection: the corpus callosum is larger in left-handers. *Science* 229:665–668.

Yanai, J. (1979). Delayed maturation of the male cerebral cortex in rats. *Acta Anatomica* 104:335–339.

Zilles, K. (1985). *The Cortex of the Rat: A Stereotaxic Atlas.* New York: Springer Verlag.

22 Experience, Perceptual Competences, and Rat Cortex

Richard C. Tees

22.1 Historical Perspective

In contemporary analysis the classic debate between nativist and empiricist points of view has become largely a matter of emphasis. There is little doubt that perceptual capacities that depend on the cortex are neither exclusively inherited nor acquired, and for the most part the task has become one of collecting relevant facts about specific competences (Tees 1976a, 1986). However, when Donald Hebb published his thesis research (1937a,b), the most influential idea about perceptual competences and their neural substrates was that they were largely inherited. Having tested rats raised from birth in the dark on visual tasks in which the stimulus targets differed in brightness, size, line orientation, or pattern, he concluded that the dark-reared (DR) rats' perception, in the absence of any prior experience, was "normal" because such animals had been able to learn each of these tasks. As he himself has pointed out (Hebb 1980), he failed to reflect on the fact that his DR rats, in acquiring the pattern discriminations, had taken six times as many trials as had the light-reared (LR) rats that Lashley (1930) had tested earlier on identical tasks. (His ability to publish this work despite his failure to test or report on performance of normally reared control animals is in itself interesting.) Later, in 1949, theorizing about perceptual development and its neural substrate, Hebb changed his views and provided an alternative not only to the nativist but also the empiricist position about perceptual capacities that depend on the cortex. As far as Hebb was concerned, mammals at birth inherited basic neurocircuitry underlying certain fundamental discriminative abilities (e.g., perception of figure from ground), whereas circuitry underlying others (e.g., perception of shape) required further elaboration, gradually emerging as a result of maturation as well as learning and experience.

At that time the use of controlled rearing emerged as the technique to help to try to expose the elements involved in the interaction between genetic and experiential factors. For instance, deprivation of sensory (e.g., visual) input from birth allowed one to investigate the competence of an older, motorically mature organism with a very limited stimulation history. Differences (or lack of differences) found in comparing a deprived animal's behavior with that of an animal reared under normal environmental conditions came to be used (rightly or wrongly) to establish the relative contribution normally played by experiential factors in the development of a specific discriminative behavior. With respect to perceptual abilities that could be measured shortly after birth, such techniques were easily adapted to help establish whether subsequent sensory experience played any role and, if so, what kind of role. Indeed experience can play very different roles in specific instances (see figure 22.1). For example, the experimental evidence may show that certain aspects *maintain* or sustain (figure 22.1F) an initially rudimentary ability. In other cases sensory experience appears to *facilitate* or sharpen an initially rudimentary perceptual ability (figure 22.1C). Changes in early stimulation history can also *induce* a qualitative and significant shift in the ontogeny of a certain aspect (figure 22.1B) of perceptual behavior (Gottlieb 1976; Tees 1976a). Although this "Gottliebian" framework for viewing experiential influences during development has added some degree of specificity to the interactional viewpoint by describing different types of developmental outcomes, there are additional matters to be dealt with beyond what initial competences are and the general role subsequent experience might play. For instance, issues regarding the timing, size, generality, and potential reversibility of any environmental influences observed in particular instances are also subjects for further analysis.

Inspecting the development of brain-behavior relations in conjunction with the controlled rearing paradigm has another important purpose. In looking at cortex and behavior during development, there are obviously vast numbers of neural and behavioral measures that change over time. Sometimes the relative independence of behavioral and neural variables can be revealed through subtle (or radical) manipulations of early stimulation history.

Since the early 1960s a great deal of evidence has been generated about the significant impact of stimulation history on the selective responsiveness of neurons within sensory systems, particularly the visual system (e.g., Mitchell and Timney 1984). At the same time unimodal deprivation and multimodal complex rearing have also been shown to produce morphological changes in both the number and structural characteristics of synapses on the cortex (Juraska, chapter 21). Although some of those involved in this research continue to assert that neural connections underlying visual abilities are determined genetically, most seem to argue that genes code only a rough outline, and the complexity of final neural connections is established in their response to environmental stimulation. The attractiveness of any such single, overarching, and general explanation has faded somewhat in recent times. Researchers now focus on describing the story with respect to specific perceptual capacities and specific aspects of neuronal circuitry.

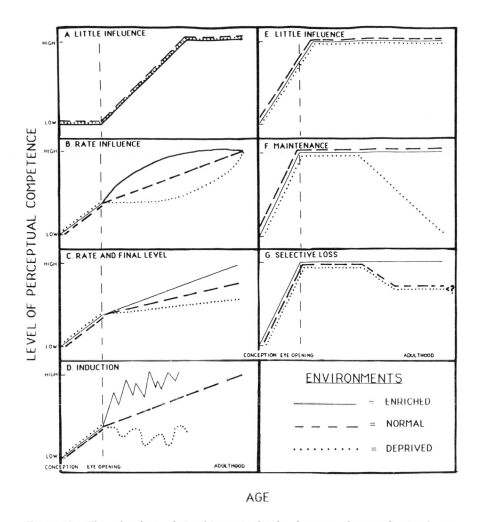

Figure 22.1 The role of stimulation history in the development of a specific visual competence (and its possibly related cortical substrate) in the case of an ability either partially (A,B,C,D) or fully developed (E,F,G) at eye opening: Some hypothetical outcomes.

There are additional complications with respect to our ability to look at the role played by experiential factors in specific competences dependent on the cortex. What sorts of new competences do the rodent's cortex make possible? Should we focus exclusively on those abilities adversely affected by adult cortical lesions (e.g., Whishaw, Dean— chapters 10 and 12, respectively)? Ideally we need to establish that neurons in designated cortical areas perform the operation essential to a specific perceptual ability and then to speculate on how these neurons execute this operation and how the function might change with age and stimulation history. In the course of this we should seriously consider the proposition that the perceptual functions of the neocortex are organized in terms of modular or independent sybsystems, as others have emphasized in their studies of primate cortex (e.g., Goldman-Rakic 1988). Unfortunately the answers currently available on these kinds of issues remain vague. For instance, Barlow (1985) has suggested that the cortex mediates behavior that requires extensive knowledge and understanding in an animal's environment. He and others suggest that the cortex enables an organism to successfully act in its own environment, to show the flexibility to learn, etc. (but see Whishaw, chapter 10). As one can see, this is only marginally helpful in providing much in the way of guideline as to what competences one should focus on. My tentative decision is to emphasize those competences that have been shown to be adversely affected by cortical lesions in rodents and to try to frame my discussion in terms of these ideals.

Specific Visual Capacities and Sensory Experience
Manipulations of a rodent's early sensory experience have involved a variety of procedures, each with its own advantages and disadvantages as well as goals (see Tees 1976a, 1986). The visual system has indeed been the focus of most controlled rearing experiments. It is obviously easier to control visual stimulation, and these attempts can be roughly subsumed under three headings: deprivation, biased rearing, and enrichment. The following sections examine the role played by experience in the development of specific and representative visual functions in rodents, notably those likely to be mediated in part by cortical neurons, such as acuity, depth, visual guidance, and form discrimination. This chapter is not intended to be an all-inclusive review or to provide a historical perspective, and some topics get only a cursory examination. The emphasis is on experiential contributions because the studies reviewed here usually involve manipulations of the environment, not genetic variables. An attempt is made to relate physiological/anatomical behavioral effects and/or to suggest some directions for future research on these important questions. A number of reviews have attempted to assess the available information on controlled rearing; their focus has been the neural and behavioral effects of controlled rearing on cats and monkeys (e.g., Mitchell and Timney 1984).

Visual Acuity

The impact of manipulations of stimulation history on the ontogeny of visual acuity in mammals has been examined quite extensively, particularly in the case of visually deprived rabbit, cat, and monkey (e.g., Mitchell and Timney 1984). One rationale for focusing on a careful assessment of visual acuity as opposed to other abilities has been the assumption that acuity is more likely than other measures to be correlated with response characteristics of single neurons. In any event work reported in this book (Dean, chapter 12) makes it clear that the ability of rats to detect stationary, high-contrast square-wave gratings of various fundamental frequencies is affected by visual cortical lesions.

Dean's observations as well as the limited physiological data available (e.g., Lennie and Perry 1981, Harnois et al. 1984) clearly emphasize the considerable similarity between rat and other mammals with respect to routing of information about stationary spatial contrasts and the parallel organization of different cell pathways in the visual system. In any event Dean's review suggests that if lesions are restricted to the striate cortex (Oc1), acuity falls to 0.7 cycle/degree, and further cortical lesions reveal that visual information carried by subcortical projection to the colliculus is limited to spatial frequencies below 0.3 cycle/degree. Virtually all of the existing behavioral and physiological studies (Legg 1984, Wiesenfeld and Branchek 1976, Hughes 1977) suggest that the vision of the normal adult hooded rat is no better than 1 cycle/degree. As Powers and Green (1978) have demonstrated, the small-eyed rodent has a large depth of focus with objects from 7 cm in front of the eye to optical infinity in equivalent focus, which means that most visual stimuli, both in the lab and in natural settings, are effectively in good focus if they are of sufficient size to be resolved. Although there are further behavioral studies of visual acuity in normally reared albino and hooded rats, no studies have focused specifically on the impact of binocular deprivation (e.g., dark rearing) on behavioral acuity or on the changes that might be observed during ontogeny. However, given the fact that adult DR rats rapidly acquire discriminations involving single interrupted and continuous lines (1°–2° in width) in various orientations (see section on form perception) and transfer effectively to new versions, it is not likely that their ability to resolve detail is dramatically affected by lack of visual experience.

We do have some evidence on the impact of environmental manipulations on other rodents' visual systems. Normal, light-reared (LR) adult hamsters, whose acuity has been estimated (behaviorally) at 0.7 cycle/degree (Emerson 1980), achieve no better levels of performance than DR adult hamsters (Chalupa 1981). Overall these results suggest that, at worst, small deficits in acuity are caused by early binocular sensory deprivation in rodents. Early selective (restrictive) exposure to lines of a single orientation also yield minor (at worse) effects on the rat's ability to resolve detail (Corrigan and Carpenter 1979). That in fact is very much the picture that has finally emerged in respect of the cat's ability to resolve detail. (Mitchell and Timney 1984), despite earlier dramatic claims to the contrary.

Interestingly, although most individuals estimate the cut-off frequency of the rat to be around 1.0 cycle/degree based on behavioral or VEP (visual evoked potential) data, Friedman and Green (1982) found that the retinal ganglion cells in normally reared and DR rats exhibit a broad range of acuities; yielding a bimodal frequency distribution with peaks at 0.3 and 0.8 cycle/degree. They also found a number of cells with acuities above 1.0 cycle/degree, with some in fact as high as 1.6 cycles/degree. Although their data showed no significant differences due to rearing condition, it is interesting that only the LR rats' retinas contained units with acuities of 1.6 cycles/degree. It is possible that visual acuity reflects the "performance" shared by a certain number of retinal ganglion cells and not a few neurons with the highest resolving capacity. Alternatively it may well be that behavioral estimations to date of rodents' ability to resolve detail as well as interpretation of electrophysiological evidence may represent an *underestimation* of the acuity of the adult experienced LR animal and the (albeit small) difference between DR and LR animals' abilities.

Although most of the work done on the effects of early monocular deprivation (MD) on the development of visual functioning has been done in species with frontal eyes and larger binocular fields, such as the cat and monkey, there is a reasonable amount of evidence from investigations that have focused on rodents. Early MD has been reported to produce anatomical/eletrophysiological abnormalities in the central representation of binocular fields of rodents similar to those seen in the MD cat and monkey, and there have also been reports of impairments in acuity in rat (Rothblat et al. 1978, Schwartz and Rothblat 1980) and hamster (Emerson et al. 1982). Although these behavioral deficits are interesting in view of the species involved (e.g., the adult rodent species involved do not have areas of markedly higher ganglion cell density around the visual axis), they shouldn't be entirely surprising. Rodents such as the rat and mouse do have large binocular fields— 80 degrees or so (Hughes 1977)—and the cortex possesses an extensive binocular segment in which the majority of cells respond to stimulation of either eye (Burne et al. 1984, Drager 1978). Most investigators emphasize that, as is the case with cat and monkey, acuity deficits observed in these studies may be attributable primarily to interocular competition mechanisms rather than visual disuse. That is to say, MD has a greater impact than does dark rearing on binocular eyelid suture.

Part of the reason for the relatively mild (but real) impact on the ability to resolve detail of the MD hamster (Emerson et al. 1982) may have to do with questions related to the effectiveness of suturing eyelids. There is considerable evidence to suggest that many cortical units can be activated visually through sutured eyelids, particularly in young animals (see Tees 1986 for a complete discussion). The eyelid of a hamster attenuates retinal illumination even less than that of a cat; thus coarse visual stimuli could activate cortical units through the deprived eye during the monocular period (Emerson et al. 1982). I would argue that the impact of MD should be considerably greater in the case of the gerbil, whose visual acuity has been estimated to be three times better than that of the hamster and the rat. Wilkinson and colleagues (1986) reported that gerbils indeed show acuity deficits with respect to the initially deprived eye that range up to 1.2 cycles/degree. In addition one month of MD (from the time of eye opening) is sufficient to induce relatively permanent acuity impairments. As is the case with other mammals, simple closure of the experienced eye for extended periods during adulthood does not necessarily reverse visual deficits. In fact Wilkinson and coworkers (1986) reported that 22 weeks of reverse monocular exposure initiated after a month or two of MD does not ameliorate the behavioral impairments observed in gerbils.

Neuroanatomical and physiological changes, which are not attributable to optical defects, have been described in other rodents after MD. These changes include (1) small shifts in the ocular dominance distribution of neurons in the binocular segment of area Oc1 toward greater control by the experienced eye in the hamster (Emerson et al. 1982) and the mouse (Drager 1978), and (2) reduced responsiveness and specificity of Oc1 neurons in the hemisphere contralateral to the deprived eye in rat (Yinon and Auerbach 1973). The evidence on the impact of DR and MD in the case of rodents is not complete. It is, however, consistent with that reported with respect to other mammals such as cat and monkey (see Tees 1986). That is to say, binocular deprivation seems to produce at best a small albeit significant difference in acuity *that is much smaller than that observed after bilateral striate lesions* (particularly those restricted to Oc1). Moreover MD does seem to produce larger effects than those produced by DR due to the competitive disadvantage the early deprived eye experiences.

Depth Perception

A great deal of research has been undertaken on the development of depth perception in rodents and the roles played by experience and by visual cortex (reviewed by Walk 1978). The work of many researchers (e.g., Bauer and Hughes 1970) makes it clear that the rat's depth perception is adversely affected by posterior cortical lesions. For example, Tees (1976b) also looked at the effect of infant and adult visual cortical lesions on a modified visual cliff apparatus in which the depth of the deep side could be varied. Depth discriminative abilities did not develop normally following the removal of the posterior cortex in infancy. Although the animals operated on in infancy did perform significantly better than did animals operated on in adulthood, they were not as good as untreated control animals when tested on such a cliff from days

20 to 160. More recently Ellard and colleagues (1986) looked at gerbils that received lesions in the visual cortex as well as in other subcortical structures. Their results (see Goodale and Carey, chapter 13) suggested strongly that the visual cortex subserved a critical aspect of the dynamic distance estimation in that the cortical-lesioned group was unable to use motion, retinal disparity, and "loom" as cues in the calibration of their jumps to a landing platform. Sinnamon and Charman (1988) have further reported that in the rat neither vertical nor horizontal head movements per se are affected by visual cortical lesions. Dean (chapter 12) argues that the evidence supports the idea that rats with large posterior lesions can in fact use self-produced as well as external movement cues.

As far as experience itself is concerned, the results of early experiments by Walk and Gibson (1961) led them to initially propose that depth perception in the rat (unlike other mammals) was innate, requiring neither experience nor maturation beyond opening. None of the early investigations attempted to study systematically performance on a cliff as a function of age, and all used the deep side on which the pattern was 50 cm to 135 cm below the glass surface—not a very sensitive measure of the limits of their ability. After systematically testing naive DR and LR rats on a modification of the cliff in which the depth of the deep side could vary, we demonstrated that the ontogeny of the rat's depth perception is a result of the collaboration between a number of sources of development (Tees 1974). Influences of the innate component is reflected in the ability of the 20-day-old rats to discriminate depth at 20 cm of differential depth. The collaboration of maturation and nonvisual experience could be seen in the improvement by the older DR animals. The influence of visual experience could be said to take two forms: (1) *facilitative*, governing sharpening or attunement, as evidenced in the decreasing differential thresholds obtained by the maturing LR animals, and (2) *maintenance*, the lack of which was seen in the decline of performance after prolonged DR. In the case of the rat DR until 90 days of age, we found that 60 days of subsequent exposure to patterned light ameliorates the serious decline of performance in the visual cliff that is normally observed after continuous DR (Tees and Midgley 1978). The visual experience not only protected the performance from decline but also yielded some evidence of improvement or partial recovery. Such a period of visual experience yielded "recovery" at most differential depths, but not at the 9-cm level, close to threshold in this particular situation (see figure 22.2). This difference might not reflect the difference in perceptual ability per se. Performance on the cliff depends on the ability to see the difference between the two sides and to "care" about the difference. In another study (Tees 1976b) visual experience was also shown to play an important role in the development of depth discriminative ability in infant-operated striate animals, as it did in unoperated animals. The performance of rats with neonatal striate

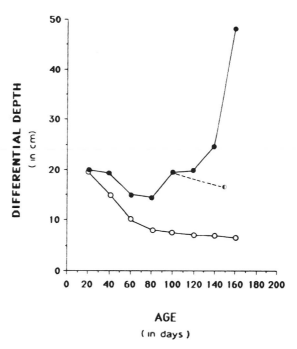

Figure 22.2 Differential visual depths at which at least 75 percent of the light-reared (open circles) dark-reared (dark circles) and dark-then-light reared (half-dark circle) rats descended to the optically shallow sides of the modified visual cliff.

lesions was adversely affected by postoperative DR. Differences were not evident at 20 days to 60 days after lesioning. Only at 80 days were the differences due to early stimulation statistically significant. (This difference is seen despite prior tests and associated visual experience.)

The effect of "cliff" or "enriched" environments on competence has been looked at in both rats and gerbils. Thiessen and colleagues (1969) looked at the impact of 50 days spent in different environments. A group of rats raised in a patterned cliff environment performed significantly better in terms of accuracy on the standard visual cliff apparatus compared with a group raised in an unpatterned, flat environment. In another study Bradley and Shea (1977) looked at gerbils tested at twenty days of age. Cliff-enriched animals rapidly discriminate depth on the visual cliff at 21 days of age, whereas all of the flat-environment–reared animals did not. At 60 days of age both animals reared in enriched and in impoverished circumstances were successful. Obviously environmental conditions appear to have accelerated the acquisition of visual depth perception rather than affected the final level of performance, at least on the standard cliff.

Extensive literature on cats' visual depth perception and the role played by experience has emerged (Mitchell and Timney 1984). An interesting story on brain-behavior relations emerges with respect to stereoscopic depth perception. Mitchell and Timney have shown that the emergence of monocular depth perception in kittens (measured behaviorally) coincides precisely with the maturation of cortical disparity-tuned neurons and that DR cats that failed to develop stereoscopic depth perception also failed to develop neural mechanisms on which they might be based.

As far as the rat is concerned, there is as yet no good comparison of binocular and monocular depth perception that might reveal evidence with respect to stereoscopic depth perception. We have some preliminary evidence from a small number of rats that DR does affect binocular depth perception. One published study (Eichengreen et al. 1966) observed that rats reared in complex environments until 21 days of age performed better monocularly than did normally raised animals, suggesting again that these early enriched circumstances had at least accelerated the emergence of depth perception. The basic notion from this study is that depth perception at 21 days of age might be relatively fragile, and thus altering the test circumstances by monocularly testing an animal and reducing information about the environment would highlight the impact of enrichment on the ability in question.

Visually Guided Behavior
For some time the argument has been made for a partial dissociation of those neural mechanisms underlying visual information processing, "perception," or discrimination and those underlying visually elicited orientation or locomotion (Schneider 1969), the geniculostriate pathway being identified with perception and the retinotectal pathway with orientation. Although such a functional dichotomy has received support from a number of studies, several investigators have suggested that orientation behavior may not be a function uniquely related to the optic tectum. Normal adult vision involves both orientational and perceptual factors acting simultaneously and/or in close interaction. One reason for questioning the dichotomy is the fact that rodents, including the rat, orient even after receiving substantial bilateral lesions of the entire superior colliculus (e.g., Midgley and Tees 1981). Goodale and Carey (chapter 13) believe that although the tectal system mediates head turns to stimuli occurring anywhere throughout the entire visual field, the output from the geniculostriate system appears to play an important part in the control of head movements to stimuli within the central part of the rodent's visual field. Although the head turn and orienting behavior of gerbils with lesions in the tectum are more disorganized than those of posterior decorticates, further lesions of cortical areas *after* bilateral tectal lesions produce animals that are further disabled with respect to orientation skills. In summary the work of Goodale and others makes several other things clear. First, ideally, orienting behavior should be analyzed as a complex response of a number of components or elements, each of which might have its own developmental history and be affected differentially by a lack of visual experience or cortical

lesions. For instance, orientation involves interruption of ongoing behavior, location of stimuli with appropriate head and postural adjustments, tracking or following the stimulus, and potentially further guided responses such as approach or avoidance. Characteristics of the stimulus itself, such as the pattern motion, distance, and size, would be expected to influence the appearance of visually related investigative sequences of behavior as well as the location (central or peripheral) of these specific stimuli.

Investigations of the consequences of experiential manipulations on the ontogeny of these visuomotor capacities have primarily focused on easily and quickly administered tasks such as perimetry, visual tracking and visual placing, and reaching. Differential responsiveness to light or dark or to a high-contrast target appears in the rat before it opens its eyes (Crozier and Pincus 1937). It is also observed in rats raised in darkness, either until their eyes are opened or until maturity, when they are tested for visual orientation (Hebb 1937a). Dark- or strobe-reared hamsters when tested as adults have been found to orient to light (as well as auditory) stimuli presented on all portions of their fields as effectively as do LR controls (Rhoades and Chalupa 1978). The failure to find differences due to lack of experience may reflect the sensitivity of the behavioral measures used. Midgley and Tees (1983) have discovered deficits in DR rodents even on a simple visuomotor response, i.e., interruption of ongoing behavior. The DR rats, beginning at 90 days of age, exhibited some neglect (lack of orientation) over a wide part of their visual field to stimuli of various degrees of complexity. Although orienting behavior is relatively preserved despite lack of visual experience, subtle aspects of visually guided behavior are influenced by these manipulations. For instance, although DR adult rats performed less ably than the LR control rats when tested on the visual cliff, they can discriminate the visual difference between shallow and deep sides of the cliff if the difference between the two sides is at least 20 cm (Tees 1974). With respect to motivational properties of heretofore missing sensory input, we have demonstrated that DR rats, tested for the first time at 90 days of age, exhibit levels of light-seeking behavior comparable to those of LR rats (Tees et al. 1980).

One oversimplification that is, however, consistent with the findings on visuomotor competence, the brain, and experience is that binocularly deprived mammals, including the rat, fail to develop these cortical mechanisms (e.g., Midgley and Tees 1983) underlying visual orientation although the retinotectal mechanisms also underlying similar competences are available to some extent to support relatively rapid recovery of these visual behaviors. The evidence on the effect of early and late lesions of the SC and cortex in both rodents and cats is certainly consistent with this idea (Finlay et al. 1980). It is the combination of dark rearing *and* SC lesions that has serious consequences for the development of visuomotor orientation skill. In terms of a speculative modularity analysis, one could easily implicate DR's adverse impact on the extrastriate (Oc2M), temporal (Te2) or posterior parietal cortex (PPC), which receive projections from SC/lateral posterior nucleus (see Dean, Goodale and Carey, and Kolb—chapters 12, 13, and 19, respectively).

A second observation about these issues has to do with competition. For example, orientation deficits observed in monkeys that are binocularly deprived for 7 to 10 months persist for months after the animals return to a normal colony situation and are much more consistent with the lack of physiological recovery in the association cortex (area 7), which, according to Kolb (chapter 19), corresponds to the PPC in the rat. Because area 7 in the monkey receives input from several systems (as does the PPC), the lack of significant input in one modality leads to very few cells being visually responsive (i.e., a decrease in its neural representation) as a result of early intermodal competition that has a significant impact on the use of orientational skills (and the use of vision) of these long-term binocularly sutured monkeys (Hyvarinen et al. 1981).

With respect to this category of visual behavior and the issues related to competitive disadvantage, the consequences of MD are particularly relevant. Although it is clear that MD results in more serious and long-lasting deficits than does binocular DR in many respects, neglect of visual arrays is probably at the heart of the visual problems that MD animals have to overcome during postdeprivation testing. We do not have as good a behavioral picture of the orientation skills of the monocularly deprived rodent as we have for the cat (see Tees 1986), but what we do have is consistent with the idea proposed with respect to MD cats. That is, these animals fail to respond to normal visual stimuli in the binocular part of their visual field when given perimetry testing with the deprived eye, and this failure persists. In all mammals examined, however, MD results in a dramatic loss of input via a binocular segment of the Y-cell pathway associated with the deprived eye (to the cortex and to the SC). According to Sherman (1979), visual neglect of monocular deprivation is a direct result of suppression of a retinotectal pathway input by the imbalanced abnormal cortical tectal pathway.

Form Perception

Posterior cortical lesions do have an adverse effect on the rat's ability to resolve details as well as to acquire various kinds of pattern discriminations (e.g., Dean, chapter 12). Even in those studies in which rats are able to acquire certain kinds of contour orientation or to discriminate possibly more complex patterns in the absence of striate cortex, the animals do not use whatever residual visual capacity they may have with respect to these kinds of discriminations without extensive training and appropriate motivation (e.g., Goldstein and Oakley 1987).

Visually deprived mammals, including the rat, required two to three times as many trials as did normally reared animals to learn discrimination, such as N versus X (Tees 1976a). Such retarded performance has been used to indicate the important contribution that visual experience plays in the development of mechanisms underlying form perception in mammals (e.g., Hebb 1949). In this regard problem difficulty per se is not critical (see figure 22.3). Visual experience plays no more of a role if the targets used are light intensities, single rectangles, or a line of dots and when near-threshold stimulus differences are used so that the task is made more difficult for a normal animal than complex pattern discriminations such as N versus X (e.g., Tees 1968, 1972, 1979).

The outcome is the same whether one looks at the relative ease or difficulty with which these animals are able to distinguish between two representative stimulus arrays or their performance during transfer or stimulus equivalence tests in which what is learned from initial exposure to specific training shapes is examined. The results of this latter kind of test are important; the key question associated with the ability to recognize a pattern is answered in terms of this basic stimulus equivalence problem (Sutherland 1968). It is the neural and psychological processes underlying the ability to recognize a pattern or object despite variations in the size or orientation and contrast that are at issue. Interestingly there is a great deal of data on the rat in this respect. After

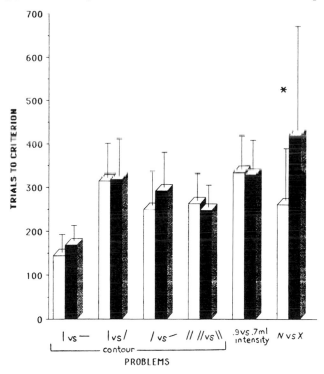

Figure 22.3 Performance (M and SDs) by separate groups of light-reared (light bars) and dark-reared (dark bars) rats in learning a complex pattern (N versus X), a near-threshold intensity discrimination, and four (line) orientation discriminations of varying degrees of difficulty in either two- or three-choice (oddity) test situations. Only performance on the complex pattern yielded significant (*) differences due to stimulation history.

Tees: Experience and Perceptual Competences

learning to discriminate a single rectangle from an equally bright target containing no rectangle, both LR and DR rats had peak generalization gradients when faced with transfer stimuli in different angular orientations (Tees 1972).

After training with two lines of dots that differ in angular orientation, both LR and DR rats transferred well to new stimulus patterns containing fewer dots, stripes, a reversal of figure-ground brightness, and so on, provided that a relative difference in orientation was maintained (Tees et al. 1978). It is important to note that each of these new versions of the original stimuli proved more (or less) difficult for LR rats to recognize as equivalent to the original stimuli, and DR rats performed *in the same manner* as their LR counterparts when confronted with each of the transfer tests (see figure 22.4A). We have even raised rats in a planetariumlike environment (Bruinsma and Tees 1977) for two hours daily from day 15 to 45, and that left the biasedly reared rats as able as LR rats in recognizing equivalences (as revealed in transfer tests). It is also important to remember that rats that are trained on discriminations between, for example, vertical and horizontal stripe stimuli that are equated for contour length and total number of dots who suffer visual (Oc1 and/or Oc2) cortical lesions (whether in one or two stages) *do not* perform as effectively as do these DR rodents (e.g., Meyer et al. 1986). That is to say, such lesioned animals take significantly longer than do control animals to learn or relearn discrimination and transfer less effectively than do visually inexperienced animals.

Our data would suggest strongly that visually naive and to some extent biasedly reared rodents seemed to possess not only the predisposition to isolate a figure from its ground (Hebb 1937a) and the capacity to respond differentially to visual vertical, oblique, and horizontal stimuli, but also to generalize from that experience to lines in different angular orientations (see figure 22.4A). On the other hand, with identifications of forms differing only in their elements' relationship to one another (e.g., N vs. X), DR animals learn more slowly and learn less than do LR rats, as evidenced in stimulus equivalence tests of these collections of lines in different orientations (Tees 1976a, 1986). This distinction is also evident when reviewing the literature on selective rearing (see Tees 1976a). Preexposure to forms such as horizontal and vertical striations is not effective in terms of later discriminative performance, although exposure to more complex patterns is (McCall and Lester 1969, Oswalt 1972).

Differences between shapes involving relational properties among sets of linear elements and the role played by visual experience in the discrimination of two of the most elementary relationships—contour separation and angular junction—have been looked at. Visually naive DR rats learned tasks in which spatial distance—i.e., the horizontal separation meeting vertical contours—was a critical feature more slowly than did their LR counterparts and performed less effectively on transfer

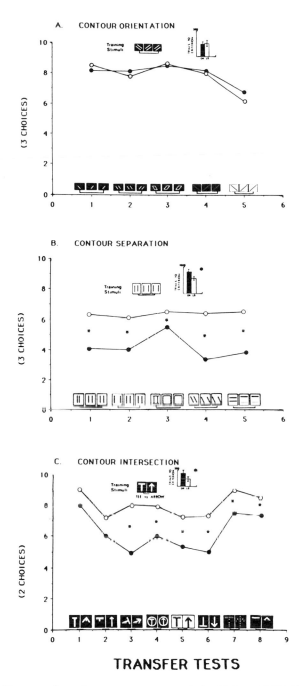

Figure 22.4 Mean number of correct responses made by 90-day-old DR (dark circles) and LR (open circles) rats to some test shapes employed during transfer testing. In B and C, LR rats transferred significantly more successfully than did DR rats even after 150 over-training trials after initial acquisition with the original training stimulus shown. In the case of A, in which the tested feature involved the orientation of line stimuli, LR rats were no more successful than were DR rats.

tests (see figure 22.4b) even after 150 trials of overtraining (Tees 1979). The same pattern of results (Tees and Midgley 1982) was observed with respect to the rat's ability to discriminate simple types of intersections between lines (see figure 22.4C). In short the capacity to perceive even the basic relation between linear elements such as contour separation of angle appears to depend on visual experience for its development. The evidence obtained from binocularly deprived rats as well as other mammals exposed to normal environments after deprivation is consistent with the above conclusion in connection with the relative importance of early experience. The deficits and the ability to recognize complex patterns and their variations during transfer testing seem most resistant to improvement during a recovery period (Tees and Midgley 1978).

The stimuli used in testing pattern recognition in LR and DR mammals so far have been relatively simple. However, we have confirmed (Sutherland and Williams 1969) that rats, having learned to discriminate the checkerboard pattern from a pattern containing an irregularity, treat as equivalent to the original (negative) stimulus a pattern containing a variety of irregularities, including a change in the shape of the checkers in both patterns (Tees 1979), and they do this at least after 150 trials of overtraining. Almost half of our DR rats (10 to 22) failed to learn the original task within 1000 trials, and the 12 that did learned it very slowly and performed very poorly on most of the transfer stimuli, even after overtraining. From the results of the transfer tests it appears that the LR rat is able to use an abstract description of the difference between the patterns and could not have been encoding a difference in spatial frequency, an exact representation of the pattern, or even a list of features. At the very least the results serve to remind us of the level of perceptual processing that must be accounted for in theories of shape recognition, even with respect to the rat and the special significance of visual experience in its development.

In the monocularly deprived rat (as is true of MD cat), there are physiological consequences due to disuse in the deprived eye's monocular cortical segment, and potentially permanent deficits in pattern discriminative abilities certainly have been reported for the MD rat (Rothblat et al. 1978). I have also argued elsewhere (Tees 1986) that these consequences are difficult to untangle from the less specific deficits related to visual attention and visuomotor skills.

In terms of speculating about the modularity of the rat visual cortex, I would like to argue that manipulations of visual experience have the greatest impact in respect of the extrastriate visual cortex (e.g., possibly Oc2L, Te2, Te3). The performance of the visually inexperienced DR rats on a variety of line orientation and complex pattern discrimination tasks resembles that of rats with selective lesions in those cortical areas (Dean, chapter 12; Meyer et al. 1986).

I have argued elsewhere (see Tees 1986 for a more complete discussion) that visual experience might play a special role in the development of *specification* (e.g., Beaulieu and Colonnier 1987) of inhibitory synaptic connections important to the development of subordinate neurons, having the veto properties that are necessary to mediate configurational discriminations. Visual experience might be viewed as changing the gating action of these neurons so that suboptimal features do exert considerable inhibition. Recent work (Gabbott and Steward 1987) on the effect of DR on the ultrastructural characteristics of synapses in rat visual cortex indicates that inhibitory S-type bouton populations are more affected by DR than are the excitatory A-type. The site of additional processing of visual pattern information must certainly involve potentially late-developing (Mayers et al. 1971) extrastriate structures (such as, for example, Oc2L and Te2, Te3); such structures either might be the potential locus of form-specific encoding developed from the line segment and/or spatial frequency information of the striate cortex or, at least, might provide a somewhat more independent transformation of the visual input in which size and position invariance is achieved (see Tees 1986). Although these are interesting speculations, there continues to be inadequate data to help support or shape these ideas. Moreover, unfortunately, the focus of research on morphological and physiological effects of changes in early visual stimulation history has been on primary (Oc1) striate cortex (see Juraska, chapter 21).

Not much information exists on the impact of a supernormal or enriched environment on pattern perceptual ability. However, there is some work reported in the current literature. For instance, rats exposed to circles and triangles and an otherwise visually sparse environment are more able than control animals to discriminate these shapes later. It appears that these early experiences with stimuli do not necessarily depend on the opportunity to manipulate the forms (Bennet et al. 1970). On the other hand Thinus-Blanc (1982) demonstrated that hamsters reared in spatially diverse environments are more able than control animals to discriminate between two cubic volumes (perceived from the inside). The learning of such discriminations by hamsters reared in standard conditions appears not to reflect the ability to take the three spatial dimensions into account equally. Only the spatially enriched animals are able to utilize cues with depth, etc., when presented with transfer stimuli in which only some of the cues are made available.

22.3 Nonvisual Capacities

Spatial Ability and Intersensory Effects
Most theoretical positions (e.g., Gibson 1969) on the development of spatial cognition seem to assign an important role to visual experience and to cortical mechanisms. Although the evidence supporting the idea that spatial competence does depend on cortical and hippocampal mechanisms (see Goodale and Carey, chapter 13), the evidence is less clear as far as experience is concerned. DR rats have been found to be

more spatially oriented than are their LR counterparts when tested on a Kretch hypothesis maze (Gamboni 1964). On the other hand rats blinded shortly after birth performed less ably than did the late-blinded rats on an auditory localization task (Spigelman and Bryden 1967). Although Sutherland and Dyck (1984) reported that neonatally enucleated rats compared well with LR animals that had been bilaterally enucleated at adulthood in trying to locate an invisible platform in the Morris water maze, they were significantly less effective in rediscovering the location of the platform when its location was shifted on probe trials. We have looked at groups of sighted and blinded LR and DR rats tested on a series of Hebb-Williams maze problems and their reversals under both repetitive and aversive reinforcement (Tees et al. 1981). LR and DR animals were also compared on a 17-arm radial maze over a 36-day period during which variations in the task were introduced. Blindness at the time of testing had a significant (adverse) impact on the performance of both LR and DR animals on all problems, but a significantly greater effect on the DR animals. Overall our visually inexperienced rats were found to be less able than were experienced control rats to acquire and store information about spatial location. Our work provided no evidence that this deficit was related to their inability to utilize visual information available to different degrees on the tasks they encountered. Lack of visual experience does retard the neural development of the visual cortex (see Juraska, chapter 21), and there is already strong evidence (Dean, chapter 12) that the visual cortex (beyond Oc1) does play an important role in the learning of complex mazes and spatial orientation when visual cues are not available. Our results certainly are consistent with the speculation that the functioning network underlying spatial ability in the rat includes structures such as the visual cortex, which are adversely affected by lack of early visual experience. In addition, in numerous studies of the behavioral and apparently related neural consequences of early rearing in complex, enriched, and multimodal sensory environments (Juraska, chapter 21), the most consistent, although not universal, behavioral finding has been the superior performance of environmentally enriched rodents in complex spatial and maze tasks. Two major and related points of controversy regarding this result involve the relative influence of visual aspects of environmental enrichment and the relative importance of particular abilities producing superior performance on such a maze task (see Tees et al. 1981).

The nature of intersensory coordination and its ontogeny are topics of related interest. This work has been concerned more generally with the perception of amodal properties or attributes, which are seen as higher-order relational stimulations, not specific to any one modality. Several individuals have speculated about the neurocircuitry that might underlie such competences as well as the role that experience might play in its development and/or maintenance (Tees 1976a, Turkewitz and

Kenny 1982). Neurons responsive to visual, tactile, and/or auditory events have been observed in both the parietal and visual cortex (as well as in the hippocampus) in normally reared rodents (e.g., Drager and Hubel 1976, Meikle 1968). Pinto-Hamuy and colleagues (1987) reported that Oc2M lesions exclusively affect visuosomatic *intermodal* tasks. Kolb (chapter 19) reports that rats with PPC lesions perform poorly on such intermodal tasks. The effect of early visual deprivation on the ability of DR and LR rats to learn temporal discriminations involving sounds and lights and their ability to abstract intersensory correspondence involving *duration* from these initial modality-specific training periods have been examined in our lab (Tees and Symons 1987). Interestingly, visually inexperienced DR rats, although somewhat less successful in acquiring initial discrimination involving visual events, were as effective as their visually experienced LR counterparts in demonstrating crossmodal transfer to signals in a new modality. One might expect developmental differences with respect to the ontogeny of crossmodal equivalences involving different dimensions. In fact we have recently found that DR rats are less able than their LR counterparts are at recognizing the correspondence between the *location* of visual and auditory events (Tees and Buhrmann 1989).

Gottlieb (1971) has pointed to a somewhat invariant sequence in which sensory systems develop in vertebrates including rodents, the auditory system becoming functional before the visual system, and tactile and olfactory systems coming on-line earlier still. Several other investigators have pointed to the fact that such differential onset results in relative independence between emerging systems (Turkewitz and Kenny 1982), thereby reducing competition, which in turn maintains normal perceptual and neural development. In the past we have focused (as have most others) on the impact of deprivation with respect to a late-developing visual system on its own development and to some extent on the development of other sensory systems. However, we have suggested (e.g., Burnstine et al. 1984) that manipulations of early sensory history may have a greater or lesser impact depending on what kind of input is being manipulated relative to this developmental sequence. For example, hypertrophy in the auditory cortex of rodents with somesthetic restrictions has been observed, although the somesthetic cortex itself is not affected by visual deprivation (Ryugo et al. 1975). The problem again is that there is virtually no direct behavioral evidence to confirm or deny these plausible notions.

Intramodal Sensory Experience and Auditory Competences
Although vision has been the chosen modality in most controlled rearing experiments, a comparable experimental design has been implemented involving manipulation of auditory experience, and several studies have examined the effects of early auditory restriction on later adult behavior and brain development in the rat. Auditory restriction

of rodents, for the most part, has involved early temporary surgical ligation of external auditory meatus, removable earplugs, or specific (permanent) damage to middle ear cochlea to restrict (monaurally or binaurally) auditory input from birth through to testing and beyond (Clopton 1986). Although the results of early studies (e.g., Batkin and Ansberry 1964) support the principles of early sensory deprivation as followed by inability to use information presented later in the affected modality, the results of these are hard to interpret. More effective and more meaningful methods of testing auditory discrimination have been used. Such tests have demonstrated that cumulative auditory experience with temporal patterns is necessary for the development of temporal integrative capacities in the rat and thus facilitates the organism's performance in learning specific auditory pattern as well as duration discriminations. On the other hand such experience does not seem to play an appreciable role in the discrimination of changes in either the intensity or frequency of auditory signals (see Tees 1967, 1967a). As is clear from Kelly's chapter (chapter 15), the role of the rat's auditory cortex in such discriminations has not been as well established as it has been in the cat. Most of the work involving manipulations of early auditory experience in the rat has looked at the neural consequences with respect to subcortical structures such as the inferior colliculus. In monaurally or binaurally deprived mice as well as rats, structural, physiological, and metabolic changes consistent with those observed in other mammals have been reported (e.g., Clopton 1986). At least in the case of early sound deprivation (Clopton and Silverman 1978, Silverman and Clopton 1977), the changes in single-unit characteristics observed in the IC are predominantly with respect to high-frequency units. In fact the physiological and behavioral responsiveness of young rats is evident only with respect to relatively low-frequency stimuli (Rubel 1985), and the ability of the developing animal to detect higher-frequency sounds emerges later during its ontogeny (Hyson and Rudy 1987). Complicating anyone's interpretation of these early-auditory-experience experiments is the fact that manipulation of early auditory experience usually involves occlusion produced by ear plugs or surgical ligation of the external meatus. Whereas the conductive loss (i.e., 25 dB) produced by earplugs has been examined using evoked potentials recording and has been found to be relatively flat across the dynamic range in the rodents in question (see Rubel 1985), internally produced and bone-conducted sounds are primarily relatively low frequencies. Occlusion of the external ear canal or filling the external auditory canal with ear plugs in fact enhances bone-conducted low-frequency sounds while attenuating high-frequency sounds. Thus the effects on neuroanatomy and on physiological responsiveness of single units throughout the system cited above could reflect the nature of the degree of control of early stimulation history. That seems to be the case. In any event we don't have good behavioral data in which, e.g., a near-threshold high-frequency discrimination test is made of binaurally deprived rats.

According to Kelly (chapter 15), auditory cortical lesions in the rat have relatively minor effects on sound localization. It is also not clear what role experience might play in the ontogeny of the ability to lateralize sounds as far as the rat is concerned, or for that matter any other creature. Preliminary evidence does suggest that auditory enrichment has a positive effect on spatial ability, as measured in the Morris water maze using two auditory beacons. Animals raised in an environment in which sound-generating toys are included in the enrichment procedure are significantly better in terms of their spatial ability than are animals raised in a silent yet enriched environment (Murdoch and Tees, in preparation).

The Impact of Intramodal Experiential Manipulations on Somesthetic Ability

In looking at the impact of restricting an early developing modality, the somatosensory system would seem to be an ideal candidate. Although the system has diverse inputs coming from a variety of unique receptor structures, most recent investigations have focused on the mystacial vibrissae of rodents (Clopton 1986). These hair-follicle receptors project to the contralateral somatosensory cortex and are well represented in the elaborate and cortical organization (Chapin and Lin, chapter 14). A great deal of physiological and anatomical evidence (Kaas et al. 1983) has accumulated on the reorganization or plasticity of the early developing system that takes place after peripheral sensory damage resulting from cauterization or removal of the vibrissae in newborn animals. Deafferentation at the periphery prevents the development of the barrel arrangement at the cortical level. There also seems to be a sensitive period for these effects with respect to cortical plasticity for peripheral changes involving a window of time possibly closing around postnatal day 7 to 10. Most attention has been paid to the changes that take place in the modality-specific neural substrate with such peripheral input restriction in developing rats. There is a little evidence that it is consistent with intermodal compensation (Gustafson and Felbain-Keramidas 1977). Cortical visual areas are increased in size in the case of early dewhiskered rats. Unfortunately there have been little useful data generated on the behavioral consequences of early vibrissae removal. Recently we have used a visual orientation/localization task along with a battery of sensorimotor tests (Symons and Tees, in press). The question was whether rats dewhiskered at birth were more attentive to visual signals and/or more able to make fine discriminations with respect to sensory inputs of other modalities. We found that animals experiencing early somatosensory restriction (by bilateral vibrissae follicle cauterization) took longer to habituate to repeated visual stimuli and were more likely to orient to subtle changes in these stimuli than were control animals. However, this was only true for animals reared with daily access to an enriched environment. In any event all early dewhiskered animals, regardless of rearing environment, displayed attenuated orientation to light tactile stimuli to the mystacial pads themselves. Rogowski and Greenough (in Burnstine et al. 1984) provided an enriched tactile (early) environment to neonatally blind and sighted mice and obtained some evidence for increased sensitivity or attention to whisker sensations. Gustafson and Felbain-Keramidas (1977) also have reported that removal of vibrissae from the first postnatal day results in rats that display different behaviors as adults. In contrast with rats with intact vibrissae and rats deprived of vibrissae as adults, rats deprived at birth and thereafter displayed faster crossings on the balance beam and less evidence of thigmotaxis in the open field. These albeit limited findings suggest that manipulations of tactile experience has functional consequences for development both for the somatosensory system and for the visual system.

22.4   Concluding Observations

I have sketched the evidence and speculated about what role experience plays in the development of the rat neocortex and competences dependent on the cortex. Table 22.1 provides a tentative and speculative sorting of some of those perceptual competences in terms of the degree to which their development is altered by manipulations of early stimulation.

The existing evidence does support the proposition that there is a common mammalian response to environmental manipulations, i.e., the rat is a useful model in most cases. One other point that emerges in my survey of the evidence is that we are in need of more and better behavioral data and a clearer picture of what "cortical operations" are involved in a rat's perceptual reactions. From the point of view of this analysis, a few of the measures taken of rats' ability at any stage of development have been chosen to be selectively sensitive to the presence or absence of particular cortical areas. Moreover the behavioral impact of complex rearing or deprivation is seldom assessed at close to the limits of normally reared rats' competence. As a consequence, with some notable exceptions, the behavioral facts about competences are limited, which makes attempts to draw inferences about potential brain-behavior relations very difficult. As far as the modularity approach to analysis of the evidence, I argue that the impact of experience (as reflected in the outcome of controlled rearing experiments) is more diffuse than that observed with specific cortical lesions. (If that is a correct assessment, it underlines the importance of a careful behavioral description of the impact of stimulation history in helping to understand cortical plasticity.) However, some "modules" are more affected by

Table 22.1 Impact of Multimodal and Unimodal Environmental Manipulations: Behavioral Evidence[a]

Limited Effect	Considerable Effect
1. Ability to resolve detail (gratings)	Ability to recognize stationary patterns on the basis of relationship between lines (contour separation, contour interaction)
2. Ability to recognize visual stimuli on the basis of *angular orientation* cues	Ability to acquire and remember spatial map of environment and to navigate to invisible targets
3. Ability to orient (respond) to external movement	
4. Ability to localize and respond to large visual stimuli	Ability to orient to spatial and temporal changes in pattern or visual events
5. Ability to recognize crossmodal attribute of *duration* and *intensity* of auditory and visual events	Ability to recognize crossmodal attribute of *location* of auditory and visual events

[a] Partial list of competences whose development is altered by multimodal complex rearing or unimodal restrictive rearing. The evidence supports the idea that the impact of early stimulation history is limited in the case of the abilities listed on the left and considerable in the case of those listed on the right.

manipulations of experience than others. Those modules that are apparently involved in competences or operations that require more information integration and are more dependent on memorial and selective attentional processes seem to be vulnerable to changes in stimulation history. All could be characterized as requiring trade-offs between an appreciation of aspects of the environment and remembering some specific features of the environment, while ignoring others. Inevitably these competences involve memory, attention, appreciation of spatial aspects of the environment and in this regard the extrastriate (Oc2M, Oc2L), parietal (PPC), and temporal (Te2) cortex would be implicated. In any event I would argue that the cortical tissue necessary for these kinds of operations could well be late developing and thus would logically be more vulnerable to manipulations of early stimulation history.

There is a reasonable alternative view to this. It could well be that controlled rearing affects every operation somewhat and equally. The more operations there are, the more modules are required to perform successfully a (perceptual) task, and the greater the impact of the controlled rearing would appear to be. Thus the small but real effects on the rat's ability to resolve detail, to orient, to process, to remember, etc., would produce cumulative and sizable effects on those cortically dependent behaviors that rely on many of these operations. The two views obviously are not mutually exclusive. I believe our ability to untangle these alternatives is somewhat limited.

One promising strategy for future research, which would allow us to better test ideas about the target of experientially induced plasticity, is the thoughtful use of specific surgical intervention in connection with manipulations of early stimulation history. If this strategy is to be effective, we need to collect anatomical as well as behavioral evidence from the same developing animals. In collecting the anatomical evidence and in the surgical interventions, we need to focus on those neural changes and structures that the behavioral evidence might be altered significantly by controlled rearing. I also would advocate the use of more broadly based behavioral measures, including tests of motor and motivational competences, which have been underutilized in the examination of experience-induced plasticity.

Acknowledgments

This chapter was written in connection with research activities supported by the Natural Sciences and Engineering Research Council of Canada (research grant APA0179). The assistance of Mirana Yu, Jordan Hanley, Michael Laycock, and Kristin Buhrmann in preparing the manuscript and figures is gratefully acknowledged.

References

Barlow, H. B. (1985). Cerebral cortex as model builder. In D. Rose and V. G. Dobson (eds.), *Models of the Visual Cortex*. Toronto: Wiley, 37–46.

Batkin, S., and Ansberry, M. (1964). Effect of auditory deprivation. *Journal of the Acoustical Society of America* 36:598.

Bauer, J. A., and Hughes, K. R. (1970). Visual and nonvisual behaviors of the rat after neonatal and adult posterior neocortical lesions. *Physiology and Behavior* 5:427–441.

Beaulieu, C., and Colonnier, M. (1987). Effect of the richness of the environment on the cat visual cortex. *Journal of Comparative Neurology* 266:478–494.

Bennet, T. L., Rickert, E. J., and McAllister, L. E. (1970). Role of tactual-kinesthetic feedback in transfer of perceptual learning for rats with pigmented irises. *Perceptual and Motor Skills* 30:916–918.

Bradley, D. R., and Shea, S. L. (1977). The effect of environment on visual cliff performance in the Mongolian gerbil. *Perception and Psychophysics* 21:171–179.

Bruinsma, Y., and Tees, R. C. (1977). The effect of bias-rearing on transfer after form discrimination training in the rat. *Bulletin of the Psychonomic Society* 10:433–435.

Burne, R. A., Parnavelas, J. G., and Lin, C. S. (1984). Response properties of neurons in the visual cortex of the rat. *Experimental Brain Research* 53:374–383.

Burnstine, T. H., Greenough, W. T., and Tees, R. C. (1984). Intermodal compensation following damage or deprivation. In C. R. Almli and S. Finger (eds.), *The behavioral biopsychology of early brain damage*. New York: Academic, 3–34.

Chalupa, L. M. (1981). Some observations on the functional organization of the golden hamster's visual system. *Behavioral Brain Research* 3:189–200.

Clopton, B. M. (1986). Neural correlates of development and plasticity in the auditory, somatosensory, and olfactory systems. In W. T. Greenough and J. M. Juraska (eds.), *Developmental neuropsychobiology*. Orlando: Academic, 364–384.

Clopton, B. M., and Silverman, M. S. (1978). Changes in latency and duration of neural responding following developmental auditory deprivation. *Experimental Brain Research* 32:39–47.

Corrigan, J. G., and Carpenter, D. L. (1979). Early selective visual experience and pattern discrimination in hooded rats. *Developmental Psychobiology* 12:67–72.

Crozier, W., and Pincus, G. (1937). Photic stimulation of young rats. *Journal of Genetic Psychology* 17:105–111.

Drager, U. C. (1978). Observations on monocular deprivation in mice. *Journal of Neurophysiology* 41:28–42.

Drager, U. C., and Hubel, D. H. (1976). Topography of visual and somatosensory projections to mouse superior colliculus. *Journal of Neurophysiology* 39:91–101.

Eichengreen, J. M., Coren, S., and Nachmias, J. (1966). Visual-cliff preference by infant rats: Effects of rearing and test conditions. *Science* 151(3712):830–831.

Ellard, C. G., Goodale, M. A., Scorfield, D. M., and Lawrence, C. (1986). Visual cortical lesions abolish the use of motion parallax in the Mongolian gerbil. *Experimental Brain Research* 64:599–602.

Emerson, V. F. (1980). Grating acuity of the golden hamster. The effects of stimulus orientation and luminance. *Experimental Brain Research* 38:43–52.

Emerson, V. F., Chalupa, L. M., Thompson, I. D., and Talbot, R. J. (1982). Behavioral, physiological, and anatomical consequences of monocular deprivation in the golden hamster (*Mesocricetus auratus*). *Experimental Brain Research* 45:168–178.

Finlay, B. L., Marder, K., and Cordon, D. (1980). Acquisition of visuomotor behavior after neonatal tectal lesions in the hamster: The role of visual experience. *Journal of Comparative and Physiological Psychology* 94(3):506–518.

Friedman, L. G., and Green, D. G. (1982). Ganglion cell acuity in hooded rats. *Vision Research* 22:411–444.

Gabbott, P. L. A., and Stewart, M. G. (1987). Quantitative morphological effects of dark-rearing and light exposure on the synaptic connectivity of layer 4 in the rat visual cortex (area 17). *Experimental Brain Research* 68:103–114.

Gamboni, W. R. (1964). Visual deprivation and hypothesis behavior in rats. *Perceptual and Motor Skills* 19:501–502.

Gibson, E. J. (1969). *Principles of perceptual learning and development.* New York: Appleton.

Goldman Rakic, P. S. (1988). Topography of cognition: Parallel distributed networks in primate association cortex. *Annual Review of Neuroscience* 11:137–156.

Goldstein, L. H., and Oakley, D. A. (1987). Visual discrimination in the absence of visual cortex. *Behavioral Brain Research* 24:181–193.

Gottlieb, G. (1971). Ontogenesis of sensory function in birds and mammals. In E. Tobach, L. R. Aronson, and E. Shaw (eds.), *The biopsychology of development.* New York: Academic, 67–128.

Gottlieb, G. (1976). The roles of experience in the development of behavior and the nervous system. In G. Gottlieb, (ed.), *Neural and behavioral specificity.* New York: Academic.

Gustafson, J. W., and Felbain-Keramidas, S. L. (1977). Behavioral and neural approaches to the function of the mystacial vibrissae. *Psychological Bulletin* 84(3):477–488.

Harnois, C., Bodis-Wollner, I., and Onofrj, M. (1984). The effect of contrast and spatial frequency on the visual evoked potential of the hooded rat. *Experimental Brain Research* 57:1–8.

Hebb, D. O. (1937a). The innate organization of visual activity. I. Perception of figures by rats reared in total darkness. *Journal of Genetic Psychology* 51:101–126.

Hebb, D. O. (1937b). The innate organization of visual acuity. II. Transfer of response in the discrimination of brightness and size by rats reared in total darkness. *Journal of Comparative Psychology* 24:277–299.

Hebb, D. O. (1949). *The organization of behavior.* New York: Wiley.

Hebb, D. O. (1980). *Essays on mind.* Hillsdale, N.J.: Erlbaum.

Hughes, M.C. (1977). Anatomical and neurobehavioural investigations concerning the thalamo-cortical organization of the rat's visual system. *Journal of Comparative Neurology* 175:311–336.

Hyson, R. L., and Rudy, J. W. (1987). Ontogenetic change in the analysis of sound frequency in the infant rat. *Development Psychobiology* 20(2):189–207.

Hyvarinen, J., Hyvarinen, L, and Linnankoski, I. (1981). Modification of parietal association cortex and functional blindness after binocular deprivation in young monkeys. *Experimental Brain Research* 42:1–8.

Kaas, J. H., Merzenich, M. M., and Killackey, H. P. (1983). The reorganization of somatosensory cortex following peripheral nerve damage in adult and developing mammals. *Annual Review of Neuroscience* 6:325–356.

Lashley, K. S. (1930). The mechanism of vision. I. A method for rapid analysis of pattern-vision in the rat. *Journal of Genetic Psychology* 37:453–460.

Legg, C. R. (1984). Contrast sensitivity at low spatial frequencies in the hooded rat. *Vision Research* 24:159–161.

Lennie, P., and Perry, V. H. (1981). Spatial contrast sensitivity of cells in the lateral geniculate nucleus of the rat. *Journal of Physiology (London)* 315:69–79.

Mayers, K. S., Robertson, R. T., Rubel, E. W., and Thompson, R. T. (1971). Development of polysensory responses in association cells of kitten. *Science* 171:1037–1038.

McCall, R. B., and Lester, M. L. (1969). Differential enrichment potential of visual experience with angles versus curves. *Journal of Comparative and Physiological Psychology* 69:644–648.

Meikle, M. B. (1968, April). *Unit activity in rat association cortex in response to auditory, visual and tactile stimulation.* Paper presented at the meeting of the Western Psychological Association, San Diego.

Meyer, P. M., Meyer, D. R., and Cloud, M. D. (1986). Temporal neocortical injuries in rats impair attending but not complex visual processing. *Behavioral Neuroscience* 100(6):845–851.

Midgley, G. C., and Tees, R. C. (1981). Orienting behavior by rats with visual cortical and subcortical lesions. *Experimental Brain Research* 41:316–328.

Midgley, G. C., and Tees, R. C. (1983). Effect of visual experience on the habituation of orienting behavior. *Behavioral Neuroscience* 97(4):624–638.

Mitchell, D. E., and Timney, B. (1984). Postnatal development of function in the mammalian visual system. In I. Darian-Smith (ed.), *Handbook of Physiology: The Nervous System III*. Bethesda, MD: American Physiological Society, 507–555.

Murdoch, L., and Tees, R. C. (in preparation). The effects of auditory enrichment on the rat's performance on the Morris water maze.

Oswalt, R. M. (1972). Relationship between level of visual pattern difficulty during rearing and subsequent discrimination in rats. *Journal of Comparative and Physiological Psychology* 81:122–125.

Pinto-Hamuy, T., Olavarria, J., Guic-Robles, E., Morgues, M., Nassal, O., and Petit, D. (1987). Rats with lesions in anteromedial extrastriate cortex fail to learn a visuosomatic conditional response. *Behavioural Brain Research* 25:221–231.

Powers, M. K., and Green, D. G. (1978). Single retinal ganglion cell responses in the dark-reared cat: Grating acuity, contrast sensitivity, and defocusing. *Vision Research* 18:1533–1539.

Rhoades, R. W., and Chalupa, L. M. (1978). Receptive field characteristics of superior colliculus neurons and visually guided behavior in dark-reared hamsters. *Journal of Comparative Neurology* 177:17–32.

Rothblat, L. A., Schwartz, M. L., and Kasdan, P. M. (1978). Monocular deprivation in the rat: evidence for an age-related defect in visual behavior. *Brain Research* 158:456–460.

Rubel, E. W. (1985). Auditory system development. In G. Gottlieb and N. A. Krasnegor (eds.), *Measurement of audition and vision in the first year of postnatal life: A methodological overview.* New Jersey: Ablex Publishing Corporation, 53–90.

Ryugo, D. K., Ryugo, R., Globus, A., and Killackey, H. P. (1975). Increased spike density in auditory cortex following visual or somatic differentiation. *Brain Research* 90:143–146.

Schneider, G. E. (1969). Two visual systems. *Science* 163:895–902.

Schwartz, M. L., and Rothblat, L. A. (1980). Long-lasting behavioral and dendritic spine deficits in the monocularly deprived albino rat. *Experimental Neurology* 68:136–146.

Sherman, S. M. (1979). Development of the lateral geniculate nucleus in cats raised with monocular eyelid suture. In R. D. Freeman (ed.), *Developmental neurobiology of vision*. New York: Plenum, 79–97.

Silverman, M. S., and Clopton, B. M. (1977). Plasticity of binaural interaction. I. Effect of early auditory deprivation. *Journal of Neurophysiology* 40:1266–1274.

Sinnamon, H. M., and Charman, C. S. (1988). Unilateral and bilateral lesions of the anteromedial cortex increase perseverative head movements of the rat. *Behavioural Brain Research* 27:145–160.

Spigelman, M. N., and Bryden, M. P. (1967). Effects of early and late blindness on auditory spatial learning in the rat. *Neuropsychologia* 5:267–274.

Sutherland, N. S. (1968). Outlines of a theory of visual pattern recognition in animals and man. *Proceedings of the Royal Society* 71:296–317.

Sutherland, N. S., and Williams, C. (1969). Discrimination of checkerboard patterns by rats. *Journal of Experimental Psychology* 21:77–84.

Sutherland, R. L., and Dyck, R. (1984). Place navigation by rats in a swimming pool. *Canadian Journal of Psychology* 38:322–347.

Symons, L. A., and Tees, R. C. (in press). An examination of the intramodal and intermodal behavioral consequences of long-term vibrassae removal in rats. *Developmental Psychobiology*.

Tees, R. C. (1967). The effects of early auditory restriction in the rat on adult duration discrimination. *Journal of Auditory Research* 7:195–207.

Tees, R. C. (1968). Effect of early restriction on later form discrimination in rat. *Canadian Journal of Psychology* 22:294–298.

Tees, R. C. (1972). Effects of visual restriction in rats on generalization along the dimension of angular orientation. *Journal of Comparative Physiological Psychology* 83:474–502.

Tees, R. C. (1974). Effect of visual deprivation on development of depth perception in the rat. *Journal of Comparative and Physiological Psychology* 86:300–308.

Tees, R. C. (1976a). Mammalian perceptual development. In G. Gottlieb (ed.), *Studies on the development of behavior and the nervous system, Vol. 3*. New York: Academic.

Tees, R. C. (1976b). Depth perception after infant and adult visual neocortical lesions in light- and dark-reared rats. *Developmental Psychobiology* 9(3):223–235.

Tees, R. C. (1979). The effect of visual deprivation on pattern recognition in the rat. *Developmental Psychobiology* 12:485–497.

Tees, R. C. (1986). Experience and visual development: Behavioral evidence: In W. T. Greenough and J. M. Juraska (eds.), *Developmental neuropsychobiology*. Orlando: Academic, 317–361.

Tees, R. C., Bruinsma, Y., and Midgley, G. (1978). The effect of visual deprivation on the rat on transfer effects after form discrimination training. *Developmental Psychobiology* 11:31–49.

Tees, R. C., and Buhrmann, K. (1989). Parallel perceptual/cognitive functions in humans and rats: Space and time. *Canadian Journal of Psychology* 43:266–285.

Tees, R. C., and Midgley, G. (1978). Extent of recovery of function after early sensory deprivation in the rat. *Journal of Comparative Physiological Psychology* 92:742–751.

Tees, R. C., and Midgley, G. (1982). Specifying the effects of visual deprivation on the rat's ability to recognize patterns. *Canadian Journal of Psychology* 36:488–498.

Tees, R. C., Midgley, G., and Bruinsma, Y. (1980). Effect of controlled rearing on the development of stimulus-seeking behaviors in rats. *Journal of Comparative and Physiological Psychology* 94:1003–1018.

Tees, R. C., Midgley, G., and Nesbit, J. C. (1981). The effect of early visual experience on spatial maze learning in rats. *Developmental Psychobiology* 14(5):425–438.

Tees, R. C., and Symons, L. A. (1987). Intersensory coordination and the effects of early sensory deprivation. *Developmental Psychobiology* 20(5):497–507.

Thiessen, D. D., Lindzey, G., and Collins, A. (1969). Early experience and visual cliff behavior in the Mongolian gerbil (*Meriones unguiculatus*): II. *Psychonomic Science* 16(5):240–241.

Thinus-Blanc, C. (1982). Selection of relevant cues in volume discrimination by golden hamsters reared in different environments. *Canadian Journal of Psychology* 36(3):520–526.

Turkewitz, G., and Kenny, P.A. (1982). Limitations on input as a basis for neural organization and perceptual development: A preliminary theoretical statement. *Developmental Psychobiology* 15:357–368.

Walk, R. D. (1978). Depth perception and experience. In R. D. Walk and H. L. Pick, Jr. (eds.), *Perception and experience*. New York: Plenum, 77–103.

Walk, R. D., and Gibson, E. J. (1961). A comparative and analytic study of visual depth perception. *Psychology Monographs* 75:1–44.

Wiesenfeld, Z., and Branchek, T. (1976). Refractive state and visual acuity in the hooded rat. *Vision Research* 16:823–827.

Wilkinson, F., Baker, A. G., and Boothroyd, K. (1986). Some effects of early monocular deprivation in the Mongolian gerbil. *Developmental Brain Research* 26:276–279.

Yinon, U., and Auerbach, E. (1973). Deprivation of pattern vision studied by visual evoked potentials in the rat cortex. *Experimental Neurology* 38:231–251.

23 Sparing and Recovery of Function

Bryan Kolb

When the cerebral cortex is damaged, there is a change in both the remaining brain and in behavior. These changes are not static but continue to evolve for months and, in the case of humans, even years. Little is known about the processes underlying postinjury change in humans, but there is a widespread belief that in view of the brain's plasticity it should be possible to affect some restitution of function. Of course control of the processes of recovery of function will require an understanding of the variables that influence both behavioral and anatomical change after brain injury. The cortex of the rat provides an excellent model for such study. One reason is that the plasticity of the rat cortex is now well documented, and more is known about the processes of plasticity in rats than in any other species. A second reason is that because there is considerable intersubject variability in the effects of brain injury in any species, large numbers of animals are needed to gauge the various factors contributing to the observed brain and behavioral changes. This is possible with animals like rats, but is impractical with larger animals such as cats or monkeys. In this chapter I review the relation between the behavioral change following cortical injury, which I refer to as *recovery* or *sparing* of function, and the change in anatomy and physiology of the remaining brain, which I call *plasticity*.

A distinction needs to be drawn between recovery and sparing of function. Recovery of function refers to behavior that was lost or disturbed by a brain injury and later returned, either wholly or partly. Sparing of function refers to behavior that was either unaffected by a lesion or that was not yet present developmentally at the time of the lesion and then appeared later.

23.1 Problems and Hunches

Evidence of sparing and recovery on the one hand and plasticity on the other has led to the assumption that recovery is mediated by plasticity, but there is still little direct proof of this. To date few experiments have been done on both behavioral and morphological changes in the same animals. Furthermore studies of both behavior and anatomy must necessarily be selective; it is not possible to study all the potential behavioral, structural, or physiological changes at once, so investigators must choose their measures and do so largely on hunches, taking advantage of the technology available to them. Thus a failure to find direct brain-behavior correlations cannot be taken as proof of their absence.

A major principle in scientific investigation is that different researchers must agree about what constitutes the phenomena they are studying. Unfortunately there is no uniform definition of what constitutes recovery. Thus behavioral recovery can refer to different things for different investigators. Figure 23.1 illustrates several different outcomes from lesions studies, each of which leads to different definitions of recovery or sparing. In outcome A there is a complete loss of function. Examples include a failure of an animal to learn some task, even with extended training, or the inability to do something, as in paralysis after a spinal cord transection. In outcome B there is a partial loss of behavior. In this case the subject might be able to perform a behavior under some conditions but not others, or it might be able to perform a task at a reduced level of efficiency. This outcome could result for several reasons, such as the interference with performance by the release of some behavior—for example, a tremor—or because the subject has learned an inefficient strategy for solving the behavioral problem. Finally, in

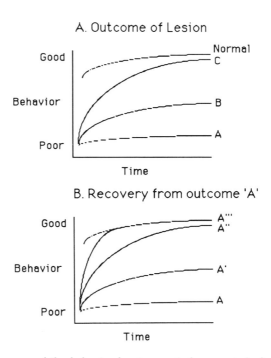

Figure 23.1 Summary of the behavioral outcomes to be expected after cortical lesions. (A) Possible effects of a lesion. There could be a complete and chronic loss of behavior (outcome A), a partial chronic loss of behavior (outcome B), a transient loss of behavior (outcome C), or no change in behavior. (B) Effects of a hypothetical treatment or variable on the different outcomes.

outcome C the subject eventually performs a behavior as well as normal animals do, although it may have sustained a substantial impairment relative to normal animals. The most common example of this occurs in studies where animals are trained to attain some performance criterion, and the lesion effect measured is the time taken to reach the criterion. Although operated animals may be impaired at reaching the criterion, they eventually do so. Note, however, that there is no guarantee that they use the same strategy to reach the performance criterion. Most demonstrations of recovery or sparing of function refer to a quantitative improvement in performance, rather than a complete return of behavior, but it is obvious from figure 23.1 that this improvement implies rather different things in different studies. Few investigators consider precisely what has occurred, making it difficult to correlate recovery with plasticity, especially across studies.

The search for answers in any area of science is guided by hunches, and the greater the ignorance, the more important such hunches become. My own thinking about recovery has been guided by a couple of simple hunches: First, one may assume that biology is conservative and that successful solutions to problems are likely to be used repeatedly. In the current context this implies that the processes of recovery will take advantage of processes utilized for other types of plastic changes in the cortex, two examples of which are learning and development. Hence it makes sense to borrow the behavioral and anatomical techniques used in these fields as we approach recovery. Second, it is clear that there is considerable localization of function in the rat cortex, much as there is in the cortex of larger-brained mammals such as humans. If recovery occurs, it leads us to question how flexible the localization is. My hunch has been that there is not a great deal of flexibility because in the absence of special treatments, there is not normally much recovery, and there are seldom changes in the afferents of the remaining cortex. Thus, if there is to be recovery of some function, we must be wary of two possibilities: The first is that a given region of cortex can process a finite number of computations, so that if a behavior appears to recover, there may be a corresponding reduction in the efficiency of other behaviors. An example of this is the observation that children with early brain injury to the language areas show restitution of language, but at the price of a general lowering of IQ. A similar phenomenon occurs in rats with posterior parietal lesions in infancy— they show improvement on some behaviors, but also a variety of behavioral changes not observed in rats operated on as adults. The second possibility is that a "recovered" behavior may not in fact be the same behavior. For example, Steele Russell (1982) found that monkeys "recovered" from lesions of the frontal eye fields by developing a strategy of moving the head instead of the eyes to track visual targets. It was only with careful observation of behavior that he found the adaptation to be a change in behavior rather than the return of a lost behavior. It is clear that the analysis of behavior must be as sophisticated as the analysis of morphology if we are to develop meaningful correlations between recovery and plasticity.

23.2 Variables Affecting Behavior after Cortical Lesions

At least eight variables influence behavioral recovery after cortical lesions: age, environment, lesion characteristics, postoperative recovery time, neuromodulators, drugs, neurotrophic factors, and choice of behavioral measures. There is a significant literature on each of these variables, so my review is necessarily selective, but tables are included that provide most of the basic references.

In studying recovery of function in the rat, researchers have tended to use one of the following different preparations: hemidecortication or hemispherectomy, bilateral (or unilateral) removal of motor cortex, or bilateral removal of visual, somatosensory, or frontal (i.e., anterior cingulate) cortex.

Age at Brain Damage
There is little doubt that the variable with the greatest effect on behavioral outcome is the age at the time of operation. It is difficult to summarize the effects of age because few systematic studies have looked at the impact of lesions at different ages during the life of the rat. These lesions are typically made either sometime during the first 10 days of life, at the age of weaning, at 90 to 120 days of age, or at 300 to 400 days of age. Behavior is normally assessed in adulthood. Because damage in the first 10 days seems to produce the most interesting effects, I focus on this period.

Table 23.1 summarizes the effects of lesions in various regions. The majority of studies have focused on sensorimotor or frontal cortex lesions, and there is nothing known about the effect of restricted lesions of visual subregions or of temporal auditory or visual areas. Eight generalizations can be made, some of which are summarized in figure 23.2:

1. There is no age at which lesions allow normal behavior, although animals may appear to be normal at performing certain tasks.

2. Bilateral damage very early (first 5 days) allows virtually no sparing, regardless of where the lesion is. The only possible exception may be in animals with relatively small lesions, but this has not been studied systematically.

3. Damage around 10 days of age yields maximal sparing. Even large lesions at that time allow significant sparing, although the amount of sparing is not the same after lesions in different regions. For instance, frontal lesions allow far better sparing than do posterior parietal lesions.

Table 23.1 Summary of the Behavioral Effects of Neonatal Lesions

Lesion	Age	Motor	Sensory	Learning	References
Unilateral lesions					
Motor	P1	PS	PS		Hicks and D'Amato 1970, 1975a,b, Whishaw and Kolb 1988
Frontal	P1			NS	Kolb et al. 1989a
Hemidecorticate	P1–7	S/PS	PS	PS	Kolb et al. 1983c, Kolb and Tomie 1988, Schallert and Whishaw 1985, Tsang 1937, Whishaw et al. 1984, 1986
Bilateral lesions					
Somato	P2		NS/PS		Finger et al. 1978, Simons and Finger 1983
Motor	P4	NS/ND		ND	Kolb and Holmes 1983
Posterior	P1		NS	NS	Bland and Cooper 1969, Schwartz 1964
Gustatory	P2–60		NS		Kiefer et al. 1984
Medial frontal	P1–5	NS		S/NS	Kolb and Nonneman 1978,
	P6–10			S/PS	Kolb and Whishaw 1985a,
	P25	NS		PS	Nonneman and
	P30–40		NS/PS		Corwin 1981,
	P60	NS		NS	Sutherland et al. 1962, Vicedomini et al. 1982
Orbital frontal	P1–5	S/NS/ND			Kolb and Nonneman 1976,
	P6–10	S		S	1978, Kolb and Whishaw
	P25	S		NS	1985a,b,
	P30–40	PS		NS	Nonneman and Corwin
	P60	NS		NS	1981
Large frontal	P1–5	NS/ND		NS/ND	Kolb 1987
	P7	NS		S/PS	Kolb and Whishaw 1981b,
	P10	PS/S		S	Kolb et al. 1983c
	P25	NS		NS/PS	
Posterior parietal	P1 5	NS/PS/ND	NS		Kolb et al. 1987,
	P10	S/ND		NS/PS	Kolb and Whishaw, 1985a
Decorticate	P1–5	NS/PS	NS	NS	Kolb and Wishaw, 1981a, Kolb et al. 1983b, Whishaw and Kolb 1984

NS = no sparing; PS = partial sparing; S = sparing; ND = new deficit; P = postnatal.

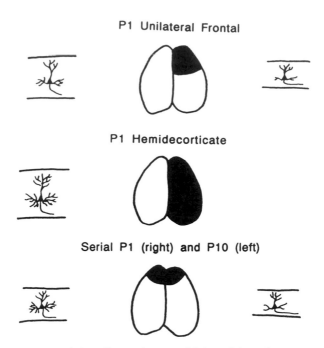

P1 Unilateral Frontal

P1 Hemidecorticate

Serial P1 (right) and P10 (left)

Figure 23.2 Summary of the effects of neonatal bilateral frontal or parietal lesions or hemidecortication on several behaviors and on brain weight. Sparing is most likely after bilateral lesions around 10 days of age or after hemidecortication at 1 day of age. In both cases sparing correlates with brain weight in the infant-operated groups, but early lesions always produce smaller brains than similar lesions in adulthood produce, even when the behavioral effects are less after the early lesions.

4. Sparing is task dependent, and as a general rule sparing is greater for learned behaviors than for species-typical behaviors. For example, in their study of rats with frontal lesions at 7 days of age, Kolb and Whishaw (1981a) found virtually complete sparing on spatial learning tasks in the same animals that were severely impaired at tests of species-typical behaviors such as food hoarding.

5. In some cases there is sparing of behaviors normally affected by lesions in adulthood, but loss or impairment of other behaviors not normally affected by equivalent adult lesions. Hence Kolb and Holmes (1983) found sparing of motor functions after infant motor cortex lesions, but at the price of impaired spatial learning.

6. The amount of sparing decreases as lesion size increases. Thus complete decortication allows no sparing, and lesions removing more than 50 percent of the cortex allow very little sparing, if any.

7. In contrast to the effects of bilateral lesions, hemidecortication allows sparing after very early lesions, but virtually none if the lesion is made at 10 days of age.

8. Lesions made around the time of weaning allow little sparing.

In sum, there is substantial variability in the behavioral effects of lesions at different ages. This variability is especially useful for studies trying to relate recovery and plasticity, for there ought to be morphological, chemical, and perhaps physiological correlates of the different behavioral outcomes.

Environment

Experimental manipulations of environments have focused on both preoperative training and environmental conditions as well as manipulations of both pre- and postoperative experience. The effects of preoperative training vary, but several generalizations are possible: First, there is better recovery of motor behaviors if animals are pretrained. For example, Whishaw (1988) has shown that rats with extensive preoperative training on a reaching task show nearly complete recovery after motor cortex lesions, whereas untrained rats with similar lesions remain chronically impaired. Second, in a recent review Braun (1988) concluded that there is no evidence for preoperative effects on the outcome of lesions in primary sensory regions. Animals with visual or somatosensory lesions nearly always take at least as long to relearn a task as they took for original learning. Third, rats are protected from the effects of frontal lesions on many tests of maze learning if they are preoperatively trained, but there is no protection of performance of delayed-response tests or tests of species-typical behaviors. In sum it appears that preoperative training may reduce the effect of lesions in motor or association regions, but it does not reduce the effect of primary sensory lesions. This may imply that there is stricter localization of function in the primary sensory regions.

There have been few studies of environmental rearing conditions on recovery from neonatal cortical lesions, but in view of the evidence that environment influences both perceptual development (Tees, chapter 22) and brain development (Juraska, chapter 21), one would predict that environment would influence brain and behavioral development after early lesions. Thus Kolb and Elliott (1987) showed that the effects of neonatal frontal lesions made at postnatal days 1 and 5 were significantly attenuated by rearing in an environment that allowed extensive locomotion and exploration of novel stimuli, as compared with rearing in standard laboratory cages. The behavioral improvement was correlated with marked changes in cortical development in the "enriched" animals because their brain was heavier and neocortex thicker than the cage-reared littermates.' Although environmental enrichment can clearly affect the behavioral outcome of cortical injury, it may not always do so. For example, Whishaw and colleagues (1984) showed that enriched housing had very little effect on rats with neonatal hemidecortications. It is unclear which factors might modulate the potential benefits of enrichment, and there needs to be a systematic study of behavior after bilateral and unilateral lesions in different cortical regions.

Postoperative Recovery Time

Behavior tends to improve "spontaneously" after cortical lesions, but there has been little systematic study of this phenomenon. Lesions produce many nonspecific changes in the brain, including edema, reduced metabolic activity and/or blood flow, shock or diaschesis, etc. In humans it is generally believed that these processes may take months to reverse themselves, but little is known about these processes in any species. The possibility that time alone will lead to recovery of function is important because treatments that enhance recovery may do so by influencing nonspecific factors such as metabolic rate rather than by leading to active changes in the brain. In my own studies I have found, for example, that frontal lesions severely disrupt spatial navigation of the Morris water maze, but the deficit declines significantly with recovery time, regardless of whether the animals are simply left in their home cage or given drug treatments such as amphetamine (e.g., Kolb et al. 1988). We simply do not know if this is due to active changes in the brain. A set of experiments by Whishaw (1988) are instructive. Whishaw trained rats to reach for food and then gave them motor cortex lesions. Some rats had gelfoam in the lesion cavity, whereas others were given cortisone and gelfoam. Another group of rats were simply sutured closed. He found that there was virtually complete and immediate recovery of reaching in rats with gelfoam and cortisone, slower recovery (a few days) with just gelfoam, and two-week recovery with no treatment at all. On the basis of histological results, he has concluded that the treatment reduced edema and thus facilitated recovery. The important message from his studies is that unless one can identify a nearly instantaneous morphological change, it is simplest to presume that nonspecific rather than an active change is influencing recovery.

Although it is tempting to think of long recovery times in the rat as being on the order of a month, Finger and colleagues (1982) reported that after somatosensory cortex lesions, there is little improvement of tactile discrimination ability at 1 month or 6 months later, but there was improvement after one or two years. Changes over such time periods are similar to those seen in people and cannot easily be attributed to the dissipation of nonspecific effects of lesions.

Lesion Characteristics

I have already alluded to the fact that larger lesions allow less recovery than do small lesions. In general, if a lesion removes an entire functional system, there typically is far less recovery than if the lesion is partial (Simons and Finger 1983). Of more interest, however, is the *serial lesion effect* (SLE), which refers to the observation that lesions incurred in multiple stages appear to allow more recovery than do single stage removals of the same size (Finger and Stein 1982). The SLE has been seen as a model of slow-growing lesions in humans and would seem to provide an ideal model to search for recovery-plasticity correlations.

Unfortunately, despite intensive study, the behavioral phenomena are still controversial. Nonetheless two conclusions appear warranted: First, I know of no instance in which a behavior that is completely lost from a single-stage lesion has been protected by a serial lesion (see table 23.2). In general the SLE appears to be restricted to recovery from outcome C in figure 23.1. Second, there may be an interaction between experience or training and the SLE. Thus in every instance of the SLE with visual cortex lesions, there was interoperative experience. In the absence of experience, the SLE failed to occur. One experiment is particularly intriguing: Scheff and Wright (1977) found an SLE with visual cortex lesions. They then removed tissue either in the frontal cortex or adjacent to the lesions and found that the latter lesions abolished the SLE. Finally, they recorded visual evoked potentials in the adjacent cortex of animals with one- or two-stage lesions and interoperative experience and found anomalous visual evoked potentials. Their data suggest that the experience produced changes in the adjacent cortex in

Table 23.2 Summary of Serial Lesion Effects (SLE) after Lesions in the Rat Cortex

Lesion	SLE	Behavioral Measure	References
SM	Yes	Tactile discrimination	Simons et al., 1975, Finger and Simons 1976, Finger et al. 1971
	No	Tactile discrimination	Walbran 1976, Finger et al. 1971
Visual	Yes[a]	Black-white discrimination	Scheff and Wright 1977, Scheff et al. 1977, Meyer et al. 1958
	Yes[a]	Pattern discrimination	Spear and Barbas 1975, Dru et al. 1975
	Yes[a]	Brightness	Petrinovich and Carew, 1968, Isaac 1964
Med Fr	Yes	Spontaneous alternation	Patrissi and Stein 1975, Nonneman and Kolb 1979, Corwin et al. 1981, 1982
	Yes	Active avoidance	Nonneman and Kolb 1979
	No	Food hoarding	Nonneman and Kolb 1979
	No	Morris water task	Kolb, unpublished[b]
	No	Spatial reversals	Kolb, unpublished

[a]The serial lesion effect only occurred in these studies if there was interoperative experience. In most studies the experience was training, although in the Isaac study the experience was total sensory stimulation.
[b]This experiment was run on four separate occasions with the same result.
Sm = somatosensory cortex; Visual = visual cortex including areas Oc1 and Oc2; Med Fr = medial frontal cortex.

the two-stage animals. Unfortunately this result has not been pursued further.

In sum the SLE remains poorly understood. Nonetheless the SLE has promise in providing a useful paradigm for studies of recovery and plasticity.

Neuromodulators

Vanderwolf (chapter 6) has shown that pharmacological blockade of neuromodulators, especially serotonin and acetylcholine, has a dramatic effect on cortical electrographic activity and behavior. Similarly there is now considerable evidence that depletion of norepinephrine (NE) in infancy blocks enrichment effects in rats (O'Shea et al. 1983, Mohammed et al. 1986), and various laboratories have shown that both NE and acetylcholine affect the development of ocular dominance in the kitten visual cortex (e.g., Bear and Singer 1986). Taken together, these data suggest that neuromodulators may influence plasticity under various conditions. There is little direct evidence of this after brain injury, however, although under some conditions NE depletion may block sparing from neonatal cortical injury (Sutherland et al. 1982, Castro et al. 1986). For instance, depleting the cortex of NE by pretreating infant rats with 6-hydroxydopamine blocks the sparing normally seen after frontal lesions at 7 days of age and potentiates the effect of early lesions on brain development (Kolb and Sutherland 1986). There is no evidence, however, that *increasing* NE in these preparations improves sparing or recovery. Amphetamine has been claimed to accelerate recovery from outcome C in figure 23.1, but I am unaware of any evidence of amphetamine-induced recovery that would not have occurred with time alone.

Pharmacological Treatments

Several drug treatments have been used to alter recovery, although the most work has been done on amphetamine. Amphetamine has a long history of use in studies of recovery, dating back at least to the 1940s, but the mechanism of action remains a mystery. Thus amphetamine improves relearning of a brightness discrimination (Braun et al. 1966), enhances the serial lesion effect (Cole et al. 1967), and accelerates recovery of locomotion after unilateral (but not bilateral) motor cortex lesions (Feeney et al. 1982). Amphetamine does not facilitate postoperative acquisition of visual learning tasks (Braun et al. 1966), however, nor does it promote recovery of behaviors that are lost after lesions (outcome A, figure 23.1), such as tongue protrusion after tongue area lesions (Kolb, unpublished data, 1989). The effect of amphetamine can be blocked with haloperidol, and it may be effective only if animals are allowed sensory experience under the drug (Feeney et al. 1982). The mechanism whereby amphetamine accelerates recovery is unknown, although its agonistic effect on catecholamines, especially NE, may be important. Several other drugs have been tried as agents to improve recovery, including apomorphine (Corwin et al. 1986), diazepam (Schallert et al. 1986), and phenobarbital (Kennard and Watson 1945), but although they appear to improve recovery under some circumstances, little is known about either the variables affecting this recovery or the mechanisms involved. In sum there are surprisingly few studies of pharmacological agents and recovery from cortical injury, and there is no evidence that any drug produces recovery that would not occur eventually. The possibility that drug treatments enhance recovery is important, however, and will likely be a subject of increasing research. In particular there is increasing evidence that the NMDA-receptor may play a role in synaptic plasticity and thus may be an important place to look in studies of recovery.

Neurotrophic and Hormonal Factors

Several neurotrophic factors, especially nerve growth factor (NGF) and GM1 ganglioside, are known to play a role in development and in the stimulation and guidance of regrowing axons in the peripheral nervous system. Similarly sex hormones, especially androgens, are known to influence neuronal growth in the central nervous system. It thus seems reasonable to expect these factors to influence recovery after cortical damage. To date there have been virtually no studies of the behavioral effects of these treatments following neocortical lesions, and the few available results are equivocal at best (Sabel et al. 1984, Attella et al. 1987).

Choice of Behavioral Tests

The choice of species to study seems to have implications for the analysis of behavioral change. Hyperbolically investigations of humans invariably use paper-and-pencil tests, those of nonhuman primates invariably use some variant of the Wisconsin General Test Apparatus, and those of rats use mazes. The choice of mazes to study rats takes advantage of the well-established ability of rats to navigate accurately through tunnels but, like the narrow choice of behavioral tests made with other species, the study of maze learning in rats results in most of the behavioral repertoire of these animals being ignored.

The reliance on maze tasks in which animals are trained to a performance criterion has led to the erronous belief that recovery and sparing of function is common after many different treatments. Two generalizations can be made. First, there is seldom sparing or recovery of species-typical behaviors, especially those that require the execution of long chains of behaviors. For example, we have consistently failed to find either recovery or sparing of nest building or food hoarding in rats or hamsters with medial frontal lesions (Kolb and Whishaw 1981b, 1985b, Nonneman and Kolb 1979), even when the same animals often showed recovery of maze learning. Second, recovery of performance on maze tests is observed only in tasks with outcome C in figure 23.1. Thus recovery occurs on tasks in which brain-damaged animals normally eventually reach criterion, although perhaps rather slowly. Recovery does not appear to occur on tests that brain-damaged animals fail (i.e., outcomes A or B in figure 23.1). For example, animals with frontal cortex lesions show a serial lesion effect when tested on tasks such as delayed alternation or active avoidance, but not on the Morris water maze (Nonneman and Kolb 1979, Kolb, unpublished data, 1989). The frontal animals normally eventually solve the former tasks, but they never perform normally on the water task.

23.3 Evidence of Plasticity after Cortical Lesions

The cortex would seem an ideal place to look for plastic changes after lesions because it is well laminated, the afferent and efferent projections have restricted terminations, and the tissue is easily accessible. Nonetheless surprisingly little is known. I have grouped the changes into several categories, including gross morphology, connections, neuropil, synaptic alterations, neurochemistry, and metabolic and blood flow changes. I consider each in turn.

Gross Morphological Changes

Gross morphological measures of brain weight, cerebral size, and cortical thickness all show reliable changes after brain damage. Table 23.3 summarizes such observations and allows several conclusions. First, when compared with adult rats' brains with equivalent damage, the brains of rats having received lesions as infants are always smaller and lighter (figure 23.2). Indeed even knife cuts reduce brain weight relative to controls. Second, cortical lesions in young rats reduce cortical thickness in the ipsilateral hemisphere relative to adult operates. Third, as a general rule, the earlier the lesion is received the greater is the loss in cortical thickness. Fourth, in contrast to partial lesions, which have little effect on the contralateral hemisphere, hemidecortication increases cortical thickness in the remaining hemisphere relative to normal controls or to adult operates, the latter of which have a reduction in cortical thickness relative to normal control animals. Fifth, in further contrast to the subtotal decortications, the earlier the hemidecortication is received, the thicker is the cortex. (Kolb 1987, Kolb and Holmes 1983, Kolb 1983a,b, Kolb and Whishaw 1981b, 1985a,b). The changes in cortical thickness have a direct correlation to behavior: The thicker the cortex, the better the sparing.

The changes in gross morphology of the brain and cortex are intriguing because they imply that plastic changes in the cortex must be responsible. Similarly, although the morphological effects of early lesions are truly massive, it seems reasonable to expect to find smaller yet parallel changes in gross morphology after adult lesions. Further it

Table 23.3 Summary of Changes in Brain Weight and Cortical Thickness after
Neonatal Lesions

Group	% Brain Weight	% CTX Thickness
P1 Decorticate	85.*	
P5 Decorticate	108.	
P1 Hemidecorticate	95.*	105.*
P2 Hemidecorticate	95.*	111.*
P5 Hemidecorticate	90.*	102.*
P10 Hemidecorticate	86.*	102.*
P1 Large frontal	73.*	77.*
P2 Large frontal	NA	78.*
P5 Large frontal	81.*	85.*
P7 Large frontal	84.*	90.*
P10 Large frontal	84.*	89.*
P25 Large frontal	97.	94.
P2 Unilateral frontal	85.*	79.* (ipsilateral)
		99. (contralateral)
P1 Motor	92.*	89.*
P4 Motor cortex		
P1 Posterior parietal	81.*	76.*
P4 Posterior parietal	92.*	NA
P5 Posterior parietal	91.*	85.*
P10 Posterior parietal	97.	98.

Numbers represent percent of normal value. Asterisks indicate significant
difference from control. CTX = cortex; NA = not available.

is reasonable to expect that these changes may reflect the effects of
different treatments on cortical plasticity. Indeed both brain weight and
cortical thickness are known to be influenced by environmental stimulation (see Juraska, chapter 21).

Changes in Cortical Connections

In 1970 Hicks and D'Amato demonstrated that if newborn rats were
given a hemispherectomy, there was a small uncrossed corticospinal
projection surviving in adulthood that was not present in adult operates. This observation led to extensive study of corticofugal projections
in rats. The general result is that neonatal hemidecortication or unilateral sensorimotor cortex lesions produce this tract, as well as producing
anomalous crossed corticopontine connections (see Castro, chapter 24,
for a detailed discussion). Similarly studies in the visual and auditory
system have shown an anomalous crossed corticotectal pathway in both
systems (Land et al. 1984, Mustari and Lund 1976, Rhoades 1981).

In addition to changes in descending cortical projections, there have
also been demonstrations of plasticity in cortical connections (see table
23.4). These include (1) increased contralateral and ipsilateral corticos-

Table 23.4 Plasticity in Cortical Connections after Cortical Injury

Anatomical Change	Representative Reference
Adult lesions	
1. Axonal regrowth from small cuts	
	Foerster 1982
2. Thalamic axonal reinnervation after callosal cuts	Vaughn and Peters 1985, Vaughn and Foundas 1982
Neonatal Lesions	
1. Anomolous uncrossed corticospinal pathway after (a) hemidecortication, (b) sensorimotor cortex	Hicks and D'Amato 1970, Leong and Lund 1973
2. Anomolous crossed corticotectal path after unilateral posterior cortex	Mustair and Lund 1976
3. Increased corticopontine projections after unilateral somatosensory lesions	Leong and Lund 1973
4. Increased ipsilateral and contralteral corticospinal projections after hemidecortication	Kolb et al. 1989
5. Anomolous nigrocortical projections after frontal lesion	Kolb and van der Koy 1985
6. Axonal regrowth (or growth) after callosal transection	Sechzer 1974
7. Reorganization of barrelfield after somatosensory lesion	Seo and Ito 1987

triatal projections following neonatal hemidecortication, (2) an anomalous nigrocortical projection to somatosensory cortex after neonatal frontal lesions; (3) axonal regrowth (or growth) after neonatal callosal transection, (4) reorganization of the barrelfield after neonatal somatosensory lesions, (5) reinnervation of layers II and III in the auditory cortex by the auditory thalamus after callosal transection in 30-day-old rats, and (6) axonal regrowth in several systems after small knife cuts. To my knowledge, none of these changes correlates with behavior.

Changes in Neuropil

Plasticity in the dendritic arbor of cortical cells has been shown convincingly after specific environmental events (see Juraska, chapter 21). Until recently, however, there has been no study of this as a mechanism of plasticity after cortical injury, but there is now evidence of changes in dendritic arborization after both neonatal and adult cortical lesions (Kolb and Gibb 1987, Kolb et al. 1989). Thus neonatal hemidecortication on P1 produces an increase in arbor in both the apical and basilar dendrites of layers II and III pyramidal cells in the motor cortex and parietal cortex, but not in the visual or temporal cortex. No changes are found in stellate cells in any of these areas. Second, frontal lesions on day P1, which allow no sparing of function, produced a decrease in both pyramidal apical and basilar dendrites as well as stellate dendrites throughout the cortex. Significantly it was these lesions that produced very thin cortex. In contrast frontal lesions on day P10, which allow significant sparing of function, produced an increase in both apical and basilar dendrites of pyramidal cells in several cortical areas (figure 23.3). Finally, both unilateral motor cortex and bilateral medial frontal cortex lesions in adulthood lead to increased arborization around the lesion border (Kolb and Whishaw, unpublished observations, 1989). In sum, it appears that changes in dendritic arbor correlate with both gross morphology (namely cortical thickness) as well as with the presence of behavioral sparing and recovery (Kolb and Whishaw 1989).

I have emphasized the changes in cortical neuropil after cortical lesions, but changes occur elsewhere as well. In particular there is a decrease in the neuropil of striatal cells after cortical lesions at any age (Kolb, unpublished data, 1989). It is reasonable to expect similar changes elsewhere too, although this has received little attention to date. For example, we have seen diencephalic atrophy after cortical lesions, especially in young animals.

Metabolic Changes
Several laboratories have shown that a unilateral cortical lesion has a significant impact on cortical glucose metabolism in the ipsilateral cortex as well as subcortically. For example, Cooper and Thurlow (1984) have suggested that discrete cortical lesions lead to a transient, temporary depression, especially in the ipsilateral hemisphere. These authors traced the return of normal metabolic activity, finding a significant return of glucose utilization in most locations by about 15 days, although changes continued for some months. Because a close relation between brain metabolism and function has been demonstrated under a variety of physiological conditions, it is reasonable to suppose that metabolic activity might correlate with recovery of function. One potential complication in research on metabolic activity is that because metabolic activity varies with behavior, a change in behavior after a lesion could produce a change in metabolic activity, rather than vice versa. Furthermore differences in postoperative behavior could contribute to the variance in postoperative metabolic activity (e.g., Colle et al. 1986). The possibility that metabolic changes may accompany recovery is intriguing and may be particularly useful in identifying regions in which to look for other morphological changes (for example, see Sharp and Evans 1983). For instance, an increase in metabolic activity may accompany the development of new connections, neuropil, or synapses.

Neurochemical Changes
There are widespread alterations in cerebral monoamine systems following focal cortical lesions in rats, and these alterations change over time, suggesting that there may be a correlation between brain chem-

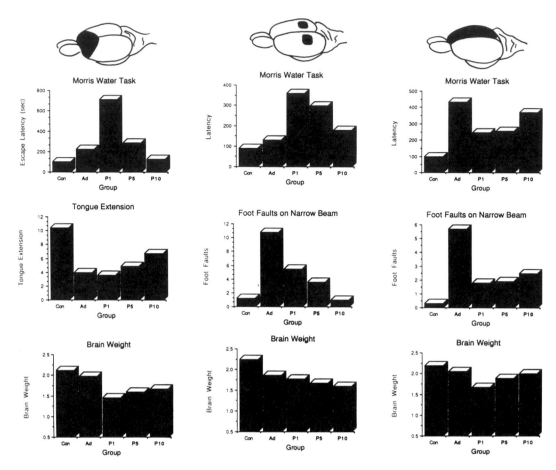

Figure 23.3 Summary of changes in dendritic arborization after neonatal lesions. (Top) A unilateral frontal lesion at P1 leads to a thinner cortex and stunted dendritic arbor ipsilateral to the lesion and no changes contralateral to the lesion. (Middle) Hemidecortication at P1 produces a thicker cortex contralaterally and an increase in dendritic arbor. (Bottom) A unilateral frontal lesion at P10 leads to an increase in dendritic arbor, whereas a similar lesion in the same rat at P1 leads to a decrease in arbor ipsilaterally.

istry and behavior. In a series of studies Robinson and colleagues have shown that small frontal lesions in the right, but not left, frontal cortex of rats produces a bilateral decrease in both NE and dopamine in the cortex and brainstem. These changes in the cortex, which are greater in the ipsilateral hemisphere, slowly reverse toward normal levels over about a 4- to 6-week period (Robinson and Coyle 1980, Robinson et al. 1980, Pearlson and Robinson 1981). The asymmetry of these effects is interesting, but is probably not a general phenomenon because we have found that larger left frontal lesions produce a chronic 50 percent drop in NE, regardless of the age at operation (e.g., Kolb et al. 1989b). Similarly we have found that neonatal frontal lesions decrease NE in the remaining cortex, although we found an *increase* in cortical NE after neonatal hemidecortication (Kolb et al. 1989b). This latter result is intriguing as we found an increase in cortical thickness in neonatal hemidecorticates as well.

The correlation between neurochemical changes and behavior is equivocal at best as no single study has done a careful examination of behavior and chemistry over time. In one study we correlated behavior (Morris water maze), cortical NE, and cortical thickness in rats with neonatal frontal lesions and found that although the morphological measures correlated with one another, chemistry did not correlate with behavior (Kolb et al. 1989b).

23.4   Integration: Sparing, Recovery, and Plasticity

Studies of plasticity and behavior seek to find a mechanism of recovery and sparing of function in the cortex. Unfortunately progress has been slow. Unequivocal evidence of sparing of function has been rare and may be restricted to the effects of lesions around 7 to 10 days for bilateral lesions and perhaps earlier for unilateral lesions. If this time-related sparing proves to be a robust result, it may provide an important clue as to when to look for significant plastic changes in the neocortex. Unequivocal evidence of recovery of function in adult animals has proved very difficult to find, however, especially when one looks for recovery from a lost behavior (outcome A in figure 23.1). Absence of evidence is most certainly not evidence of absence, however, and there are several promising lines of work that has just begun. In particular the pharmacological, neuromodulator, and metabolic approaches may be the most fruitful because there is now compelling evidence of cortical plasticity after cortical injury. Nonetheless there is an important point to consider in the evaluation of these studies: Although it has proved relatively easy to demonstrate morphological changes after brain damage, it has been more difficult to correlate these changes with behavior. Unequivocal demonstrations of recovery and plasticity will not be found until there is a recognition of both the nature of behavioral change after brain injury (figure 23.1) and the complex nature of behavioral assessment. It is not sufficient to demonstrate a quantitative difference in performance between groups of brain-damaged rats studied on a single behavioral task. Behavior is at least as difficult to measure as morphology, and behavioral assessment requires a battery of behavioral tests. No competent neuropsychologist would presume to assess human cortical function with a single behavioral test, and the same rule applies to the study of behavior in the rat.

Another major obstacle in correlating plasticity and behavior is that there is an assumption that changes in the brain are responsible for observed changes in behavior. Thus, for example, if an increase in cortical thickness is associated with improved performance on a learning task, it is reasonable to assume that the behavioral change results from the thicker cortical mantle. What is not considered, however, is that there may have been a prior change in behavior, such as increased exploratory activity, that caused the brain to change. In this case the increased exploration may have both the brain and improved performance in a maze task. Similarly a demonstration of a correlation between cortical NE or regional metabolic activity and improved maze learning does not imply causation because a change in locomotor behavior could be responsible for changes in neurochemistry, metabolism, or maze performance. This complex two-way nature of brain-behavior relations is seldom considered in behavioral neuroscience, but it is nonetheless important. Consider, too, Vanderwolf's demonstration (chapter 6) that behavior alters both cortical electroencephalograms and evoked potentials.

Perhaps the best brain-behavior correlations to date have been found in studies of rats with early lesions, both because the behavioral and anatomical differences following damage at different ages are so large and because the outcomes include both a worsening and an improvement in behavior, depending on the precise age at which the brain is damaged. The large variance in behavioral outcome has thus made it easier to find anatomical correlates of the behavior, including changes in cortical connections, cortical thickness, and dendritic arbor, each of which appears to predict the behavioral outcomes.

The results of studies on the cortex of rats are of interest in themselves, but they will be especially significant if they accord well with what is known about brain-behavior relations in primates, especially humans. It is clear that although significant sparing can occur in humans or nonhuman primates with early cortical injuries, there are clear limits to sparing that are similar to those observed in rats. For example, although damage to the neocortex of infants allows significant sparing of certain functions, such as language, this sparing is partial and is often associated with other unexpected deficits (see Kolb and Whishaw 1985c, 1989 for details). Furthermore, if the damage occurs in the first year or so, the lesions may have more severe effects on general intellectual functioning than if the lesions occur later in early childhood.

These results parallel those observed in rats. Studies of recovery in humans or other primates are few in number and not especially encouraging to date (see Kolb and Whishaw 1985c). Nevertheless there are now clinical trials of amphetamine as a postinjury treatment, a result based directly on work done first with rats. More is known about postinjury plasticity in monkeys than in humans, but again most work has focused on early brain injuries (e.g., Goldman-Rakic et al. 1983, Rakic 1984), and in general the results parallel those observed in rats. To my knowledge, there have been no studies of changes in neuropil after infant lesions in any primate species, however, but our results in rats suggest that this would be a profitable course to pursue.

Acknowledgment

This research was supported by a grant from the Medical Research Council of Canada.

References

Attella, M. J., Nattinville, A., and Stein, D. G. (1987). Hormonal state affects recovery from frontal cortex lesions in adult female rats. *Behavioral and Neural Biology* 48:352–367.

Bear, M. F., and Singer, W. (1986). Modulation of visual cortical plasticity by acetylcholine and nonreadrenaline. *Nature* 320:172–176.

Bland, B., and Cooper, R. M. (1969). Posterior neodecortication in the rat: age at operation and experience. *Journal of Comparative and Physiological Psychology* 69:345–354.

Braun, J. J. (1988). Experimental amnestic sensory agnosia. In J. Schulkin (ed.), *Preoperative events: Their effect on behavior following brain damage.* Hillsdale, N.J.: Lawrence Erlbaum.

Braun, J. J., Meyer, P. M., and Meyer, D. R. (1966). Sparing of a brightness habit in rats following visual decortication. *Journal of Comparative and Physiological Psychology* 61:79–82.

Castro, A. J., Kartje-Tillotson, G., Barnes, D., and Swenson, R. D. (1986). Disruption of corticospinal plasticity by 6-hydroxydopamine as measured by intracortical microstimulation in rats. *Developmental Brain Research* 24:295–298.

Cole, D., Sullins, W. R., and Isaac, W. (1967). Pharmacological modification of the effects of spaced occipital ablations. *Psychopharmacologia* 11:311–316.

Colle, L. M., Holmes, L. J., and Pappius, H. M. (1986). Correlation between behavioral status and cerebral glucose utilization in rats following freezing lesion. *Brain Research* 397:27–36.

Cooper, R. M., and Thurlow, G. A. (1984). 2-deoxyglucose uptake in the thalamus of awake rats after neocortical ablations. *Experimental Neurology* 86:261–271.

Corwin, J. V., Nonneman, A., and Goodlett, C. (1981). Limited sparing of function on spatial delayed alternation after two-stage lesions of prefrontal cortex in the rat. *Physiology and Behavior* 26:763–771.

Corwin, J. V., Kanter, S., Watson, R. T., Heilman, K. M., Valenstein, E., and Hashimoto, A. (1986). Apomorphine has a therapeutic effect on neglect produced by unilateral dorsomedial prefrontal cortex lesions in rats. *Experimental Neurology* 94:683–698.

Corwin, J. V., Vicedomini, J. P., Nonneman, A. J., and Valentino, L. (1982). Serial lesion effect in rat medial frontal cortex as a function of age. *Neurobiology of Aging* 3:69–76.

Dru, D., Walker, J. P., and Walker, J. B. (1975). Self-produced locomotion restores visual capacity after striate lesions. *Science* 187:265–266.

Feeney, D. M., Gonzalez, A., and Law, W. A. (1982). Amphetamine, haloparidol, and experience interact to affect rate of recovery after motor cortex injury. *Science* 217:855–857.

Finger, S., Hart, T., and Jones, E. (1982). Recovery time and sensorimotor cortex lesions effects. *Physiology & Behavior* 29:73–78.

Finger, S., and Stein, D. G. (1982). *Brain Damage and Recovery: Research and Clinical Perspectives.* New York: Academic Press.

Finger, S., Marshak, R. A., Cohen, M., Scheff, S., Trace, R., and Niemand, D. (1971). Effects of successive and simultaneous lesions of somatosensory cortex on tactile discrimination in the rat. *Journal of Comparative and Physiological Psychology* 77:221–227.

Finger, S., and Simons, D. (1976). Effects of serial lesions of somatosensory cortex and further neodecortication on retention of a rough-smooth discrimination in rats. *Experimental Brain Research* 25:183–197.

Finger, S., Simmons, D., and Posner, R. (1978). Anatomical, physiological and behavioral effects of neonatal sensorimotor cortex ablation in the rat. *Experimental Neurology* 60:347–373.

Foerster, A. P. (1982). Spontaneous regeneration of cut axons in adult rat brain. *Journal of Comparative Neurology* 210:335–356.

Goldman-Rakic, P. S., Isseroff, A., Schwartz, M. L., and Bugbee, N. M. (1983). The neurobiology of cognitive development. In P. Mussen (ed.), *Handbook of Child Psychology: Biology and Infant Development.* New York: Wiley.

Hicks, S. P., and D'Amato, C. J. (1970). Motor-sensory and visual behavior after hemispherectomy in newborn and mature rats. *Experimental Neurology* 29:416–438.

Hicks, S. P., and D'Amato, C. J. (1975a). Motor-sensory cortex-corticospinal system and developing locomotion and placing in rats. *American Journal of Anatomy* 143:1–42.

Hicks, S. P., and D'Amato, C. J. (1975b). Functional adaptation after brain injury and malformation in early life in rats. In *Abberant development in infancy.* London: Wiley, 27–47.

Isaac, W. (1964). Role of stimulation and time in the effects of spaced occipital ablations. *Psychological Reports* 14:151–154.

Kennard, M. A., and Watson, C. W. (1945). The effect of anticonvulsant drugs on recovery of function following cerebral cortical lesions. *Journal of Neurophysiology* 8:221–231.

Kiefer, S. W., Cabral, R. J., and Garcia, J. (1984). Neonatal ablations of the gustatory neocortex in the rat: Taste aversion learning and taste reactivity. *Behavioral Neuroscience* 98:804–812.

Kolb, B. (1987). Recovery from early cortical damage in rats. I. Differential behavioral and anatomical effects of frontal lesions at different ages of neural maturation. *Behavioral Brain Research* 25:205–220.

Kolb, B., Day, J., Gibb, R., and Whishaw, I. Q. (1989b). Recovery from early cortical lesions in rats. 6. Cortical noradrenaline depletion following frontal lesions is correlated with reduced cortical thickness but not with spatial learning. *Psychobiology,* in press.

Kolb, B., and Elliott, W. (1987). Recovery from early cortical damage in rats. II. Effects of experience on anatomy and behavior following frontal lesions at 1 or 5 days of age. *Behavioral Brain Research* 26:47–56.

Kolb, B., and Gibb, R. (1987). Dendritic proliferation as a mechanism of recovery and sparing of function. *Society for Neuroscience Abstracts* 13:1430.

Kolb, B., Gibb, R., and van der Kooy, D. (1989). Cortical development after neonatal cortical lesions. I. Effects of hemidecortication. (Submitted for publication.)

Kolb, B., and Holmes, C. (1983). Neonatal motor cortex lesions in the rat: absence of sparing of motor behaviors and impaired spatial learning concurrent with abnormal cerebral morphogenesis. *Behavioral Neuroscience* 97:697–709.

Kolb, B., Holmes, C., and Whishaw, I. Q. (1987). Recovery from early cortical lesions in rats. III. Neonatal removal of posterior parietal cortex has greater behavioral and anatomical effects than similar removals in adulthood. *Behavioral Brain Research* 26:119–137.

Kolb, B., and Nonneman, A. J. (1976). Functional development of the prefrontal cortex continues into adolescence. *Science* 193:335–336.

Kolb, B., and Nonneman, A. J. (1978). Sparing of function in rats with early prefrontal cortex lesions. *Brain Research* 157:135–148.

Kolb, B., Reynolds, B., and Fantie, B. (1988). Frontal cortex grafts have different effects at different postoperative recovery times. *Behavioral and Neural Biology* 50:193–206.

Kolb, B., and Sutherland, R. J. (1986). A critical period for noradrenergic modulation of sparing from neocortical parietal cortex damage in the rat. *Society for Neuroscience Abstracts* 12:322.

Kolb, B., Sutherland, R. J., and Whishaw, I. Q. (1983a). Abnormalities in cortical and subcortical morphology after neonatal neocortical lesions in rats. *Experimental Neurology* 79:223–244.

Kolb, B., Sutherland, R. J., and Whishaw, I. Q. (1983b). A comparison of the contributions of the frontal and parietal association cortex to spatial localization in rats. *Behavioral Neuroscience* 97:13–27.

Kolb, B., Sutherland, R. J., and Whishaw, I. Q. (1983c). Neonatal hemidecortication or frontal cortex ablation produces similar behavioral sparing but opposite effects on morphogenesis of remaining cortex. *Behavioral Neuroscience* 97:154–158.

Kolb, B., and Tomie, J. (1988). Recovery from early cortical damage in rat. IV. Effects of hemidecortication at 1, 5 or 10 days of age on cerebral anatomy and behavior. *Behavioral Brain Research* 28:259–274.

Kolb, B., and van der Kooy, D. (1985). Early cortical lesions alter cerebral morphogenesis and connectivity in the rat. *Society for Neuroscience Abstracts* 11:989.

Kolb, B., and Whishaw, I. Q. (1981a). Decortication in rats in infancy or adulthood produced comparable functional losses on learned and species-typical behaviors. *Journal of Comparative and Physiological Psychology* 95:468–483.

Kolb, B., and Whishaw, I. Q. (1981b). Neonatal frontal lesions in the rat: sparing of learned but not species-typical behavior in the absence of reduced brain weight and cortical thickness. *Journal of Comparative and Physiological Psychology* 95:863–879.

Kolb, B., and Whishaw, I. Q. (1985a). Earlier is not always better: behavioral dysfunction and abnormal cerebral morphogenesis following neonatal cortical lesions in the rat. *Behavioral Brain Research* 17:25–43.

Kolb, B., and Whishaw, I. Q. (1985b). Neonatal frontal lesions in hamsters impair species-typical behaviors and reduce brain weight and neocortical thickness. *Behavioral Neuroscience* 99:691–706.

Kolb, B., and Whishaw, I. Q. (1985c). *Fundamentals of Human Neuropsychology.* 2nd ed. New York: Freeman & Co.

Kolb, B., and Whishaw, I. Q. (1989). Plasticity in the neocortex: mechanisms underlying recovery from early brain damage. *Progress in Neurobiology* 32:235–276.

Kolb, B., Zaborowski, J., and Whishaw, I. Q. (1989a). Recovery from early cortical damage in rats: 5. Unilateral lesions have different behavioral and anatomical effects than bilateral lesions. *Psychobiology* (in press).

Land, P. W., Rose, L. L., Harvey, A. R., and Liverman, S. A. (1984). Neonatal auditory cortex lesions result in aberrant crossed corticotectal and corticothalamic projections in rats. *Developmental Brain Research* 12:126–130.

Leong, S. K., and Lund, R. D. (1973). Anomalous bilateral corticofugal pathways in albino rats after neonatal lesions. *Brain Research* 62:218–221.

Meyer, D. R., Isaac, W., and Maher, B. (1958). The role of stimulation in spontaneous reorganization of visual habits. *Journal of Comparative and Physiological Psychology* 51:546–548.

Mohammed, A. K., Johsson, G., and Archer, T. (1986). Selective lesioning of forebrain noradrenaline neurons at birth abolishes the improved maze learning performance induced by rearing in complex environment. *Brain Research* 398:6–10.

Mustari, M. J., and Lund, R. D. (1976). An aberrant crossed visual corticotectal pathway in albino rats. *Brain Research* 112:37–44.

Nonneman, A. J., and Corwin, J. F. (1981). Differential effects of prefrontal cortex ablation in neonatal, juvenile, and young adult rats. *Journal of Comparative and Physiological Psychology* 95:588–602.

Nonneman, A. J., and Kolb, B. (1979). Functional recovery after serial ablation of pre-frontal cortex in the rat. *Physiology and Behavior* 22:895–901.

O'Shea, L., Saari, M., Pappas, B. A., Ings, R., and Stange, K. (1983). Neonatal 6-hydroxydopamine attenuates the neural and behavioral effects of enriched rearing in the rat. *European Journal of Pharmacology* 92:43–47.

Patrissi, G., and Stein, D. G. (1975). Temporal factors in recovery of function after brain damage. *Experimental Neurology* 47:470–480.

Pearlson, G. D., and Robinson, R. G. (1981). Suction lesions of the frontal cerebral cortex in the rat induce asymmetrical behavioral and catecholaminergic responses. *Brain Research* 218:233–242.

Petrinovich, L., and Carew, T. J. (1968). Interaction of neocortical lesion size and interop experience in retention of a learned brightness disc. *Journal of Comparative and Physiological Psychology* 68:451–454.

Rakic, P. (1984). Defective cell-to-cell interactions as causes of brain malformations. In E. S. Gollin (ed.), *Malformations of development: Biological and psychological sources and consequences.* New York: Academic Press.

Rhoades, R. W. (1981). Expansion of the ipsilateral visual corticotectal projection in hamsters subjected to partial lesions of the visual cortex during infancy: Anatomical experiments. *Journal of Comparative Neurology* 197:425–445.

Robinson, R. G., and Coyle, J. T. (1980). The differential effect of right versus left hemispheric cerebral infarction on catecholamines and behavior in the rat. *Brain Research* 188:63–78.

Robinson, R. G., Shoemaker, W. J., and Schlumpf, M. (1980). Time course of changes in catecholamines following right hemispheric cerebral infarction in the rat. *Brain Research* 181:202–208.

Sabel, B. A., Dunbar, G. L., and Stein, D. G. (1984). Gangliosides minimize behavioral deficits and enhance structural repair after brain injury. *Journal of Neuroscience Research* 12:429–443.

Schallert, T., Hernandez, T. D., and Barth, T. M. (1986). Recovery of function after brain damage: Severe and chronic disruption by diazepam. *Brain Research* 379:104–111.

Schallert, T., and Whishaw, I. Q. (1985). Neonatal hemidecortication and bilateral cutaneous stimulation in rats. *Developmental Psychobiology* 18:501–514.

Scheff, S., Bernardo, L., and Cotman, C. (1977). Progressive brain damage accelerates axon sprouting in the adult rat. *Science* 197:795–797.

Scheff, S. W., and Wright, D. C. (1977). Behavioral and electrophysiological evidence for cortical reorganization of function in rats with serial lesions of the visual cortex. *Physiological Psychology* 5:103–107.

Schulkin, J. (1988). *Preoperative events: their effects on on behavior following brain damage.* Hillsdale, N.J.: Erlbaum.

Schwartz, S. (1964). Effect of neonatal cortical lesions and early environmental factors on adult rat behavior. *Journal of Comparative and Physiological Psychology* 57:72–77.

Sechzer, J. A. (1974). Axonal regeneration or generation after corpus callosum section in the neonatal rat. *Experimental Neurology* 45:186–188.

Seo, M. L., and Ito, M. (1987). Reorganization of rat vibrissa barrelfield as studied by cortical lesioning on different postnatal days. *Experimental Brain Research* 65:251–260.

Sharp, F., and Evans, P. (1983). Bilateral [14C]2-deoxyglucose uptake by motor pathways after unilateral neocortex lesions in the rat. *Developmental Brain Research* 6:1–11.

Simons, D. J., and Finger, S. (1983). Neonatal vs. adult sensorimotor cortex damage: The ability to use spared cortical fragments of target tissue to guide tactile learning. *Physiological Psychology* 11:29–34.

Simons, D., Puretz, J., and Finger, S. (1975). Effects of serial lesions of somatosensory cortex and further neodecortication on tactile retention in rats. *Experimental Brain Research* 23:353–365.

Spear, P. D., and Barbas, H. (1975). Recovery of pattern discrimination ability in rats receiving serial or one-stage visual cortex lesions. *Brain Research* 94:337–346.

Steele Russell, I. (1982). Some observations on the problem of recovery of function following brain damage. *Human Neurobiology* 1:68–72.

Sutherland, R. J., Kolb, B., Becker, J. B., and Whishaw, I. Q. (1982). Cortical noradrenaline depletion eliminates sparing of spatial learning after neonatal frontal cortex damage in the rat. *Neuroscience Letters* 32:125–130.

Tsang, Y. C. (1937). Maze learning in rats hemidecorticated in infancy. *Journal of Comparative Psychology* 24:221–248.

Vaughn, D. W., and Foundas, S. (1982). Synaptic proliferation in the auditory cortex of young adult rat following callosal lesions. *Journal of Neurocytology* 11:29–51.

Vaughn, D. W., and Peters, A. (1985). Proliferation of thalamic afferents in cerebral cortex altered by callosal deafferentation. *Journal of Neurocytology* 14:705–716.

Vicedomini, J. P., Corwin, J. V., and Nonneman, A. J. (1982). Role of residual anterior neocortex in recovery from neonatal prefrontal lesions in the rat. *Physiology and Behavior* 28:797–806.

Walbran, B. B. (1976). Age and serial ablations of somatosensory cortex in the rat. *Physiology and Behavior* 17:13–17.

Whishaw, I. Q. (1988). Factors affecting recovery from motor cortex damage in rats. Talk presented at the Canadian Psychological Association, Montreal, Quebec.

Whishaw, I. Q., and Kolb, B. (1984). Behavioral and anatomical studies of rats with complete or partial decortication in infancy: functional sparing, crowding or loss and cerebral growth or shrinkage. In R. Almli and S. Finger (eds.), *Recovery of Function*, Vol. 2. New York: Academic Press, 117–138.

Whishaw, I. Q., and Kolb, B. (1988). Sparing of skilled forelimb reaching and corticospinal projections after neonatal motor cortex removal or hemidecortication in the rat: Support for the Kennard doctrine. *Brain Research* 451:97–114.

Whishaw, I. Q., Sutherland, R. J., Kolb, B., and Becker, J. B. (1986). Effects of neonatal forebrain noradrenaline depletion on recovery from brain damage: Performance on a spatial navigation task as a function of age of surgery and postsurgical housing. *Behavioral and Neural Biology* 46:285–307.

Whishaw, I. Q., Zaborowski, J., and Kolb, B. (1984). Postsurgical enrichment aids adult hemidecorticate rats on a spatial navigation task. *Behavioral and Neural Biology* 42:183–190.

24   Plasticity in the Motor System

Anthony J. Castro

Neuroanatomical plasticity after central nervous system (CNS) injury has been clearly demonstrated in numerous studies over the past fifteen to twenty years. In mammals, as particularly demonstrated by studies on rats, hamsters, cats, and, to a much lesser extent, monkeys, this response is expressed typically by a qualitative and/or quantitative alteration of axonal connections that were not damaged by the injury. Because plasticity is commonly more prominent if lesions occur perinatally, it is often proposed to explain why functional recovery may be more pronounced after CNS lesions in the newborn in comparison with lesions occurring at maturity, i.e., the *Kennard principle*. However, direct evidence for a causal relation between plasticity and recovery is generally lacking (Finger and Almli 1985, Goldberger 1986). In fact the evidence is sometimes contradictory. For example, plasticity found in the developing hamster visual system after tectal lesions has been associated with a maladaptive response to a visual stimulus (Schneider 1979, Finlay et al. 1979). Similarly the possibility that the spasticity that occurs after spinal cord lesions may be mediated by the observed sprouting of dorsal root afferents (Chambers et al. 1973, Goldberger and Murray 1985) does not represent a return of normal function, even though it might provide a basis for functional recovery (Goldberger and Murray 1978, 1985). Such observations may therefore challenge the usefulness of anatomical plasticity to the behaving animal. Nonetheless they suggest that remodeled connections may indeed be functional, albeit with negative consequences as far as an animal's ability to perform specific tasks is concerned.

Accounts of the possible negative effects of neuroanatomical plasticity on recovery support several reports that have redefined the Kennard principle by employing behavioral tasks that revealed more prominent deficits after lesions occurring shortly after birth (Schneider 1979, Stein et al. 1983, Kolb and Whishaw 1985, Kolb 1987, Kolb and Elliott 1987, Kolb et al. 1987). In serving to qualify the unreserved application of the Kennard principle, such studies demonstrate that (1) the testing methods used in assessing function, (2) the time of lesion placement within the developmental sequence, (3) the postoperative time of testing, and

(4) the postoperative environmental experience of the animals are variables that significantly affect the outcome of lesions occurring at various ages.

Extensive analysis demonstrating some of these variables included testing of rats on a variety of motor functions, such as tongue extension, grooming, beam walking, swimming, and spatial navigation (Kolb 1987, Kolb and Tomie 1988). In this work rats receiving *bilateral* frontal cortical lesions at 10 days of age performed better than did rats receiving lesions as adults, whereas rats receiving the same lesions at 5 days of age performed similar to adult operates on most tests, and those sustaining bilateral frontal cortical lesions at 1 day of age showed more impairment than all other groups. In comparison rats receiving *unilateral* cortical lesions at the younger ages performed better than did the adult lesion group. Moreover those receiving the earliest unilateral lesions performed best. In further work animals receiving unilateral cortical lesions at birth showed less impairment than an adult lesion group showed when tested on a skilled forelimb task that required rats to reach between cage bars to grasp food pellets (Whishaw and Kolb 1988). In demonstrating the importance of age and testing methods as well as the extent of the lesions, the results obtained after unilateral cortical lesions support other reports that are also in accordance with the Kennard principle. For example, testing on a series of complex motor and behavioral tests showed greater recovery after unilateral cortical hemispherectomy in neonatal cats as compared with adult operates (Burgess and Villablanca 1986, Burgess et al. 1986, Villablanca et al. 1986).

In view of findings showing greater recovery of motor function after lesions in newborn animals, this chapter is intended to examine the lesion-induced remodeling of motor pathways in relation to functional recovery.

24.1 The Structural-Functional Analysis of Plasticity

The possible relation of neuroanatomical plasticity to functional recovery, as extensively reviewed by Steward (1982), is difficult to assess because several criteria must be satisfied to demonstrate a cause-effect correlation. *First* and foremost among these criteria is the necessity for demonstrating that the measured behavior is directly related to the neuronal systems or structures under examination. Although this appears to be an obvious prerequisite, the specific functions of particular regions within the CNS are often not well understood. For example, although numerous experiments demonstrating the lesion-induced remodeling of hippocampal pathways have led to important insights concerning the principles guiding neuronal plasticity (Cotman and Nieto-Sampedro 1982), the complex nature of hippocampal-related functions make structural-functional associations very difficult. *Second*, the observed plasticity should be consistent with known data on normal projections. A lesion-induced reorganization of connections that departs from normal topography or that results in projections to areas generally not associated with the system under study can lead to highly speculative interpretations. An example of this derives from interesting studies that show the development of anomalous retinal projections to the medial geniculate nucleus after ablation of the retina's principal targets (the superior colliculus and dorsolateral geniculate nucleus) and the medial geniculate's principal input (ascending auditory pathways) in newborn hamsters (Frost 1982). These abnormal projections, which showed evidence of a retinotopic distribution, raise intriguing questions concerning the usefulness of visual information being relayed to the auditory cortex (Frost 1982).[1] *Third,* the remodeled connections should establish synaptic contacts that are electrophysiologically viable. Although electron microscopic analysis has often provided anatomical evidence of synaptic plasticity, the electrophysiological viability of these connections may be more difficult to evaluate. This is particularly true when remodeling may involve the redistribution of synapses to different regions of the postsynaptic neuron, as has been observed with corticorubral remodeling after cerebral cortical lesions (Kosar et al. 1985, Tsukahara 1985). Electrophysiological relevance may be further clouded in cases where axonal remodeling results in a novel innervation pattern presenting neurotransmitter-containing pathways that are atypical for a particular region within the CNS. In this regard several studies have shown the remodeling of cholinergic septohippocampal projections in response to lesions that alter noncholinergic hippocampal afferents (Cotman and Nieto-Sampedro 1982, Zimmer et al. 1986).

24.2 The Corticospinal Tract and Related Pathways as a Model System

The analysis of plasticity in accordance with the conditions presented above necessitates several experiments using wide-ranging techniques. However, many of the difficulties in correlating plasticity with recovery may be simplified by using an experimental model with well-defined behavioral and physiological functions. In this regard the rodent corticospinal tract (CST) may serve as a model system for study. Similar to that of the primate, the rodent CST is associated with the control of precise, individual limb and digit movements (Castro 1972, Kalil and Schneider 1975, Lawrence and Kuypers 1968a, Reh and Kalil 1982). Accordingly the sparing of purposeful limb and digit movements after a CNS injury would indicate that the CST system is intact and working properly or that other systems have adapted to support some of the functions normally subserved by the CST.

Studies showing less impairment of a skilled forelimb-reaching task after unilateral cortical lesions in neonatal rats as compared with adults with similar lesions (Whishaw and Kolb 1988) indicate that the newborn

Castro: Plasticity in the Motor System

rat possesses recovery mechanisms that are not operative in the adult nervous system. Assuming that the animals are not using different behavioral strategies to accomplish the task, this finding suggests that either different neuronal pathways have altered the ability to recover CST-mediated functions or that the CST projection from the spared hemisphere has somehow compensated for the unilaterally ablated pathway. The latter possibility is supported by the general observation that bilateral lesions—which, in the case of the sensorimotor cortex, would disrupt the CST bilaterally—are more debilitating than unilateral lesions (Kolb 1987, Kolb and Tomie 1988, also see Kolb, chapter 23). Additionally the finding that bilateral cortical lesions produce *greater* behavioral deficits when performed in the perinatal period rather than in adolescence or adulthood suggests that the spared hemisphere may be responsible for the marked sparing of function after unilateral lesions in the newborn. Indeed several studies, as detailed below, have demonstrated bilateral CST projections originating from the spared hemisphere after unilateral cortical lesions in the newborn, but not the adult, rat. The presence of bilateral CST projections, which is clearly different from the normal contralateral distribution, provides the anatomical framework enabling one cortical hemisphere to exert direct control over limbs on both sides of the body.

Although discrete, skilled movements may be controlled primarily by the CST, the activity of this pathway operates in concert with many other neuronal projections that are involved in orienting and posturing the body to perform even the simplest of motor acts. Considered in this light, CST plasticity after neonatal cortical lesions is likely to reflect one component of an extensive pattern of remodeling involving several pathways. This chapter therefore focuses on the remodeling of corticospinal and cortico-brainstem pathways observed after cerebral cortical lesions. Remodeling found after other lesions is included when it serves to illustrate further the use of the CST as a model system to study plasticity or to demonstrate the remodeling of other pathways generally considered to affect motor output. The possible role of plasticity in recovery of function is indirectly considered by examining remodeling in relation to the conditions or parameters outlined in the preceding section. As a general rule the plasticity described in this report is attributed to the lesion-induced growth or axonal sprouting of existing connections rather than to the abnormal persistence of developmentally transient projections (Mihailoff et al. 1984, Nah et al. 1980, Schreyer and Jones 1982).

Although much of the work described in this chapter has been done on rats, the use of the rodent CST as a model system to study plasticity is supported by studies of remodeling using other species. For example, work on cats demonstrated an increase of ipsilateral cortical projections to the spinal cord and dorsal column nuclei after unilateral cerebral hemispherectomy sustained shortly after birth (Gomez-Pinella et al.

1986). Also unilateral prefrontal cortical lesions made at six weeks before birth in monkeys resulted in an increase of cortical projections from the unablated hemisphere to the contralateral caudate nucleus (Goldman 1978). Additional work on monkeys did not reveal cortical efferent remodeling in response to unilateral motor or sensorimotor cortical lesions made between 7 days and 3 months of age (Sloper et al. 1983). However, this absence of remodeling was attributed to the relative maturity of the newborn monkey brain compared with that of the rat.

24.3 Corticospinal Plasticity

Cerebral Cortical Lesions
The CST in rodents as well as in other mammals is primarily a crossed projection, although a small ipsilateral component has been reported (Vahlsing and Feringa 1980). However, after unilateral sensorimotor cerebral cortical lesions in newborn rats, a quantitative increase in ipsilateral CST fibers originating from the unablated hemisphere has been described in several papers (Hicks and D'Amato 1970, Leong and Lund 1973, Castro 1975) (figure 24.1). Comparable remodeling of the unablated CST was also observed after unilateral medullary pyramidotomy in the newborn rat (Castro 1978a). These anomalous ipsilateral CST fibers, abnormal in the sense of being more numerous than those found in normal mature rats, were not observed in response to cortical lesions made beyond postnatal day 17 (Hicks and D'Amato 1970, Leong 1976a). In initial studies the abnormal CST fibers were found traversing the base of the ipsilateral dorsal funiculus, similar in course to the normal rodent CST, but on the opposite side. Recent work using more sensitive tracing methods described an additional anomalous CST projection within the ipsilateral ventral funiculus (Reinoso and Castro 1986). These ipsilateral fibers appeared to terminate within areas of the spinal cord

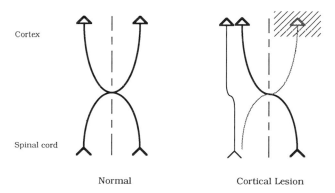

Figure 24.1 Corticospinal tract remodeling after a unilateral cortical lesion in the newborn. In this and subsequent figures, the hatched area indicates a neonatal lesion, and the shaded line represents axonal degeneration.

Castro: Plasticity in the Motor System

gray matter that corresponded to the normal crossed CST projections. Electron microscopic studies indicated that these projections make normal synaptic contacts, suggesting a functional viability (Leong 1976b, McClung and Castro 1975).

Characteristically, normal CST projections from fore- and hindlimb areas of the motor cortex project topographically to cervical and lumbar spinal cord levels (Wise et al. 1979, Ullan and Artieda 1981, Miller 1987). This somatotopy reflects the precise motor control associated with the CST system. Recent work involving the use of retrograde transported fluorescent dyes demonstrated a similar topography for the anomalous ipsilateral CST projections (Reinoso and Castro 1989) (figure 24.2). This study also showed that the ipsilateral CST fibers arise not as collateral branches of normal crossed projections but from a separate neuronal population (Reinoso and Castro 1989). These findings thus indicate the correct anatomical framework for the control of independent limb movement by the ipsilateral CST pathway.

Cerebral cortical control of limb movements via the CST is demonstrated in several reports that examined movements evoked by intracortical microstimulation at low current intensities (see Neafsey, chapter 8). These low-threshold, evoked movements were not found after medullary pyramidal lesions that transected CST fibers (Asanuma et al. 1981, Kartje-Tillotson et al. 1987). Using the microstimulation procedure in normal adult rats, low current intensities evoked only contralateral limb movements corresponding to the predominantly crossed CST projection. However, intracortical microstimulation of the unablated hemisphere in mature rats that sustained unilateral cortical lesions at birth

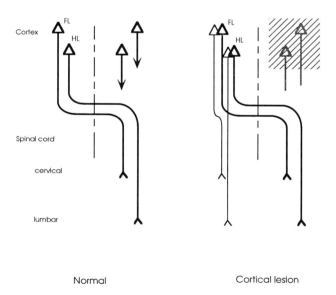

Figure 24.2 Topographic distribution of forelimb (FL) and hindlimb (HL) corticospinal tract projections after neonatal cortical lesion

evoked bilateral limb movements at low current thresholds (Kartje-Tillotson et al. 1985). Disruption of the evoked movements by medullary pyramidotomy indicated that these movements were mediated by corticospinal rather than corticobulbar fibers. However, the question remains as to the possible role of normal crossed CST fibers in controlling anomalous ipsilateral movements. A better test of the physiological function of the ipsilateral CST would be to examine the effects of a specific lesion of the anomalous CST fibers. Unfortunately, although the ipsilateral fibers course separately from normal fibers within the base of the spinal cord dorsal funiculus, their proximity to normal CST projections and to dorsal column pathways makes such a lesion improbable.

Spinal Cord and Medullary Pyramidal Lesions
Evidence of a greater remodeling after neonatal rather than adult lesions is often explained in terms of an intrinsic plasticity associated with developing systems. Accordingly CST remodeling after unilateral, neonatal cortical ablation appears to correspond to the protracted postnatal development of this pathway (Donatelle 1977, Schreyer and Jones 1982, Kort et al. 1985). The predominantly postnatal development of this system, which at birth only extends to the upper cervical spinal cord, makes it a particularly useful model for studying axonal growth and plasticity after spinal cord damage as well as plasticity after cortical lesions. For example, developing CST axons have been observed to grow around partial midthoracic spinal cord lesions made in newborn to 6-day-old rats (Bernstein and Stelzner 1983, Schreyer and Jones 1983). Although not observed after lesions made at older ages (Bernstein and Stelzner 1983), CST growth around lesions made in 6-day-old rats suggests that transected growing axons may regenerate. Recent work demonstrating the survival of CST neurons after spinal cord axotomy (Bates and Stelzner 1987) supports this possibility. In this work retrograde fluorescent tracers were injected into the upper thoracic cord of 3 to 4-day-old rats, followed by a cervical spinal cord transection at postnatal day 6. Subsequent histological examination at weaning demonstrated numerous fluorescently labeled cortical neurons, suggesting that they survived axotomy. However, whether this corresponds to proximal axonal sprouting or to regeneration distal to the lesion remains to be determined.

Studies of CST growth around medullary pyramidal lesions made in newborn hamsters also suggest the regeneration of growing CST fibers that were transected during their growth phase (Kalil 1984, Kalil and Reh 1979, 1982). However, similar findings after pyramidotomy in kittens were attributed not to axonal regeneration but rather to the continued growth of later-developing CST axons that were not transected by the lesion (Tolbert and Der 1987). Using methods similar to those in the study by Bates and Stelzner (1987), feline CST neurons labeled by spinal cord injections of the retrograde tracer fast blue (FB) at 2 to 5 days of age did not survive axotomy by pyramidotomy 7 to 8 days later (Tolbert and Der 1987). Although these findings present rather convincing evidence that CST plasticity after medullary pyramidal lesions in kittens does not represent axonal regeneration, the possibility remains that transected axons not labeled by the FB injection may have survived and regenerated.

Further studies on the effects of partial spinal lesion on newborn rats examined limb movements evoked by intracortical microstimulation (Dauzvardis et al. 1985, Dauzvardis and Castro 1986). In this work hindlimb movements evoked by cortical stimulation were observed after lesions that led to a rerouting of CST fibers, but they were not observed in an adult lesion group that did not demonstrate CST remodeling. Suggesting the electrophysiological integrity of CST fibers that grew around partial spinal cord lesions, this possibility could be further tested by examining the effects of medullary pyramidotomy, which would transect the CST fibers and therefore likely abolish or raise the current intensity needed to evoke the limb movements.

Possible behavioral correlates of CST remodeling after partial spinal cord lesions at birth derive from studies in rats and cats. Testing for postural reflexes and locomotor tasks after midthoracic hemisection made in rats at birth or at maturity demonstrated deficits that were task dependent, but generally less pronounced in animals receiving lesions at birth (Prendergast et al. 1982). Like the rat, the late-developing feline CST (Goldberger 1986, Tolbert and Der 1987) was also observed to grow caudally beyond partial spinal cord lesions made on the day of birth (Bregman and Goldberger 1982, 1983c). Also similar to results obtained using rats, extensive behavioral analysis comparing the effects of spinal cord lesion in newborn and adult cats demonstrated that the degree of recovery exhibited between the newborn and adult lesion groups varied according to the particular test (Bregman and Goldberger 1983a,b). However, the reported sparing of CST-mediated tactile-placing responses in neonatal as compared with adult operates corresponded to the CST remodeling observed only in the neonatal lesion group (Goldberger 1986). Similarly in hamsters that sustained medullary pyramidotomy at birth, the ability to manipulate sunflower seeds digitally, a skill particularly associated with an intact CST (Reh and Kalil 1982), corresponded to observed CST plasticity.

24.4 Brainstem Plasticity

Many experiments, as described below, have demonstrated a lesion-induced plasticity of corticofugal projections to several areas of the brainstem, including the pontine gray, red nucleus, and thalamus. This remodeling of fibers originating from the unablated cortical hemisphere occurs after the same cerebral cortical lesions that promote CST plasticity, and, like the CST response, this remodeling was more prominent after lesions made shortly after birth (Leong 1976a). Also like CST plasticity, cortico-brainstem remodeling of projections from the unablated hemisphere is expressed in terms of an increase of projections to areas deprived of their normal afferent inputs by the cortical lesion. Although the precise functions of these cortico-brainstem pathways are not clearly understood, their apparent involvement with motor functions is inferred from their origins in the motor and somatosensory cortex. Furthermore their contribution to CST-related functions is indicated by studies, done primarily on cats, that demonstrate that these connections are partly formed as axonal collaterals of CST fibers (Catsman-Berrevoets and Kuypers 1981, Rustioni and Hayes 1981, Keizer and Kuypers 1984, Ugolini and Kuypers 1986, Keizer et al. 1987).

Pontine Gray

Cerebral Cortical Lesions

Corticopontine fibers originate from widespread areas of the cerebral cortex, but are most dense from the motor and somatosensory areas that give rise to the CST (Wiesendanger and Wiesendanger 1982a). A major corticopontine contingent also arises from the visual cortex with a minor projection from the auditory cortex. Axonal tracing studies revealed a medial to lateral succession of ipsilateral termination fields from the motor, somatosensory, and visual cortex, respectively (Wiesendanger and Wiesendanger 1982b). Within this general plan corticopontine fibers originating from electrophysiologically defined forelimb and hindlimb areas, as well as from the face region of the motor and somatosensory cortex-demonstrated a precise topographic distribution pattern (Kartje-Tillotson et al. 1986, Kosinski et al. 1986, Mihailoff et al. 1985) that is reminiscent of CST topography. Developmentally these projections demonstrate an intense wave of synaptic proliferation within the pontine gray at postnatal days 6 through 13 (Mihailoff et al. 1984, Mihailoff and Bourell 1986).

Similar to the CST the postnatal developmental schedule of corticopontine fibers suggests an intrinsic capacity for remodeling in response to lesions occurring within the developmental period. Reflecting this capacity for remodeling, several studies have demonstrated an increase in the normally sparse crossed corticopontine projections after unilateral cerebral cortical lesions in the newborn rat (figure 24.3) (Castro and Mihailoff 1983, Leong and Lund 1973, Leong 1976a, 1978). Similar to CST plasticity the anomalous corticopontine fibers originating from fore- and hindlimb cortical areas demonstrated a topographic distribution that resembled normal uncrossed projections (Kartje-Tillotson et al. 1986). Although not examined electrophysiologically, electron microscopic data of corticopontine plasticity demonstrated the presence of synaptic terminals (Leong 1976b, Mihailoff and Castro 1981), which

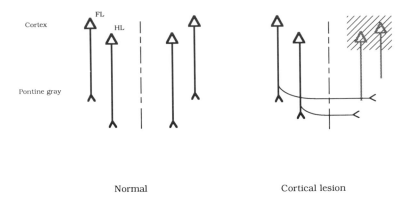

Normal   Cortical lesion

Figure 24.3 Topographic distribution of forelimb (FL) and hindlimb (HL) corticopontine projections after neonatal cortical lesion

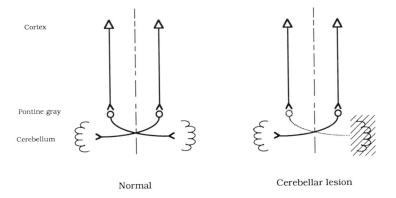

Normal   Cerebellar lesion

Figure 24.4 Corticopontine remodeling after neonatal hemicerebellectomy

presumably contacted receptor sites made available by the removal of normal inputs secondary to the neonatal cerebral cortical lesion. In further studies electrical stimulation of the unablated hemisphere in adult rats that sustained cerebral cortical lesions at birth produced a bilateral increase in uptake within the pontine gray and several other subcortical areas of systemically administered [^{14}C]2-deoxyglucose (Sharp and Evans 1983), providing evidence of functional activity. This bilateral response was not observed in animals sustaining a cortical lesion at 30 days of age.

Cerebellar Lesions
Corticopontine remodeling has also been observed after cerebellar lesions in newborn rats (Leong 1977a, 1978, Castro and Mihailoff 1983) (figure 24.4). Unlike the corticopontine and CST remodeling seen after cerebral cortical lesions, which deprive the pontine gray and spinal cord of normal cortical inputs, cerebellar lesions result in a substantial neuronal loss within the pontine gray contralateral to the lesion. Reflecting

this loss of target neurons within the pontine gray, the observed increase of crossed corticopontine fibers demonstrates the ability of axons growing into the reduced target area to establish alternate synaptic contacts, in this case within the opposite pontine gray (Leong 1980). The crossed axons were therefore apparently able to successfully compete for synaptic sites with normal ipsilateral afferents. In further work the combination of cerebellar lesions with cerebral cortical lesions was found to further increase the plasticity over that seen after single lesions, presumably by eliminating the competition from corticopontine afferents for synaptic sites (Castro and Mihailoff 1983). The concept that developing pathways deprived of their normal target areas may compete for alternative synaptic sites was described in prior studies on the hamster visual system (Schneider 1973). In this work unilateral tectal lesion in the newborn induced retinotectal fibers to establish projections to the spared tectum, and this projection was increased by additional lesions, depriving the spared tectum of its normal afferents.

The function of normal corticopontine projections, much less of remodeled corticopontine fibers, is not clearly understood except that they represent a pathway whereby the cerebral cortex can exert a strong influence on cerebellar activity. However, considering the density of corticopontine projections from the motor and somatosensory cortex as a measure of their importance to motor function, the remodeling of this system as part of the overall response to cortical lesions would logically represent a necessary component of recovery mechanisms.

Regarding corticopontine remodeling (and corticorubral plasticity, as described below) after cerebellar lesions, behavioral studies have implicated the cerebral cortex in recovery from cerebellar damage occurring in young rats (Smith et al. 1974). In this work secondary cerebral cortical lesions made at maturity caused a reinstatement of deficits that had been compensated for after earlier cerebellar lesions. Further evidence of cerebral cortical participation in recovery from cerebellar lesion deficits was suggested by electrophysiological experiments (O'Donoghue et al. 1986). In this study intracortical microstimulation evoked bilateral, low-threshold limb movements in adult rats that sustained unilateral hemicerebellar lesions at young ages. As in normal control rats, only contralateral limb movements could be elicited at low current thresholds after lesions in older animals.

Red Nucleus

Corticorubral Projections
Cortical efferents from the motor and sensory cortex project ipsilaterally to the rodent red nucleus (Brown 1974, Naus et al. 1985). However, anomalous contralateral corticorubral projections were observed in rats that sustained sensorimotor *cortical lesions* at birth (Nah and Leong 1976a,b, Naus et al. 1985, 1986a) (figure 24.5). Similar to normal fibers,

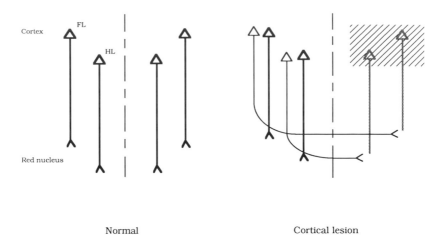

Cortex

FL

HL

Red nucleus

Normal   Cortical lesion

Figure 24.5 Remodeling of forelimb (FL) and hindlimb (HL) corticorubral projections after a neonatal cortical lesion

these abnormal crossed fibers were distributed within the rostral parvicellular region of the red nucleus, but they were not formed from axonal collaterals of normal ipsilateral projections (Naus et al. 1986a). Ultrastructurally the abnormal crossed projections as well as the normal uncrossed projections contacted the distal dendrites of rubral neurons (Nah and Leong 1976b, Naus et al. 1987). Similar corticorubral remodeling after cortical lesions in kittens has also been found (Villablanca et al. 1982, Kosar et al. 1985, Leonard and Goldberger 1987) and described using electrophysiological methods to distribute in a topographic pattern resembling normal fore- and hindlimb corticorubral projections (Tsukahara et al. 1983, Tsukahara 1985).

Corticorubral remodeling has also been observed after unilateral *cerebellar lesions* in the newborn rat (Shieh et al. 1985). From this electron microscopic study, ipsilateral corticorubral fibers that normally terminate on distal dendrites appeared to expand their terminal fields to replace cerebellar afferents that terminate closer to the neuronal soma (figure 24.6). A similar corticorubral remodeling to reinnervate deafferented rubral neurons was found after cerebellar lesions in adult cats (Tolbert et al. 1982).

Studies on adult cats have demonstrated remodeling of corticorubral projections in response to a *classical conditioning paradigm* rather than in response to a lesion (Tsukahara 1985). This work paired electrical stimulation of the cerebral peduncle (the conditioned stimulus) with forelimb electric shock (the unconditioned stimulus). Animals learned to avoid the shock by flexing their forelimb to the conditioned stimulus by the seventh day of training. Further analysis demonstrating a new fast-rising component in monosynaptic corticorubral dendritic excitatory postsynaptic potentials provided electrophysiological evidence of corticorubral sprouting. In addition to demonstrating remodeling in the

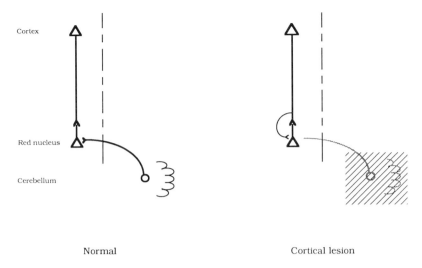

Cortex

Red nucleus

Cerebellum

Normal   Cortical lesion

Figure 24.6 Corticorubral remodeling after neonatal hemicerebellectomy

intact brain, these findings using the red nucleus as a model system further support the notion of a causal relationship between anatomical and behavioral plasticity. Nonetheless the possible functional significance of rubral remodeling after cortical lesion is still unknown. However, considering the generally accepted concept that the corticorubrospinal system works in cooperation with the CST system to control limb musculature (Lawrence and Kuypers 1968a,b), remodeling of corticorubral projections after cortical lesions would be expected to accompany CST remodeling. This seems particularly logical because cortical lesions in the newborn did not cause a remodeling of the rubrospinal tract itself (Castro et al. 1977).

Cerebellar Efferent Projections

Cerebral cortical lesions in the newborn rats cause the remodeling of cerebellorubral fibers that appear to recover synaptic sites left vacant by cerebral cortical lesions (Shieh et al. 1984) (figure 24.7). Cerebellorubral remodeling was also observed after cortical hemispherectomy in adult cats (Olmstead et al. 1983). Electrophysiological confirmation of this feline remodeling was derived from intracellular recording techniques (Tolbert et al. 1982, Tsukahara 1985).

Hemicerebellar lesions in newborn rats also led to a remodeling of cerebellar efferents originating from the unablated cerebellar hemisphere (Lim and Leong 1975, Leong 1977b, Castro 1978b, Haroian and Campellone 1986) (figure 24.8). Coursing through the superior cerebellar peduncle, these primarily crossed, late-developing (Naus et al. 1986b) projections demonstrated a bilateral distribution to several areas, including the red nucleus and ventral thalamus. Projecting to areas deprived of normal inputs by hemicerebellectomy, the anomalous ip-

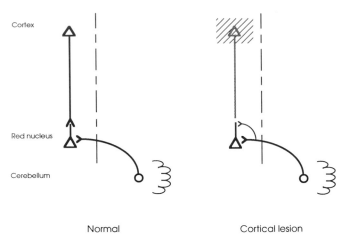

Figure 24.7 Cerebellorubral remodeling after cerebral cortical lesion

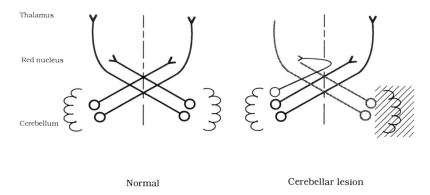

Figure 24.8 Cerebellorubral remodeling after neonatal hemicerebellectomy

silateral thalamic afferents were derived mainly from axonal branches of normal crossed cerebellothalamic fibers (Molinari et al. 1986), whereas abnormal cerebellorubral fibers were not collaterals of normal projections (Gramsbergen and Ijkema-Paassen 1982). Similar to normal crossed projections, these anomalous ipsilateral cerebellorubral projections contacted the soma and proximal dendrites of magnocellular rubral neurons (Naus et al. 1987). Although these anomalous connections have been confirmed electrophysiologically (Kawaguchi and Yamamoto 1981), chronic recording of extracellular rubral activity in sleeping and active rats demonstrated abnormal electrical activity in association with these pathways (Gramsbergen et al. 1984). These findings were suggested to represent a causal relation between the abnormal activity within the red nucleus and the more severe locomotor deficits that have been reported after cerebellar lesions at 5 or 10 days of age compared with similar lesions made at 30 days of age (Gramsbergen 1981).

Of particular interest concerning cerebellar efferent remodeling is the apparent regeneration of transected fibers traversing the superior cerebellar peduncle, as observed anatomically and electrophysiologically in kittens (Kawaguchi et al. 1981, Kawaguchi et al. 1986).

Thalamus

Bilateral corticothalamic projections, which are more extensive and more dense ipsilaterally, have been described in normal rats (Sharp and Gonzalez 1986a, Molinari et al. 1985). However, an increase in crossed projections originating from the unablated hemisphere was observed after unilateral cortical lesions in newborn (Neumann et al. 1982, Sharp and Gonzalez 1986a) and in adult rats (Pritzel and Huston 1981) as well as after unilateral cerebral cortical hemispherectomy in kittens (Villablanca and Gomez-Pinilla 1987) (figure 24.9). Concerning lesions in newborn rats, these contralateral projections were not attributed to a lesion-induced persistence of developmentally transient projections, but were believed to represent the collateral sprouting of normal ipsilateral corticothalamic fibers that crossed the midline at the level of the thalamus (Neumann et al. 1982). This issue has not been resolved in cats (Villablanca and Gomez-Pinilla 1987).

The reported increase in crossed corticothalamic projections, observed to occur in rats by 7 days postlesion, was found to coincide with the cessation of lesion-induced spontaneous turning behavior in both neonatal and adult lesion groups (Pritzel and Huston 1981, Neumann et al. 1982). However, it should be noted that the cessation of turning additionally coincided with the development of anomalous crossed substantia nigral projections to the deafferented thalamus (Huston et al. 1985). These anomalous nigrothalamic projections were observed after large, unilateral telencephalic lesions were made in both infant (7-day-old) and adult rats. Although the temporal correlations between cortico-

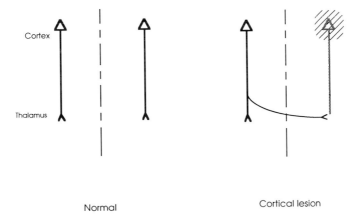

Figure 24.9 Corticothalamic remodeling after neonatal cortical lesion

and nigrothalamic plasticity and the cessation of abnormal turning behavior may suggest a causal relation (Huston et al. 1985), the possible contributions of many other pathways that also remodel after cortical lesions must be considered (Villablanca and Gomez-Pinilla 1987).

Despite the observed plasticity of several cortical efferent pathways, remodeling of thalamocortical projections to the unablated cortical hemisphere was not observed after unilateral cerebral cortical lesions in the newborn (Sharp and Gonzalez 1986a) (figure 24.10). Similarly, in light of the extensive thalamic atrophy observed ipsilateral to cerebral cortical lesions (Kolb et al. 1983, Sharp and Gonzalez 1986b), the absence of medial lemniscal remodeling to the opposite thalamic nuclei (Kosinski 1984) (figure 24.10) was surprising, although remodeling of dorsal column nuclear projections to the pontine gray was observed (Kosinski et al. 1987). Electrophysiological analysis of cortical activity evoked by cutaneous stimulation in adult rats that sustained cortical lesions at birth also revealed no evidence of remodeling corresponding to ascending projections to or from thalamic nuclei (Kosinski 1984).

24.5 Summary

Unilateral lesions involving the sensorimotor cortex of the newborn rat result in the widespread remodeling of several cortical projections originating from the opposite, unablated hemisphere (figure 24.11). Although the remodeling described in this chapter has focused on the more extensively studied cortical pathways to the spinal cord, pontine gray, red nucleus, and thalamus, corticofugal remodeling to the superior colliculus, pretectum, medullary reticular formation, and dorsal column

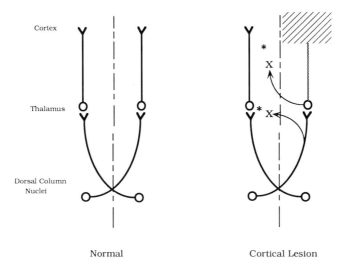

Figure 24.10 Absence (*) of thalamocortical and medial lemniscal remodeling after neonatal cortical lesions

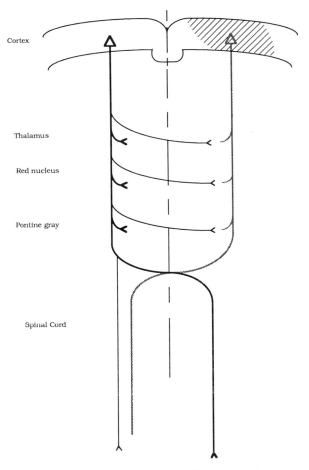

Figure 24.11 Summary of corticofugal remodeling after unilateral cortical lesions in newborn rats

nuclei has also been reported (Leong and Lund 1973, Leong 1976a,b). In general, lesion-induced cortical efferent plasticity represents a less dense but topographic mirror image of normal projections and reflects an anomalous growth of axons into areas deprived of their normal afferent inputs. In many cases the anomalous projections demonstrated a normal ultrastructural synaptology that appeared to be functional electrophysiologically. A similar plasticity of cerebellar efferents coursing through the superior cerebellar peduncle to areas deprived of normal inputs after unilateral cerebellar lesion has also been found (figure 24.12). Additionally corticopontine and corticorubral remodeling have also been observed after hemicerebellar lesions. In conclusion, the extensive remodeling of motor pathways found after unilateral cerebral or cerebellar lesions suggests that the spared cerebral or cerebellar hemisphere may assume a bilateral function.

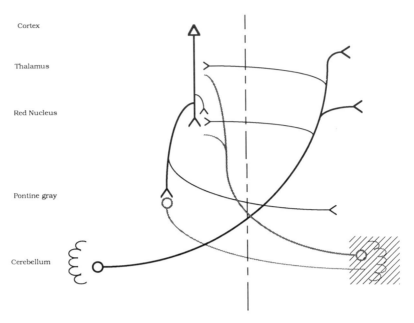

Cortex

Thalamus

Red Nucleus

Pontine gray

Cerebellum

Figure 24.12 Summary of cerebellofugal remodeling after neonatal hemicerebellectomy

Notes

The author gratefully acknowledges the helpful comments of Dr. Rand Swenson and the assistance of Mr. Thomas Hogan in preparing the figures. This study was supported by NIH Grant NS13230.

1. In this chapter the terms *abnormal* and *anomalous* are used synonymously in reference to neural projections that deviate from the (normal) connectivity found in control animals. For example, if pathway A, which normally only projects unilaterally to nucleus B (on the right side of the neuraxis), is found also to project to nucleus B∝ (on the left side) in response to a lesion, then the input to B∝ represents an abnormal projection. However, if this input to B∝ resembles normal projections in all ways except for laterality, one might interpret this to be an appropriate, albeit abnormal, connection, given the experimental circumstances. If, however, lesion-induced remodelling causes pathway A to project to a completely novel site, nucleus C, this would objectively represent an abnormal projection that may be considered inappropriate. The main point is that the normality of connections should be judged according to the objective criterion of the norm, whereas the appropriateness of connections represents a subjective analysis of the given facts.

References

Asanuma, H., Babb, R. S., Mori, A., and Waters, R. S. (1981). Input-output relationships in cat's motor cortex after pyramidal section. *Journal of Neurophysiology* 46:694–703.

Bates, C. A., and Stelzner, D. J. (1987). Do corticospinal projection neurons die after spinal transection in the neonatal rat? *Society for Neuroscience Abstracts* 13:921.

Bernstein, D., and Stelzner, D. J. (1983). Plasticity of the corticospinal tract following midthoracic spinal injury in the postnatal rat. *Journal of Comparative Neurology* 221:382–400.

Bregman, B. S., and Goldberger, M. E. (1982). Anatomical plasticity and sparing of function after spinal cord damage in neonatal rats. *Science* 217:553–555.

Bregman, B. S., and Goldberger, M. E. (1983a). Infant lesion effect: I. Development of motor behavior following neonatal spinal cord damage in cats. *Developmental Brain Research* 9:103–117.

Bregman, B. S., and Goldberger, M. E. (1983b). Infant lesion effect: II. Recovery of function after spinal cord damage in newborn and adult cats. *Developmental Brain Research* 9:119–135.

Bregman, B. S., and Goldberger, M. E. (1983c). Infant lesion effect: III. Anatomical correlates of sparing and recovery of function after spinal cord damage in newborn and adult cats. *Developmental Brain Research* 9:137–154.

Brown, L. T. (1974). Corticorubral projections in the rat. *Journal of Comparative Neurology* 154:149–168.

Burgess, J. W., and Villablanca, J. R. (1986). Recovery of function after neonatal or adult hemispherectomy in cats. II. Limb bias and development, paw usage, locomotion and rehabilitative effects of exercise. *Behavioral Brain Research* 20:1–18.

Burgess, J. W., Villablanca, J. R., and Levine, M. S. (1986). Recovery of functions after neonatal or adult hemispherectomy in cats. III. Complex functions: Open field exploration, social interactions, maze and holeboard performances. *Behavioral Brain Research* 20:217–230.

Castro, A. J. (1972). Motor performance in rats. The effects of pyramidal tract section. *Brain Research* 44:313–323.

Castro, A. J. (1975). Ipsilateral corticospinal projections after large lesions of the cerebral hemisphere in neonatal rats. *Experimental Neurology* 47:343–352.

Castro, A. J. (1978a). Analysis of corticospinal and rubrospinal projections after neonatal pyramidotomy in rats. *Brain Research* 144:155–158.

Castro, A. J. (1978b). Projections of the superior cerebellar peduncle in rats and the development of new connections in response to neonatal hemicerebellectomy. *Journal of Comparative Neurology* 178:611–628.

Castro, A. J., Clegg, D. A., and McClung, J. R. (1977). The effect of large unilateral cortical lesions on rubrospinal tract sprouting in newborn rats. *American Journal of Anatomy* 149:39–46.

Castro, A. J., and Mihailoff, G. A. (1983). Corticopontine remodelling after cortical and/or cerebellar lesions in newborn rats. *Journal of Comparative Neurology* 219:112–123.

Catsman-Berrevoets, C. E., and Kuypers, H. G. J. M. (1981). A search for corticospinal collaterals to thalamus and mesencephalon by means of multiple retrograde fluorescent tracers in cat and rat. *Brain Research* 218:15–33.

Chambers, W. W., Liu, C. N., and McCouch, G. P. (1973). Anatomical and physiological correlates of plasticity in the central nervous system. *Brain, Behavior and Evolution* 8:5–26.

Cotman, C. W., and Nieto-Sampedro, M. (1982). Brain function, synapse renewal and plasticity. *Annual Review of Psychology* 33:371–401.

Dauzvardis, M. F., and Castro, A. J. (1986). Cortically-evoked hindlimb movements in adult rats that sustained partial mid-thoracic spinal cord lesions at 6-8 days of age. *Neuroscience Abstracts* 12:510.

Dauzvardis, M. F., Kartje-Tillotson, G., and Castro, A. J. (1985). Cortically-evoked movements in rats that sustained neonatal spinal cord lesions. *Neuroscience Abstracts* 11:1286.

Donatelle, J. M. (1977). Growth of the corticospinal tract and the development of placing reactions in the postnatal rat. *Journal of Comparative Neurology* 175:207–232.

Finger, S., and Almli, C. R. (1985). Brain damage and neuroplasticity: mechanisms of recovery or development? *Brain Research Reviews* 10:177–186.

Finlay, B. L., Wilson, K. G., and Schneider, G. (1979). Anomalous ipsilateral retinotectal projections in Syrian hamsters with early lesions: topography and functional capacity. *Journal of Comparative Neurology* 183:721–740.

Frost, D. O. (1982). Anomalous visual connections to somatosensory and auditory systems following brain lesions in early life. *Developmental Brain Research* 3:627–635.

Goldberger, M. E. (1986). Mechanisms contributing to sparing of function following neonatal damage to spinal pathways. *Neurochemical Pathology* 5:289–307.

Goldberger, M. E., and Murray, M. (1978). Recovery of movement and axonal sprouting may obey some of the same laws. In C. W. Cotman (ed.), *Neuronal Plasticity*. New York: Raven Press, 73–96.

Goldberger, M. E., and Murray, M. (1985). Recovery of function and anatomical plasticity after damage to the adult and neonatal spinal cord. In C. W. Cotman (ed.), *Synaptic Plasticity*. New York: Guilford Press, 77–110.

Goldman, P. S. (1978). Neuronal plasticity in primate telencephalon: anomalous projections induced by prenatal removal of frontal cortex. *Science* 202:768–770.

Gomez-Pinella, F., Villablanca, J. R., Sonnier, B. J., and Levine, M. S. (1986). Reorganization of pericruciate cortical projections to the spinal cord and dorsal column nuclei after neonatal or adult cerebral hemispherectomy in cats. *Brain Research* 385:343–355.

Gramsbergen, A. (1981). Locomotor behavior after cerebellar lesions in the young rat. In H. Flohr and W. Precht (eds.), *Lesion-Induced Neuronal Plasticity in Sensorimotor Systems*. New York: Springer Verlag, 324–336.

Gramsbergen, A., and Ijkema-Paassen, J. (1982). CNS plasticity after hemicerebellectomy in the young rat. Quantitative relations between aberrant and normal cerebellorubral projections. *Neuroscience Letters* 33:129–134.

Gramsbergen, A., Schuling, F. H., and Vos, J. E. (1984). Electrical activity in the red nuclei of rats and the effects of hemicerebellectomy at young ages. *Behavioral Brain Research* 12:91–98.

Haroian, A. J., and Campellone, A. D. (1986). A quantitative analysis of the ipsilateral cerebellothalmic projection following hemicerebellectomy in neonatal rats. A retrograde HRP study. *Developmental Brain Research* 26:69–78.

Hicks, S. P., and D'Amato, C. J. (1970). Motor-sensory and visual behavior after hemispherectomy in newborn and mature rats. *Experimental Neurology* 29:416–438.

Huston, J. P., Morgan, S., and Steiner, H. (1985). Behavioral correlates of plasticity in substantia nigra efferents. In B. E. Will, P. Schmitt, and J. C. Dalrumple-Alford (eds.), *Brain Plasticity, Learning, and Memory*. New York: Plenum Press, 383–395.

Kalil, K. (1984). Development and regrowth of the rodent pyramidal tract. *Trends in Neuroscience* 7:394–398.

Kalil, K., and Reh, T. (1979). Regrowth of severed axons in the neonatal central nervous system: establishment of normal connections. *Science* 205:1158–1161.

Kalil, K., and Reh, T. (1982). A light and electron microscopic study of regrowing pyramidal tract fibers. *Journal of Comparative Neurology* 211:265–275.

Kalil, K., and Schneider, G. E. (1975). Motor performance following unilateral pyramidal tract lesions in the hamster. *Brain Research* 100:170–174.

Kartje-Tillotson, G., Neafsey, E. J., and Castro, A. J. (1985). Electrophysiological analysis of motor cortical plasticity after cortical lesions in newborn rats. *Brain Research* 322:103–111.

Kartje-Tillotson, G., Neafsey, E. J., and Castro, A. J. (1986). The topography of corticopontine plasticity after cortical lesions in newborn rats. *Journal of Comparative Neurology* 250:206–214.

Kartje-Tillotson, G., O'Donoghue, D. L., Dauzvardis, M. F., and Castro, A. J. (1987). Pyramidotomy abolishes abnormal movements evoked by intracortical microstimulation in adult rats that sustained neonatal cortical lesions. *Brain Research* 415:172–177.

Kawaguchi, S., Miyata, H., and Kato, N. (1986). Regeneration of the cerebellofugal projection after transection of the superior cerebellar peduncle in kittens: morphological and electrophysiological studies. *Journal of Comparative Neurology* 245:258–273.

Kawaguchi, S., Miyata, H., Kawamura, M., and Harada, Y. (1981). Morphological and electrophysiological evidence for axonal regeneration of axotomized cerebellothalamic neurons in kittens. *Neuroscience Letters* 24:13–18.

Kawaguchi, S., and Yamamoto, T. (1981). Reorganization of the cerebello-cerebral projection following hemicerebellectomy or cerebral cortical ablation. In H. Flohr and W. Precht (eds.), *Lesion-Induced Neuronal Plasticity in Sensorimotor Systems*. New York: Springer Verlag, 314–323.

Keizer, K., and Kuypers, H. G. J. M. (1984). Distribution of corticospinal neurons with collaterals to lower brainstem reticular formation in cat. *Experimental Brain Research* 54:107–120.

Keizer, K., Kuypers, H. G. J. M., and Ronday, H. K. (1987). Branching cortical neurons in cat which project to the colliculi and to the pons: a retrograde fluorescent double-labeling study. *Experimental Brain Research* 67:1–15.

Kolb, B. (1987). Recovery from early cortical damage in rats. I. Differential behavioral and anatomical effects of frontal lesions at different ages of neural maturation. *Behavioral Brain Research* 25:205–220.

Kolb, B., and Elliott, W. (1987). Recovery from early cortical damage in rats. II. Effects of experience on anatomy and behavior following frontal lesions at 1 or 5 days of age. *Behavioral Brain Research* 27:47–56.

Kolb, B., Holmes, C., and Whishaw, I. Q. (1987). Recovery from early cortical damage in rats. III. Neonatal removal of posterior parietal cortex has greater behavioral and anatomical effects than similar removals in adulthood. *Behavioral Brain Research* 26:119–137.

Kolb, B., Sutherland, R. J., and Whishaw, I. Q. (1983). Abnormalities in cortical and subcortical morphology after neonatal neocortical lesions in rats. *Experimental Neurology* 79:223–244.

Kolb, B., and Tomie, J.-A. (1988). Recovery from early cortical damage in rats. IV. Effects of hemidecortication at 1, 5 or 10 days of age on cerebral anatomy and behavior. *Behavioral Brain Research* 23:259–274.

Kolb, B., and Whishaw, I. Q. (1985). Earlier is not always better: behavioral dysfunction and abnormal cerebral morphogenesis following neonatal cortical lesions in the rat. *Behavioral Brain Research* 17:25–43.

Kort, E. J. M., Gribnau, A. A. M., van Aanholt, H. T. H., and Nieuwenhuys, R. (1985). On the development of the pyramidal tract in the rat. *Anatomy and Embryology* 172:195–204.

Kosar, E., Fujito, Y., Mukrakami, F., and Tsukahara, N. (1985). Morphological and electrophysiological study of sprouting of corticorubral fibers after lesions of the contralateral cerebrum in kitten. *Brain Research* 347:217–224.

Kosinski, R. (1984). *The distribution of dorsal column nuclear efferents to the basilar pontine gray in normal and neonatally brain damaged rats.* Doctoral dissertation, Loyola University of Chicago.

Kosinski, R. J., Neafsey, E. J., and Castro, A. J. (1986). A comparative topographical analysis of dorsal column nuclear and cerebral cortical projections to the basilar pontine gray in rats. *Journal of Comparative Neurology* 244:163–173.

Kosinski, R. J., Neafsey, E. J., and Castro, A. J. (1987). Remodeling of dorsal column nuclear efferents to the basilar pontine gray after cortical ablations in newborn rats. *Brain Research* 406:302–307.

Lawrence, D. G., and Kuypers, H. G. J. M. (1968a). The functional organization of the motor system in the monkey. I. The effects of bilateral pyramidal lesions. *Brain* 91:1–18.

Lawrence, D. G., and Kuypers, H. G. J. M. (1968b). The functional organization of the motor system in the monkey. II. The effects of lesions of the descending brain-stem pathways. *Brain* 91:15–36.

Leonard, C. T., and Goldberger, M. E. (1987). Consequences of damage to the sensorimotor cortex in neonatal and adult cats. II. Maintenance of exuberant projections. *Developmental Brain Research* 32:15–30.

Leong, S. K. (1976a). An experimental study of the corticofugal system following cerebral lesions in the albino rats. *Experimental Brain Research* 26:235–247.

Leong, S. K. (1976b). A qualitative electron microscopic investigation of the anomalous corticofugal projections following neonatal lesions in the albino rats. *Brain Research* 107:1–8.

Leong, S. K. (1977a). Sprouting of the corticopontine fibers after neonatal cerebellar lesion in the albino rat. *Brain Research* 123:164–169.

Leong, S. K. (1977b). Plasticity of cerebellar efferents after neonatal lesion in albino rats. *Neuroscience Letters* 7:281–289.

Leong, S. K. (1978). Effects of deafferenting cerebellar or cerebral inputs to the pontine and red nuclei in the albino rat. *Brain Research* 155:357–361.

Leong, S. K. (1980). A qualitative electron microscopic study of the corticopontine projections after neonatal cerebellar hemispherectomy. *Brain Research* 194:299–310.

Leong, S. K., and Lund, R. D. (1973). Anomalous bilateral corticofugal pathways in albino rats after neonatal lesions. *Brain Research* 62:218–221.

Lim, K. H., and Leong, S. K. (1975). Aberrant bilateral projections from the dentate and interposed nuclei in albino rats after neonatal lesions. *Brain Research* 96:306–309.

McClung, J. R., and Castro, A. J. (1975). An ultrastructural study of ipsilateral corticospinal fibers in the rat. *Brain Research* 89:327–330.

Mihailoff, G. A., Adams, C. E., and Woodward, D. J. (1984). An autoradiographic study of the postnatal development of sensorimotor and visual components of the corticopontine system. *Journal of Comparative Neurology* 222:116–127.

Mihailoff, G. A., and Bourell, K. W. (1986). Synapse formation and other ultrastructural features of postnatal development in the basilar pontine nuclei of the rat. *Developmental Brain Research* 28:195–212.

Mihailoff, G. A., and Castro, A. J. (1981). Autoradiographic and electron microscopic evidence for axonal sprouting in the rat corticopontine system. *Neuroscience Letters* 21:267–273.

Mihailoff, G. A., Lee, H., Watt, C. B., and Yates, R. (1985). Projections to the basilar pontine nuclei from face sensory and motor regions of the cerebral cortex in the rat. *Journal of Comparative Neurology* 237:251–263.

Miller, M. W. (1987). The origin of corticospinal neurons in rat. *Experimental Brain Research* 67:339–351.

Molinari, M., Bentivoglio, M., Granato, A., and Minciacchi, D. (1986). Increased collateralization of the cerebellothalamic pathway following neonatal hemicerebellectomy. *Brain Research* 372:1–10.

Molinari, M., Minciacchi, D., Bentivoglio, M., and Macchi, G. (1985). Efferent fibers from the motor cortex terminate bilaterally in the thalamus of rats and cats. *Experimental Brain Research* 57:305–312.

Nah, S. H., and Leong, S. K. (1976a). An ultrastructural study of the anomalous corticorubral projection following neonatal lesions in the albino rat. *Brain Research* 111:162–166.

Nah, S. H., and Leong, S. K. (1976b). Bilateral corticofugal projection to the red nucleus after neonatal lesions in the albino rat. *Brain Research* 107:433–436.

Nah, S. H., Ong, L. S., and Leong, S. K. (1980). Is sprouting the result of a persistent neonatal connection? *Neuroscience Letters* 19:39–44.

Naus, C., Flumerfelt, B. A., and Hrycyshyn, A. W. (1985). An anterograde HRP-WGA study of aberrant corticorubral projections following neonatal lesions of the rat sensorimotor cortex. *Experimental Brain Research* 59:365–371.

Naus, C. G., Flumerfelt, B. A., and Hrycyshyn, A. W. (1986a). Contralateral corticorubral fibers induced by neonatal lesions are not collaterals of the normal ipsilateral projection. *Neuroscience* 70:52–58.

Naus, C. G., Flumerfelt, B. A., and Hrycyshyn, A. W. (1987). Ultrastructural study of remodeled rubral afferents following neonatal lesions in the rat. *Journal of Comparative Neurology* 259:131–139.

Naus, C. G., Hrycyshyn, A. W., and Flumerfelt, B. A. (1986b). Quantitative analysis of rubral degeneration following neonatal deafferentation. *Experimental Neurology* 94:359–367.

Neumann, S., Pritzel, M., and Huston, J. P. (1982). Plasticity of cortico-thalamic projections and functional recovery in the unilateral detelencephalized infant rat. *Behavioral Brain Research* 4:377–388.

O'Donoghue, D. L., Kartje-Tillotson, G., Neafsey, E. J., and Castro, A. J. (1986). A study of forelimb movements evoked by intracortical microstimulation after hemicerebellectomy in newborn, young and adult rats. *Brain Research* 385:311–320.

Olmstead, C. E., Villablanca, J. R., Sonnier, B. J., McAllister, J. P., and Gomez, F. (1983). Reorganization of cerebellorubral terminal fields following hemispherectomy in adult cats. *Brain Research* 274:336–340.

Prendergast, J., Shusterman, R., and Phillips, T. (1982). Comparison of the effect of midthoracic spinal hemisection at birth or in adulthood on motor behavior in the adult rat. *Experimental Neurology* 78:190–204.

Pritzel, M., and Huston, J. P. (1981). Unilateral ablation of telencephalon induces appearance of contralateral cortical and subcortical projections to thalamic nuclei. *Behavioral Brain Research* 3:43–54.

Reh, T., and Kalil, K. (1982). Functional role of regrowing pyramidal tract fibers. *Journal of Comparative Neurology* 211:276–283.

Reinoso, B. S., and Castro, A. J. (1986). Anomalous ventral corticospinal projections after unilateral cerebral cortical lesions in newborn rats. *Neuroscience Abstracts* 12:510.

Reinoso, B. S., and Castro, A. J. (1989). A study of corticospinal remodelling using retrograde fluorescent tracers in rats. *Experimental Brain Research* 74:387–394.

Rustioni, A., and Hayes, N. L. (1981). Corticospinal tract collaterals to the dorsal column nuclei of cats. *Experimental Brain Research* 43:237–245.

Schneider, G. E. (1973). Early lesions of the superior colliculus: factors affecting the formation of abnormal retinal projections. *Brain, Behavior and Evolution* 8:73–109.

Schneider, G. E. (1979). Is it really better to have your brain lesion early? A revision of the "Kennard Principle." *Neuropsychologia* 17:557–583.

Schreyer, D. J., and Jones, E. G. (1983). Growing corticospinal axons by-pass lesions of neonatal rat spinal cord. *Neuroscience* 9:31–40.

Schreyer, D. J., and Jones, E. G. (1982). Growth and target finding by axons of the corticospinal tract in prenatal and postnatal rats. *Neuroscience* 7:1837–1853.

Sharp, F. R., and Evans, K. L. (1983). Bilateral [14C]2-deoxyglucose uptake by motor pathways after unilateral neonatal cortex lesions in the rat. *Developmental Brain Research* 6:1–11.

Sharp, F. R., and Gonzalez, M. F. (1986a). Adult rat motor cortex connections to thalamus following neonatal and juvenile frontal cortical lesions: WGA-HRP and amino acid studies. *Developmental Brain Research* 30:169–187.

Sharp, F. R., and Gonzalez, M. F. (1986b). Fetal cortical transplants ameliorate thalamic atrophy ipsilateral to neonatal frontal cortex lesions. *Neuroscience Letters* 71:247–251.

Shieh, J. Y., Leong, S. K., and Wong, W. C. (1984). An electron microscopic study of the cerebellorubral connections after neonatal lesions in the sensorimotor and adjacent cortex in the albino rat. *Brain Research* 324:1–10.

Shieh, J. Y., Leong, S. K., and Wong, W. C. (1985). An electron microscopic study of the corticorubral fibers after neonatal deep cerebellar nuclear lesions in albino rats. *Brain Research* 335:201–206.

Sloper, J. J., Brodal, P., and Powell, T. P. S. (1983). An anatomical study of the effects of unilateral removal of sensorimotor cortex in infant monkeys on the subcortical projections of the contralateral sensorimotor cortex. *Brain* 106:707–716.

Smith, R. L., Parks, T., and Lynch, G. (1974). A comparison of the role of the motor cortex in recovery from cerebellar damage in young and adult rats. *Behavioral Biology* 12:177–198.

Stein, D. G., Finger, S., and Hart, T. (1983). Brain damage and recovery: problems and perspectives. *Behavioral and Neural Biology* 37:185–222.

Steward, O. (1982). Assessing the functional significance of lesion-induced neuronal plasticity. *International Review of Neurobiology* 23:197–254.

Tolbert, D. L., and Der, T. (1987). Redirected growth of pyramidal tract axons following neonatal pyramidotomy in cats. *Journal of Comparative Neurology* 260:299–311.

Tolbert, D. L., Marshall, C. A., and Murphy, M. G. (1982). Collateral sprouting of somatosensory corticofugal axons into the cerebellar deafferented red nucleus. *Brain Research* 237:473–478.

Tsukahara, N. (1985). Synaptic plasticity in the red nucleus and its possible behavioral correlates. In C. Cotman (ed.), *Synaptic Plasticity*. New York: Guilford Press, 201–229.

Tsukahara, N., Fujito, Y., and Kubota, M. (1983). Specificity of the newly-formed corticorubral synapses in the kitten red nucleus. *Experimental Brain Research* 51:45–56.

Ugolini, G., and Kuypers, H. G. J. M. (1986). Collaterals of corticospinal and pyramidal fibres to the pontine grey demonstrated by a new application of the fluorescent fibre labelling technique. *Brain Research* 365:211–227.

Ullan, J., and Artieda, J. (1981). Somatotopy of the corticospinal neurons in the rat. *Neuroscience Letters* 21:13–18.

Vahlsing, H. L., and Feringa, E. R. (1980). A ventral uncrossed corticospinal tract in the rat. *Experimental Neurology* 70:282–287.

Villablanca, J. R., and Gomez-Pinilla, F. (1987). Novel crossed corticothalamic projections after neonatal cerebral hemispherectomy. A quantitative autoradiography study in cats. *Brain Research* 410:219–231.

Villablanca, J. R., Burgess, J. W., and Olmstead, C. E. (1986). Recovery of function after neonatal or adult hemispherectomy in cats: I. Time course, movement, posture and sensorimotor tests. *Behavioral Brain Research* 19:205–226.

Villablanca, J. R., Olmstead, C. E., Sonnier, B. J., McAllister, J. P., and Gomez, F. (1982). Evidence for a crossed corticorubral projection in cats with one cerebral hemisphere removed neonatally. *Neuroscience Letters* 33:241–246.

Whishaw, I. Q., and Kolb, B. (1988). Sparing of skilled forelimb reaching and corticospinal projections after neonatal motor cortex removal or hemidecortication in the rat: Support for the Kennard doctrine. *Brain Research* 451:97–114.

Wiesendanger, R., and Wiesendanger, M. (1982a). The corticopontine system in the rat. I. Mapping of corticopontine neurons. *Journal of Comparative Neurology* 208:215–226.

Wiesendanger, R., and Wiesendanger, M. (1982b). The corticopontine system in the rat. II. The projection pattern. *Journal of Comparative Neurology* 208:227–238.

Wise, S. P., Murray, E. A., and Coulter, J. D. (1979). Somatotopic organization of corticospinal and corticotrigeminal neurons in the rat. *Neuroscience* 4:65–78.

Zimmer, J., Laurberg, S., and Sunde, N. (1986). Non-cholinergic afferents determine the distribution of the cholingeric septohippocampal projection: a study of the AChE staining pattern in the rat facia dentata and hippocampus after lesions, X-irradiation, and intracerebral grafting. *Experimental Brain Research* 64:158–168.

25 Neural Transplantation in the Cerebral Cortex

Stephen B. Dunnett

Neural transplantation in the cerebral cortex is a powerful experimental technique that is currently being used to investigate a variety of issues related both to the transplantation paradigm itself and to the intrinsic anatomy, development, plasticity, repair, and functional organization of the cerebral cortex. Because the technique is still in its infancy, we are confronted by a mixture of ignorance and the fascination of potential developments rather than a body of established knowledge. This overview of recent studies is therefore organized in terms of the variety of outstanding experimental issues relating to cortical development, organization, and function onto which neural transplantation offers the prospect of casting new light. By far the greatest majority of these studies have been conducted on the species that is the subject of this book: the laboratory rat.

25.1 Techniques of Neural Transplantation

Since the earliest attempts at transplantation of neural tissues in the mammalian brain, the neocortex has been a key source of donor tissue and a target site for transplantation. In 1890 Thompson took cortical tissue from adult cats and implanted the tissue pieces into the neocortex of adult dogs. Although Thompson reported clear survival of those transplanted tissues for a period of several weeks in the host brain, it is likely that only glial and meningeal cells—rather than neurons—survived the transplantation process.

The first unequivocal cases of successful transplantation of mammalian brain tissue were reported by Elizabeth Dunn in 1917. She implanted wedges of cortical tissue taken from neonatal rat pups into cavities made in the neocortex of littermates. Although the success rate was less than 10 percent, her four successful cases all involved exposure of the lateral ventricles and apposition of the graft tissue to the choroid plexus, with its rich vascular supply, to provide nutrients for the isolated graft tissue. A second factor in her success was almost certainly the identification of the developing brain as a suitable source for donor tissue, with greater growth capacity and tolerance of anoxia than that of mature neurons (Stenevi et al. 1976).

In the subsequent decades further sporadic studies can be identified in the literature. Thus, for example, Le Gros Clark (1940) transplanted fetal rabbit cortex to 6-week-old hosts, using a cannula/plunger technique that is still widely used, with considerable success. The embryonic tissue in many cases continued to grow and differentiate. Neurons within the grafts developed toward a mature cytologic phenotype and were seen in a number of cases to become organized in clusters or layers of cells of particular types in "a somewhat indistinct laminar pattern . . . characteristic of the normally developed cerebral cortex." Glees (1940) confirmed this capacity of embryonic cortical neuroblasts to continue differentiation when implanted onto the host cortical surface under the pia and observed one cortical graft to develop many features of the normal cortical organization. For example, a wedge-shaped zone within this case was composed of a narrow compact layer of pyramidal cells lying in immediate relation to a parallel row of small granular cells.

It may seem surprising that these remarkable studies attracted so little attention at the time. However, within the general zeitgeist derived from Cajal and others that all regeneration in the adult mammalian central nervous system is abortive, these early graft studies may have been considered bizarre anomalies rather than illustrative of general principles for growth and regeneration worthy of active investigation. Following the demonstration by Raisman (1969) of collateral sprouting of synaptic connections in the mature CNS, the prospect of remodeling and regeneration of connections in the mammalian nervous system began to appear more plausible, and the viability of transplantation of neural tissues in the brain was confirmed by three separate research groups in the early 1970s. First, Das and Altman (1971, 1972) showed reliable survival of neonatal cerebellum transplanted to the cerebellum of neonatal hosts and migration of thymidine-labeled granule cells from the grafts into the host brain. Second, Olson and colleagues showed that sympathetic (Olson and Malmfors 1970) or central (Olson and Seiger 1972) noradrenergic neurons grafted to the anterior eye chamber had the capacity not only to survive but also to provide an extensive and appropriately organized noradrenergic reinnervation of the host iris. Third, Björklund and colleagues observed that central catecholaminergic axons would sprout and reinnervate appropriate target tissues, such as muscle or iris, when grafted into the brain (Björklund and Stenevi 1971, Svendgaard et al. 1975).

These early studies led to the identification and systematic characterization of the parameters and conditions for obtaining reliable survival of neural tissue grafts in the brain (Stenevi et al. 1976), which in essence involve (1) use of graft tissue taken from donors at the particular embryonic or neonatal age when the cells of interest are just completing final cell division, and (2) selection of graft placement and transplantation procedure to optimize the rapid vascularization and cerebrospinal fluid drainage of the grafted cells in the host brain. A variety of different transplantation techniques that have been used to study cortical grafts are illustrated in figure 25.1.

In the subsequent decade the neocortex has provided one convenient model system for the development of transplantation techniques both as a source of donor tissues and as a suitable transplantation site. Thus, for example, embryonic cortical tissues become rapidly revascularized within approximately 24 hours by extension of the fine capillaries from the host brain into the grafts, whether placed in the neocortex (Smith and Ebner 1986), the cerebellum (Rosenstein 1987), or the hippocampus (Lawrence et al. 1984) of the host brain. The fate of the dividing embryonic cortical cells in the host brain can be followed by labeling in utero with tritiated thymidine (Jaeger and Lund 1980a, Floeter and Jones 1984, Alexandrova et al. 1985) or in culture with fluorescent dyes (McConnell 1985, Colombo et al. 1987) or leucoagglutinin (Kamo et al. 1987) as cell markers before transplantation. Cortical tissue can be frozen and stored for up to four months and retain viability for subsequent transplantation (Houle and Das 1980). Additionally cross-species grafting between human and rat has been studied in the development of human fetal cortical tissue in the anterior eye chamber of rats (Olson et al. 1987). Conversely the rat neocortex has been used as a transplantation site for other human tissues, including fetal spinal cord (Kamo et al. 1987) and pathological cortical tissue from Alzheimer's patients' brains (van den Bosch de Aguilar et al. 1984).[1]

25.2   Intrinsic Organization of Cortical Grafts

Labeled cortical cells implanted into the neocortex of the neonatal ferret (a species that is particularly immature at birth) undergo extensive migration to an appropriate laminar level in the host cortex (McConnell 1985). However, the majority of studies have employed hosts at a more mature stage of development, including the neonatal rat, and in such cases cortical grafts are generally seen to be clearly demarcated from the host brain. Thus Jaeger and Lund (1980a) labeled embryonic cortical tissue with thymidine before implantation in the occipital cortex of the neonatal rat and found that labeled neurons were only observed within the grafts up to 12 weeks later, although a few labeled glial cells were seen to have migrated short distances into adjacent areas of host cortex. Similarly Lindsay and Raisman (1984) found that thymidine-labeled glial cells migrated considerable distances into the host hippocampus, whereas labeled neurons remained contained within the borders of the hippocampal grafts. In general the graft tissue is readily distinguishable in the host brain in Nissl-stained sections, with a variable degree of gliosis at the graft-host border that may be sparse or almost completely absent (Dunnett et al. 1987a, Floeter and Jones 1984, Stein and Mufson

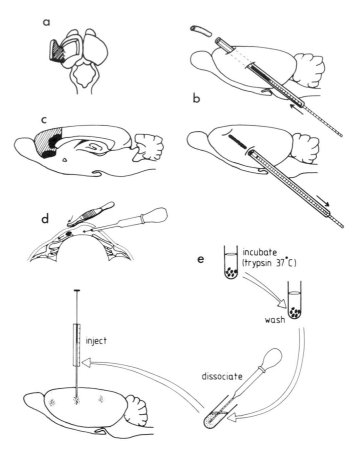

Figure 25.1 Techniques for grafting cortical tissues in the neocortex or anterior eye chamber of rats. (a) Dissection of embryonic neocortex. (b) Cannula/plunger technique of Smith and Ebner (1986), in which a core of cortical tissue is removed by penetration of the cannula, and the embryonic graft tissue is ejected as it is withdrawn. (c) Delayed transplantation technique of Stenevi and colleagues (1980), in which an aspirative lesion of the neocortex is made 1 to 6 weeks before implantation of the graft tissue. (d) Intraocular technique of Olson and Malmfors (1970), in which graft tissue is ejected onto the host iris in the anterior chamber of the eye. (e) Dissociated cell suspension technique of Björklund and coworkers (1983a), in which graft tissue pieces are incubated in trypsin, washed, and mechanically dissociated, and 2–3μl aliquots are stereotaxically injected in one or several sites in the host brain. The illustrations are based on Seiger 1985, Smith and Ebner 1986, Olson et al. 1984, and Dunnett 1987.

1987), but may in some cases completely encapsule the graft (Krüger et al. 1986). Although a major gliotic scar is generally not apparent in Nissl-stained material to isolate the graft from the host brain, immunohistochemical staining using glial fibrillary acidic protein and vimentin antibodies indicates the continuing presence of an abnormal astrocytic reaction at the graft-host interface (Smith and Ebner 1986, Björklund et al. 1983a, 1984).

As mentioned above, in the early studies using general cell body stains Glees (1940) and Le Gros Clark (1940) both noted the differentiation of large pyramidal cells and small to medium-sized granule cells within their grafts of cortical tissue and the occasional aggregation of the cells into somewhat diffuse layers. Golgi staining of neurons in the grafts has confirmed the occurrence of large pyramidal and both spiny and aspiny medium-sized neurons characteristic of the types seen in the intact neocortex (Jaeger and Lund 1981, Floeter and Jones 1984). However, a clear laminar organization in cortical grafts is only rarely observed. A more common pattern is for grafted cortical cells to become organized into clusters (Floeter and Jones 1984, Jaeger and Lund 1980b, 1981, Stein and Mufson 1987). These clusters may be separated by bands of myelinated fibers in the depths of the graft and cell-poor zones reminiscent of a molecular layer, particularly at the graft-host border, so that the neuronal clusters appear layered, but a clear lamination of cells within the grafts is generally denied. Although the majority of studies have used solid grafts implanted into cortical cavities or as plugs into cortical or subcortical sites, a similar reaggregation of neurons into disorganized clusters is seen when the graft is implanted as a dissociated suspension of embryonic cortical cells (Floeter and Jones 1984, Sofroniew et al. 1986). To the extent that the cells within the grafts develop a laminar organization, the layers do not show a particular alignment with the host neocortical laminae unless the graft has been carefully implanted so as to maintain the normal orientation (Andres and Van der Loos 1985, Chang et al. 1986).

Several recent studies have used immunocytochemical staining to identify specific populations of neurons within cortical grafts implanted in the neocortex, including glutamic acid decarboxylase, choline acetyltransferase, NADPH-diaphorase, vasoactive intestinal polypeptide, neuropeptide Y, cholecystokinin, pancreatic polypeptide, and somatostatin immunoreactive neurons (Ebner et al. 1984, Floeter and Jones 1985, Gonzalez and Sharp 1987, Sharp et al. 1987, Stein and Mufson 1987), all of which are characteristic of normal cortex. In parallel, receptors for neuropeptides, including vasoactive intestinal polypeptide and bombesin, have been detected autoradiographically in the grafts (Getz et al. 1987). Conversely antibodies against other peptides that have not been found in the intact neocortex, including substance P, α-melanocyte- or corticotropin-stimulating hormones, β-endorphin or arginine-vasopressin, do not label cells in the cortical grafts (Ebner et al. 1984). Grafts of other neuronal populations implanted in the neocortex retain their characteristic cell populations. Thus, for example, Fine and colleagues (1985b) implanted cholinergic rich basal forebrain neurons into the neocortex of cholinergically depleted rats and confirmed good survival of choline acetyltransferase immunoreactive neurons. In this case somatostatin, enkephalin, and neuropeptide Y immunoreactivity was observed within the basal forebrain grafts, but not staining for substance P, neurotensin, or vasoactive intestinal polypeptide, the last of which is characteristic of the normal neocortex.

Thus a variety of morphological and immunohistochemical markers indicate that many different types of neurons included in the tissue graft retain predetermined expression of particular neurotransmitters, independent of whether those cell types are characteristically found in the normal cortex, whereas cortical tissues themselves develop the apparently full range of normal basic cell types. However, abnormal enzyme expression in the grafts has been observed under some circumstances. In particular embryonic cortical neurons develop tyrosine hydroxylase immunoreactivity when transplanted from early embryos (Park et al. 1986), although this enzyme is absent in intact cortex. It is likely that tyrosine hydroxylase expression is inhibited in normal development by local influences that are not available to the grafted cells in the adult brain, because a similar expression of the enzyme is observed in cortical neurons in in vitro culture (Iacovitti et al. 1987).

25.3 Connectivity of Cortical Grafts

Afferent and efferent connectivity of cortical tissue grafts and cortical graft placement has been considered using a variety of techniques, including neuroanatomical tracers, tissue- or neurotransmitter-specific markers, and electrophysiological methods.

When implanted into the neocortex of neonatal rats, cortical tissues have been observed to establish extensive connections with the host brain. For example, injection of HRP or fluorescent tracers into the grafts reveals extensive retrograde labeling in the thalamus and contralateral neocortex (Chang et al. 1984, Castro et al. 1985) and in a variety of monoaminergic subcortical regulatory nuclei including the locus coeruleus, raphe nucleus, and basal forebrain (Castro et al. 1988). Similarly anterograde labeling with HRP or injection of retrograde labels into target areas has revealed efferent connections in the pyramidal tract (Stanfield and O'Leary 1985, Castro et al. 1987), thalamus, and striatum (Chang et al. 1984).

In several studies similar patterns of reafferentation have been observed when the grafts are implanted in adult hosts. Thus the grafts are seen to be reinnervated by NADPH-diaphorase fibers from the host cortex (Sharp et al. 1986) and by acetylcholinesterase-positive fibers of presumed basal forebrain origin (Dunnett et al. 1987a, Gibbs and Cotman 1987, Sofroniew et al. 1986, Stein and Mufson 1987). HRP labeling of the grafts has revealed retrograde labeling of cells in the contralateral cortex and in subcortical thalamic, basal forebrain, locus coeruleus, and raphe nuclei (Dunnett et al. 1987a, Gibbs et al. 1985, Labbe et al. 1983). Clear demonstration of reciprocal efferent connections of cortical grafts implanted in the adult nervous system are sparse, but projections to the thalamus, amygdala, and hippocampus have been suggested by both anterograde and retrograde HRP labeling (Dunnett et al. 1987a, Gibbs et al. 1985, Gonzalez et al. 1988). Conversely extensive outgrowth from subcortical monoaminergic grafts implanted in the adult cortex has been well established by histochemical and immunohistochemical labeling, both for dopamine-rich (Dunnett et al. 1985a, Herman et al. 1986) and cholinergic-rich graft tissues (Fine et al. 1985b, Dunnett et al. 1986, Clarke and Dunnett 1986).

25.4 Electrophysiological Function of Cortical Grafts

Electrophysiological techniques have been widely used to study intrinsic organization and functional connectivity of neuronal grafts in the neocortex. Attempts have been made to determine the degree to which intrinsic activity in the grafts is organized similarly to that observed in the intact cortex. Moreover, as an adjunct to anatomical tracing techniques, physiological recording permits the determination of the degree to which patterned information can be relayed between grafts and the host brain.

In one remarkable series of studies, Bragin (1986a,b, Bragin et al. 1987) made aspirative lesions of the barrelfield of adult rats' somatosensory cortex followed by transplantation of isotopic embryonic cortex to the lesion cavity. Microelectrodes were implanted into the grafts 2 to 3 months later to allow time for host-graft connections to become established. Background activity of cells in the graft consisted of low-frequency, randomly distributed discharges similar to those observed in the contralateral intact cortex. More dramatically cells in the grafts responded by bursts of firing to vibrissae stimulation, indicating the convergence of inputs from peripheral receptors into the grafts. The main difference with intact neocortex was not the pattern of firing per se, but that grafted cells had larger receptive fields, compatible with the histological observations that grafted cells were not organized into detectable barrellike zones. Confirmation of these observations has recently been obtained by Levin and coworkers (1987) using 2-deoxyglucose autoradiography to determine metabolic activity. They demonstrated that cortical grafts located in somatosensory cortex showed focal areas of increased 2-deoxyglucose uptake (by approximately 43 percent) in response to vibrissae stimulation. The specificity of this effect was demonstrated by the use of control grafts of noncortical tissue in the somatosensory cortex or of cortical tissue in nonsomatosensory sites, both of which failed to show any detectable response to stimulation.

In addition to the study of cortical tissue grafts, other tissues that normally innervate or are innervated by the neocortex have also been seen to reestablish functional connections with the host cortex following transplantation. For example, Hamasaki and coworkers (1987a,b) demonstrated reciprocal connections between lateral geniculate nucleus grafts and the host occipital cortex by electrical stimulation and recording in slice preparations. Similarly Harvey and colleagues (1982) found that when tectal tissue was implanted over the superior colliculus, electical stimulation of the host occipital cortex orthodromically excited 25 of 214 single units within the grafts at latencies (< 15 ms, mean 7.3 ms), suggesting a monosynaptic input. In both of these studies the implants were made into neonatal hosts. However, even in adult hosts physiologically effective sprouting of cortical neurons has been observed into striatal grafts (Rutherford et al. 1987).

25.5 Manipulation of Cortical Development

Neural transplantation provides a powerful means of identification and manipulation of a variety of factors involved in neural development. This strategy can be illustrated with three examples.

Development of Parietal Cortex in Oculo

Olson and colleagues (1983, 1984) have employed the anterior eye chamber as a site that will provide effective protection, nutrition, and support for the in vivo culture of developing neural tissues. Seiger and Olson (1975) provided the first detailed description of cortical graft development in oculo, with a lack of distinct layering and a cell-poor outer molecular layer similar to the normal developing neocortex. Such grafts do not grow large in size, but develop an abnormal degree of gliosis (Björklund and Dahl 1982, Björklund et al. 1984), which is progressively more severe and associated with progressively more pathological vascularization as the age of the host animal at the time of transplantation increases (Eriksdotter-Nilsson et al. 1986). Olson and colleagues (1983, 1984) suggest that such abnormalities of development in isolated cortex are attributable in part of a loss of trophic influences from contacts with other brain areas. When cortex is transplanted to the eye chamber along with sympathetic ganglia or locus coeruleus tissue, the cograft establishes an extensive noradrenergic reinnervation of the cortex graft (Olson et al. 1979, 1984). Moreover cografts of locus coeruleus or tectum induce a marked stimulation of growth and reduction in reactive gliosis to normal cortical levels in the cortical grafts (Björklund et al. 1983b). On electrophysiological investigation only the locus coeruleus–stimulated cortical grafts showed spontaneous patterns or slow sustained discharge similar to that observed in the normal parietal cortex, and this response was augmented by local application of glutamate or acetylcholine (Palmer et al. 1983). By contrast, isolated cortical grafts fired in abnormal sporadic high-frequency bursts and were insensitive to transmitter application. These obervations indicate the importance of extrinsic inputs for the normal development and organization of neocortical tissues.

Visual System Development

Lund and colleagues (1982, 1987) have employed neural transplantation to systematically evaluate a series of questions related to normal visual system development, such as why the axons grow to the right places in the brain, how they stop growing when they reach appropriate targets, and why a similar pattern of regrowth is not observed after injury. Within this global strategy the development, extent, and specificity of connections have been evaluated between retinal, tectal, or cortical tissues implanted in the visual cortex (Chang et al. 1984, McLoon and Lund 1984, Sharkey et al. 1987), between occipital cortex grafts implanted over the tectum (Jaeger and Lund 1980b), and between the intact cortex and tectal or other grafts implanted over the tectum (Lund and Harvey 1981, Harvey and Lund 1981; see also Harvey et al. 1982). These studies have demonstrated the continuing differentiation of an appropriate internal organization within the grafts and a remarkable degree of specificity for areas of the host brain to grow into and receive projections from the grafts of each type (Lund et al. 1982). The developmental status of the host is important, such that extensive reformation of afferent and efferent connections is only seen when implants are placed in the neonatal brain, whereas relatively sparse connectivity has been observed in the adult host brain (McLoon and Lund 1983). In particular axonal growth is frequently observed to follow an abnormal route to reach an appropriate target, suggesting that growth depends on a variety of neurotropic mechanisms rather than passively following particular cellular or molecular substrates (Lund et al. 1987; see also Matthews 1985). Moreover the timetable of events is relatively normal, even where appropriate connectivity is not established. For example, normal ganglion cell death is observed after transplantation of retinal aggregates to the occipital cortex, even though the retinal cells in this site do not innervate thalamic or tectal targets. This suggests that cell death is an intrinsic developmental property of retinal ganglion cells, rather than depending on interactions with established terminals (Lund et al. 1987).

Topographic Development of Cortical Connections

It has already been noted that embryonic cortical tissue implanted into the neonatal cortex establishes afferent connections from the host thalamus (Chang et al. 1984, Castro et al. 1985) and efferent pyramidal tract projections (Stanfield and O'Leary 1985). The establishment of such connections appears to be determined by the topographic location of the graft in the developing host neocortex, rather than by the area of embryonic cortex from which the graft was dissected. Thus, for example, Chang and colleagues (1986) implanted different embryonic cortical areas into the occipitoparietal region of the neonatal cortex and observed that the grafts all received inputs from the thalamic nuclei that normally innervate the cortical areas adjacent to the graft placement (see also Floeter and Jones 1985). Similarly embryonic frontal (Castro et al. 1987), parietal (Floeter and Jones 1984), or occipital (Stanfield and O'Leary 1985, Porter et al. 1987) cortical areas can all develop pyramidal tract projections at least as far as the spinomedullary junction (and in the Castro et al. 1987 study, to the level of the cervical spinal cord) when transplanted to the rostral motor cortex area of neonatal rats. These observations support the hypothesis that the precise patterns of cortical connectivity are in part determined by "supragenomic factors" involving extensive growth potential and selective collateral elimination (Stanfield 1984).

25.6   Inhibition and Repair of Degenerative Damage

Retrograde Degeneration in the Thalamus

Neonatal lesions of the frontal or occipital cortex result in developmental atrophy of the corresponding afferent nuclei of the thalamus. Haun and Cunningham (1984, 1987) found that five days after transplanting embryonic neocortex into the cavity formed by a neonatal occipital lesion, atrophy in the corresponding dorsal lateral geniculate nucleus of the host was markedly attenuated. Noncortical (cerebellar) control grafts were ineffective in preventing the lesion-induced atrophy. In these studies, using cell-suspension grafts of the cortical cells, the protection was only temporary. However, Sharp and Gonzalez (1986) have achieved permanent prevention of retrograde thalamic atrophy using cortical implants into neonatal frontal cortical lesions. Although the two groups employed different cortical lesion sites, Sharp and Gonzalez considered that the most likely reason for more lasting protection in their study was due to the use of solid tissue implants. These observations indicate that the trophic interactions necessary for the survival of developing neurons and lost by the removal of appropriate targets can be reestablished by transplant-derived replacement of those targets. It may be necessary for developing host thalamic neurons to innervate the grafts to achieve such protection, although it cannot at present be excluded that the influence is entirely attributable to diffusable neurotrophic factors.

Retrograde Degeneration in the NBM

If transplants can provide trophic support in a developmental context, it is of interest to consider whether similar trophic support can be provided against retrograde degeneration following axotomy or target removal in adulthood. This has been investigated in the magnocellular cholinergic cells of the nucleus basalis, which atrophy in response to extensive loss of cortical targets by mechanical devascularization or excitotoxic lesion (Sofroniew et al. 1983, Sofroniew and Pearson 1985). Cortical cell suspensions implanted in the damaged cortex completely prevented this retrograde atrophy of the cholinergic neurons of the host nucleus basalis system, which sprouted to extensively reinnervate the cortical tissue grafts (Sofroniew et al. 1986). These observations support the notion that target-derived trophic factors are necessary for the maintenance of neural connections in the mature central nervous system as well for their normal development and can be substituted by neural tissue grafts.

25.7 Functional Repair of Cortical Denervation

In view of the complex precision of the columnar organization that has been thought to underlie the functional processing subserved by the neocortex (Mountcastle 1979), one of the most dramatic findings of recent research has been the apparent capacity of cortical grafts to ameliorate some complex learning deficits resulting from cortical damage. Stein and colleagues first showed that rats' abilities to learn a delayed alternation task in a T maze, which is disrupted by aspirative lesions of the frontal cortex, could be substantially restored after transplantation of embryonic cortical tissue into the lesion cavity (Labbe et al. 1983, Stein et al. 1988). Similar effects after transplantation of embryonic cortical tissues have been reported on the recovery of visual brightness (Stein et al. 1985) and pattern (Haun et al. 1985) discrimination following occipital cortex lesions, of taste aversion learning after gustatory neocortex lesions (Bermudez-Rattoni et al. 1987), and of spatial maze learning after allocortical (hippocampal) lesions (Kimble et al. 1986).

Such dramatic recovery on complex learning tasks, when taken together with the observed formation of afferent and efferent connections between cortical grafts and the damaged host brain, makes it tempting to suggest that the grafts influence recovery by means of a functional reconstruction of damaged cortical neural circuitries. However, this conclusion is premature. Björklund and coworkers (1987), have reviewed a variety of mechanisms by which grafted tissues can influence the behavioral capacities of the host animal. These include

1. *Nonspecific or negative consequences of the implantation surgery.* These may include graft-growth–inducing, space-occupying lesions; cyst and scar formation; changes in the blood-brain barrier; or induction of further degenerative changes in the host brain.

2. *Trophic actions on the host brain.* The acute secretion of trophic factors

and the migration of glial cells into the host brain may reduce lesion-induced cell death or promote functional reorganization and recovery within the host brain, independent of any sustained effect of the grafted neurons.

3. *Diffuse release of hormones or transmitters.* The grafted cells may provide a chronic secretion of deficient neuroactive chemicals such as hormones or neurotransmitters to the host brain.

4. *Reformation of afferent and/or efferent connections between the graft and the host brain.* Only in this case do the formation and activity of neuronal connections between the graft and host brain subserve functional changes observable in the behavior of the host animal.

Evidence for each of these mechanisms of action has been observed in other model systems for neural transplantation (Björklund et al. 1987, Dunnett and Björklund 1987) and consequently must be considered in the case of the effects on more complex behaviors of grafts in the neocortex. Thus Stein and colleagues (1985) found that frontal but not occipital cortical tissue grafts were effective in ameliorating the visual discrimination deficits associated with occipital lesions, suggesting the importance of some feature of the embryonic tissue other than the selection of the appropriate population of neurons to replace those damaged by the lesion. Moreover the timing of transplantation and behavioral testing have turned out to be critical. First, recovery is only observed when the graft surgery is conducted within 7 to 14 days of the lesions, and not at either shorter or longer intervals (Dunnett et al. 1987a, Kesslak et al. 1986a, Stein et al. 1988). Second, the grafts are effective only in studies where behavioral testing commences within a few days of transplantation, before sufficient time has elapsed for the growth of any graft-host connections, and not when behavioral testing is delayed by 6 weeks or more (Dunnett et al. 1987a, Stein et al. 1985). Indeed Dunnett and colleagues (1987a) demonstrated one group of animals receiving transplants 7 days after frontal cortex lesion that were significantly improved with respect to the rats with lesions alone when testing commenced 1 week later, but significantly impaired when re-tested after a 6-month interval.

These observations suggest that although the cortical graft tissue may come to form connections with the host brain, this does not underlie the functional recovery that is often observed. Rather the rapid sequence of the behavioral changes indicates that the grafts stimulate or secrete neurotrophic substances that promote functional recovery in the host brain (Kesslak et al. 1986, Stein 1987). Indeed Kesslak and coworkers (1986a,b) demonstrated that a similar pattern of recovery could be induced by the implantation of purified cultured astrocytes or of adult tissue grafts predominantly comprised of glia. Conversely once healthy embryonic grafts establish connections with the host brain, functional deficits over and above those induced by the lesions have been observed

(Dunnett et al. 1987a). In this latter case it has not been resolved whether the long-term impairments are due to inhibition of long-term recovery in the host brain, to the grafts developing space-occupying lesions, or to graft-derived inputs adding noise to the remaining intact host cortex.

25.8 Functional Repair of Cortical Deafferentiation

A conceptually different approach to the possibility of functional repair in the cortex relates to the replacement by transplantation of diffuse afferent systems of the isodendritic core. Analogous to the regulatory control of the basal ganglia by ascending mesencephalic dopamine neurons, which has provided the most powerful system for studying the functional capacity of neural transplants (Brundin and Björklund 1987, Dunnett et al. 1985a, Lindvall et al. 1987), the neuronal circuitry of the neocortex receives inputs from a variety of subcortical monoaminergic nuclei. These afferents arise from subcortical and brainstem cholinergic, catecholaminergic, and sertonergic nuclei; are widely arborized; and are believed to provide for the general regulatory control of information processing in the cortical circuitries (Björklund and Lindvall 1986, Richardson and DeLong 1988, Segal and Bloom 1978). Recently particular attention has focused on the neocortical cholinergic innervation arising in the basal forebrain nucleus basalis magnocellularis (NBM) after the demonstration of degeneration of this system in association with the cognitive and memory failures of aging and Alzheimer's dementia (Bartus et al. 1982, Coyle et al. 1983).

In a widely studied model system for Alzheimer's disease, many studies have demonstrated impairments in learning and/or memory functions in rats with bilateral lesions of the NBM (Dean and Bartus 1985, Collerton 1986, Dunnett and Barth, in press, Fisher and Hanin 1986, Smith 1988). More recently several groups have indicated that such impairments can be substantially ameliorated by cholinergic-rich basal forebrain grafts implanted in multiple neocortical sites in tasks ranging from active and passive avoidance (Arendash and Mouton 1987, Dunnett et al. 1985b, Fine et al. 1985a), spatial navigation in a water maze (Dunnett et al. 1985b), T maze alternation learning (Welner et al. 1988), and operant delayed matching to sample (Dunnett 1987). These observations raise several issues of specificity.

Is the Recovery Related to Cholinergic Cell Replacement?
Fine and colleagues (1985b) used a range of histochemical markers to determine that in addition to the choline acetyltransferase–immunoreactive neurons of primary interest, several types of peptidergic neurons were also present in the basal forebrain grafts. However, only the cholinergic cells were seen to give rise to any extensive reinnervation of the host brain in the animals that showed functional recovery on the passive avoidance and water maze tasks (Dunnett et al. 1985b). Addi-

tionally several of the studies in which recovery was seen have employed control grafts of noncholinergic tissues, and in these animals no behavioral recovery was observed (Fine et al. 1985a, Welner et al. 1988). Because NBM lesions damage considerably more than just the magnocellular cholinergic neurons of the basal forebrain, it has been difficult to determine from lesion studies whether the effects of NBM damage are specifically due to cortical cholinergic deafferentation (Abrogast and Kozlowski 1988, Dunnett et al. 1987b, Everitt et al. 1987). The transplantation studies, however, provide considerable support for the hypothesis that cortical cholinergic systems are critically involved in at least those tasks on which recovery is observed.

Is the Recovery Specific to Memory Functions?
NBM lesions make deafferent wide areas of the neocortex of its regulatory cholinergic inputs. In particular the most extensive cholinergic depletion in rats is in the dorsolateral quadrant of the neocortex throughout its rostrocaudal extent. These areas subserve primary sensory and motor functions in addition to including the parietal association cortex, whereas prefrontal and temporal cortical areas are left relatively intact. It would be premature to suppose that the primary disturbances following such a pattern of cortical deafferentation are restricted to higher cognitive, learning, and memory functions. Indeed several reports have indicated a variety of neurological, regulatory, and sensorimotor deficits after NBM lesions, and in one study cortical cholinergic grafts have been seen to significantly ameliorate several of the rats' sensorimotor deficits (Dunnett et al. 1985b).

Is the Model System Applicable to the Memory Dysfunctions Associated with Aging?
It has been well established in several studies that cholinergic grafts implanted in the hippocampus of old rats can ameliorate age-related deficits in spatial navigation abilities (Gage et al. 1984). However, only recently has this issue been addressed with regard to cortical cholinergic systems. Dunnett and associates (1988) trained rats on a delayed nonmatching to sample task to assess short-term memory capacities. Whereas 24-month-old rats forgot sooner than did young controls, memory was significantly improved in old rats with cholinergic grafts placed bilaterally into either hippocampal or neocortical sites. It has yet to be confirmed that this particular effect is specific to the use of cholinergic tissues. If so, however, it will be particularly interesting to determine whether combined graft placements into both neocortical and allocortical sites can yield improvement greater than from either placement alone. Along similar lines Arendt and colleagues (1988) have recently shown that cholinergic graft placement into combined hippocampal and cortical sites does provide a greater amelioration of deficits

in radial maze learning in rats with prolonged alcohol intoxication than is seen in rats with either single-graft placement.

25.9 Summary and Conclusions

The techniques are now well established for the viable transplantation of cortical and other neural tissues into the neonatal and adult cortex, at least in the laboratory rat. Under appropriate conditions such grafts survive well and can establish reciprocal connections with the host brain. On this basis neural transplantation has become a powerful technique for the study of mechanisms involved in the development of the central nervous system and its capacity for regeneration after injury. Moreover a variety of anatomical, electrophysiological, and behavioral techniques suggest that grafted neural tissue may sustain functional interactions with the host brain. It remains undetermined whether such experimental observations may ever acquire therapeutic application.

Note

1. No survival of neurons was seen in this latter study, as expected for mature donor tissue, whereas the pathological twisted neurofilaments of the grafts appeared to become incorporated within the gliotic reaction induced in the host rat cortex. The authors therefore proposed such cortical transplantation as providing a model for the role of transmissible agents in the course of the human disease, but the observations may reflect no more than the highly insoluble nature and hence poor phagocytic removal of pathological neurofibrillary proteins.

References

Abrogast, R. E., and Kozlowski, M. R. (1988). Quantitative morphometric analysis of the neurotoxic effects of the excitotoxin, ibotenic acid, on the basal forebrain. *Neurotoxicology* 9:39–46.

Alexandrova, M. A., Polezhaev, L. V., and Cherkasova, L. V. (1985). Transplantation of dissociated embryonic brain cells in the brain of adult normal rats and rats subjected to hypoxia. *Journal für Hirnforschung* 26:275–279.

Andres, F. L., and Van der Loos, H. (1985). Removal and reimplantation of the parietal cortex of the neonatal mouse: consequences for the barrelfield. *Developmental Brain Research* 20:115–121.

Arendash, G. W., and Mouton, P. R. (1987). Transplantation of nucleus basalis magnocellularis cholinergic neurons into the cholinergic-depleted cerebral cortex. *Annals of the New York Academy of Science* 495:431–443.

Arendt, T., Allen, Y., Sinden, J., Schugens, M. M., Marchbanks, R. M., Lantos, P. L., and Gray, J. A. (1988). Cholinergic-rich brain transplants reverse alcohol-induced memory deficits. *Nature* 332:448–450.

Bartus, R. T., Dean, R. L., Beer, B., and Lippa, A. S. (1982). The cholinergic hypothesis of geriatric memory dysfunction. *Science* 217:408–417.

Bermudez-Rattoni, F., Fernandez, J., Sanchez, M. A., Aguilar-Roblero, R., and Drucker-Colin, R. (1987). Fetal brain transplants induce recuperation of taste aversion learning. *Brain Research* 416:147–152.

Björklund, A., and Lindvall, O. (1986). Catecholaminergic brain stem regulatory systems. *Handbook of Physiology—The Nervous System IV,* American Physiological Association, Washington, D.C., 155–235.

Björklund, A., and Stenevi, U. (1971). Growth of central catecholamine neurones into smooth muscle grafts in the rat mesencephalon. *Brain Research* 31:1–20.

Björklund, A., Lindvall, O., Isacson, O., Brundin, P., Wictorin, K., Strecker, R. E., Clarke, D. J., and Dunnett, S. B. (1987). Mechanisms of action of intracerebral neural implants: studies on nigral and striatal grafts to the lesion striatum. *Trends in Neuroscience* 10:509–516.

Björklund, H., and Dahl, D. (1982). Glial disturbances in isolated neocortex: evidence from immunohistochemistry of intraocular grafts. *Developmental Neuroscience* 5:424–436.

Björklund, H., Dahl, D., Haglid, K., Rosengren, L., and Olson, L. (1983a). Astrocytic development in fetal parietal cortex grafted to cerebral and cerebellar cortex of immature rats. *Developmental Brain Research* 9:171–180.

Björklund, H., Dahl, D., and Olson, L. (1984). Morphometry of GFA and vimentin positive astrocytes in grafted and lesioned cortex cerebri. *International Journal of Developmental Neuroscience* 2:181–192.

Björklund, H., Seiger, Å., Hoffer, B. J., and Olson, L. (1983b). Trophic effects of brain areas on the developing cerebral cortex. I. Growth and histological organization of intraocular grafts. *Developmental Brain Research* 6:131–140.

Bragin, A. G. (1986a). Neuronal responses of embryonic rat somatosensory neocortex grafted into adult rat barrelfield (in Russian). *Neurophysiologia* 18:833–836.

Bragin, A. G. (1986b). Involvement of neurones of the grafted embryonial neocortex of rats in host's neocortical sensory functions. [Russian] *Journal of Higher Nerve Operations* 5:929–938.

Bragin, A. G., Bohne, A., and Pavlik, V. D. (1987). Electrophysiological indexes of the degree of grafted neural tissue integration with the host brain (in Russian). *Neurophysiologia* 19:498–504.

Brundin, P., and Björklund, A. (1987). Survival, growth and function of dopaminergic neurons grafted to the brain. *Progress in Brain Research* 71:293–308.

Castro, A. J., Tonder, N., Sunde, N. A., and Zimmer, J. (1987). Fetal cortical transplants in the cerebral hemisphere of newborn rats: a retrograde fluorescent analysis of connections. *Experimental Brain Research* 66:533–542.

Castro, A. J., Tonder, N., Sunde, N. A., and Zimmer, J. (1988). Fetal neocortical transplants grafted to the cerebral cortex of newborn rats receive afferents from the basal forebrain, locus coeruleus and midline raphe. *Experimental Brain Research* 69:613–622.

Castro, A. J., Zimmer, J., Sunde, N. A., and Bold, E. L. (1985). Thalamic afferents to fetal cortical tissue transplanted to the cerebral cortex of neonatal rats. *Society of Neuroscience Abstracts* 11:65.

Chang, F. L., Steedman, J. G., and Lund, R. D. (1984). Embryonic cerebral cortex placed in the occipital region of newborn rats makes connections with the host brain. *Developmental Brain Research* 13:164–166.

Chang, F. L., Steedman, J. G., and Lund, R. D. (1986). The lamination and connectivity of embryonic cerebral cortex transplanted into newborn rat cortex. *Journal of Comparative Neurology* 244:401–411.

Clarke, D. J., and Dunnett, S. B. (1986). Ultrastructural organization of choline acetyltransferase-immunoreactive fibres innervating the neocortex from embryonic ventral forebrain grafts. *Journal of Comparative Neurology* 250:192–205.

Collerton, D. (1986). Cholinergic function and intellectual decline in Alzheimer's disease. *Neuroscience* 19:1–28.

Columbo, J. A., Almeida, J. I., and Molina, S. (1987). In vitro culture and labelling of neural cell aggregates followed by transplantation. *Exp. Neurol.* 98:606–615.

Coyle, J. T., Price, J. T., and DeLong, M. R. (1983). Alzheimer's disease: a disorder of cortical cholinergic innervation. *Science* 219:1184–1190.

Das, G. D., and Altman, J. (1971). Transplanted precursors of nerve cells: their fate in the cerebellums of young rats. *Science* 173:637–638.

Das, G. D., and Altman, J. (1972). Studies on the transplantation of developing neural tissue in the mammalian brain. I. Transplantation of cerebellar slabs into the cerebellum of neonatal rats. *Brain Research* 38:233–249.

Dean, R. L., and Bartus, R. T. (1985). Animal models of geriatric cognitive dysfunction: evidence for an important cholinergic involvement. In J. Traber and W. H. Gispen (eds.), *Senile Dementia of the Alzheimer Type*. Heidelberg: Springer Verlag, 269–282.

Dunn, E. H. (1917). Primary and secondary findings in a series of attempts to transplant cerebral cortex in the albino rat. *Journal of Comparative Neurology* 27:565–582.

Dunnett, S. B. (1987). Anatomical and behavioral consequences of cholinergic-rich grafts to the neocortex of rats with lesions of the nucleus basalis magnocellularis. *Annals of the New York Academy of Science* 495:415–429.

Dunnett, S. B., and Barth, T. (in press). Animal models of Alzheimer's disease and dementia (with an emphasis on cortical cholinergic systems). In P. Wilner (ed.), *Behavioural Models in Psychopharmacology*. Cambridge: Cambridge University Press.

Dunnett, S. B., and Björklund, A. (1987). Mechanisms of function of neural grafts in the adult mammalian brain. *Journal of Experimental Biology* 132:265–289.

Dunnett, S. B., Badman, F., Rogers, D. C., Evenden, J. L., and Iversen, S. D. (1988).

Cholinergic grafts in the neocortex or hippocampus of aged rats: reduction of delay-dependent deficits in the delayed non-matching to position task. *Experimental Neurology* 102:57–64.

Dunnett, S. B., Björklund, A., Gage, F. H., and Stenevi, U. (1985a). Transplantation of mesencephalic dopamine neurons to the striatum of adult rats. In A. Björklund and U. Stenevi (eds.), *Neural Grafting in the Mammalian CNS.* Amsterdam: Elsevier, 451–469.

Dunnett, S. B., Ryan, C. N., Levin, P. D., Reynolds, M., and Bunch, S. T. (1987a). Functional consequences of embryonic neocortex transplanted to rats with prefrontal cortex lesions. *Behavioral Neuroscience* 101:489–503.

Dunnett, S. B., Toniolo, G., Fine, A., Ryan, C. N., Björklund, A., and Iversen, S. D. (1985b). Transplantation of embryonic ventral forebrain neurons to the neocortex of rats with lesions of nucleus basalis magnocellularis. I. Sensorimotor and learning impairments. *Neuroscience* 16:787–797.

Dunnett, S. B., Whishaw, I. Q., Bunch, S. T., and Fine, A. (1986). Acetylcholine-rich neuronal grafts in the forebrain of rats: effects of environmental enrichment, neonatal noradrenaline depletion, host transplantation site and regional source of embryonic donor cells on graft size and acetylcholinesterase-positive fibre outgrowth. *Brain Research* 378:357–373.

Dunnett, S. B., Whishaw, I. Q., Jones, G. H., and Bunch, S. T. (1987b). Behavioural, biochemical and histochemical effects of different neurotoxic amino acids injected into nucleus basalis magnocellularis of rats. *Neuroscience* 20:653–669.

Ebner, F. F., Olschowska, J. A., and Jacobowitz, D. M. (1984). The development of peptide-containing neurons within neocortical transplants in adult mice. *Peptides* 5:103–113.

Eriksdotter-Nilsson, M., Björklund, H., Dahl, D., and Olson, L. (1986). Growth and development of intraocular fetal cortex cerebri grafts in rats of different ages. *Developmental Brain Research* 28:75–84.

Everitt, B. J., Robbins, T. W., Evenden, J. L., Marston, H. M., Jones, G. J., and Sirkiä, T. E. (1987). The effects of excitotoxic lesions of the substantia innominata, ventral and dorsal globus pallidus on the acquisition and retention of a conditional visual discrimination: implications for cholinergic hypotheses of learning and memory. *Neuroscience* 22:441–469.

Fine, A., Dunnett, S. B, Björklund, A., and Iversen, S. D. (1985a). Cholinergic ventral forebrain grafts into the neocortex improve passive avoidance memory in a rat model of Alzheimer disease. *Proceedings of the National Academy of Science of the USA* 82:5227–5230.

Fine, A., Dunnett, S. B., Björklund, A., Clarke, D., and Iversen, S. D. (1985b). Transplantation of embryonic ventral forebrain neurons to the neocortex of rats with lesions of nucleus basalis magnocellularis. I. Biochemical and anatomical observations. *Neuroscience* 16:769–786.

Fisher, A., and Hanin, I. (1986). Potential animal models for senile dementia of Alzheimer's type, with emphasis on AF64A-induced toxicity. *Annual Review of Pharmacology and Toxicology* 26:161–181.

Floeter, M. K., and Jones, E. G. (1984). Connections made by transplants to the cerebral cortex of rat brains damaged *in utero*. *Journal of Neuroscience* 4:141–150.

Floeter, M. K., and Jones, E. G. (1985). Transplantation of fetal postmitotic neurons to rat cortex: survival, early pathway choices and long-term projections of outgrowing axons. *Developmental Brain Research* 22:19–38.

Gage, F. H., Björklund, A., Stenevi, U., Dunnett, S. B., and Kelly, P. A. T. (1984). Intrahippocampal septal grafts ameliorate learning impairments in aged rats. *Science* 225:533–536.

Getz, R. L., Moody, T. W., and Rosenstein, J. M. (1987). Neuropeptide receptors are present in fetal neocortical transplants. *Neuroscience Letters* 79:97–102.

Gibbs, R. B., and Cotman, C. W. (1987). Factors affecting survival and outgrowth from transplants of entorhinal cortex. *Neuroscience* 21:699–706.

Gibbs, R. B., Harris, E. W., and Cotman, C. W. (1985). Replacement of damaged cortical projections by homotypic transplants of entorhinal cortex. *Journal of Comparative Neurology* 237:47–65.

Glees, P. (1940). The differentiation of the brain and other tissues in an implanted portion of embryonic head. *Journal of Anatomy* 75:239–247.

Gonzalez, M. F., and Sharp, F. R. (1987). Fetal frontal cortex transplanted to injured motor/sensory cortex of adult rats. I. NADPH-diaphorase neurons. *Journal of Neuroscience* 7:2991–3001.

Gonzalez, M. F., Sharp, F. R., and Loken, J. E. (1988). Fetal frontal cortex transplanted to injured motor/sensory cortex of adult rats: reciprocal connections with host thalamus demonstrated with WGA-HRP. *Experimental Neurology* 99:154–165.

Hamasaki, T., Hirakawa, K., and Toyama, K. (1987a). Electrophysiological and histological study of synaptic connections between lateral geniculate transplant and host visual cortex. *Applied Neurophysiology* 50:463–464.

Hamasaki, T., Komatsu, Y., Yamamoto, N., Nakajima, S., Hirakawa, K., and Toyama, K. (1987b). Electrophysiological study of synaptic connections between a transplanted lateral geniculate nucleus and the visual cortex of the host rat. *Brain Research* 422:172–177.

Harvey, A. R., and Lund, R. D. (1981). Transplantation of tectal tissue in rats. II. Distribution of host neurons which projects to transplants. *Journal of Comparative Neurology* 202:505–520.

Harvey, A. R., Golden, G. T., and Lund, R. D. (1982). Transplantation of tectal tissue in rats. III. Functional innervation of transplants by host afferents. *Experimental Brain Research* 47:437–445.

Haun, F., and Cunningham, T. J. (1984). Cortical transplants reveal CNS trophic interactions in situ. *Developmental Brain Research* 15:290–294.

Haun, F., and Cunningham, T. J. (1987). Specific neurotrophic interactions between cortical and subcortical visual structures in developing rat: in vivo studies. *Journal of Comparative Neurology* 256:561–569.

Haun, F., Rothblat, L. A., and Cunningham, T. J. (1985). Visual cortex transplants in rats restore normal learning of a difficult visual pattern discrimination. *Investigations in Opthalmology and Visual Science* 26 (supplement 3): 288.

Herman, J. P., Choulli, K., Geffard, M., Nadaud, D., Taghzouti, K., and LeMoal, M. (1986). Reinnervation of the nucleus accumbens and frontal cortex of the rat by dopaminergic grafts and effects on hoarding behavior. *Brain Research* 372:210–216.

Houle, J. D., and Das, G. D. (1980). Freezing of embryonic neural tissue and its transplantation in the rat brain. *Brain Research* 192:570–574.

Iacovitti, L., Lee, J., Joh, T. H., and Reis, D. J. (1987). Expression of tyrosine hydroxylase in neurons of cultured cerebral cortex: evidence for phenotypic plasticity in neurons of the CNS. *Journal of Neuroscience* 7:1264–1270.

Jaeger, C. B., and Lund, R. D. (1980a). Transplantation of embryonic occipital cortex to the brain of newborn rats: an autoradiographic study of transplant histogenesis. *Experimental Brain Research* 40:265–272.

Jaeger, C. B., and Lund, R. D. (1980b). Transplantation of embryonic occipital cortex to the tectal region of newborn rats: a light microscopic study of organization and connectivity of the transplants. *Journal of Comparative Neurology* 194:571–597.

Jaeger, C. B., and Lund, R. D. (1981). Transplantation of embryonic occipital cortex to the tectal region of newborn rats: a Golgi study of mature and developing transplants. *Journal of Comparative Neurology* 194:571–597.

Kamo, H., Kim, S. U., McGeer, P. L., Araki, M., Tomimoto, H., Kimura, H. (1987). Transplantation of cultured human spinal cord cells into the rat motor cortex: use of phaseolus vulgaris leucoagglutinin as a cell marker. *Neuroscience Letters* 76:163–167.

Kesslak, J. P., Brown, L., Steichen, C., and Cotman, C. W. (1986a). Adult and embryonic front cortex transplants after frontal cortex ablation enhance recovery on a reinforced alternation task. *Experimental Neurology* 94:615–626.

Kesslak, J. P., Nieto-Sampedro, M., Globus, J., and Cotman, C. W. (1986b). Transplants of purified astrocytes promote behavioral recovery after frontal cortex ablation. *Experimental Neurology* 92:377–390.

Kimble, D. P., Bremiller, R., and Stickrod, G. (1986). Fetal brain implants improve maze performance in hippocampal-lesioned rats. *Brain Research* 363:358–363.

Krüger, S., Sievers, J., Hansen, C., Sadler, M., and Berry, M. (1986). Three morphologically distinct types of interface develop between adult host and fetal brain transplants: implications for scar formation in the adult central nervous system. *Journal of Comparative Neurology* 249:103–116.

Labbe, R., Firl, A., Mufson, E. J., and Stein, D. G. (1983). Fetal brain transplants: reduction of cognitive deficits in rats with frontal cortex lesions. *Science* 221:470–472.

Lawrence, J. M., Huang, S. K., and Raisman, G. (1984). Vascular and astrocytic reactions during establishment of hippocampal transplants in the adult host brain. *Neuroscience* 12:745–760.

Le Gros Clark, W. E. (1940). Neuronal differentiation in implanted foetal cortical tissue. *Journal of Neurology and Psychiatry* 3:263–272.

Levin, B. E., Dunn-Meynell, A., and Sced, A. F. (1987). Functional integration of fetal cortical grafts into the afferent pathway of the rat somatosensory cortex (SmI). *Brain Research Bulletin* 19:723–734.

Lindsay, R. M., and Raisman, G. (1984). An autoradiographic study of neuronal development, vascularization and glial cell migration from hippocampal transplants labelled in intermediate explant culture. *Neuroscience* 12:513–530.

Lindvall, O., Dunnett, S. B., Brundin, P., and Björklund, A. (1987). Transplantation of catecholamine-producing cells to the basal ganglia in Parkinson's disease: experimental and clinical studies. In F. C. Rose (ed.), *Parkinson's Disease: Clinical and Experimental Advances.* London: John Libbey, 189–206.

Lund, R. D., and Harvey, A. R. (1981). Transplantation of tectal tissue in rats. I. Organization of transplants and pattern of distribution of host afferents within them. *Journal of Comparative Neurology* 201:191–209.

Lund, R. D., Rao, K., Hankin, M. H., Kunz, H. W., and Gill, T. J. (1987). Transplantation of retina and visual cortex to rat brains of different ages. *Annals of the New York Academy of Science* 495:227–241.

Lund, R. D., Harvey, A. R., Jaeger, C. B., and McLoon, S. C. (1982). Transplantation of embryonic neural tissue to the tectal region of newborn rats. In *Changing Concepts of the Nervous System.* New York: Academic Press, 361–375.

McConnell, S. K. (1985). Migration and differentiation of cerebral cortical neurons after transplantation into the brains of ferrets. *Science* 229:1268–1271.

McLoon, S., and Lund, R. D. (1983). Development of fetal retina, tectum, and cortex transplanted to the superior colliculus of adult rats. *Journal of Comparative Neurology* 217:376–389.

McLoon, S., and Lund, R. D. (1984). Loss of ganglion cells in fetal retina transplanted to rat cortex. *Developmental Brain Research* 12:131–135.

Matthews, M. A. (1985). Transplantation of fetal lateral geniculate nucleus to the occipital cortex: connectivity with host's area 17. *Experimental Brain Research* 58:473–489.

Mountcastle, V. B. (1979). An organizing principle for cerebral function: the unit module and the distributed system. In F. O. Schmitt and F. G. Worden (eds.), *The Neurosciences Fourth Study Program.* Cambridge, MA: MIT Press, 21–42.

Olson, L., and Malmfors, T. (1970). Growth characteristics of adrenergic nerves in the adult rat. Fluorescence histochemical and ^{3}H-noradrenaline uptake studies using tissue tranplantation to the anterior chamber of the eye. *Acta Physiologica Scandinavica supplementum* 348:1–112.

Olson, L., and Seiger, Å. (1972). Brain tissue transplanted to the anterior chamber of the eye. I. Fluorescence histochemistry of immature catecholamine and 5-hydroxytryptamine neurons innervating the rat iris. *Zeitschrift für Zellforchung* 195:175–194.

Olson, L., Björklund, H., and Hoffer, B. J. (1984). Camera bulbi anterior: new vistas on a classical locus for neural tissue transplantation. In J. R. Sladek and D. M. Gash (eds.), *Neural Transplants: Development and Function*. New York: Plenum Press, 125–165.

Olson, L., Björklund, H., Seiger, Å, and Hoffer, B. J. (1983). Brain transplants in oculo: anatomical and physiological insights. In A. Björklund and U. Stenevi (eds.), *Neural Grafting in the Mammalian CNS*. Amsterdam: Elsevier, 365–387.

Olson, L., Seiger, Å, Hoffer, B. J., and Taylor, D. (1979). Isolated catecholaminergic projections from substantia nigra and locus coeruleus to caudate, hippocampus and cerebral cortex formed in intraocular sequential double brain grafts. *Experimental Brain Research* 35:47–67.

Olson, L., Strömberg, I., Bygdeman, M., Granholm, A.-Ch., Hoffer, B., Freedman, R., and Seiger, Å. (1987). Human fetal tissues grafted to rodent hosts: structural and functional observations of brain, adrenal and heart tissues in oculo. *Experimental Brain Research* 67:163–178.

Palmer, M., Björklund, H., Olson, L., and Hoffer, B. (1983). Trophic effects of brain areas on the developing cerebral cortex. II. Electrophysiology of intraocular grafts. *Developmental Brain Research* 6:141–148.

Park, J. K., Joh, T. H., and Ebner, F. F. (1986). Tyrosine hydroxylase is expressed by neocortical neurons after transplantation. *Proceedings of the National Academy of Sciences of the USA* 83:7495–7498.

Porter, L. L., Cedarbaum, J. M., O'Leary, D. D. M., Stanfield, B. B., and Asanuma, H. (1987). The physiological identification of pyramidal tract neurons within transplants in the rostral cortex taken from the occipital cortex during development. *Brain Research* 436:136–142.

Raisman, G. (1969). Neuronal plasticity in the septal nuclei of the adult rat. *Brain Research* 14:25–48.

Richardson, R. T., and DeLong, M. R. (1988). A reappraisal of the functions of the nucleus basalis of Meynert. *Trends in Neuroscience* 11:264–267.

Rosenstein, J. M. (1987). Neocortical transplants in the mammalian brain lack a blood-brain barrier to macromolecules. *Science* 235:772–774.

Rutherford, A., Garcia-Munoz, M., Dunnett, S. B., and Arbuthnott, G. W. (1987). Electrophysiological demonstration of host cortical inputs to striatal grafts. *Neuroscience Letters* 83:275–281.

Segal, M., and Bloom, F. E. (1978). The action of norepinephrine in the rat hippocampus. IV. The effects of locus coeruleus stimulation on evoked hippocampal unit activity. *Brain Research* 107:517–525.

Seiger, Å. (1985). Preparation of immature central nervous system regions for transplantation. In A. Björklund and U. Stenevi (eds.), *Neural Grafting in the Mammalian CNS*. Amsterdam: Elsevier, 71–77.

Seiger, Å, and Olson, L. (1975). Brain tissue transplanted to the anterior chamber of the eye. III. Substitution of lacking central noradrenaline input by host iris sympathetic fibers in the isolated cerebral cortex developed *in oculo*. *Cell and Tissue Research* 159:325–338.

Sharkey, M. A., Steedman, J. G., Lund, R. D., and Dom, R. M. (1987). Tectal transplants into the occipital cortex of the newborn rat. *Developmental Brain Research* 31:119–123.

Sharp, F. R., and Gonzalez, M. F. (1986). Fetal cortical transplants ameliorate thalamic atrophy ipsilateral to neonatal frontal cortex lesions. *Neuroscience Letters* 71:247–251.

Sharp, F. R., Gonzalez, M. F., Ferriero, D. M., and Sagar, S. M. (1986). Injured adult neocortical neurons sprout fibres into surviving fetal frontal cortex: evidence using NADPH-diaphorase staining. *Neuroscience Letters* 65:204–208.

Sharp, F. R., Gonzalez, M. F., and Sagar, S. M. (1987). Fetal frontal cortex transplanted to injured motor/sensory cortex of adult rats. II. VIP-, somatostatin-, and NPY-immunoreactive neurons. *Journal of Neuroscience* 7:3002–3015.

Smith, G. (1988). Animal models of Alzheimer's disease: experimental cholinergic denervation. *Brain Research Reviews* 13:103–118.

Smith, L. M., and Ebner, F. F. (1986). The differentiation of non-neuronal elements in neocortical transplants. In G. D. Das and R. B. Wallace (eds.), *Neural Transplantation and Regeneration*. New York: Springer Verlag, 81–101.

Sofroniew, M. V., and Pearson, R. C. A. (1985). Degeneration of cholinergic neurons in the basal nucleus following kainic acid or N-methyl-D-aspartic acid application to the cerebral cortex in the rat. *Brain Research* 339:186–190.

Sofroniew, M. V., Isacson, O., and Björklund, A. (1986). Cortical grafts prevent atrophy of cholinergic basal nucleus neurons induced by excitotoxic cortical damage. *Brain Research* 378:409–415.

Sofroniew, M. V., Pearson, R. C. A., Eckstein, F., Cuello, A. C., and Powell, T. P. S. (1983). Retrograde changes in cholinergic neurons in the basal forebrain of the rat following cortical damage. *Brain Research* 289:370–374.

Stanfield, B. B. (1984). Postnatal reorganization of cortical projections: the role of collateral elimination. *Trends in Neuroscience* 7:37–41.

Stanfield, B. B., and O'Leary, D. D. M. (1985). Fetal occipital cortical neurones transplanted to the rostral cortex can extend and maintain a pyramidal tract axon. *Nature* 313:135–137.

Stein, D. G. (1987). Transplant-induced functional recovery without specific neuronal connections. *Progress in Research, American Paralysis Association* 18:4–5.

Stein, D. G., and Mufson, E. J. (1987). Morphological and behavioral characteristics of embryonic brain tissue transplants in adult, brain-damaged subjects. *Annals of the New York Academy of Science* 495:444–463.

Stein, D. G., Labbe, R., Attella, M. J., and Rakowsky, H. A. (1985). Fetal brain tissue transplants reduce visual deficits in adult rats with bilateral lesions of the occipital cortex. *Behavioral and Neural Biology* 44:266–277.

Stein, D. G., Palatucci, C., Kahn, D., and Labbe, R. (1988). Temporal factors influence recovery of function after embryonic brain tissue transplants in adult rats with frontal cortex lesions. *Behavioral Neuroscience* 102:260–267.

Stenevi, U., Björklund, A., and Dunnett, S. B. (1980). Functional reinnervation of the denervated neostriatum by nigral transplants. *Peptides* 1 (supplement 1): 111–116.

Stenevi, U., Björklund, A., and Svendgaard, N.-Aa. (1976). Transplantation of central and peripheral monoamine neurons to the rat brain: techniques and conditions for survival. *Brain Research* 114:1–20.

Sevendgaard, N.-Aa., Björklund, A., and Stenevi, U. (1975). Regenerative properties of central monoamine neurons as revealed in studies using iris transplants as targets. *Advances in Anatomy, Embryology and Cell Biology* 51:1–77.

Thompson, W. G. (1890). Successful brain grafting. *New York Medical Journal* 51:701–702.

van den Bosch de Aguilar, P., Langhendries-Weverberg, C., Goemaere-Vanneste, J., Flament-Durand, J., Brion, J. P., and Couck, A. M. (1984). Transplantation of human cortex with Alzheimer's disease into rat occipital cortex: a model for the study of Alzheimer's disease. *Experientia* 40:402–403.

Welner, S. A., Dunnett, S. B., Salamone, J. D., MacLean, B., and Iversen, S. D. (1988). Transplantation of embryonic ventral forebrain grafts to the neocortex of rats with bilateral lesions of nucleus basalis magnocellularis ameliorates a lesion-induced deficit in spatial memory. *Brain Research* 463:192–197.

Author Index

Dawson, D. R., 345, 372
Dawson, G. D., 355, 372
Dawson, T. M., 134, 135, 140
Day, J., 557
Deacon, T. W., 25, 27, 31, 90, 104, 462, 468
Deakin, J. F. W., 132, 139
Dean, P., 101, 279, 282, 283, 284, 286, 287, 288, 289, 290, 291, 293, 294, 296, 300, 301, 306, 309, 323, 331, 332, 338
Dean, R. L., 314, 601, 604, 605
de Belleroche, J., 126, 140
de Bruin, J. P. C., 57, 65, 66, 68, 69, 73, 74, 443, 447, 449, 452, 458
De Courten, C., 68
Deems, D. A., 427
DeFelipe, J., 105
Dekker, J. J., 105
de Lacoste, M. C., 501
de Lacoste-Utamsing, C., 483, 499
DeLong, M. R., 233, 601, 605, 610
Dement, W. C., 189
Demeter, S., 483, 499
Denenberg, J. O., 499
Denenberg, V. H., 72, 499
Deniau, J. M., 316, 332
Dennis, S. G., 32, 141
Der, T., 104, 569, 570, 588
Derer, P., 36, 67
de Reuck, A. V. S., 403
Desban, M., 148, 332
Descarries, L., 131, 134, 135, 138, 140
Descartes, R., 239, 263
Deschenes, M., 187
Desimone, R., 300
Desmond, M. M., 31
De Souza, E. B., 136, 140
DesRosiers, M. H., 149
Detari, L., 160, 181
Deutch, A. Y., 125, 140
Devine, J. V., 218, 237
DeVoogd, T. J., 501
De Vries, G. J., 65, 66, 68, 69, 74
Dewhurst, W., 187
Dewson, J. H., III, 396, 399
De Yoe, E. A., 275, 276, 297, 299, 301
Diamond, I. T., 6, 14, 15, 197, 203, 207, 297, 298, 301, 313, 322, 332, 335, 395, 396, 399, 403
Diamond, M. C., 55, 56, 57, 67, 74, 485, 486, 489, 492, 493, 499, 500, 501, 503
DiCara, L. V., 259, 263, 429

Di Chiari, G., 316, 330, 332
Dierker, M. L., 380
DiLorenzo, P. M., 417, 425
DiMattia, B. V., 464, 468, 469
Dimitrios, A., 209
Dimond, S., 236
Dineen, J., 297, 303
Dinopoulos, A., 50, 67
Diop, L., 133, 140
Dittmer, D. S., 75
Divac, I., 23, 31, 84, 88, 89, 104, 107, 112, 134, 140, 150, 160, 181, 307, 340, 437, 438, 440, 441, 443, 444, 446, 452, 455, 456, 458, 460, 469, 471
Dizio, P., 336
Dobson, V. G., 530
Dolbakyan, E., 228, 234
Dom, R. M., 611
Domesick, V. B., 28, 31, 84, 104, 333
Domich, L., 187
Donatelle, J. M., 569, 582
Dorner, G., 66
Donoghue, J. P., 26, 29, 31, 33, 83, 90, 91, 94, 97, 98, 104, 197, 207, 211, 228, 230, 238, 320, 332, 350, 353, 355, 372, 373, 453
Dori, 67
Doty, R. W., 286, 301, 499
Doucet, G., 131, 132, 134, 138, 140
Douglas, A., 354, 373
Douglas, R. M., 208, 335
Dowling, G. A., 499
Doyle, A. C., 158, 181
Drager, U. C., 324, 332, 512, 513, 525, 531
Dray, A., 316, 333
Dreher, B., 102, 110, 276, 277, 282, 286, 297, 306, 309, 311, 312, 333
Droogleever Fortuyn, A. B., 77, 104, 341, 373
Dru, D., 545, 556
Drucker-Colin, R., 604
Druga, R., 384, 399, 404
Drysdale, D. B., 503
Dubois, B., 144
Dudar, J. D., 159, 181
Dunbar, G. L., 559
Dunn, E. H., 605
Dunn, J. D., 204, 208
Dunn, L. T., 413, 425
Dunnett, S. B., 189, 238, 330, 333, 478, 591, 592, 594, 595, 599, 600, 601, 602, 604, 605, 606, 607, 609, 610, 612

Dunn-Meynell, A., 609
Durham, D., 121, 141
Dutar, P., 183, 375
Dyck, R., 524, 534
Dyer, R. S., 322, 333
Dykes, R. W., 353, 373, 375, 402
Dyson, S. E., 307

Eadie, L. A., 67
Ebert, A., 66
Ebner, F. F., 50, 51, 65, 66, 104, 353,
354, 372, 375, 591, 592, 593, 606,
610, 611
Eccles, J. C., 179
Eckenstein, F., 125, 135, 141, 146, 149
Eckmann, K. W., 31, 104, 425, 453,
468
Eckstein, F., 611
Edelman, G. M., 404
Edmunds, S. M., 52, 71
Edvinsson, L., 136, 141, 144
Edwards, S. B., 333
Edwards, S. G., 313
Egger, M. D., 364, 378
Egyhazi, E., 232, 235
Ehlert, J., 499
Eichenbaum, H., 31, 104, 410, 425,
447, 453, 468
Eichengreen, J. M., 516, 531
Eichler, A. J., 441, 453
Elde, R. P., 148
Elger, C. E., 354, 373
Ellard, C. G., 292, 301, 321, 322, 324,
325, 333, 334, 514, 531
Ellen, P., 453
Elliott, C., 502
Elliott, W., 543, 557, 563, 584
Ellison, G. D., 241, 266
Elul, R., 159, 181
Emerson, V. F., 511, 512, 513, 531
Emmers, R., 408, 425
Emson, P. C., 128, 129, 132, 134, 137,
141, 142, 143, 187, 441, 453
Enna, S. J., 179
Epstein, A. N., 69, 207, 243, 266, 424,
426
Erickson, R. P., 272, 274, 411, 415,
421, 425, 428
Eriksdotter-Nilsson, M., 596, 606
Esclapez, M., 130, 141
Espinoza, S. G., 101, 103, 105, 276,
277, 278, 295, 296, 301, 307, 460, 469
Essman, W. B., 188
Evans, K. L., 572, 587

Evans, P., 551, 560
Evarts, E. V., 230, 238, 372
Evenden, J. L., 215, 219, 226, 234,
605, 606
Everitt, B. J., 413, 425, 602, 606
Evrard, P., 43, 45, 47, 67
Ewer, R. F., 287, 301
Ewert, J.-P., 298, 301

Fahrbach, S. E., 204, 208
Fahrenkrug, J., 143, 149
Fairbanks, M. K., 184
Fairen, A., 45, 67, 80, 105
Falk, D., 264
Falk, U., 426
Fallon, J. H., 137, 141
Fantie, B., 557
Farb, C., 402
Farber, N., 424
Faull, R. L. M., 28, 31, 84, 91, 107,
316, 333, 340
Fauman, B., 160
Fauman, M., 181
Fawcett, J. W., 50, 52, 66, 67, 74
Faye-Lund, H., 203, 208, 384, 399
Feder, R., 159, 181
Fedoroff, S., 73
Feeney, D. M., 330, 333, 546, 556
Feher, J., 316, 332
Fekete, D. M., 376
Fekete, M. I. K., 146
Felbain-Keramidas, S. L., 527, 528,
532
Feldhaus, S., 36, 71
Feldman, J. L., 209
Feldman, M. L., 80, 82, 105, 108, 109,
135, 141
Feldman, S. C., 136, 143
Felleman, D. J., 376
Feltz, P., 316, 333
Feng, A. S., 391, 400
Ferger, J., 316, 332
Feringa, E. R., 354, 378, 588
Ferino, F., 203, 208, 453
Ferino, G., 28, 31, 441
Fernandez, J., 604
Fernandez, V., 107, 337
Ferreira, A., 443, 447, 449, 453
Ferrier, J. M. R., 452
Ferrier, R. J., 290, 300, 301
Ferriero, D. M., 611
Fibiger, H. C., 148, 160, 183, 185,
450, 457
Field, J., 428

Subject Index